WALLS OF CONTAINMENT

THE ARCHITECTURE AND LANDSCAPES OF LUNACY

WALLS OF CONTAINMENT

THE ARCHITECTURE AND LANDSCAPES OF LUNACY

by

PATRICK QUINLAN

Published by
UNIVERSITY COLLEGE DUBLIN PRESS
PREAS CHOLÁISTE OLLSCOILE BHAILE ÁTHA CLIATH

2021

First published 2021

by
University College Dublin Press
UCD Humanities Institute,
Room H103, Belfield,
Dublin 4

www.ucdpress.ie

ISBN 978-19-1-08207-42 hb

CIP data available from the British Library

The support of the following donors has been gratefully received:

Grangegorman Development Agency
Gníomhaireacht Forbartha Ghráinseach Ghormáin

TU Dublin
Ollscoil Teicneolaíochta Bhaile Átha Cliath
Technological University Dublin

Seirbhís Sláinte Níos Fearr á Forbairt | Building a Better Health Service

Designed in Ireland by
Kende Creative | www.kende.ie

Printed in Scotland on acid-free paper by
Bell & Bain Ltd
Burnfield Road, Thornliebank, Glasgow, G46 7UQ, UK

Dedication

To my parents, Anne and Victor

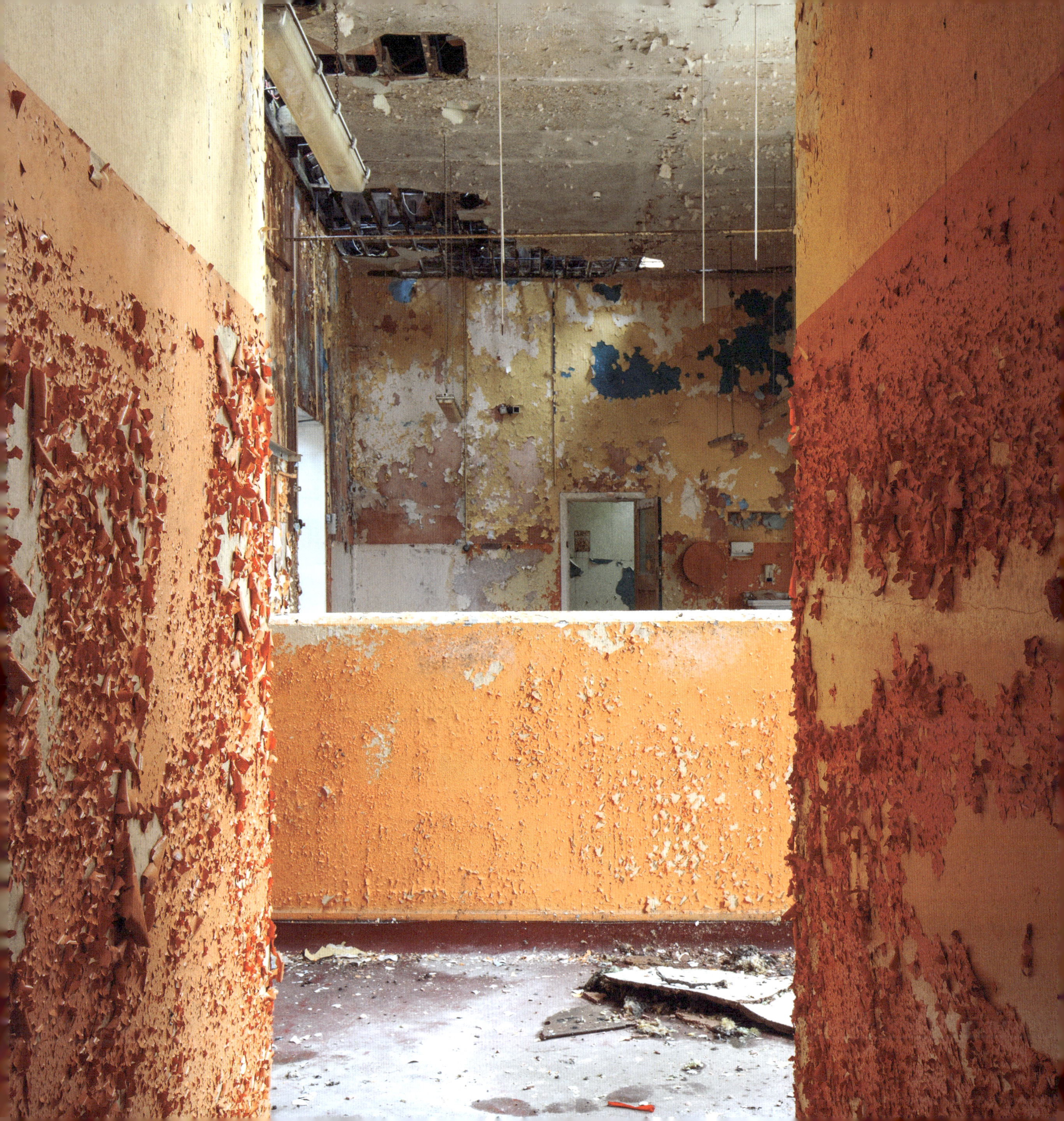

Contents

Acknowledgements

Despite the socially mandated silence that long shrouded them, there are few families in Ireland who do not have some connection with the institutions described in this book. For my part, I started this project thinking myself well placed to tackle the subject matter from the safe distance of dispassionate detachment. It was only during the journey that I learned that my eponymous 'mad [grand-]uncle' departed this life in one of the buildings described herein – albeit after a stay of days rather than decades. On the other hand, I also learned that my great-grandfather – decades earlier – chaired a fateful committee meeting that decided to repurpose a redundant workhouse as a cheaper alternative to constructing the new buildings so urgently needed at the same hospital. In this, as in so many other aspects of Irish social history that are now being aired, researcher and reader alike are forced to think of the actors we encounter throughout these stories not as a remote and alien 'they' but as an intimately related 'we'.

The late, great Maeve Binchy once quipped that she relished redrafting her will, for it allowed her to indulge in pleasant thoughts about those on whom she might lavish her generosity. Composing acknowledgements at the end of a project is a similar experience – an opportunity to fondly recall all of those whose contributions have enriched the journey. Enduring early influences, such as the after-school local history classes hosted by Clonmel librarian Marie Boland, are no less part of this journey than the impromptu walk around Portrane with Chris Shaw, which gave me my first glimpse of the fascinating complexity of the asylum typology. This interest blossomed into a thesis for the award of Master of Urban and Building Conservation under the supervision of Dr Finola O'Kane in the UCD School of Architecture – a course of study and research that I was only able to undertake with the liberal support (financial, practical, moral and intellectual) of my then-employer, conservation architect Margaret Quinlan.

The logistics of arranging access to every former asylum would have been formidable without the good offices of Eleanor Masterson in HSE Estates, and my former colleague Donal Blake of Scott Tallon Walker Architects, who opened the door that opened the doors. I am grateful in turn to the dozens of regional and local HSE staff who facilitated our visits in one way or another, including: Howard Beardmore, Mike Bermingham, John Browne, Grainne Cahill, Gerry Carroll, Margaret Caulfield, Caroline Coakley, Terry Clarke, Kieran Cronin, Brendan Cuskelly, Liam Fahy, Edward Falvey, Ed Fennell, Paul Flood, Marion Geary, Anthony Gyves, Brian Haran, Gerry Hardiman, Seamus Halvey, Paul Hayden, Clodagh Hanratty, Brian Haran, Caroline Higgins, Nora Higgins, David Hogan, Joe Hoare, Laurence

Kane, Mark Kane, Selina Kavanagh, Tim Keogh, Tracy Lanigan, Pat Marks, Ger McCormack, Paul McCormack, Pat McDermott, Martin McGrath, Angela McNamara, Patrick Meade, Brendan Mulligan, Paul Mullins, Michael Mulvey, Christy Murphy, Brian O'Brien, Alan O'Connell, Terry O'Connor, Gerard O'Meara, George O'Neill, Damian O'Reilly, John Power, Bernard Pierce, Brendan Redington, Dominic Roarty, Joe Scales, and Trevor Vaughan. Amidst this list are very many individuals – some recalled from retirement – who personally guided either myself or David around the buildings and whose warm welcomes never failed to revive after many hours on the road. Their recollections of a working lifetime could repopulate cold and empty spaces with sights and sounds, people and personalities, but their contribution to this work goes far beyond reminisce and anecdote. Theirs is a real and valuable knowledge of the inner workings of an institution not to be found in any archives and which academics and historians of many stripes would do well to cherish while they still can. For it was the knowledge gleaned during those early conversations that taught me how to actually see what lay in front of me, and which created a foundation of understanding on which the rest of this edifice has been built. And to any whose names have fallen between the cracks of my filing system, I offer also my apologies.

I am grateful to individuals at other sites for facilitating our photographic expeditions, including Eamon Galavan at Enniscorthy, David Lee at GMIT Castlebar, and Caroline Millar at the Clayton Hotel, Sligo; also, to Stephen Hamilton, for sharing his infectious enthusiasm for the history of Purdysburn. Professors Harry Kennedy and Damien Mohan of the Central Mental Hospital were kind enough to share their fascinating experiences of operating that most unique of institutions, and also allowed me the rare privilege of exploring the 'secret garden' that flourishes, unbeknownst to most, behind the great wall of Dundrum. Governor Martin O'Reilly of Castlerea Prison was similarly generous with his time and knowledge of the institution under his charge. Conversations with Dr Aisling Campbell, Consultant Psychiatrist, and John Farrelly, CEO of the Mental Health Commission, added nuance to my views on contemporary psychiatric spaces and practices.

Dr Liz Twohig has been a longstanding friend and valued mentor in my many ventures, always on hand with wise counsel to help discern a course through the mists that occasionally obscure the way. Dr Gill Allmond has been kind enough to critique my work on Purdysburn; likewise, Una Sugrue of the Grangegorman Development Agency who, in addition to reviewing an early draft of the manuscript, has been ever-generous in sharing the latest invaluable insights arising from her own work on the legacy buildings at

Grangegorman. My current PhD supervisor, Professor Leslie Topp of Birkbeck, University of London, while stimulating my latest line of research, has inspired insights and avenues of inquiry that have directly benefitted this text. I am deeply indebted to both external readers – Professor Gary Boyd of Queen's University, Belfast, and Dr Richard Butler of the University of Leicester – for returning a wealth of astute observations and constructive comments, and for challenging me to refine and clarify the core objective of the work. I wish to thank Noelle Moran in UCD Press for her enthusiasm and encouragement throughout the long journey from draft to final product, and Daniel Morehead for his sterling work in meeting and exceeding the high quality of production and graphics to which we all aspired. Needless to say, any errors and omissions are entirely my own.

I have been privileged to enjoy a fruitful collaboration with David Killeen, whose extraordinary artistic and technical talents behind the lens speak for themselves from the pages of this volume. David's original commission was to visit just four sites, but he undertook it as his sacred mission to record every one of these places as they stand today, often on the cusp of an uncertain future. Come what may, his work will endure as both an artistic achievement and an invaluable record for decades to come. Many other individuals and organisations have been generous in facilitating the reproduction of graphic material and are credited where relevant, but particular thanks are due to Patricia Fallon at the National Archives of Ireland, Colum O'Riordan and his team at the Irish Architectural Archive, and to Paul Ferguson of the Trinity Map Library, for their special willingness to assist in every way possible.

Every minute spent researching and writing is one minute less spent on some other aspect of life. I am therefore blessed in my wife, Katya, who has shared both her husband and her home with this project for many years, and has been unfailing in her support, encouragement, and constructive engagement, while simultaneously expanding our family from nought to two in less time than it has taken me to deliver a single book. But the greatest thanks are reserved for my parents, Anne and Victor who, amongst everything else, identified my interests in history and historic buildings from an unreasonably early age and nourished them with Sunday outings to every historic site within a hundred-mile radius. This book is dedicated to them.

Patrick Quinlan,
May 2021

Photographic Reflections

It is seldom that one has an opportunity to photograph such an intriguing subject, and on such a large scale; to delve into a piece of Irish history, long hidden from view. In many respects, these buildings speak of a darker side of our past – places of lost souls, forgotten by society. But as Patrick describes elsewhere within this book, the whole story is often more complex.

Numerous photographers have documented institutions such as these from different perspectives, but all too often it is with an unhealthy focus on the more stygian aspects of these places. From the outset, I wished to achieve a more balanced view, to record the subtleties and the nuances, the flashes of colour and texture, the moments of unexpected beauty. Yet on the whole, I cannot deny that the combination of grand scale and unwieldy layout made for a weighted atmosphere verging on the oppressive, a sensation encountered to a greater or lesser extent in each of these buildings.

Today, the buildings are husks of their former selves: the patients and staff who once animated them are now gone, leaving only remnants of an institution that once was. I felt motivated by a particular sense of urgency to document as much as possible within the narrow window still open to us, before many of these buildings deteriorate past the point of no return.

I wish to record my special thanks to all of the on-site caretakers and managers who brought me around each facility, many of whom started their careers when the hospitals were still large and vibrant entities. They were able to give me a precious insight into how these institutions functioned and what life was like within their walls.

The experience of undertaking this commission and spending two years documenting these spaces has left a profound mark on me. Whatever becomes of these buildings, I am glad to have played a role in preserving their story. I would like to thank Patrick for the opportunity to work with him and I am very proud to have been part of this project.

David Killeen,
January 2021

David Killeen Photography
www.davidkilleen.com

List of Illustrations

Chapter 3

Chapter 4

Chapter 5

Chapter 6

Chapter 7

Chapter 8

Chapter 9

Conclusion

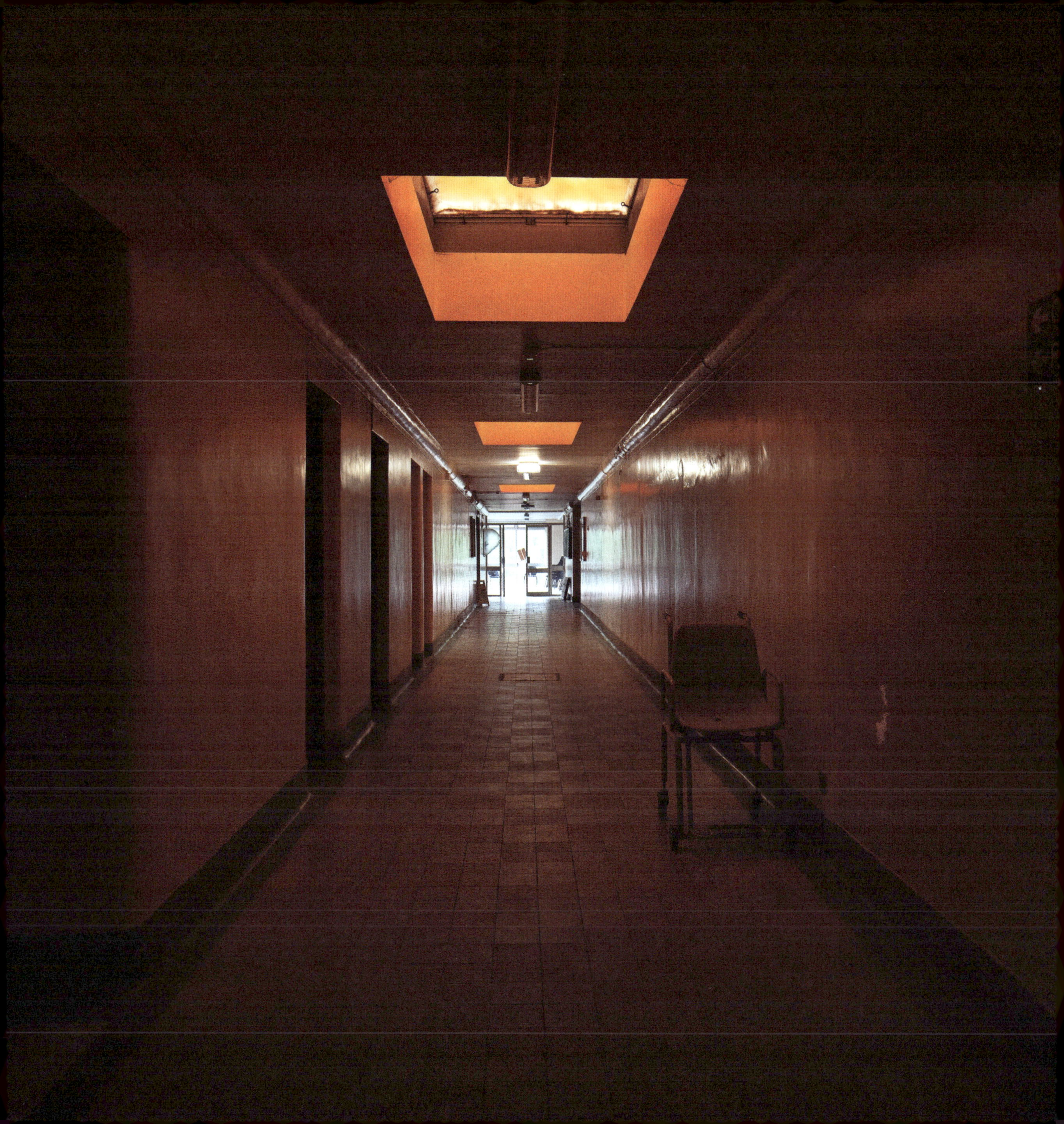

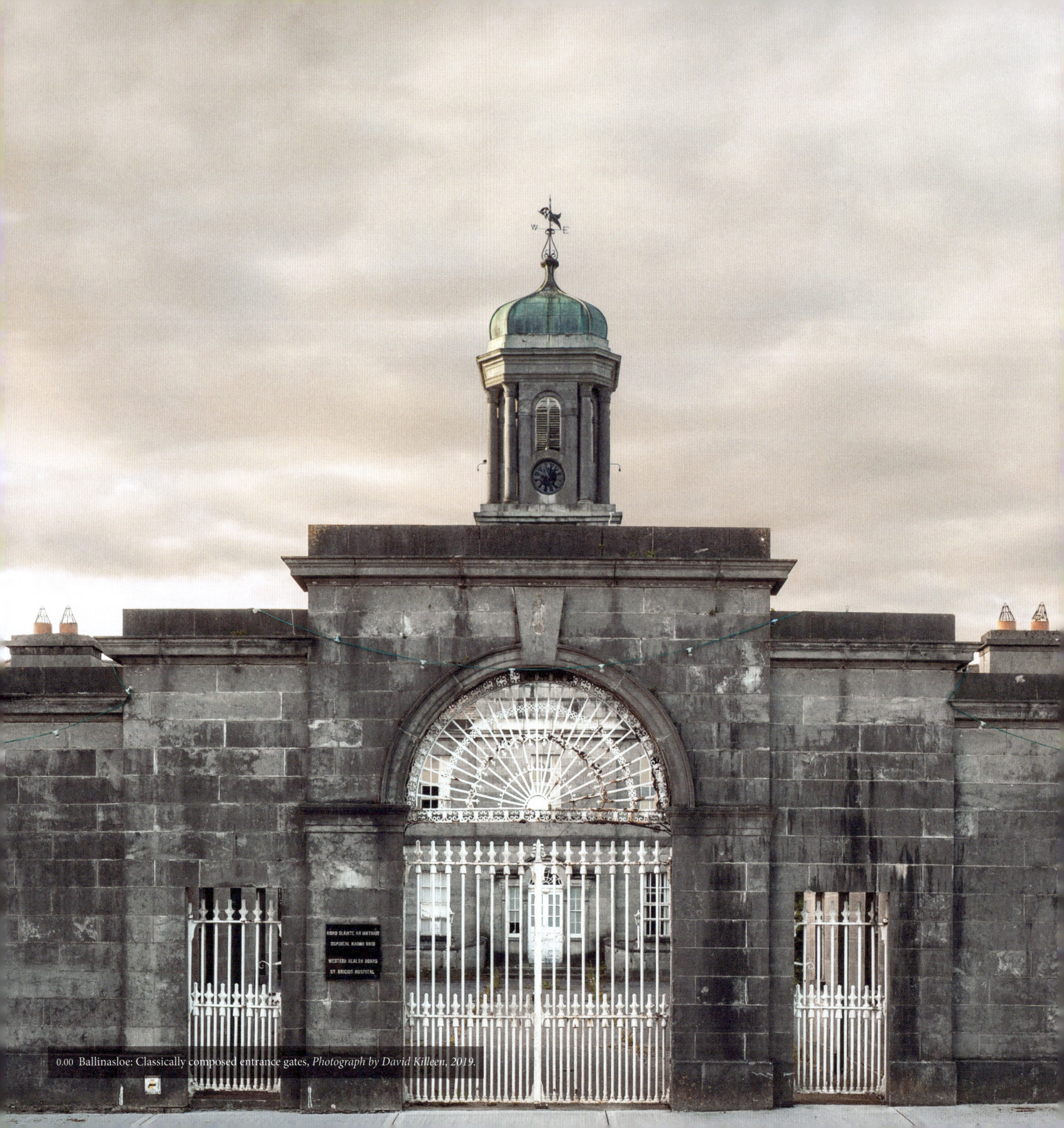

0.00 Ballinasloe: Classically composed entrance gates, *Photograph by David Killeen, 2019.*

Introduction

> *the great advance made in the interests of humanity... by the erection of the new asylums, whereby the sad condition of the insane poor has been so materially alleviated. Ample and convenient sites have generally been purchased, on healthy, elevated positions, and commanding views of the most beautiful scenery. A pleasing and not necessarily expensive style of architecture has been adopted and carried out in a manner highly creditable to the architects engaged, and ornamental to the country.*[1]

The journey that led to this book started in a north Dublin field, nine years ago. The field in question was to become the site for Ireland's new national forensic mental hospital – the largest single investment in the mental health sector in over a century. But my attention that soft May morning was drawn to another structure nearby – one that not only laid claim to the same title in its day, but that ranked as the largest publicly funded civilian building project undertaken during the period of British rule in Ireland.[2] The Portrane Asylum was also, by the time of my visit, the largest empty building in Ireland, its last patients having departed just a few months before. It soon became apparent that Portrane was not the only empty asylum in Ireland. The decommissioning of these buildings was a matter of public policy, informed by contemporary best practice and pursued vigorously by the Mental Health Commission.[3] However, the structured plan to close the asylums has not been matched by any vision for their future, leaving a challenging legacy of unwanted, unused and, in some cases, unusable buildings. Thus began a 2,500 kilometre pilgrimage to document the 27 surviving asylum sites on the island of Ireland as they stood on the threshold of an uncertain future: a journey traced annually by the Inspectors of Lunacy prior to Irish independence, but seldom travelled by any individual since.

The term 'asylum' infers many meanings. In the abstract it conveys an idea of refuge and sanctuary. In current affairs it is most usually paired with 'seeker' to refer to those who have sought refuge on our shores, and whose experience of Ireland's latter-day institutional landscape is far from a source of civic pride. In recent history it became synonymous with residential institutions for the insane. In our towns and cities it is that place that today retains a lingering sense of otherness. The imperative to provide 'asylum' for 'poor lunatics' led to the creation of specific organisations for their care, which in turn demanded specialised facilities to carry out their work. For much of the period considered in this book, the idea, the institution and the place

1. *Copy of Treasury Minute... 10 August 1855*, HC 1856 [9] LIII.367, p. 4.
2. In terms of both built footprint (ca. 24,000 m^2) and total floor area (ca. 37,000 m^2) within a single building, Portrane is without peer. By way of comparison, the largest government-funded building in Dublin, Sir Aston Webb's Royal College of Science on Merrion Street (now Government Buildings), had a footprint of less than 5,000 m^2 and a total area less than 25,000 m^2. It is difficult to identify a precise a single figure for the cost of the new asylum at Portrane, but it certainly exceeded £370,000 (see Case Study 25) compared to the £225,000 cost of the College of Science buildings. *Public Offices Site (Dublin) Act 1903, Account 1919–20*, HC [3] xix, p. 365.
3. Mental Health Commission, *Under the Clock Towers: An Overview of Remaining Nineteenth-Century Public Psychiatric Hospitals Due for Closure* (Dublin, 2011).

existed as an undivided trinity whose identity was charged with meaning and whose organisational structure exercised almost unlimited power over its subjects. This book will trace the history of the asylum as an *idea*, its evolution as an *institution*, but most of all its legacy as a physical *place* that retains a powerful hold on our collective consciousness to this day.

The language of lunacy

The terms 'lunatic', 'idiot', 'imbecile' and 'inmate' are today regarded as politically incorrect, outdated terms whose use may be seen as pejorative or humiliating to persons with a mental illness or intellectual disability. However, their use throughout this book should not be interpreted in this way. These words represent the commonly accepted medical and legal terminology in the period before the introduction of the 1945 Mental Treatment Act, and are therefore used as a reflection of the authentic language within particular historic periods. Even the less loaded term 'handicapped', in use into the late twentieth century, has in turn come to be seen as insensitive, but again is used where appropriate in its historic context.

The names of the institutions themselves also changed repeatedly, from 'District Lunatic Asylums' to 'District Mental Hospitals' in 1925, enjoying a very brief interlude as 'Psychiatric Hospitals' before being re-christened after various saints by whose names most of the institutions remain known to this day.[4] While the full and historically appropriate name may occasionally be invoked when discussing a particular institution, for consistency and brevity I will by default refer to each institution only by the name of the town or city in which it is situated. Brevity also dictates that the objects of this study are referred to collectively as asylum buildings or sites, with occasional exceptions when pointedly discussing those twentieth-century sites at Ardee, Castlerea and Derry, which were purpose-built after the term 'lunatic asylum' had fallen out of use. And while the English language offers no collective noun for asylums in the plural, I might on a lighter note propose '*an alienation of asylums*' as my semantic contribution to the field.[5]

At its simplest this book is about the buildings and landscapes of Ireland's lunatic asylums. More precisely, it focuses on those lunatic asylums that were purpose-built, at public expense, in the period after 1814. It covers all asylums in the Republic of Ireland and Northern Ireland that were built prior to partition, and includes the three new greenfield 'mental hospitals' – asylums in all but name – erected thereafter.

Architectural historians act as interpreters for the stories that buildings have to tell. The very act of building, of committing limited resources to achieve a particular end, is the point at which high-minded idealism collides with the real world, when words take flesh as brick and mortar and live among us. Internationally, researchers have long been attracted to asylum architecture by the alluring notion that these were not mere containers but essential tools through which cures could be achieved; buildings were invested with the power to 'mend muddled minds'. But such buildings can also tell other stories. Thomas Markus[6] reveals how organisational power structures embedded within the asylum's physical fabric invite closer comparison with schools and prisons than with the contemporary medical hospitals found in Jeremy

4. The changing political landscape pre- and post-Independence sees 'Maryborough' become 'Portlaoise', 'The Richmond' become 'Grangegorman', and 'Eglinton' become 'Cork'.
5. The earliest psychiatrists were known variously as asylum doctors or 'alienists': practitioners who cared for those whose mental state had 'alienated' them from normal society.
6. Thomas Markus, *Buildings and Power: Freedom and Control in the Origin of Modern Building Types* (Oxon, 1993).
7. Jeremy Taylor, *Hospital and Asylum Architecture in England 1840–1914: Building for Health Care* (London, 1991).
8. Leslie Topp, *Freedom and the Cage: Modern Architecture and Psychiatry in Central Europe, 1890–1914* (Pennsylvania, 2017).
9. Christine Stevenson, *Medicine and Magnificence: British Hospital and Asylum Architecture, 1660–1815* (New Haven, 2000).
10. Carla Yanni, *The Architecture of Madness: Insane Asylums in the United States* (Minneapolis, 2007).
11. Although, in identifying how architecture accommodated clinical best practice, Reuber perhaps underplays the instances where it pointedly diverged. Reuber's clinical justifications for later design trends are also perhaps less convincing than those for the earliest radial buildings. Markus Reuber, *Staats- und Privatanstalten in Irland, Irre, Artze und Idioten 1600–1900* (Koln, 1994); Ibid., 'The architecture of psychological management: The Irish Asylums, 1801–1922', in *Psychological Medicine*, no. 26 (1996), pp 1179–89; Ibid., 'Moral management and the "Unseen Eye", Public Lunatic Asylums, 1800–1845', in Elizabeth Malcolm and Greta Jones (eds), *Medicine, Disease and the State in Ireland, 1650–1940* (Cork, 1999), pp 209–29.

Taylor's[7] defining survey of English hospital and asylum architecture. Leslie Topp's[8] work on 'caged freedom' explores the inevitable paradoxes of early twentieth-century efforts to afford asylum patients greater freedom – or at any rate to create an image of freedom – a theme that has challenged designers of mental health facilities from William Tuke's day to our own. Christine Stevenson[9] explored the propaganda value of the façade of London's infamous Bethlem Hospital, showing how designers could choose to conceal or reveal the nature of the institution within, while also reflecting changing perceptions of what level of architectural splendour is appropriate when building for charity. Carla Yanni's[10] study of the American asylum typology feels familiar on this side of the Atlantic, albeit with some interesting variations.

Yet Irish asylum architecture remains the subject of very little serious scholarship. It took the curiosity of a German psychiatrist working in Ireland in the 1990s, Markus Reuber, to trace the development of the historic buildings through which he conducted his clinical rounds. In revealing how the buildings of each age reflected prevailing clinical principles, Reuber's detailed plan-form analysis has hardly been bettered.[11] Frederick O'Dwyer composed a succinct history of the entire typology as part of a wider survey of hospital architecture[12] and revisits the subject in the context of other 'administrative' histories, as well as meticulously detailed construction accounts of individual asylums at Killarney[13] and Enniscorthy.[14] Most of the buildings are described within one or more architectural surveys – in summary by the National Inventory of Architectural Heritage, in finer detail within the Pevsner series of architectural guides[15] and with greater wit in Jeremy Williams' gazetteer[16] – but are seldom adequately contextualised with respect to social, political or medical matters. Beyond these works, many of the largest and most complex buildings ever built in this country have remained below the radar of the architectural historian.[17]

The decisions that a society makes about where, when and how to erect new buildings are seen as reliable indicators of its priorities. As Reuber put it:

> *These buildings represent well-considered responses to charters formulated by politicians, doctors, architects and societal pressures. They are thus important historical artefacts, and it is surprising how little of this source material has been used in the analysis of institutional management.*[18]

I have sought to address this gap by setting out a historic account of the Irish asylum system from its inception to the present day, told via the story of its buildings and landscapes. In exploring the architectural legacy of the asylum project, by tracing changing spatial, stylistic or technical approaches and by identifying the instances where rhetoric and reality diverge, it is hoped to offer some modest reflections on wider trends and theories that may contribute to the ongoing historical debate about the nature of the asylum as idea, institution and place.

'Built with… solidity to express the notions of their day',[19] our architectural journey around Ireland's asylums will reveal the paradoxes embedded in the very fabric of the buildings as architects grappled with the competing priorities of cure and containment, of aspiration and economy, of internal functionality and external

12. Frederick O'Dwyer, *Irish Hospital Architecture: A Pictorial History* (Department of Health and Children, 1997), pp 10–13, 49–55. An updated version of this text featured in 'Lunatic Asylums, 1800 – 1939', in Rolf Loeber, Hugh Campbell, Livia Hurley, John Montague and Ellen Rowley (eds), *Art and Architecture of Ireland, Volume IV* (Dublin, 2015), pp 212–14.
13. Frederick O'Dwyer, *The Architecture of Deane and Woodward* (Cork, 1997), pp 89–107.
14. O'Dwyer, 'Architectural Heritage Impact Assessment Report, St Senan's Hospital Enniscorthy' (Unpublished report, 2019).
15. **Omagh**: Alistair Rowan, *The Buildings of Ireland: North West Ulster* (London, 1979), p. 447; **Ardee**: Christine Casey and Alistair Rowan, *The Buildings of Ireland: North Leinster* (London, 1993), p. 119; **The Richmond**: Christine Casey, *The Buildings of Ireland: Dublin* (London, 2005), pp 256–60; **Armagh**: Kevin V. Mulligan, *The Buildings of Ireland: South Ulster* (London, 2013), pp 137–8. **Monaghan**: Ibid., pp 479–80.
16. Jeremy Williams, *A Companion Guide to Architecture in Ireland, 1837–1921* (Dublin, 1994).
17. The asylum as a typology received the briefest mention in Craig's definitive introduction to Irish Architecture – Maurice Craig, *The Architecture of Ireland from Earliest Times to 1880* (Dublin, 1982), p. 173 – but has otherwise fallen into a gap between much better studied areas of elite, monumental, ecclesiastical and Georgian architecture on the one hand, and domestic or vernacular buildings on the other. Indeed, of all of the urban typologies that combined civic and practical functions, only Ireland's courthouses and prisons have belatedly received the level of attention they are due. A number of historians from other disciplines have ventured to interpret the architectural legacy of individual institutions, but seldom entirely successfully.
18. Markus Reuber, 'The architecture of psychological management: The Irish asylums, 1801–1922', in *Psychological Medicine*, no. 26 (1996), p. 1179.
19. Enoch Powell MP, Address to the National Association of Mental Health Annual Conference, 9 Mar. 1961.

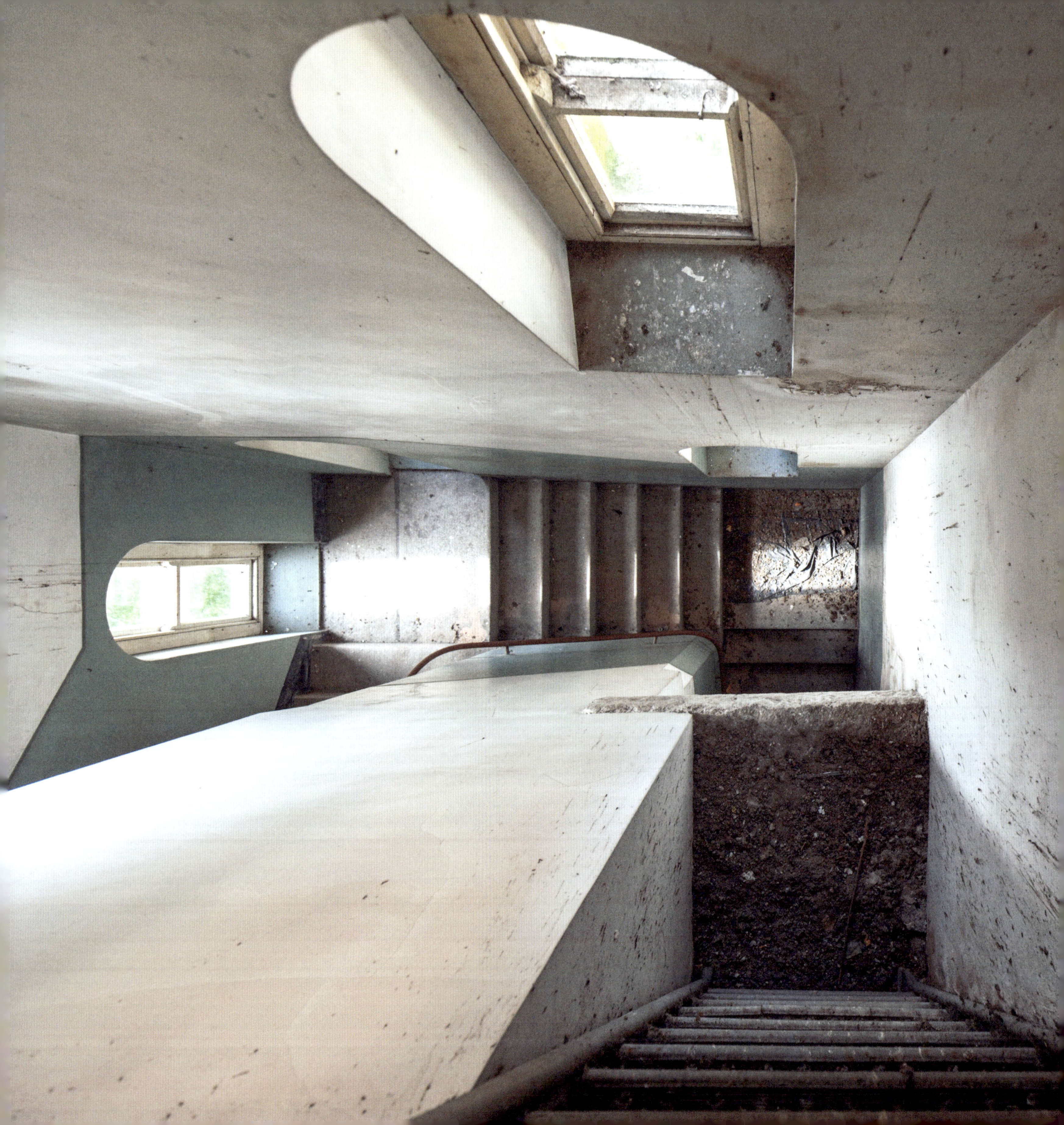

0.01 Enniscorthy: Interior of stair tower, *Photograph by David Killeen, 2019.*

0.02 Clonmel: The cupola or clocktower would become an iconic image of asylumdom, *Photograph by David Killeen, 2019.*

0.03 Cork: The second phase of asylums were architecturally ambitious, but prone to problems, *Photograph by David Killeen, 2019.*

0.04 Portrane: By the close of the nineteenth century, new asylums were akin to small towns in their own right, *Image courtesy of the National Library of Ireland (NPA MOR2149).*

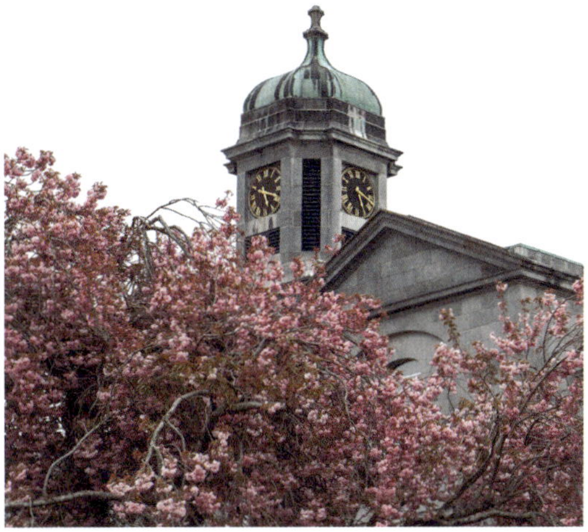

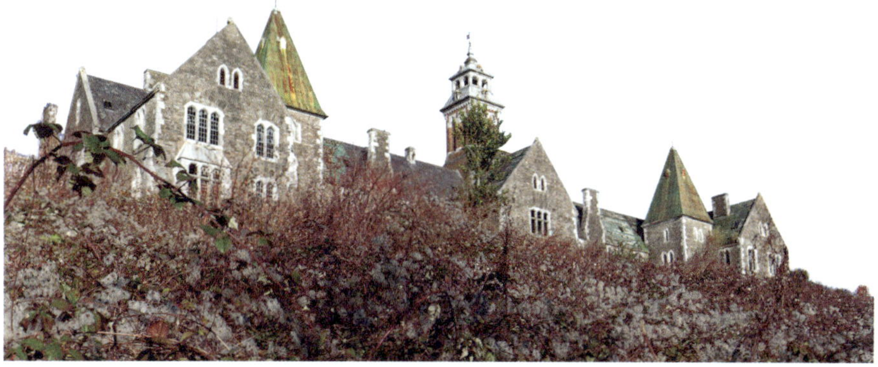

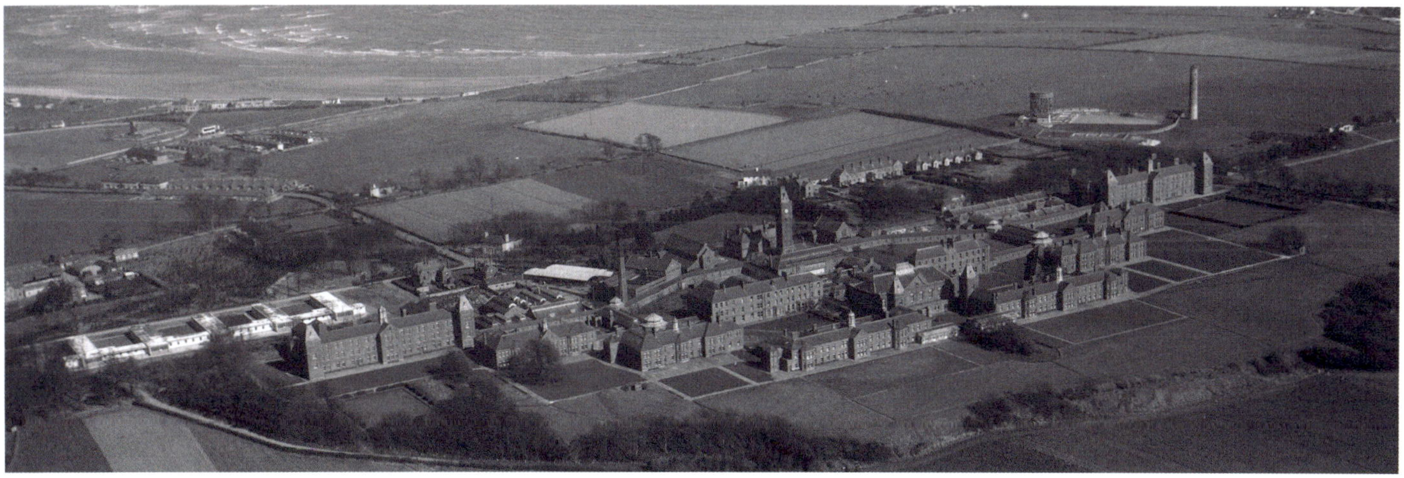

appearance. And whereas traditional architectural-historical approaches often limit their inquiry to the novel buildings of the age, we cannot hope to understand the challenging and sometimes contradictory status of these places in contemporary Ireland without studying their long and complex evolution.[20] This author concurs with McCullough's observation that 'the tradition of change, albeit inimical to the idea of art as a perfect form, has its own strong patterns and traditions' which are no less worthy of our understanding.[21]

20. It is notable that the discipline of historical archaeology has demonstrated a greater willingness than that of architectural history to explore the reciprocal relationships between buildings and their users over time. Readers interested in the long story of another challenging carceral site on the island of Ireland may enjoy: Laura McAtackney, *An Archaeology of the Troubles: The Dark Heritage of Long Kesh/Maze Prison* (Oxford, 2014).

21. Niall McCullough, *Palimpsest: Change in the Irish Building Tradition* (Dublin, 1994).

Chapter structure and gazetteer

This book is structured in two parts: a historic narrative and a gazetteer. The chronological narrative spans nine chapters, each one addressing a key phase of development of the asylum system. Generalisations are inevitable when telling a story that spans 29 individual institutions, 200 years of history and 3 legal jurisdictions, but they are based on a broad foundation of new empirical knowledge: a study of the buildings and landscapes of every single asylum site. I have also taken this knowledge as licence to offer critical commentary on the relative architectural merits of various buildings – value judgements that are inevitably subjective but that may help readers to winnow the architectural wheat from the chaff. The history and evolution of every individual asylum is revealed in the individual case studies in the gazetteer section of the book, which it is hoped will satisfy the thirst of communities to understand how their local institution fits into the wider history of the type. These are not intended to be exhaustive – and could not compete with the substantial histories that already exist for many individual institutions – but rather aim to reveal aspects of the buildings and landscapes that are exemplary, exceptional, or sometimes just mildly entertaining.

Returning to the main chronology, the first chapter offers some necessary historical context before introducing Ireland's first purpose-built public lunatic asylum – The Richmond in Dublin. In Chapter Two we will see how legislative reform catapulted Ireland from relative laggard to become the first jurisdiction in the world to implement a statutory, centrally planned, nationwide infrastructure of institutional care for the mentally ill. Through this and two subsequent chapters, we explore the main phases of construction that transformed the institutional landscape, including a detailed architectural dissection of the distinctly different building types that emerged from each era. We will trace a journey from the earliest asylums, which embodied both pioneering theories and regressive attitudes, through impressive architectural set-pieces designed by the leading architects of the era, to enormous receptacles for the hopeless that demonstrated technical ingenuity in accommodating historically unprecedented numbers of people in a single building. All were set within attractively landscaped sites that in some cases bear stronger witness to the curative aspirations of the institution than the buildings themselves.

Readers will discern a shift in emphasis in Chapters Five and Six, from new green-field structures to an exploration of how existing asylum sites were adapted to meet the insatiable demand for accommodation and the increasingly complex needs of the institution. By now, the *idea* of the asylum had been laid to rest amidst the pauper graves of those whom it had failed to cure, but its existence as an *institution* had put down deep roots, and the *places* adapted continuously to suit. I will argue that the less glamorous but far more numerous building projects of this era are relevant to understanding prevailing priorities and attitudes, not least the conflicts and compromises that were inevitable within a system trying to accommodate a patient growth curve that resembled a slow-motion epidemic. And even in a time when local committees of management seemed more concerned with buying farmland than building wards, we do encounter worthy initiatives in several localities that appear to have fallen below the radar of Irish psychiatric history to date.

Asylum provision in most western nations expanded exponentially between 1850 and 1950, but Ireland's similar growth in this period took place against the unique backdrop of a continuously falling population. In boasting the world's highest number of psychiatric beds per capita by the 1950s, 'institution-prone' Ireland seemed determined to fulfil Dean Swift's satirical observation that 'no nation wanted it so much'. In Chapters Seven and Eight we see the system peak and begin its long, slow decline amidst the shifting sands of mental health policy and a wider turn away from relying on institutional solutions to solve societal problems. A shrinking system needed few new buildings but even so, institutional history does not stop evolving and existing buildings (mostly) do not stop standing. In something of a break from conventional architectural-history approaches, I have continued to trace the story of Ireland's asylums through these years, revealing that decisions *not* to build, *not* to maintain, and even to *demolish*, are more relevant to understanding present perceptions of these places than the unfulfilled promises of shiny new buildings from a distant past. Pursuit of the architectural story right up to the present day has thrown a slightly more critical light on existing accounts of progress in the rollout of new models of care – but this is a baton better carried forward by historians of other stripes.

By Chapter Nine we will find that the asylum as an *idea* and as an *institution* is no more. Of the original trinity, only the *places* remain: buildings and landscapes that evoke complex and sometimes conflicting responses in the hearts and minds of the communities they were built to serve. Today, approximately half of these sites have a clear future. For the others, a slow decline from abandonment, through decay, to ultimate dereliction, is already playing out. Visiting these places, 'majestic, imperious, brooding', it is impossible not to be awestruck their scale, their complexity, their embodiment of societies in microcosm. But most powerful of all is the profound emptiness of places that resonate with the memories of thousands of lives lived under an institutional regime that long outlived the ideals on which it was founded.

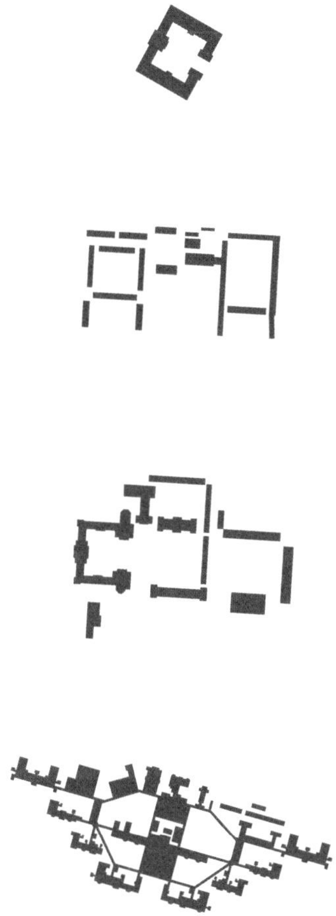

0.05 Comparative figure ground plans, c.1900, of the Royal College of Science (latterly Government Buildings), The Royal Barracks (latterly Collins Barracks), Trinity College Dublin, and Portrane Lunatic Asylum. *Drawn by the author.*

Methodology and sources

The fieldwork on which this book is based was originally undertaken during the period 2012–14 while writing a major thesis for the award of Master of Urban and Building Conservation at University College Dublin. At that time, I was conscious that the window of opportunity to experience many of these places as living entities rather than archaeological artefacts was narrow and closing rapidly, provoking my self-imposed challenge to visit and record every site in the Republic of Ireland as

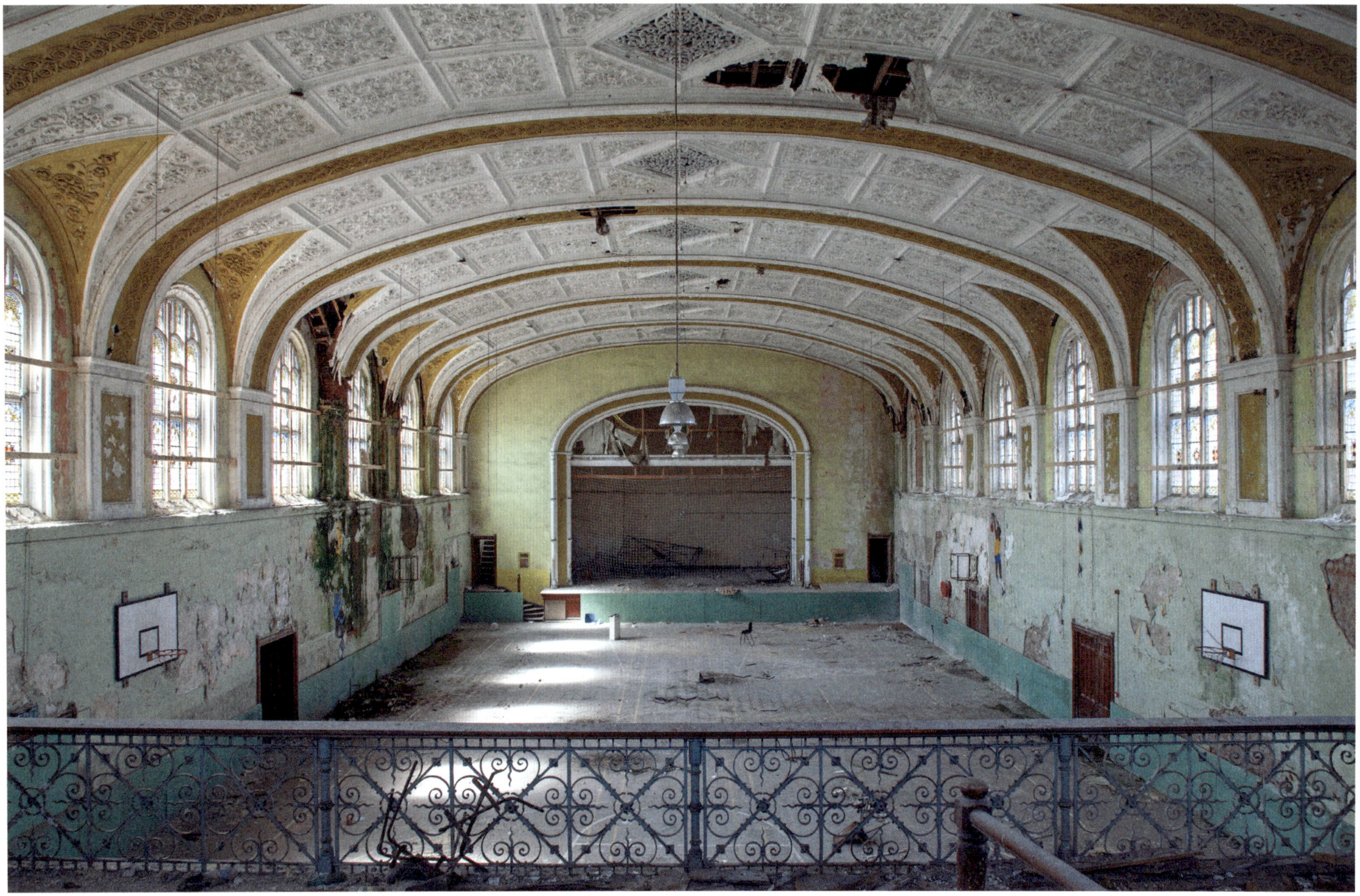

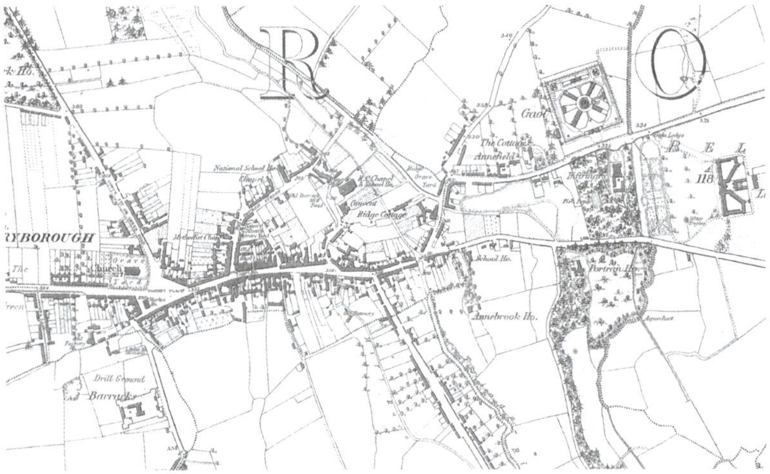

National School Ho.
The Cottage
Annefield
School Ho.
Annebrook Ho.
Drill Ground
Barracks

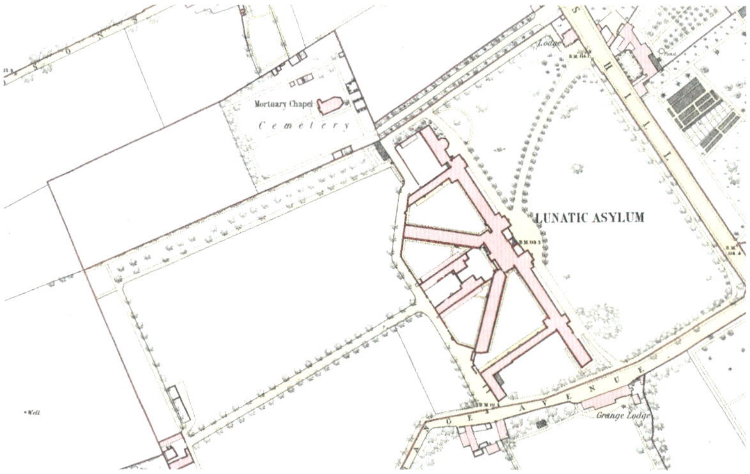

Mortuary Chapel
Cemetery
LUNATIC ASYLUM
Grange Lodge

0.06 Portrane: The ever-expanding range of ancillary spaces included recreation halls on a vast scale, *Photograph by David Killeen, 2019.*

0.07 Maryborough / Portlaoise: Location of asylum on the eastern outskirts, close to county goal and infirmary, *Reproduced courtesy of Trinity College Dublin (OS-Laois-10560-Sheet 13-1841).*

0.08 Waterford: Early asylum governors showed a firm commitment to landscaping, *Reproduced courtesy of Trinity College Dublin (OS-Waterford City-1056-Sheet 9:99-1872).*

0.09 Gransha: The therapeutic value of daylight and ventilation would return to prominence between the 1930s and 50s, *Photograph by author, 2020.*

0.10 Dundrum: The lush gardens offer a hint of how the majority of asylum sites must have looked at their peak, *Photograph by David Killeen, 2019.*

0.11 Limerick: As the institutions contracted through the later twentieth century, peripheral wards were abandoned, *Photograph by David Killeen, 2019.*

0.12 Killarney: The nostalgia that attaches to abandoned spaces should not blind us to the fact these were worlds of locked doors and constrained lives, *Photograph by David Killeen, 2019.*

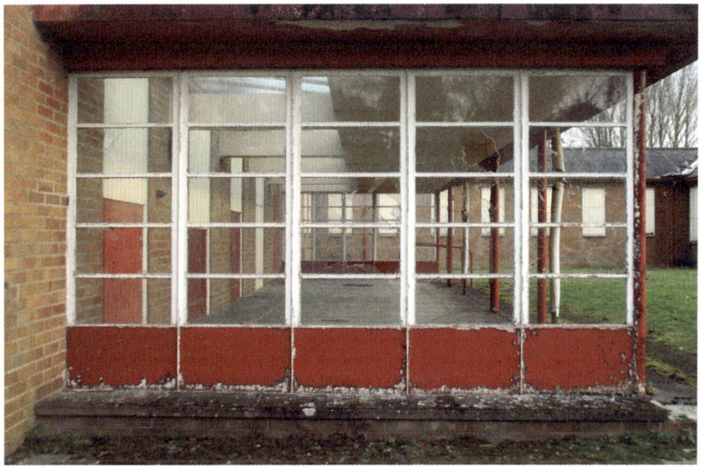

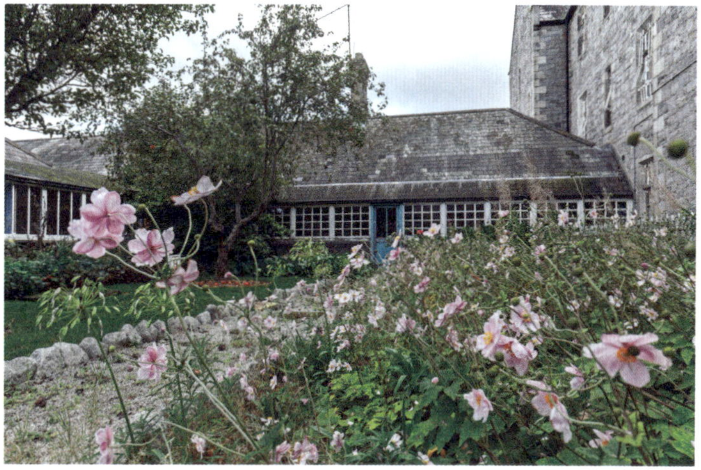

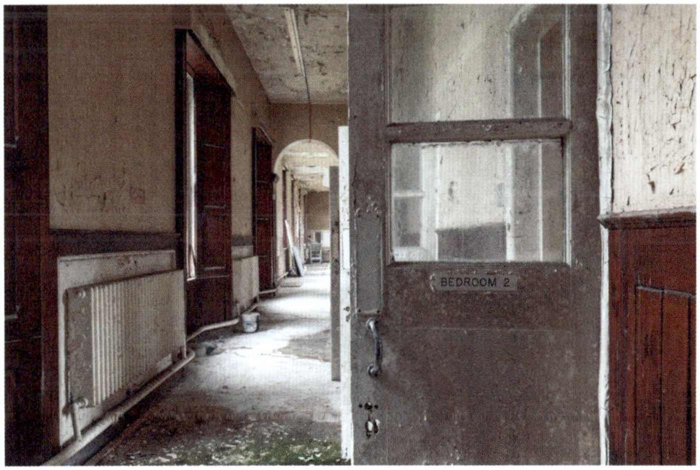

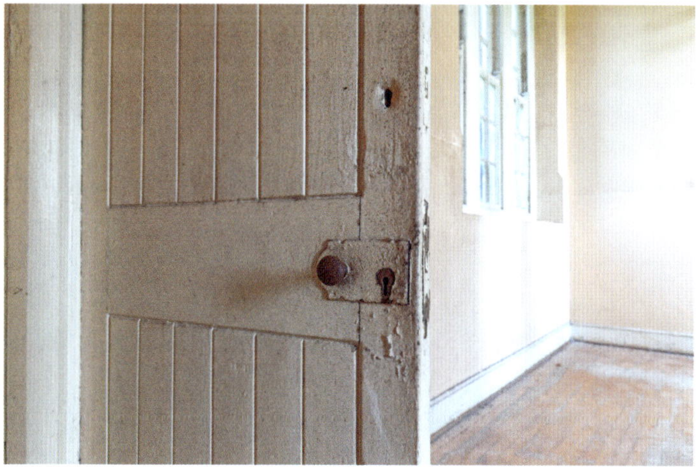

it stood on the cusp of an uncertain future. This resulting national inventory now comprises a database of some 1,000 data points identifying the prevalence, condition and age of almost 40 architectural and landscape features across 27 extant sites. Revisions, corrections and updates were made arising from further fieldwork and archival research carried out during 2019–20, at which time the geographic scope was extended to include asylum sites in Northern Ireland. Despite efforts to redress the balance, it is acknowledged that the text continues to place greater emphasis on later twentieth-century developments south of the border.

From the international asylum literature, it is clear that few scholars have had the privilege of being able to study every institution across an entire nation, much less the naivety to attempt to do so across a timeframe spanning from inception to present day. Such an approach doubtless has many flaws, but its unique strength is that it allows findings of fact to be made about the relative influence of various architectural trends and the prevalence of specific features. In this way it is hoped that this work will provide a broad platform of knowledge for future scholars who choose to delve more deeply into the buildings and landscapes of individual institutions, and offer a solid context against which to compare their findings. It is also hoped that book will encourage those of a non-architectural persuasion researching social, medical or political aspects of Ireland's institutional legacy to recognise the influence of buildings and landscapes on the objects of their study. And insofar as I occasionally venture to corroborate or refute wider revisionist conceptions of the asylum, it is based on the humble but firm evidence of what actually got built on this island.

The founding fathers of asylumdom described their ventures in almost utopian terms: an opportunity to create a perfect alternative society within which the mad could be restored to their senses.[22] In the space of little more than a generation, this alluring vision succeeded in convincing a whole society, from pauper families to political leaders, that the asylum was the best place to cure the insane in their midst. The medical profession who came to command the asylum project then succeeded in perpetuating this myth, even as living evidence of their shortcomings accumulated around them in ever more crowded institutions. In terms of the life and death of the *idea* of the asylum, Ireland's history broadly reflects the international experience.

Historians of the asylum typology enjoy an embarrassment of documentary riches. Readers will encounter quotations from nineteenth-century practitioners such as William Hallaran,[23] William Stark,[24] Samuel Tuke,[25] William Browne,[26] John Connolly[27] and Eyre C. Kenny,[28] whose publications offer invaluable representations of contemporary theories and attitudes. As a focus for intensive political debate over many decades, repeated reform of lunacy law spawned innumerable select committees and commissions, entities whose reports and minutes of evidence provide a superb insight into the trending concerns that stimulated legislative change. The Inspectors of Lunacy, their predecessors and successors, have generated two centuries of annual reports in almost unbroken run, including a description of the state of every institution alongside an ever-increasing array of statistics, supplemented by reports from other bureaucracies such as the Commissioners of Public Works and

22. Andrew Scull (ed.), *The Asylum as Utopia: W. A. F. Browne and the Mid-Nineteenth Century Consolidation of Psychiatry* (Hove, 2014).
23. William Saunders Hallaran, *An Inquiry Into the Causes Producing the Extraordinary Addition to the Number of Insane* (Cork, 1810); Hallaran, *An Inquiry into the Causes and Cure of Insanity* (Cork, 1818).
24. William Stark, *Remarks on the Construction of Public Hospitals for the Cure of Mental Derangement; Read to a Committee of Inhabitants of the City of Glasgow* (Glasgow, 1810).
25. Samuel Tuke, *Practical Hints on the Construction and Economy of Pauper Lunatic Asylums* (London, 1815).
26. William Browne, *What Asylums Were, Are and Ought to Be* (Edinburgh, 1837).
27. John Connolly, *The Construction and Government of Lunatic Asylums* (London, 1847).
28. Eyre E. C. Kenny, *Short Hints and Observations on the Arrangement and Management of Lunatic Asylums* (Dublin, 1848).

the Local Government Board. The sheer breadth of material can be a mixed blessing, demanding discipline to ensure that any conclusions remain temporally and spatially relevant, while also remaining critically conscious of their limitations in representing only professional, officially sanctioned, 'top-down' views of the asylum system. Documented 'views from below', sadly, are few and far between, and in this work they will be encountered only in the reflections of a handful of contemporary authors such as Hanna Greally and Kate Millett.

Scholars of medical and social history are shedding new light on the nuances of the asylum system through prolonged immersion in the minute books, correspondence and patient case files of individual institutions, but such a fine-grained, manuscript-based approach was not compatible with the geographic ambition of this research. Instead, the buildings themselves are my primary source. In visiting and documenting each site I recorded observations about their design, construction, evolution, condition, use and future challenges, and took copious photographs to inform later plan-form and façade analysis. Online Ordnance Survey maps for the entire island of Ireland allowed me to undertake historic map analysis for every asylum, clarifying the unique spatial evolution of each building ensemble and landscape which in turn informed broader observations around architecture, siting, orientation and landscape design. *The Dublin Builder*, its successor the *Irish Builder*, and other documentary sources cited within Irish Architectural Archive's *Dictionary of Irish Architects*, helped to clarify details and fill chronological gaps, albeit as industry periodicals; they are very far from infallible. This empirical approach, combining contemporary fieldwork with primary architectural and topographical sources as the basis for detailed architectural and spatial analysis, represents a significant original contribution to the field, and a robust base from which to affirm or challenge the dominant documentary records of 'smug officialdom'.

I have accessed some 300 manuscript drawings in the Irish Architectural Archive and National Archives of Ireland and dozens of historic photographs in the National Photographic Archive. No one collection offers complete coverage of a single asylum through all periods of its evolution, but material of some description exists for close to four-fifths of sites. Drawings may therefore be found to represent key building types from all but the most recent era, and at all scales from ironmongery fittings to site plans, collectively creating a very comprehensive picture. Analysis of this rich seam of material helps to reveal the original design intent, changes in approach during the design and construction process, and subtleties that have been lost or altered over time, many of which would merit far more detailed investigation than I have been able to give. In considering the evolution of psychiatric spaces in the later twentieth century, I have also been able to draw upon the views of those working in or retired from the psychiatric service and Mental Health Commission. But most importantly of all, on many sites I was privileged to be guided by long-serving staff members who generously shared their intimate knowledge of the places to which they had committed a working lifetime. Years spent in the archives could not have matched what I learned from spending a couple of hours in the company of each. This story is immeasurably richer for it.

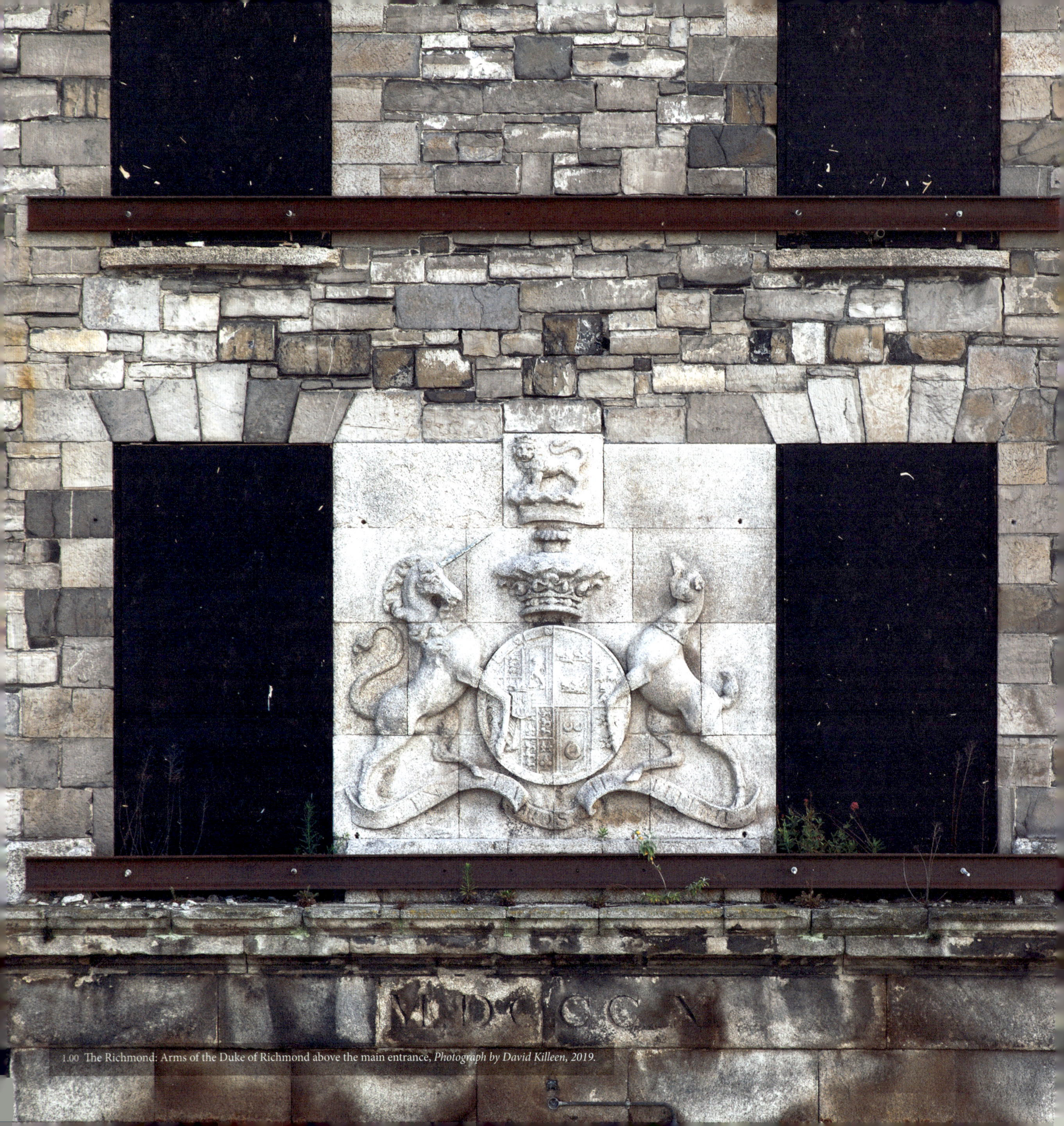

1.00 The Richmond: Arms of the Duke of Richmond above the main entrance, *Photograph by David Killeen, 2019.*

The Lunatic at Large

A house for fools and mad[1]

Until the middle of the eighteenth century specialist institutional care for the insane was all but unknown in Ireland. Mentally ill persons were cared for at home or in the homes of their extended families or social peers. Those too fractious or violent to be cared for in family settings, or for whom social or economic disadvantage had ruptured support networks, were left to wander as vagrant lunatics. Some, by virtue of criminal conviction or 'outrageous conduct', ended up as inmates within an expanding infrastructure of houses of industry, bridewells and prisons – institutions whose governors had neither the resources nor the expertise to manage the challenging behaviour of the distressed and disturbed.[2] The plight of such 'poor fools and lunatics' came to be seen as especially piteous, suffering the combined traumas of their own illness, egregious physical restraint, and unsanitary and overcrowded conditions alongside 'criminals, vagabonds, prostitutes' and the other detritus of eighteenth-century society.[3]

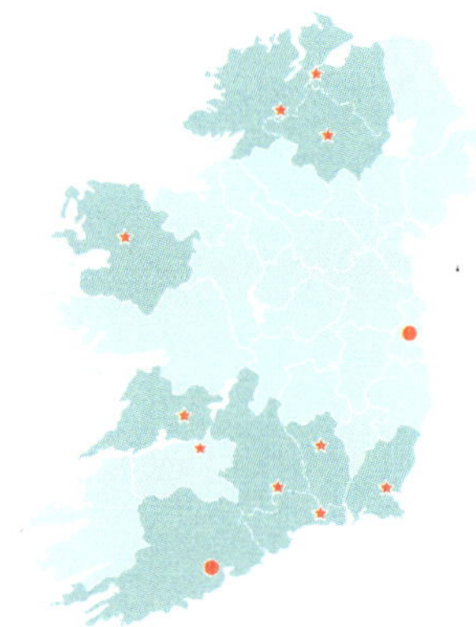

Asylum distribution in Ireland, **1815**, *Drawn by the author.*

Even internationally, institutional precedents were few. The most prominent, London's Bethlem (Bethlehem) Hospital, had its roots in a thirteenth-century monastic foundation, and was reconstructed in 1676 on a palatial scale to become the largest civil building of a new London rising from the ashes of the Great Fire.[4] It would become one of the most infamous buildings in Britain, entering the lexicon via its colloquial name 'Bedlam' as a synonym for chaos. Magnificent in architecture but often scandalous in governance, Bethlem would become a 'model for its successors either to imitate or deliberately avoid' for more than a century after its erection.[5]

Ireland's first purpose-built specialist institution for the insane, St Patrick's Hospital, Dublin, ranked as a very early imitator. Author, social satirist and Dean of Dublin's St Patrick's Cathedral, Jonathan Swift, had served as a governor of Bethlem since 1714 and was inspired by his knowledge of that institution to found a similar facility for 'fools and mad' in Ireland, leaving a bequest in his will for the purpose. St Patrick's Hospital received its royal charter in 1746 and opened in 1757, becoming only the fourth purpose-built public or voluntary institution for the care of the mentally ill in all of Great Britain and Ireland.[6] Architect George Semple's plan was but a fraction of the size of its illustrious forbear, but replicated its basic features of cell-lined galleries for male and female patients flanking a central block reserved for the master of the institution.

1. Jonathon Swift, *Verses on the Death of Dr Swift* (Dublin, 1739).
2. The increased tendency to 'contain' such individuals within institutional settings is argued by Foucault and others to stem from the diminishing tolerance of 'rational' societies for behaviour that deviated from more narrowly defined norms.
3. Joseph Robins, *Fools and Mad: A History of the Insane in Ireland* (Dublin, 1986), pp 32–7.
4. Only St Paul's Cathedral and the Tower of London were longer. Scaled by author from Ogilby and Morgan's map of London, 1677.
5. Leonard Smith, 'The architecture of confinement: Urban public asylums in England, 1750–1820', in Leslie Topp, James Moran and Jonathon Andrews (eds), *Madness, Architecture and the Built Environment* (New York & Oxon, 2007), p. 42.
6. Between Bethlem (1676) and St Patrick's (1757), Norwich's small Bethel Hospital opened in 1713 and London's St Luke's Hospital for the Insane opened in 1751.

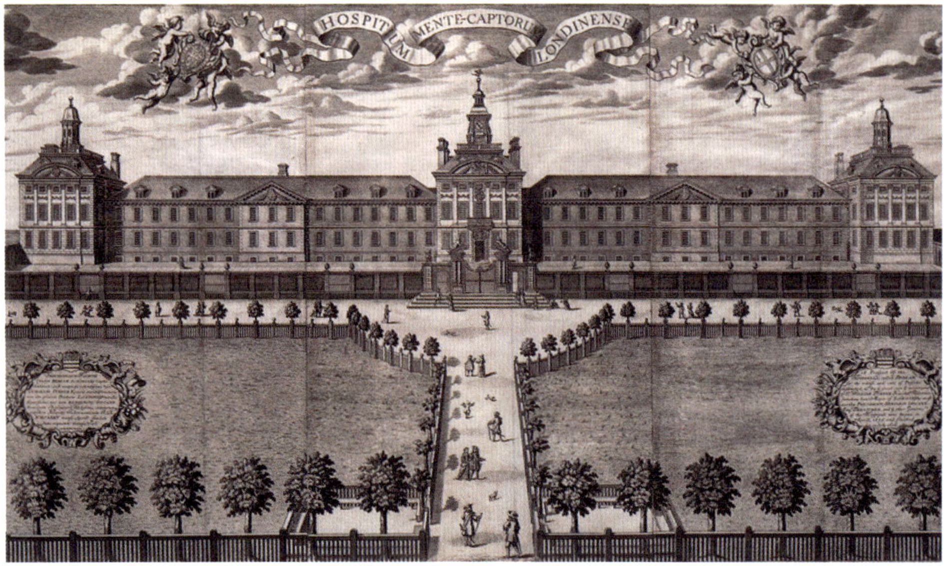

1.01 Robert Hooke's 1676 Bethlem Hospital invited comparisons with royal palaces, *Wellcome Collection (Engraving by Robert White, 1677).*

However, Swift's early vision did not naturally evolve into a widening of institutional provision in Ireland. Even as towns and cities across England in the later eighteenth century began to erect purpose-built institutions for the care of the indigent insane supported by voluntary subscription,[7] few Irish urban centres had the interest or means to follow suit. Even in metropolitan Dublin efforts to elicit subscriptions to support St Patrick's continued operation proved largely unsuccessful, indicating that the plight of 'poor lunatics' was slow to gain traction in the intimate circles of Ireland's upper class.[8] Meanwhile – and in contrast with Georgian England[9] – private sector madhouses in Ireland remained few in number, small in scale and, in the absence of research to the contrary, limited in impact.[10]

The lunatic cells

Wider public provision for the insane would instead emerge in the form of 'lunatic cells' within the Houses of Industry, such as those erected at Dublin (1776) and Limerick (1777). Surviving drawings show the lunatic cells at Dublin as little more than single-storey sheds, laid out in back-to-back rows enclosing small courtyards, but lacking even the most rudimentary comforts.[11] If historians still quibble over the validity of generalising the Georgian madhouse as a place of 'shit, straw and stench',[12] so far as the sanitary arrangements can be deduced from the surviving drawings of the Dublin cells, they could hardly have been otherwise.

An Act of Parliament in 1787 empowered (but did not oblige) grand juries – the predecessors of modern county councils – to attach dedicated lunatic wards to the houses of industry in their counties. By the 1820s lunatic departments established under this legislation could be found adjacent to houses of industry or county infirmaries in Clonmel, Cork, Derry, Ennis and Waterford, some by now in receipt of co-funding from voluntary subscriptions. Former county goals at Lifford, Roscommon

7. Smith, *The Architecture of Confinement*, p. 42.
8. Christine Stevenson, *Medicine and Magnificence: British Hospital and Asylum Architecture, 1660–1815* (New Haven, 2000), p. 97. See also Robins, *Fools and Mad*, p. 50. The level of private subscriptions would improve towards the turn of the nineteenth century, especially in Cork, but was also driven by contributions from the Quaker communities. *Report from the Select Committee on the Lunatic Poor in Ireland*, HC 1817 [430] viii, p. 13.
9. In England, revelations of scandals in unregulated private madhouses provided the impetus for legislative reform on more than one occasion. Kathleen Jones, *Asylums and After: A Revised History of the Mental Health Services from the Early 18th Century to the 1990s* (London, 1999), p. 55, pp 90–1.
10. Eighteenth century private provision is under-researched. Reports of the Inspectors of Prisons between the 1820s and 40s note between five and ten private establishments, generally holding fewer than 200 patients. See also Alice Mauger, '"Confinement of the Higher Orders": The social role of private lunatic asylums in Ireland, c. 1820–60', in *Journal of the History of Medicine and Allied Sciences*, 67:2, (2012), pp 281–317.
11. Joseph Reynolds, *Grangegorman: Psychiatric Care in Dublin since 1815* (Dublin, 1992), p. 9, p. 23. These cells bear some resemblance to the 'loges' for the insane built at the famous Paris asylum of Salpêtrière in the 1780s, which would form the typological precedent for asylum development in France. Irish Architectural Archive (hereafter IAA), Murray Collection, 1806–15, Hardwicke Lunatic Cells, 92/46, Sheets 0402, 0403; John D. Thompson and Grace Goldin, *The Hospital: A Social and Architectural History* (New Haven & London, 1975), pp 54–6.
12. Andrew Scull's pithy and oft-cited summary of the Georgian madhouse was later criticised by Roy Porter as being 'at best partially true, and taken over from nineteenth century reformist sloganizing'. Roy Porter, *Mind-Forg'd Manacles: A History of Madness in England from the Restoration to the Regency* (London, 1987), p. 276.

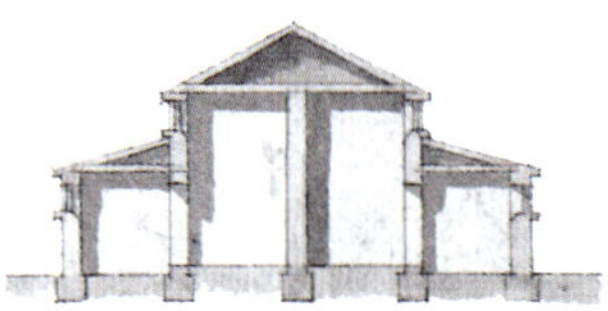

1.02 Dublin House of Industry Cells, 1817, *Image courtesy of the Irish Architectural Archive (RIAI Murray Collection 92/46: 405).*

and Wexford – condemned as unfit for prisoners – were adapted to contain lunatics, along with a dedicated section of Omagh's (operational) goal.[13] However, the county gaols still accommodated significant numbers of lunatics amidst their general inmate population, a situation that would continue to challenge all concerned with asylum and prison reform for many decades to come.[14]

One of the latest and most technically advanced local asylums established under this early legislation was at Kilkenny's House of Correction. Four courtyards allowed for the separation and classification of male and female 'enraged' and 'convalescent' patients, watched over by an octagonal central 'Keeper's House'. The entire complex was to have been enclosed within a starkly blank wall relieved only by a sombre classical gateway. If the architectural language was drawn directly from contemporary prison architecture, significant improvements were at least evident compared to the comfortless character of earlier lunatic cells: such improvements included under-floor heating flues, a lavish ratio of eight privies for only twenty patients, and 'a particular contrivance' that allowed the cells to be 'well lighted and well ventilated, or the contrary, at the option of the attendant physician'.[15]

The framework of an institutional infrastructure was thus emerging across most parts of the island, albeit providing a standard of accommodation somewhere between primitive and punitive, often banished both physically and psychologically to the rear of a larger institution and offering little or nothing in the way of treatment or cure. And if these cells would in turn become the object of horror and indignation, it is worth observing that the capitation grant received for the care of lunatics therein was up to three times that payable for other unfortunate inmates of the same institution.[16]

The relatively modest provisions of the 1787 Act would pale in comparison with the ambitious institutional expansion to come, but in one important respect its influence resonates to this day. The act mandated a process of external oversight and inspection of facilities for the insane – initially by the Inspectors General of Prisons – a principle that has endured for over 230 years and is continued today by the Mental Health Commission. Thus, conditions that prevailed in even the most secluded quarters would become both a matter of public record and, in due course, evidence that could be weaponised in the hands of the reform-minded.

Moral management

By the dawn of the nineteenth century 'moral management', or 'moral treatment', was emerging as the dominant theory in the treatment of insanity.[17] The classic narrative identifies Philippe Pinel as the pioneer who, in striking the manacles from insane prisoners at the Bicetre Asylum in Paris in 1793, proved that the insane could respond favourably to care and kindness. But in terms of publicity and influence in the English-speaking world, it would be a family of York Quakers to whom most credit is given for furthering the cause of humanitarian treatment of the mentally ill in the early nineteenth century. In response to the abuses revealed in the nearby York Asylum, William Tuke established 'The Retreat' in 1796 to offer an alternative vision of care for the insane in line with his Quaker principles.[18] The Tuke family's successful implementation of 'moral management' at York resonated with Enlightenment ideals

13. *Annual Report of the Inspectors General of Prisons 1824*, HC 1824 [294] xxii, p. 70. See also Richard J. Butler, *Building the Irish Courthouse and Prison: A Political History, 1750–1850* (Cork, 2019), p. 159, p. 246.
14. Some were present by virtue of a conviction – 'criminal lunatics' – but others were committed by magistrates on account of non-criminal disturbed behaviour or 'outrageous conduct'. The latter category were worthy objects for sympathetic treatment, how best to deal with the former became a recurring challenge for legislative reformers.
15. From historic map analysis, it appears that only one half of the complex was built as planned, so the imposing gateway may actually never have existed. At time of writing, the octagonal Keeper's House is still standing within a radically altered context, its former role long forgotten. *Report from the Select Committee on the Lunatic Poor in Ireland*, HC 1817 [430] viii, pp 43–4.
16. At Clonmel in 1820, grants of 18 shillings per head were paid in respect of the 39 lunatics in the house. The other 164 inmates including old and infirm, prostitutes, vagrants and petty criminals yielded grants of 6 shillings per head. Rev. William Burke, *A History of Clonmel* (Waterford, 1907), p. 199.
17. It is notable at this time that the term 'moral' could be interpreted in either psychological/mental or ethical terms.
18. Irish Quakers operated institutions at Donnybrook and Hampton House, but their history, regime and influence are as yet insufficiently understood. Catherine Cox, *Negotiating Insanity in the Southeast of Ireland, 1820–1900* (Manchester, 2012), p. 15.

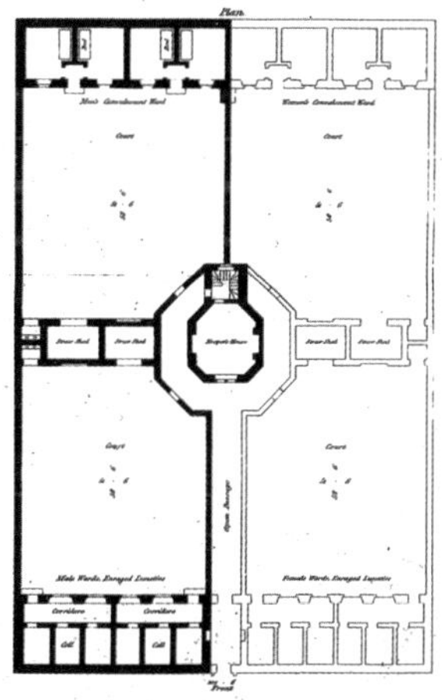

1.03 Kilkenny City and County Lunatic Asylum, 1816, *Image courtesy of ProQuest LLC (ProQuest House of Commons Parliamentary Papers, HC 1817 (430) viii, pp 44).*

around humanity, reason and progress, and was upheld as an exemplar in contrast to the restraint, punishment and harsh discipline that had typified the treatment of insanity in the eighteenth century. The Retreat would achieve widespread renown, not least as the source for an 1815 treatise published by his grandson Samuel, *Practical Hints on the Construction and Economy of Pauper Lunatic Asylums*, which would prove highly influential to parliamentary committees considering legislative reform in both Ireland and England.[19] Further research – sadly beyond the scope of this book – is merited to fully reveal the role of the Irish Quaker community in spreading the 'new gospel' of moral management in Ireland. Dublin's Quaker community founded at least one institution in Donnybrook along the lines of 'The Retreat', while it was observed that 'the exertions and sacrifices of time and of money [by] Quakers of independent fortune and station' were instrumental in founding and subsidising the operation of the house of industry lunatic departments across the south of Ireland.[20]

It was becoming more widely recognised that 'the attention and care necessary for the effectual relief of these distressed poor objects' could not be given in facilities not built for that purpose, and that some form of specialised public provision for poor lunatics was required.[21] It had been a core tenet of 'The Retreat' that 'the building and its design would create a healing space [that would] also instil… a new set of habits allowing the patient to become a new person: a sane person.'[22] This optimistic and compelling premise would inspire a generation of reformers to expend unprecedented sums of public money in the construction of a new generation of specialised residential institutions. And while the later evolution of the asylum project may be seen to drift far from these benevolent roots, it is also worth observing that even Tuke's ideal asylum is founded on several concepts that may not be seen as unequivocally benign today, including the imperative to securely segregate those deemed insane away from sane society, and the replacement of obvious, outward signs of physical coercion and bodily restraint with more subtle, submerged measures designed to achieve similarly effective moral and psychological control by acting upon the mind.[23]

Returning to Ireland, the lunatic department at the Cork House of Industry seems to have been the first to make the transition from mere annex to discrete institution. Under the direction of physician William Saunders Hallaran, whose reported emphasis on individual treatment and engagement with each patient anticipated the tenets of moral management, 'Cork City and County Lunatic Asylum' came into being around 1791 with the construction of a building measuring 288 x 18 feet.[24] Further extensions brought the total capacity up to 300 patients by 1822,[25] in a structure that appears to survive to the present day, submerged within the warren of buildings that comprise the South Infirmary and Victoria University Hospital.[26] The built form of the Cork asylum adhered to a model recognisable from Bethlem and St Patrick's Hospital: a symmetrical building arranged as male and female patient wings flanking a central administration block. Within these wings, small cells for individual patients opened onto galleries that doubled as day spaces. Unlike St Patrick's, whose layout was forever compromised by the tiny 1¼ acre site within which architect George Semple had to shoe-horn his design,[27] sufficient space existed at Cork to provide a walled, landscaped garden – itself another portent of things to come.

19. Pinel and Tuke were both specifically cited by Sir John Leslie Foster as key influences in the new approach adopted at the Richmond Asylum in his evidence at the committee hearings. *Report from the Select Committee on the Lunatic Poor in Ireland*, HC 1817 [430] viii, p. 11; Samuel Tuke, *Practical Hints on the Construction and Economy of Pauper Lunatic Asylums* (London, 1815).
20. *Report from the Select Committee on the Lunatic Poor in Ireland*, HC 1817 [430] viii, p. 13.
21. *Report from the select committee appointed to consider… making provision for the care of lunatics and idiots by Grand Jury presentments 1804*, HC 1803/4 [109] p. iv.
22. Barry Edington, 'A space for moral management: The York Retreat's influence on asylum design', in Leslie Topp, James Moran and Jonathon Andrews (eds), *Madness, Architecture and the Built Environment* (New York & Oxon, 2007), p. 86, p. 90, p. 100.
23. Michel Foucault, *Madness and Civilisation* (tr. Richard Howard; New York, 1965), p269; Foucault, *Discipline and Punish* (tr. Alan Sheridan; New York, 1977), p. 172.
24. William Saunders Hallaran, *An Inquiry Into the Causes Producing the Extraordinary Addition to the Number of Insane* (Cork, 1810), p. 11.
25. Robins, *Fools and Mad*, pp 57–9.
26. 'A Plan of the City & Suburbs of Cork according to the latest improvements by William Beauford, 1801', and 'Plan of the City and Suburbs of Cork, Surveyed and Drawn by Thomas Holt, 1832', www.corkpastandpresent.ie/mapsimages/corkcityinoldmaps/, accessed on 30 Nov. 2020.
27. Elizabeth Malcolm, *Swift's Hospital: A History of St Patrick's Hospital, Dublin, 1746–1989* (Dublin, 1989), pp 33–41.

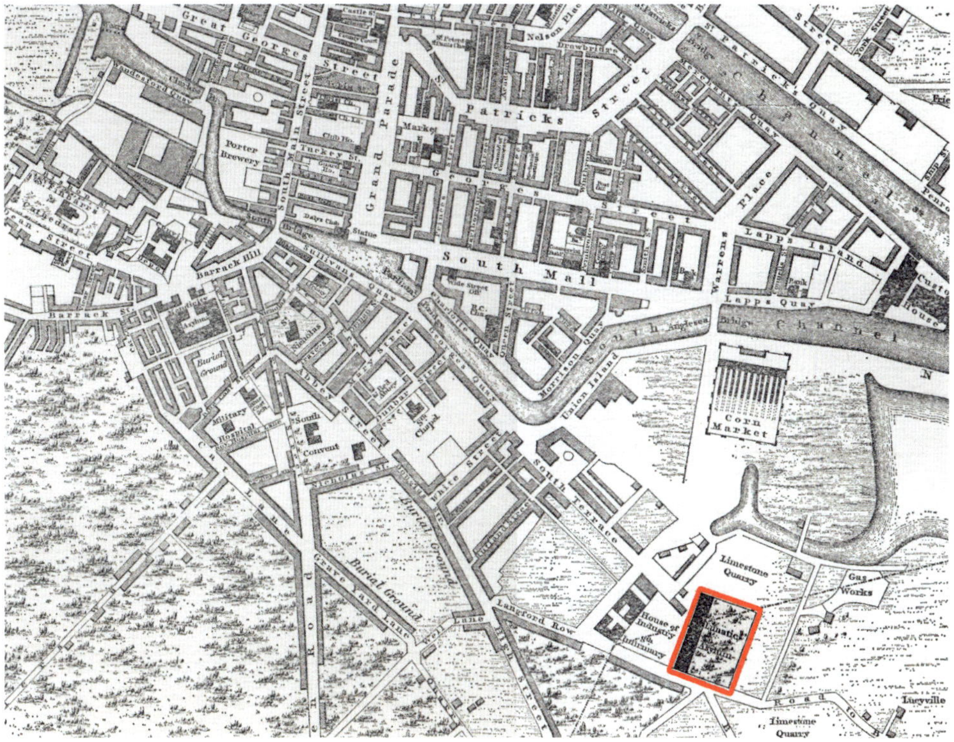

1.04 Plan of the City and Suburbs of Cork, Surveyed and Drawn by Thomas Holt, 1832. 'Lunatic Asylum' and walled garden shown separately from the House of Industry, *Image courtesy of Cork City Libraries.*

Meanwhile in 1804 with the scars from the dissolution of Ireland's own parliament still fresh (and the controversial project of 'Union' arguably in need of tangible vindication), a House of Commons Select Committee was established at Westminster to investigate 'making provision for the care of lunatics and idiots by Grand Jury presentments'. A bill 'for establishing provincial asylums for lunatics in Ireland',[28] was prepared but never enacted, even as a similar permissive act was passed for England in 1808.[29] It would take a petition from the Governors of the Dublin House of Industry, which claimed to be inundated with lunatics and idiots sent from all over the country, to prompt the establishment of a parliamentary Commission of Enquiry in 1808. The Commission's 1809 report led in short order to the construction of a large, specialist facility for the insane adjacent to the existing house of industry complex on the north-east fringes of Dublin city.[30] The building opened to patients in 1814 and was formally established under statute the following year as the 'Richmond Lunatic Asylum… [for]… the reception of lunatics from all parts of the kingdom', ushering in the era of publicly funded institutional provision for the insane that would persist for almost two centuries.[31]

The Richmond Lunatic(k) Asylum

The Richmond Asylum was designed by Board of Works architect Francis Johnston and named in honour of the incumbent Lord Lieutenant, the Earl of Richmond, whose arms adorn its entrance. Johnston would have been familiar with St Patrick's Hospital, having trained under Thomas Cooley, who was responsible for extensions to that

28. *Select Committee appointed to consider… making provision for the care of lunatics and idiots by Grand Jury presentments* HC 1803/4 [109] iv; *Bill for establishing provincial asylums for lunatics in Ireland 1805*, HC 1805 [61] i.
29. *Act for the better Care and Maintenance of Lunatics, being Paupers or Criminals in England 1808*. 48 Geo. 3, c.96.
30. Reynolds, *Grangegorman*, pp 20–1.
31. *Richmond Lunatic Asylum (Ireland) Act 1815*, 55 Geo. 3, c. 107.

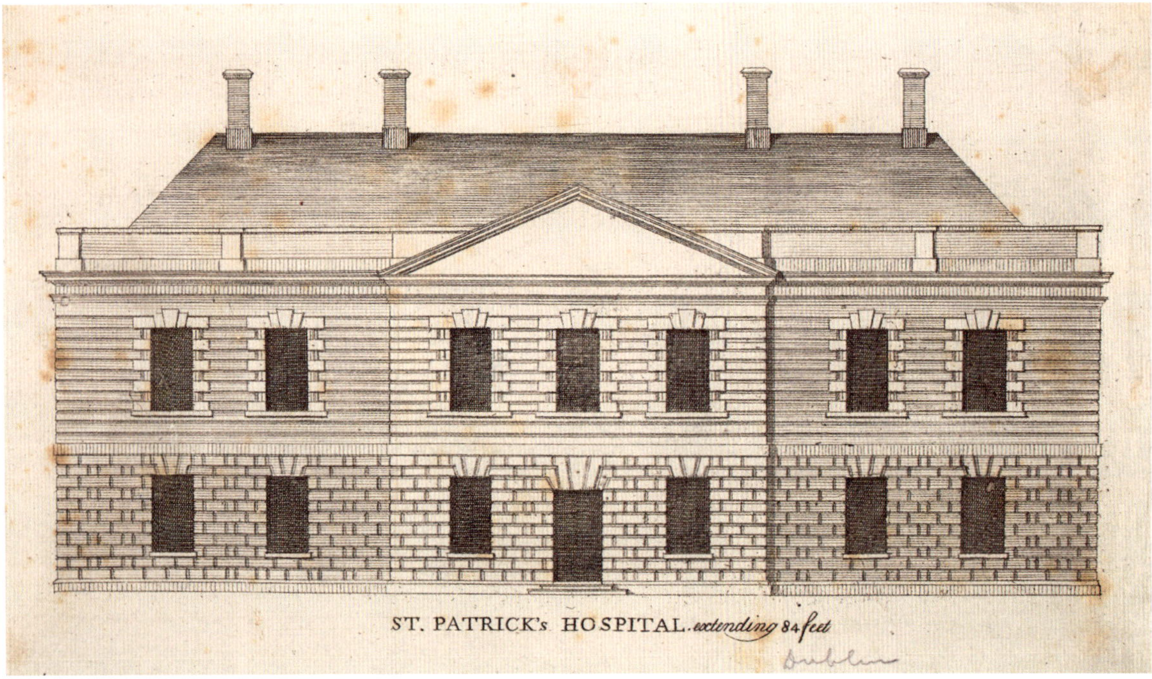
ST. PATRICK's HOSPITAL. extending 84 feet

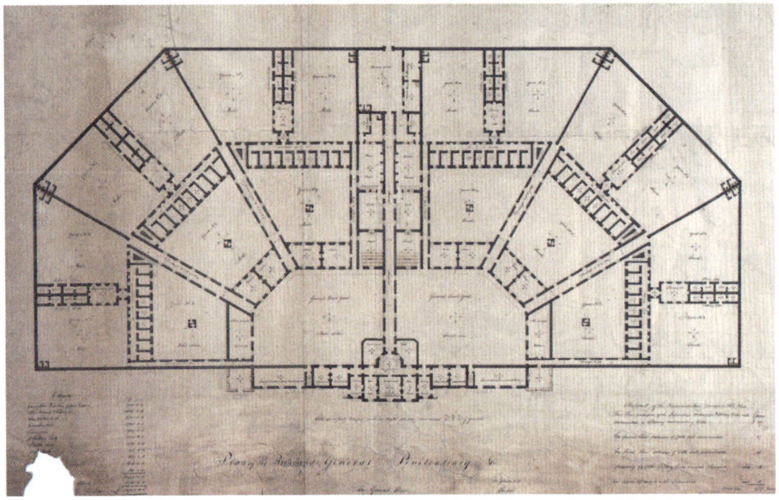

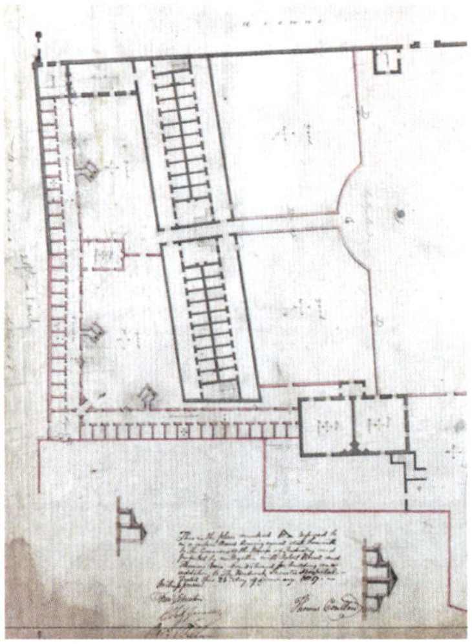

1.05 George Semple's design for St Patrick's Hospital, 1757, repeated the principles of Bethlem, albeit behind a much more modest façade, *Image courtesy of the National Library of Ireland (ET A320).*

1.06 Richmond Penitentiary: Ground floor plan, 1811, *Image courtesy of the Irish Architectural Archive (RIAI Murray Collection 92/46: 427).*

1.07 Plans to extend the Hardwicke 'lunatic cells' at the Dublin House of Industry, 1817. Note the absence of any facilities beyond the serried ranks of cells, *Image courtesy of the Irish Architectural Archive (RIAI Murray Collection 92/46: 405).*

1.08 Clonmel's former House of Industry, with its lunatic department to rear, was later adapted in its entirety as an auxilary to the main asylum, *Reproduced courtesy Trinity College Dublin (OS-Clonmel-500-Sheets 13,19-1876).*

1.09 Richmond Asylum, Dublin: 'Lunatick Asylum' inscription recently discovered to parapet, *Photograph by Grangegorman Development Agency, 2015.*

1.10 Richmond Asylum, Dublin: Entrance front, *Photograph by David Killeen, 2019.*

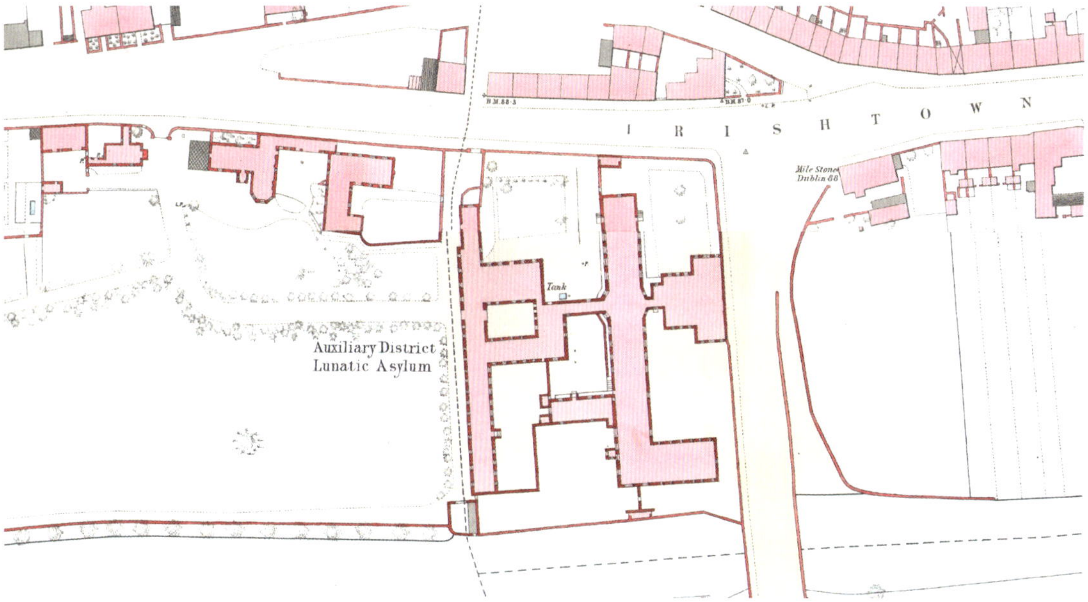

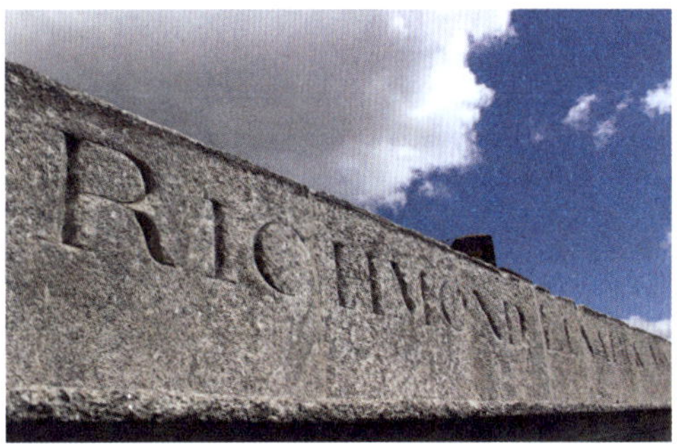

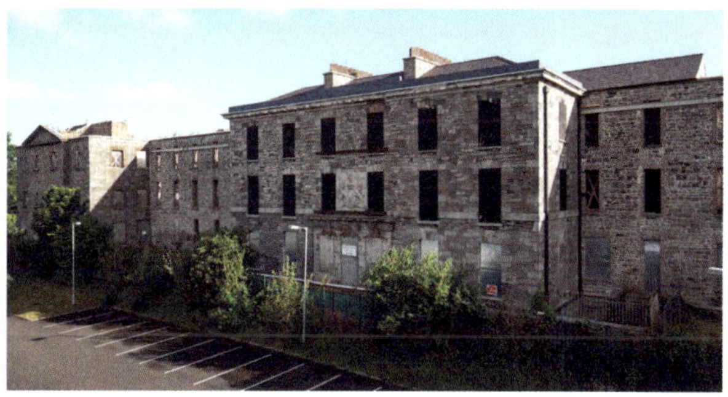

building between 1778 and 1783.[32] However, while Johnston was one of the most accomplished architects of his era, his relatively primitive design for the Richmond Asylum cannot be counted as one of his better works. Accommodation, as already encountered at Bethlem, St Patrick's and most asylums that would follow, featured a central administration block flanked by male and female wards composed mainly of single cells opening onto galleries. But unlike these others, Johnston arranged the wards around a quadrangular courtyard – a layout that appears more closely related to a seventeenth-century alms-house or an eighteenth-century house of industry than to the curative potential of emerging asylum design.[33] If anything, it is inferior to all of these in being fully enclosed on all sides and rising to a third story to the detriment of effective ventilation and creating what was condemned as a 'veritable trap for foul miasma'.[34] Recent works to rescue the building's surviving southern range from ruin have revealed a previously hidden inscription on the parapet proclaiming the building's function as a 'Lunatick Asylum', the archaic spelling reinforcing the sense that this building was more a relic of the eighteenth century than a pioneer for the nineteenth.[35]

In at least one respect Johnston anticipated progressive asylum design by facilitating the strict segregation of different categories of patients – something increasingly seen as critical to achieving cures. In these matters, Johnston may have been influenced by Dr Alexander Jackson, physician to the house of industry and a keen proponent of the curative potential of moral management. In 1813 Jackson travelled to York and Bethlem, where he likely gained insights into emerging trends as described by Tuke and others to which Johnston himself may not yet have been exposed.[36] This was a particularly interesting time in Johnston's career, a moment when, in addition to the asylum, his drawing board was strewn with designs for no fewer than three different carceral institutions. Arising from a prison reform act of 1810, he was tasked with producing a model prison design 'upon which all new Gaols in Ireland may be built, varying… only according to the size which may be suitable to the extent of [each] county'. His model prison design of August 1810 and his design for the unrelated Richmond Bridewell were both archaic courtyard schemes in the manner of the Richmond Asylum, with the Bridewell notable only for the carved inscription that admonished all who entered its sombre portals: 'Cease to do Evil, Learn to do Well.'[37]

The third commission was for a new government-sponsored penitentiary on a site immediately adjacent to the asylum – a politically significant project that predated London's equivalent Millbank Penitentiary by several years and which had the obvious potential to serve as an exemplar for prison reform in Ireland.[38] Whatever influences came to bear on Johnston between August 1810 and January 1811 resulted in a dramatically different design from his earlier efforts: a novel and highly complex layout that facilitated the separation of multiple classes of prisoners. Butler argues that in combining elements of two different design approaches to prison design – the radial and the polygonal – but without quite understanding the underlying principles of either, Johnston 'managed to eliminate the usefulness of both'. The functional shortcomings of the new penitentiary quickly became apparent, leading this much

32. Reuber, 'Moral management and the "Unseen Eye"', p. 209; Malcolm, *Swift's Hospital*, p. 73.

33. O'Dwyer suggested that Johnston's plan for the Richmond may have been based on Robert Reid's design for the Morningside Asylum in Edinburgh published in 1807, but Richmond resembles Morningside only superficially as a quadrangular building with a courtyard quartered by communicating corridors. Morningside is a radically different building and more architecturally developed in many respects – not least the disposition of its wings as three-storey blocks linked to corner pavilions by single-storey wings (facilitating ventilation), its design for phased construction, the integration of spaces for collective activity, and the use of double- rather than single-loaded galleries. Casey concurs. Christine Casey, *The Buildings of Ireland: Dublin* (London, 2005). Others have interpreted the Richmond's connecting corridors (and central privy block) as an early example of panoptic design, which they most assuredly were not.

34. The 'miasma' theory held that diseases such as cholera were spread by foul air, and thus preventable by effective ventilation.

35. I am grateful to Una Sugrue of the Grangegorman Development Agency, for sharing this insight. While popular spelling may not have been standardised until later in the nineteenth century, Johnston was already out of step with his government client, whose parliamentary papers and official reports consistently use the modern spelling of 'Lunatic' through the whole century.

36. Reuber, 'Moral management and the "Unseen Eye"', p. 213. Late design changes also followed, probably on Jackson's advice, to create the corridor connection between the blocks, which had all previously been independently accessed in the manner of barrack blocks, and which also formed separate airing yards to complete the programme of segregation of patients. IAA, Murray Collection, 1814, Richmond Asylum, 92/46, Sheets 0411, 0412, 0413.

37. Bernadette Goslin, 'The *Murray Collection* of architectural drawings' (unpublished MA thesis, 1990), p. 156; Butler, *Building the Irish Courthouse and Prison*, pp 197–8.

38. Robin Evans, *The Fabrication of Virtue: English Prison Architecture, 1750–1840* (Cambridge, 1982), p. 278, p. 291.

vaunted experiment in central-government-sponsored prison-building to be judged as a very expensive failure.[39] But what is more significant for our purposes is that Johnston had at last begun to engage with a core philosophy of the contemporary reform movement: that the power and potential of architecture to influence moral character lay not in slogans carved in stone, but in the rational disposition of spaces and the projection of central power through the act of 'seeing without being seen'.[40]

While early prison-reform themes of security, classification and ventilation owed much to the work of John Howard, the concept of planning buildings to facilitate centralised surveillance had its roots in the late eighteenth-century work of social reformer and utilitarian philosopher Jeremy Bentham. Bentham spent a long career promoting his 'Panopticon' concept – that institutions planned around a central 'all-seeing eye' had the power to reform the wayward. Initially conceived as a model penitentiary, he later extended the principle to 'any Sort of Establishment, in which Persons of any Description are to be kept under Inspection', including poorhouses, madhouses, factories, schools and much else besides.[41] Though Bentham himself failed to see his most pioneering designs executed, his arguments for the potential of centralised inspection found wider traction in two distinct forms, albeit neither was a perfect facsimile of the original highly transparent 'panopticon'. In radially planned

39. Butler's conclusion takes account of the views of Henry Heaney and Edward McParland, the latter having revised his earlier opinion of the building as one of considerable innovation. Butler, *Building the Irish Courthouse and Prison*, pp 189–97.

40. Jeremy Bentham, *Panopticon, or the Inspection-House* (Dublin, 1791) p. 23.

41. Ibid.

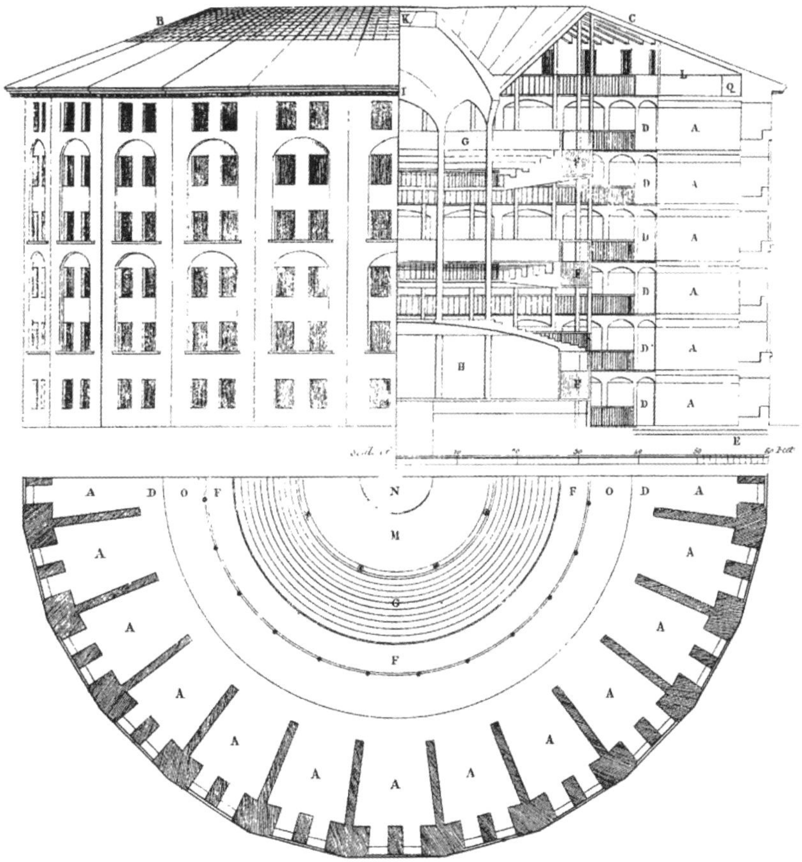

1.11 Plan of Jeremy Bentham's panopticon prison, *drawn by Willey Reveley in 1791, Public Domain Mark 1.0*

buildings, cell wings radiate from a central block, from which the interior of each wing (though not the interior of each cell) could be monitored. In polygonal buildings, cells wings were arranged around a perimeter that enclosed the airing yards, the central block principally supervising the exterior yards rather than the interior of the buildings. And if today we find it hard to dissociate this concept of centralised surveillance from its near-universal application in prison design, it may come as a surprise to discover that it was in the lunatic asylums of Ireland, under the hand of Francis Johnston, that elements of Bentham's theory would first be put into practice at a national scale.

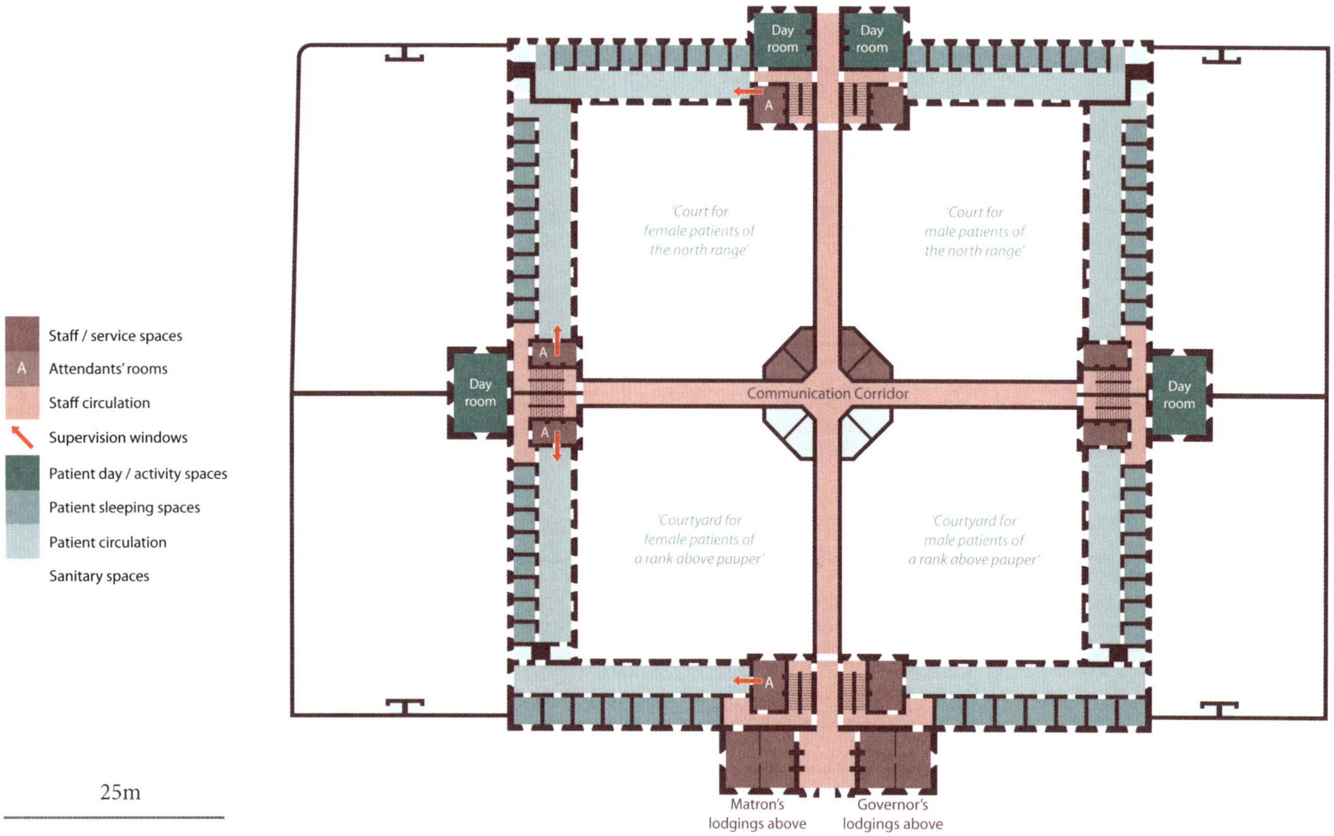

1.12 Plan diagram of The Richmond with key spaces annotated. Note the lack of internal connections between the four blocks which the central communication corridor sought to rectify. *Drawn by the author.*

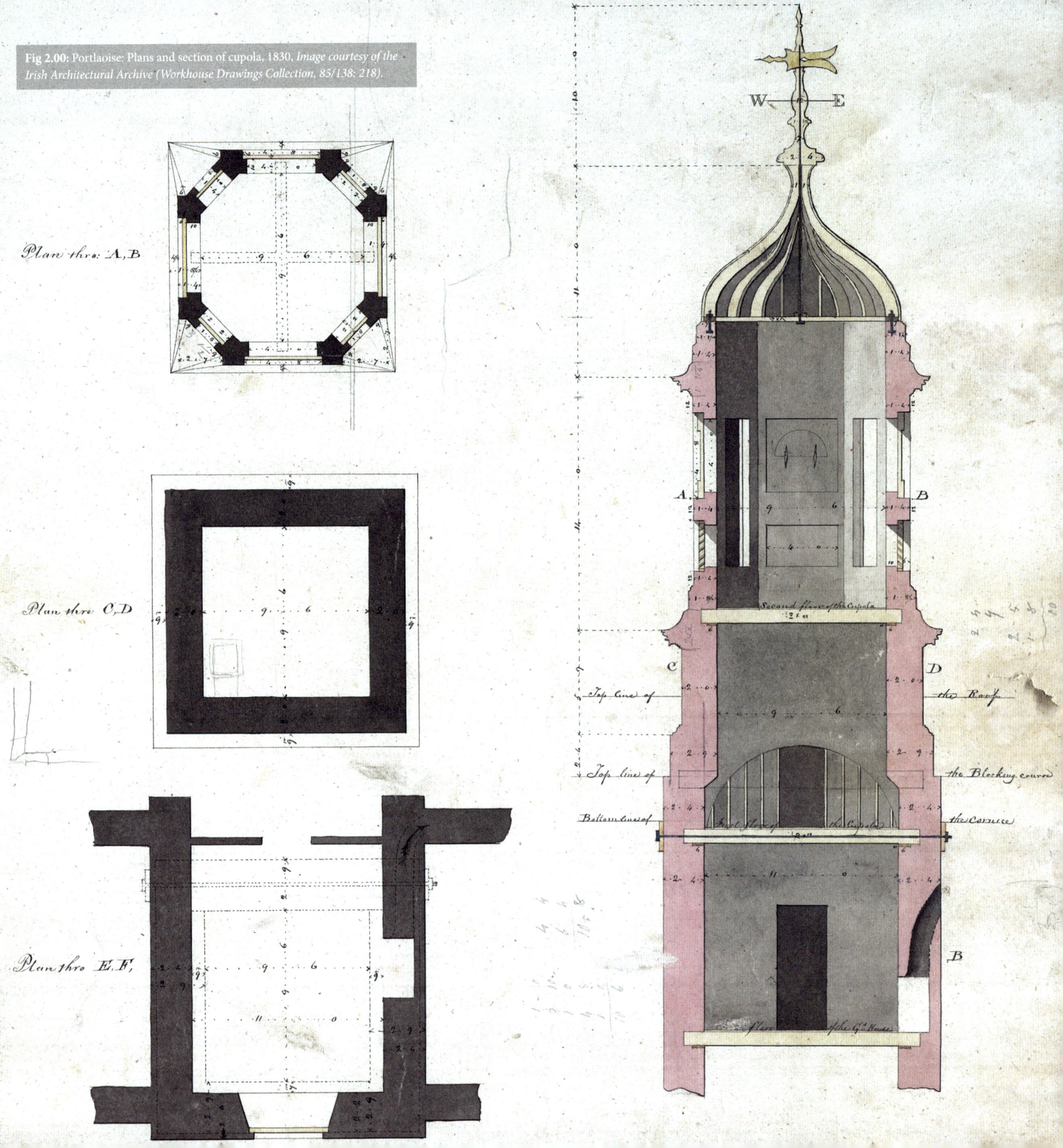

Fig 2.00: Portlaoise: Plans and section of cupola, 1830, *Image courtesy of the Irish Architectural Archive (Workhouse Drawings Collection, 85/138: 218).*

Designing for Moral Management

establish a species of espionage [1]

The Richmond was designed to house some 200 patients, but was full within two years of opening. Plans were prepared to add new convalescent wings to east and west, but it was already clear that the institution would never be able to serve the needs of its national catchment.[2] Meanwhile a parliamentary committee established in 1815 to examine the state of English madhouses digressed into matters across the Irish Sea, concluding that 'the necessity of making some further provision for Insane Persons [in Ireland] appears to be more urgent even than in this part of the United Kingdom.'[3] A further select committee was thus established in 1817 to enquire specifically into the 'expediency of making provision for the relief of the lunatic poor in Ireland'.[4] Oral evidence was heard from members familiar with the conditions prevailing in different parts of the country and from prominent reformers including John Leslie Foster and Thomas Spring Rice, along with documentary evidence from others, such as Alexander Jackson, who were involved in the day-to-day operation of the existing institutions.

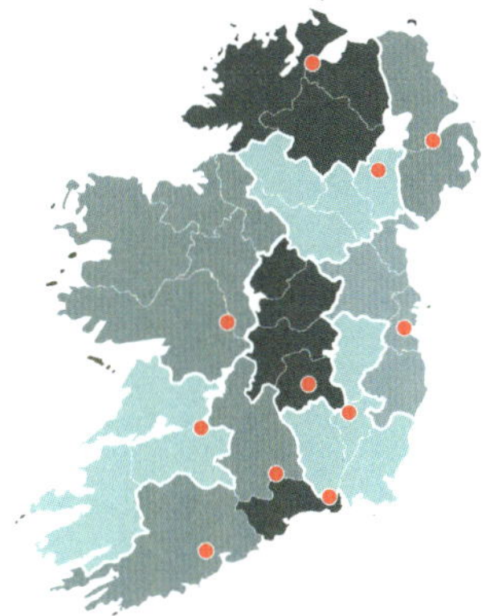

Asylum distribution in Ireland showing district boundaries, 1835, *Drawn by the author.*

The committee paid relatively less attention to conditions in society at large, beyond the infamous claim that profoundly deranged individuals in pauper households were managed by 'making a hole in the floor of the cabin not high enough for the person to stand up in, with a crib over it to prevent his getting up, the hole is about five feet deep, and they give this wretched being his food there, and there he generally dies.'[5] Instead inquiries focused on the existing state of institutional care, revealing an uneven geographical distribution of institutions of starkly contrasting quality. At one end of the spectrum the achievements of Dr Hallaran at Cork and Alexander Jackson at The Richmond were lauded; at the other extreme patients in Limerick were described as chained in filthy cells and as being exposed to freezing winter conditions resulting in frostbitten and amputated limbs.

On balance, the substance of the proceedings would seem to justify the committee's claim to be motivated by 'benevolent intentions… to contribute to the cure of malady and the alleviation of wretchedness'. But even at this early point in

1. Samuel Tuke, *Practical Hints on the Construction and Economy of Pauper Lunatic Asylums* (London, 1815), p. 28.
2. Irish Architectural Archive (hereafter IAA), Murray Collection, 1814, Richmond Asylum, 92/46, Sheets 0411, 0412, 0413; Joseph Robins, *Fools and Mad: A History of the Insane in Ireland* (Dublin, 1986), pp 63–4.
3. *Report from the Committee on Madhouses in England* (hereafter *1815 Select Committee Report*), HC 1814–15 [296] pp 4–5, p. 24
4. *Report from the Select Committee on the Lunatic Poor in Ireland*, HC 1817 [430], viii.
5. Ibid, p. 23.

our story it is worth noting the categorical assumption that such 'wretchedness' could only be alleviated within the confines of an institutional model. And beneath the surface, a latent desire to maintain public order by coercive means can occasionally be detected: 'There were a great many idiots about the streets of Wexford, and there are none now, so that from that I should think it is sufficient.'[6] Between the extreme versions of a highly centralised national institution and a geographically dispersed model of county-based asylums, the committee ultimately recommended the erection of 'four or five' new district asylums around the country, to be operated on the principles of moral management and funded from local taxation levied jointly on the counties of which each district was composed.[7] But in shining a light on the plight of the insane, the reformers had unwittingly initiated a process that would see institutional provision grow more than one-hundred-fold in less than a century.[8]

A legislative first

While English reforms foundered on political fears of increasing the power of central government,[9] Irish (Whig) members of parliament campaigned for and passed an Act 'to provide for the establishment of asylums for the lunatic poor in Ireland'.[10] Various explanations have been posited to explain Ireland's success in passing mandatory legislation that was not palatable in England, including suggestions that it was a feature of colonial social policy or part of a wider trend of 'experimenting with new ideas in social management before implementing them in England'.[11] Yet the true reasons may be altogether more pragmatic. The new asylums would need to serve districts comprised of three, four or five counties, and it was highly unlikely that so many grand juries could be relied upon to voluntarily co-ordinate their actions. Grand juries of adjacent cities and counties already duplicated prisons and courthouses that should logically have been combined, while numerous scandals and delays in implementing prison reforms revealed them to be incompetent, corrupt and unfit agents for the delivery of new public buildings.[12] As so many grand juries had already failed to make provision for the insane under existing (voluntary) legislation, central government was justifiably sceptical that their goals could be achieved other than by mandatory legislation. Understanding this context slightly tempers the pride implicit in the oft-repeated statement that Ireland was the first country in the world to establish a statutory national public asylum system. But whatever the motivation, further amendments to the original 1817 legislation in 1820, 1821, 1825 and 1826 demonstrated that successive (Tory) governments were committed to ensuring that shortcomings in statute could not be used as an excuse for inaction.

The 1817 Act assigned responsibility for designing and constructing the new asylums to a centralised 'Commission of Control and Correspondence' (Board of Control), acting on the instructions of the Lord Lieutenant. The Act left decisions regarding the number and location of asylums to the discretion of the Lord Lieutenant, who was soon inundated with representations from various interest groups seeking to influence the location of new asylums. Further details on the associated political machinations may be encountered within the individual institutional histories in the second part of this book; suffice here to note that the end

6. *Report from the Select Committee on the Lunatic Poor in Ireland*, HC 1817 [430], viii.
7. In weighing the inevitable trade-offs between quality and accessibility of care, it was considered that the single asylum in Dublin was too inaccessible, but that individual counties could not sustain specialist skills to deliver high-quality care. There is nothing new in contemporary disputes that seek to retain (often underperforming) local hospital services in opposition to a policy of creating fewer 'centres of excellence'. Ibid, p. 10.
8. Damien Brennan, *Irish Insanity, 1800–2000* (Oxon, 2014), p. 124. Table A1: Total asylum population reached 22,138 in 1902 and 25,180 by 1915.
9. Scull, *The Most Solitary of Afflictions*, (New Haven & London, 1993); Markus Reuber, 'The architecture of psychological management: The Irish asylums, 1801–1922', in *Psychological Medicine*, no. 26 (1996), p. 1181.
10. Lunatic Asylums (Ireland) Act 1817, 57 Geo iii c106. Brennan and Reuber both concur that Ireland was the first jurisdiction in the world to roll out a national asylum network, but this was also in the context of meagre public provision and an almost non-existent private or voluntary sector in Ireland. What is perhaps more significant in the international historical context is that the new asylums were specifically intended to operate in accordance with the principles of moral management from the outset.
11. Brennan, *Irish Insanity*, p. 1; Niall McCullough and Valerie Mulvin, *A Lost Tradition: The Nature of Architecture in Ireland* (Dublin, 1987), p. 115. Markus also cites the potential of Ireland as a testing ground for policy, albeit in the context of educational reform. In the context of educational reform, see also Thomas Markus, *Buildings and Power: Freedom and Control in the Origin of Modern Building Types* (London and New York, 1993), p. 75.
12. The cities and counties of Galway, Cork and Waterford erected duplicate courthouses, prisons, or both, sometimes on adjacent sites. Butler also reveals the repeated failure of many grand juries to comply with central edicts on reformed prison designs. Richard J. Butler, *Building the Irish Courthouse and Prison, A Political History, 1750–1850* (Cork, 2019), pp 176–234.

result was a geographically uneven distribution of asylums that included Armagh, Belfast and Londonderry in Ulster; Limerick, Waterford and Clonmel in Munster; Carlow and Maryborough in Leinster; and a single asylum at Ballinasloe to serve all of Connaught.[13] And far from the 'nimby' attitudes familiar to a modern audience, a new asylum was a potentially desirable addition to the civic landscape, and not only as a monument to the benevolence and enlightenment of the local ruling elites.[14] It doubtless helped that the initial capital cost was met by a Treasury loan, repayable from local taxation (county cess) levied across all of the counties comprising the asylum district. The initial construction and ongoing operation of a new asylum therefore conferred economic benefits on the immediate locality in which it was located, at the expense of the landowners and occupiers of neighbouring counties.

Adopting moral management

Kindness and one-to-one care were essential requisites of this new approach of 'moral treatment'. Patients, segregated by degree of insanity, would be free from physical restraint but encouraged to exercise 'internal restraint, generated by the religious family environment and the patients' wish to earn the superintendent's esteem', under whose constant, benevolent supervision they lived.[15] Samuel Tuke's argument that the design of the building could improve the treatment and cure of the patient helped to establish the fundamental assumption that asylums should be housed in purpose-built rather than adapted premises:

> *how great a degree, the prevention of abuses, and the compatibility of comfort with security, must depend on the construction of their abodes… The regulations of an asylum should establish a species of espionage… this cannot be effected in an ill constructed building.*[16]

The 1817 Committee's commitment to moral management thus proved incompatible with their rather less inspired suggestion that disused barracks could be appropriated for use as asylums.[17] Extending the benign 'moral influence' of the governor to a larger cohort of patients demanded new architectural responses that prioritised simplicity of superintendence, a brief readily answered by Jeremy Bentham's 'panopticon' principle. William Stark was the first to apply the concept to the design of a major asylum at Glasgow: his ideas were circulating in print from 1807 even though the building itself was not completed until 1814.[18] Stark's rigorous panoptic plan seemed to offer the holy grail of combining simplicity of supervision with a high degree of classification: patients were segregated by gender, 'rank in life' and degree of insanity, arranged in four arms radiating from, and under the direct surveillance of, the governor's quarters at the centre. The concept was refined and slightly softened by the Quaker architect James Bevans, whose contributions would dominate the architectural discourse at the parliamentary Committee on Madhouses in England in 1815. Bevans' connection to the acclaimed York Retreat entitled him to some standing,[19] but the highly developed panoptic designs he submitted to the committee demonstrate conceptual sophistication and technical competence far

13. *Fourteenth Report of the Inspectors-General of Prisons*, HC 1836 [118] xxxv.
14. Enthusiasm was evident in trying to secure a new asylum for the county or city – the actual selection of a specific site within the urban area could still give rise to local objections, as seen in the multiple submissions made regarding prospective sites for the Waterford asylum. National Archives of Ireland: Chief Secretary's Office, 1832, Correspondence relating to the new lunatic asylum in Waterford city, CSO/RP/1832/2119.
15. Markus Reuber, 'Moral management and the "Unseen Eye": Public Lunatic Asylums, 1800–1845', in Elizabeth Malcolm and Greta Jones (eds), *Medicine, Disease and the State in Ireland, 1650–1940* (Cork, 1999), p. 211.
16. The word 'espionage', in this context, is simply taken to mean supervision, without any political overtones. Samuel Tuke, *Practical Hints on the Construction and Economy of Pauper Lunatic Asylums* (London, 1815), pp 23–4, p. 28.
17. *Report from the Select Committee on the Lunatic Poor in Ireland*, HC 1817 [430] viii, p. 4.
18. William Stark, *Remarks on the Construction of Public Hospitals for the Cure of Mental Derangement: Read to a Committee of Inhabitants of the City of Glasgow* (Glasgow, 1810). First edition published 1807.
19. Of which his father John, is generally cited as architect. Reuber, 'Moral management and the "Unseen Eye"', p. 232. Bevans Junior admitted of certain deficiencies in the design of *The Retreat*. His role as surveyor saw him visit almost every private madhouse in London over a four-year period, as well St Luke's and Bethlem Hospitals. His very specific criticisms of the latter directly influenced the Committee's final recommendations for changes to that building. *1815 Select Committee Report*, pp 6–7, 32–3. Interestingly, Markus also notes that James Bevans collaborated directly with Jeremy Bentham in 1815 in the design of a school for the latter's own children. Markus, *Buildings and Power*, p. 67.

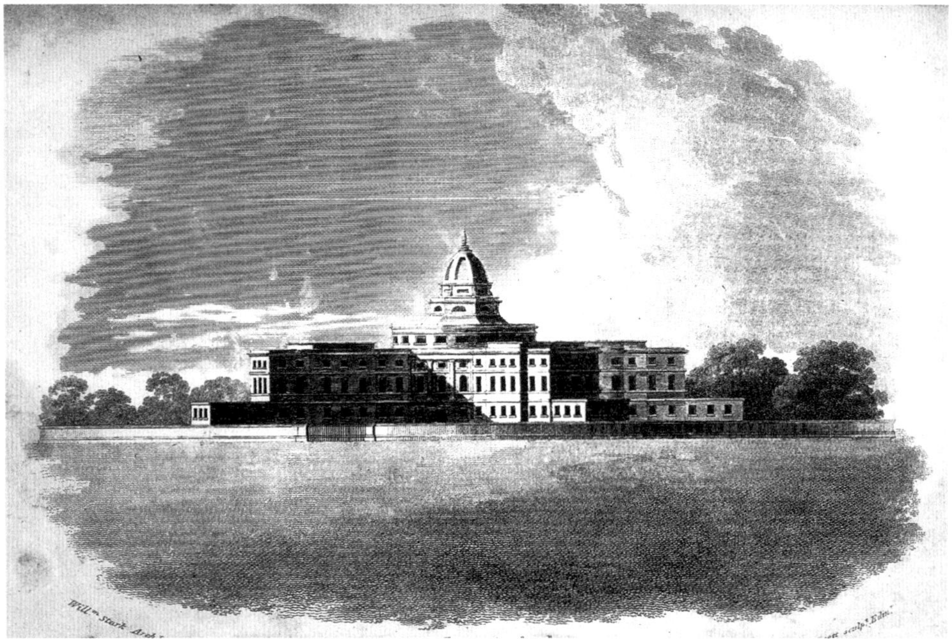

2.01 Elevation of William Stark's Glasgow Asylum, 1807, *Wellcome Collection (William Stark, 1807) Attribution 4.0 International (CC BY 4.0).*

beyond the simple domesticity of The Retreat.[20] Between 1817 and 1818, both Bevans and Johnston submitted draft plans for standard asylums to the Irish Board of Control. Bevans' reputation and expertise may have preceded him in London, but in Ireland proved insufficient to dislodge the incumbent designer of the Richmond Asylum and architect to the Board of Works. Johnston secured the commission, but his apparent incorporation of several aspects of Bevan's designs caused the latter to complain that his designs were being used without authorisation or payment.[21]

Inspection and classification

It is easy to forget that meanings and associations change over time. Today, we have to be reminded that the word 'hospital' once applied to a wide range of 'hospitable' institutions, not solely a centre for the practice of medicine. While a modern audience may similarly struggle to conceive of a radial building designed for ease of supervision as anything other than 'prison-like', at the dawn of the nineteenth century panoptic architecture seemed to offer the potential to reform many of the ills of society, not merely the criminal. As the logical product of a rational, scientific approach, it represented a profound physical manifestation of Enlightenment thinking. So even if later commentators criticised Johnston's standard designs asylums as being too 'prison-like', we must not rush to ascribe penal motives to his efforts.

In summary, Johnston's plans for both the smaller (100-bed) and larger (150-bed) asylums feature a central block containing administration and officers' apartments, from which radiate four wings of one or two storeys (sometimes over basement), each containing between ten and thirteen patient cells of vaulted masonry, with a nurses room and day room on each floor, all opening off single-loaded vaulted corridors or 'galleries'. Separate airing yards were provided for each ward, flanked by 'airing sheds'

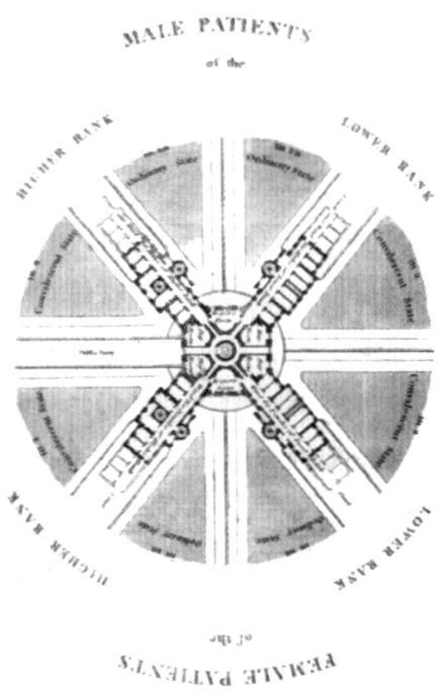

2.02 Annotated plan of Glasgow Asylum, 1807, showing classification by gender, rank and degree of insanity, *Wellcome Library (William Stark, 1807) Attribution 4.0 International (CC BY 4.0).*

20. *1815 Select Committee Report*, p. 91, p. 150, pp 160–3, Plates I to VI.
21. Bevans presented various designs, including proposals for the new Wakefield Asylum, which, with two centres of inspection rather than one, could invite the moniker 'biopticon'. However, it is his generic design for a pauper asylum for 70 patients, specifically prepared by order of the committee, which provides the most obvious link to the Irish asylums that followed.

or 'walking sheds' which ensured that the Irish weather would be no impediment to patients partaking of a daily constitutional. Convalescent patients, accommodated in shared rooms on the first floor, were permitted access to the open airing shed to the front of the building and the extensive grounds beyond.

Internal windows – potentially copied from Bevan's design – allowed the governor or matron to inspect the patient galleries and dayrooms from the comfort of their own quarters or adjacent 'inspection lobbies' – to see without being seen.[22] For patients, the ever-present possibility of unseen vigilance was supposed to encourage the self-restraint on which the theory of moral management was substantially founded. No less importantly, their keepers (as nurses and attendants were originally known) laboured under the same sense of potential surveillance, designed to deter them from abusing patients in the manner that had proven all too common in earlier institutions for the insane. Compared to the outmoded courtyard of the Richmond Asylum, Johnston's new prototypes demonstrated a good grasp of the latest theories in the treatment of insanity, even if they were tainted by a lingering whiff of plagiarism. He also exercised more sensitivity in execution than Stark, whose ruthlessly efficient Glasgow asylum so closely resembled the programme of a contemporary prison that Tuke, originally a proponent of panoptic design principles, rued that 'it is therefore possible to carry our views of easy inspection too far; and I think it would be doing so to adopt some of the panopticon plans.'[23]

Reuber has already demonstrated how Johnston's plans answered the demands of moral management, though he had less to say about their shortcomings. Johnston's design included self-contained annexes for refractory or 'noisy' patients at the extremities of the building, each containing six cells, a day room and separate airing yard. Examination of the basement plans reveal a further 12 subterranean cells, lit and ventilated by tiny slit windows. While the drawings do not officially ascribe any use, in practice the temptation to use them for the detention of 'very dirty and ungovernable patients' must have been hard to resist.[24] From a utilitarian point of view, physically isolating the most challenging cases did at least have the benefit of sparing other patients from daily exposure to profoundly disturbed behaviour, but Tuke had specifically warned against succumbing to the exclusionary impulse, and with good reason: 'the evil of noise is not so great as those of filth, starvation, and cruelty.'[25] This design decision meant that patients in greatest need of therapeutic relief were lodged in spaces that denied them the benefits of the supposedly curative gaze of the 'unseen eye'. Worse, consigning such patients out of sight and sound also risked them slipping out of mind and back into the netherworld of 'shit, straw and stench' that these exemplary institutions were supposed to have banished.

A carefully cultivated image

If the architectural plan governs the practical operation and daily experience of those who use the building, the facade is the medium through which its sense of purpose is communicated to outsiders. As in so many other respects, the facade of London's newly reconstructed Bethlem Hospital (1676) became something of a cause célèbre. The new hospital was a source of civic pride immediately after its construction and

22. While Bevans' specific proposals to the Irish Commissioners are not known to survive, the similarities between his previously published designs and Johnston's ultimate design are clear. *Minutes of Commissioners for General Control and Correspondence for Superintending… the Erection… of Asylums for the Lunatic Poor*, 25 Sep. 1817 – Apr. 1818, cited in Katherine Fennelly, 'Out of sound, out of mind: Noise control in early nineteenth-century lunatic asylums in England and Ireland', in *World Archaeology* 26:3 (2014), p. 421. Fennelly states that Bevans was originally invited to submit plans by Robert Peel, then secretary to the Lord Lieutenant, before being side-lined in favour of Johnston. Una Sugrue notes that Francis Johnston's library contained a copy of Stark's 1807 *Remarks*, and Watson and Pritchett's 1819 *Plans, Elevations, Sections and Designs/Drawings of the Pauper Lunatic Asylum at Wakefield, York*, from which he could have drawn inspiration directly without relying upon Bevans' intermediation.
23. *1815 Select Committee Report*, Plate VI.
24. Tuke, *Practical Hints*, p. 33. Tuke's book instead included plans of the proposed Wakefield Asylum.
25. *Annual Asylum Report 1844*, HC 1845 [645] xxvi, p. 20.

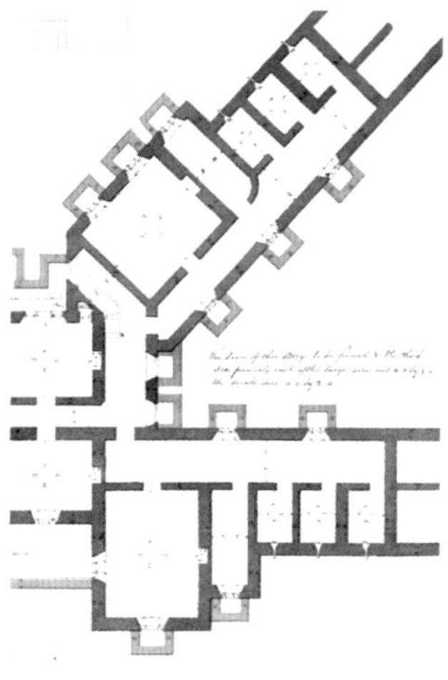

2.03 Carlow: Basement plan, 1829. Note banks of three cells lit and ventilated only by a narrow slit. *Image courtesy of the Irish Architectural Archive (RIAI Murray Collection 92/46: 123).*

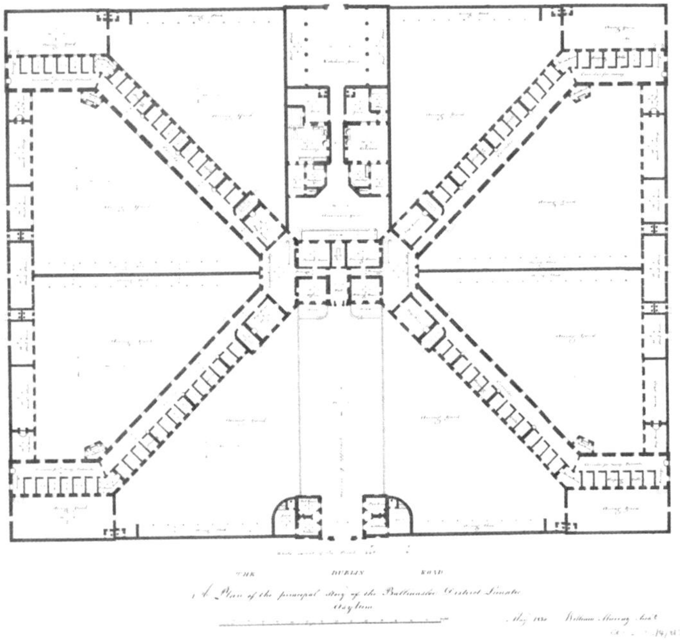
THE DUBLIN ROAD

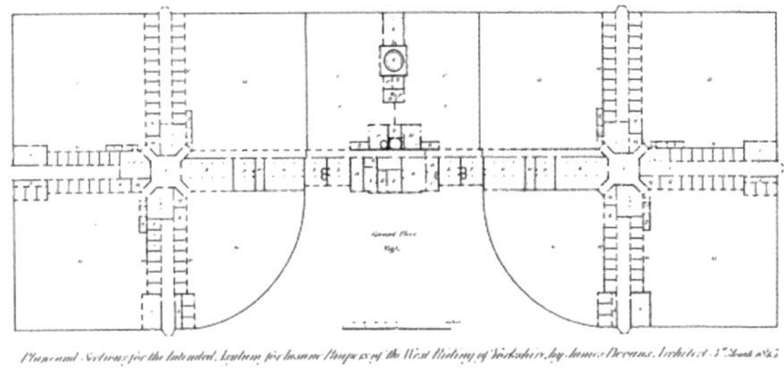
Ground Floor
Plans and Sections for the Intended Asylum for Insane Paupers of the West Riding of Yorkshire, by James Bevans, Architect

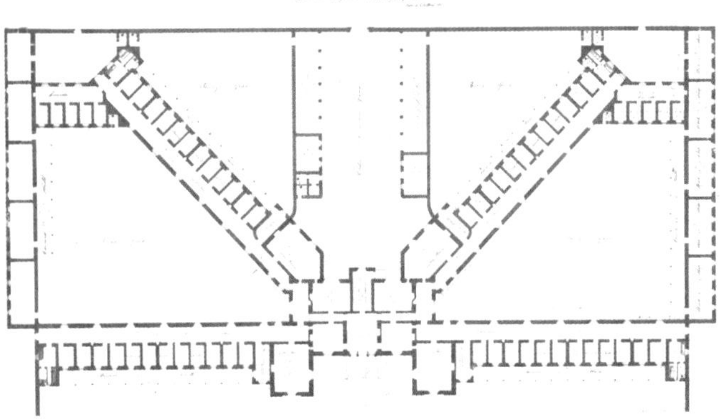

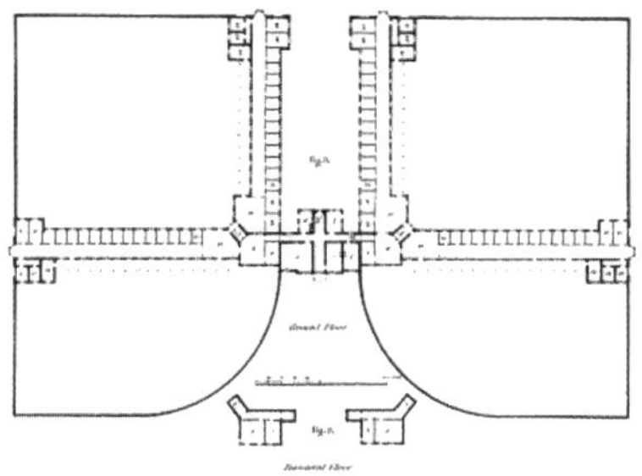
Ground Floor

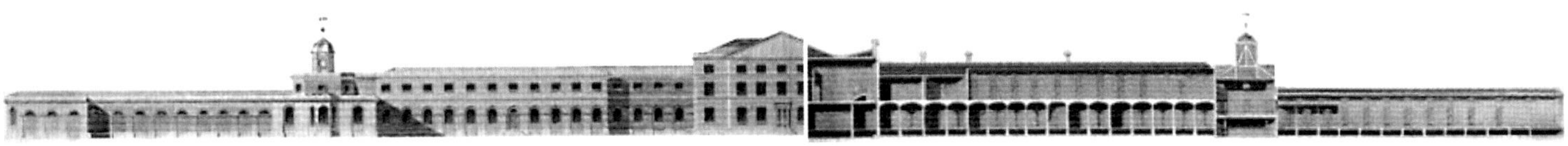

Fig. 1.

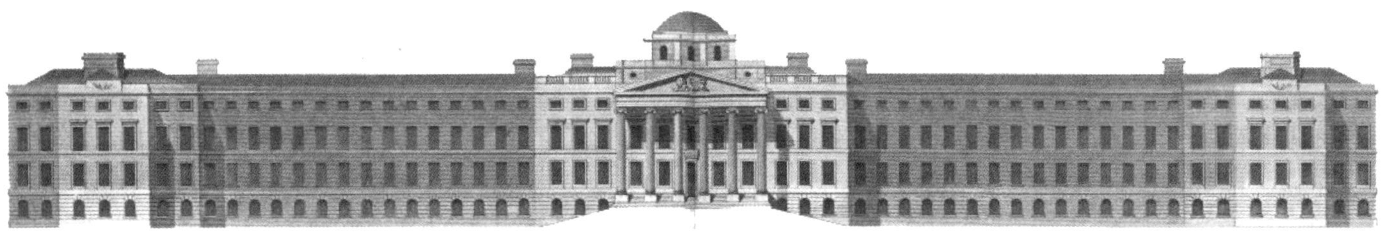

2.04 Ballinasloe: Ground floor plan of 'First Class asylum for 150 patients.' William Murray implemented several minor modifications compared to the earlier Limerick asylum., *Image courtesy of the National Archives of Ireland (Office of Public Works Collection, OPW/5HC/4/883: 2).*

2.05 Plan of James Bevans' proposal for Wakefield Asylum, 1815, *Image courtesy of ProQuest LLC (ProQuest House of Commons Parliamentary Papers, HC 1814-15 [296], Plate V).*

2.06 Armagh: Ground floor plan of Francis Johnston's 'Second Class asylum for 100 patients,' 1825, *Image courtesy of the Irish Architectural Archive (RIAI Murray Collection 92/46: 65,70).*

2.07 Plan of James Bevans' 'Design for an asylum for 70 Insane Paupers, 1815, including all of the key features which would later be found in Johnston's standard design for the Irish asylums, *Image courtesy of ProQuest LLC (ProQuest House of Commons Parliamentary Papers, HC 1814-15 [296], Plate VI).*

2.08 Elevation and section of James Bevans' proposal for Wakefield Asylum, 1815, *Image courtesy of University of Southampton Digital Scholarship Team (HC 1814-15 [296], Plate IV.*

2.09 Bethlem: The third Bethlem Hospital, opened 1817, was no less palatial than its predecessor, and its operation no less prone to scandal, *Image courtesy of University of Southampton Digital Scholarship Team (HC 1814-15 [296], Plate VII.*

2.10 Belfast: Elevation and sections showing differentials in floor level and partially blocked cell windows, *Image courtesy of the Irish Architectural Archive (RIAI Murray Collection 92/46: 108).*

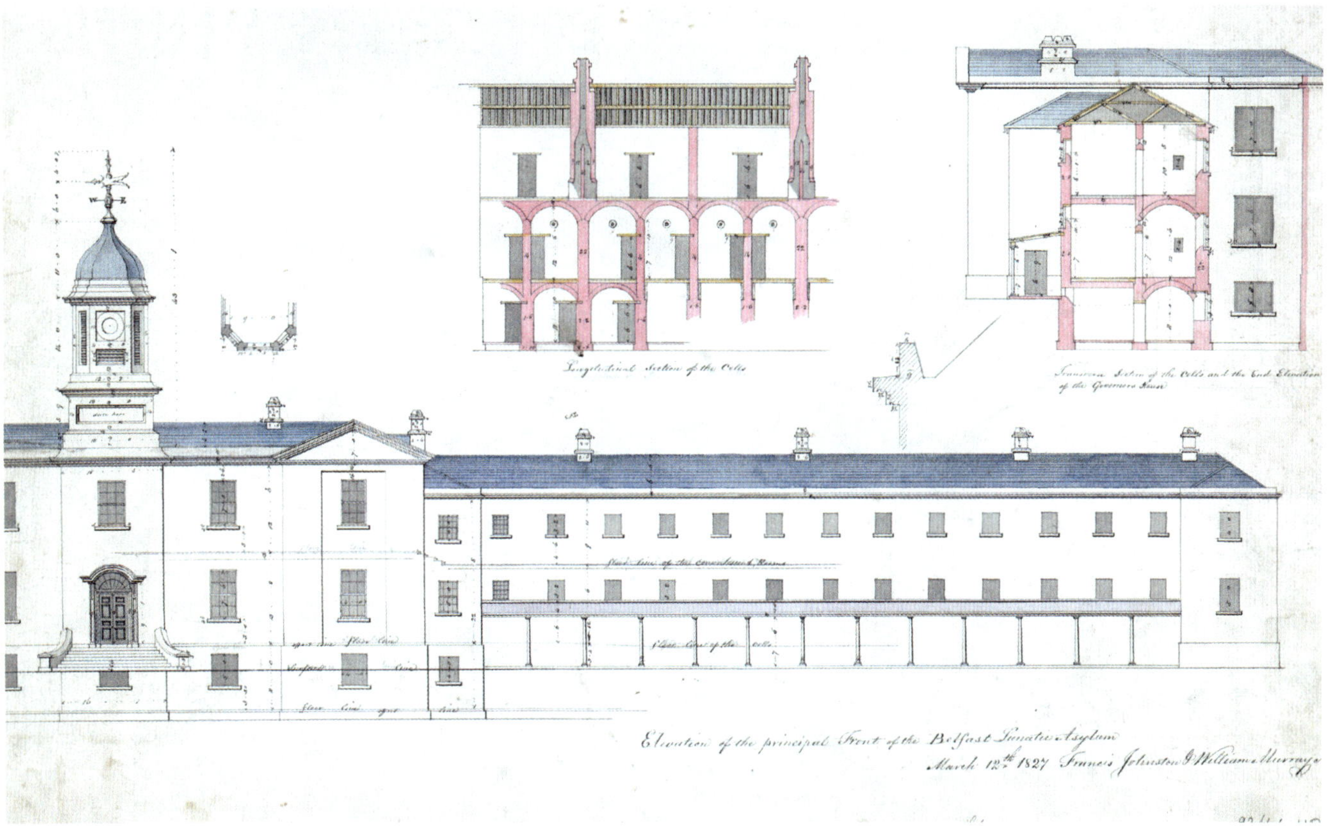

26. Tuke, *Practical Hints*, p. 20.
27. Thomas Brown 1730, cited in Christine Stevenson, *Medicine and Magnificence: British Hospital and Asylum Architecture, 1660–1815* (New Haven, 2000), pp 88–90.
28. Albeit a much more modest dome than the monumental version that now surmounts the building in its current incarnation as Britain's Imperial War Museum.

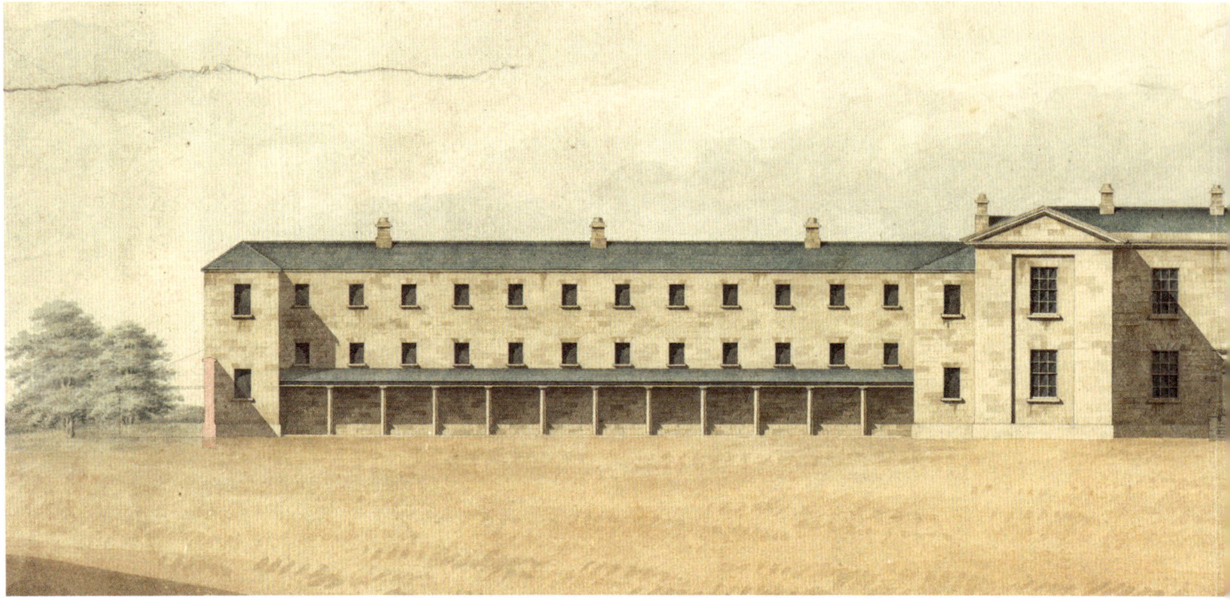

2.11 Armagh: Elevation, 1825. Note domestic disposition of central block, prior to addition of cupola. *Image courtesy of the Irish Architectural Archive (RIAI Murray Collection 92/46: 66).*

bore favourable comparison with London's royal palaces, but the presence of such a grandiose façade on a charitable institution soon came to be seen as a wasteful, immoral or even insane use of resources.

> *Bedlam is a pleasant Piece, that it is, and abounds with Amusements; the first of which is the building so stately a Fabrick for Persons wholly unsensible of the Beauty and Use of it: The Outside is a perfect Mockery to the Inside, and Admits of two Amusing Queries, Whether the Persons that ordered the Building of it, or those who inhabit it, were the maddest?*[26]

Bethlem's replacement building, four storeys in height, fifty-five bays in length and dominated by a grandiose classical portico and central dome,[27] was no less externally extravagant than its predecessor, and would prove no less prone to scandal within. Nearing completion as the 1815 Select Committee convened, Bevans was invited to critique the building. Amidst many highly practical criticisms he condemned the 'excessive expense' of a building whose grand portico rendered the rooms behind 'extremely gloomy'.[28]

It is in this context that Johnston's designs for the first phase of asylums in Ireland should be understood. Any sense of extravagance was to be avoided, yet the building's external countenance needed to be expressive of the enlightened curative regime carried out within. It should be recognisable as an important public building, yet retain some sense of being a domestic setting for the 'moral family'. This was a challenge that Johnston was well equipped to handle. By contrast with his inexperience in prison design, Johnston's portfolio was laden with civic and residential projects – schools and courthouses, modest glebes and aristocratic mansions. The predisposition of architects of 'the long eighteenth century' to employ traditional

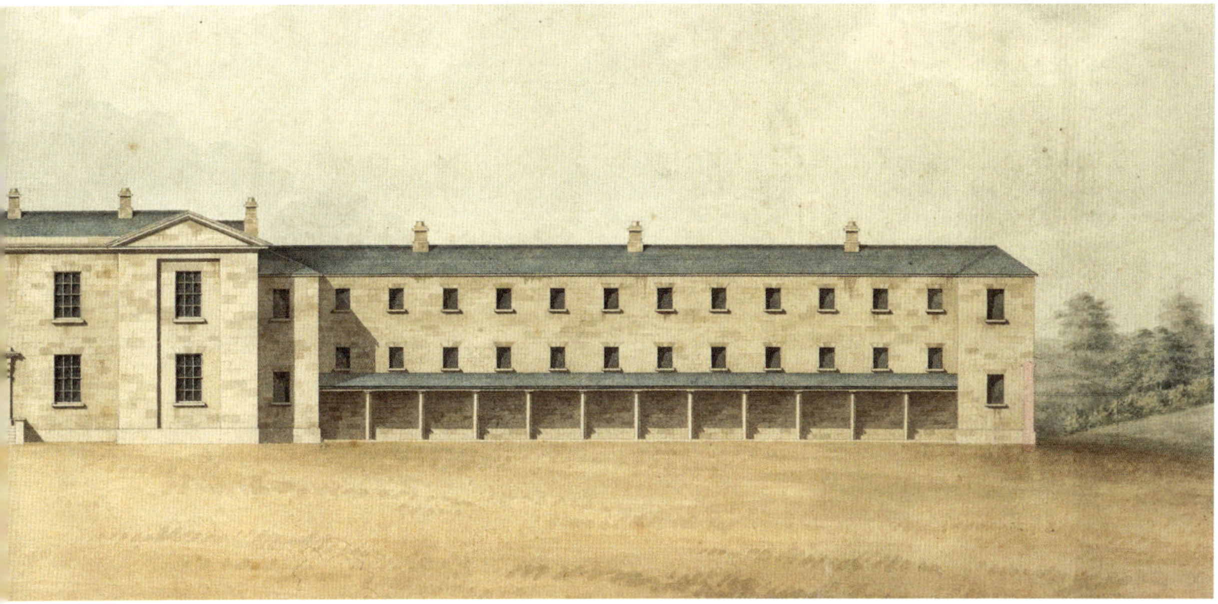

domestic precedents when designing new charitable institutions was therefore entirely compatible with the visual expression of moral management.

The centrepiece of Johnston's design reflected the scale and features of a comfortable Georgian home but nevertheless included several visual clues as to its true purpose. The execution of the entire frontage in crisp limestone ashlar (granite at Carlow) of the highest quality conveyed that this was a building of dignity and substance.[29] A sternly classical cupola – similar to those used by Johnston at his Penitentiary and Bridewell – was appended during the construction of the first standard asylum at Armagh and became an indispensable feature of the type thereafter.[30] The cupola was universally understood as a marker of a public building[31] and had the benefit of being visible even above high boundary walls, negating the need to inscribe 'Lunatic Asylum' in the central parapet as Johnston had originally proposed.[32] While housing nothing more sinister than a clock and designed in a manner that made its use as a look-out physically impossible, the cupola unambiguously identifies the governor's house as the seat of authority. From there it would take little imagination on behalf of generations of patients and staff to transform a blind and harmless clocktower into a potent symbol of the 'all-seeing supervision machine' over which it presided.[33] It seems reasonable to infer that Johnston and his peers also saw the cupola as an architectural signifier of the authority of central control, just as Stark and Bevans almost invariably marked the inspection nodes of their panoptic designs with domes or cupolae, respectively.[34]

If the layout of the spaces reveals the ingenious means by which the principles of 'moral management' were embodied in the very fabric of the building, and the elevations represent the expression of these values to the wider world, the architectural sections conceal secrets of their own. The first thing we notice is that the individual cells and long galleries of the ground floor are entirely constructed of

29. An elevation is included as an appendix to the *1815 Select Committee Report*, HC 1814–15 [296] Plate VII.
30. This high-quality ashlar externally, and the solid vaulted masonry structure internally, meant that the first phase of asylums would prove to be the most expensive, on a per-bed basis, of any era of construction. See Chapter Four.
31. Frederick O'Dwyer, *Irish Hospital Architecture: A Pictorial History* (Dublin, 1997), p. 10.
32. Clocktowers and cupolae on buildings of public charity enjoyed a long lineage, as seen from the Royal Hospital, Kilmainham, through various almshouses and Dr Steeven's Hospital, to Richard Cassel's Lying-in Hospital (The Rotunda). Only the cupola on the latter distinguished it from Dublin's pre-eminent private mansion, Kildare (later Leinster) House, also by Cassels. Edward McParland, *Public Architecture in Ireland 1680–1760* (New Haven & London, 2001) pp 53–89.
33. By now, the intention was to state 'lunatic' rather than 'lunatick', but the point is moot as the entablature would instead bear the date in Roman numerals. IAA, Murray Collection, 1820, Armagh District Lunatic Asylum, 92/46, Sheet 0066; ibid., 1828, Belfast District Lunatic Asylum, 92.46, Sheet 0118.
34. The symbolic power of the domineering water tower (or clocktower, as the functions were usually combined) was later cemented in the modern imagination by Enoch Powell's speech of 1961, which we will encounter at greater length in Chapter Seven.

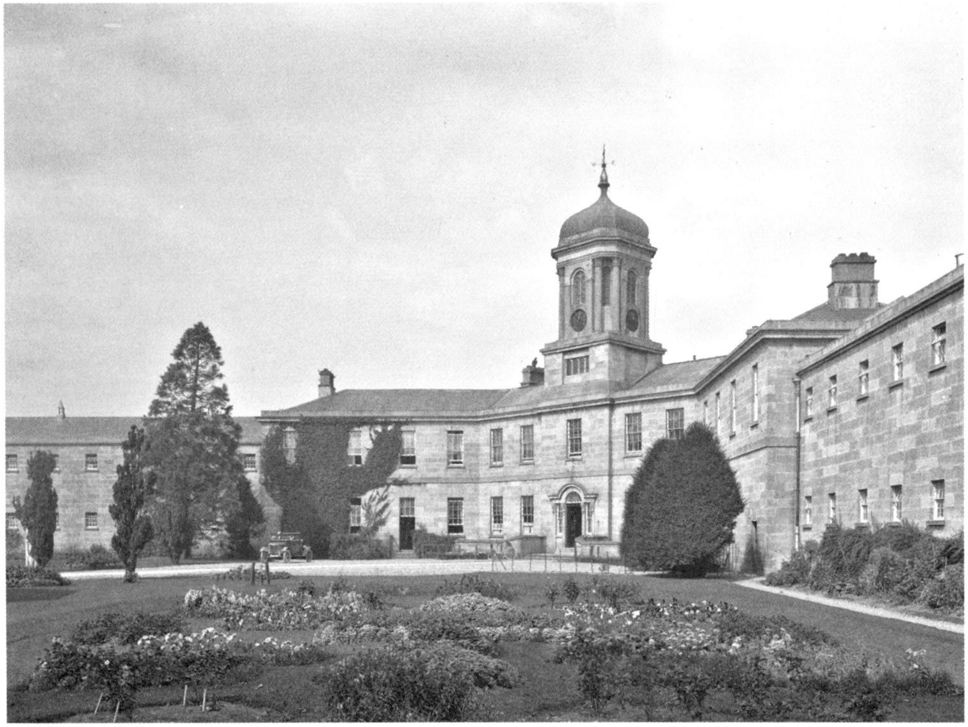
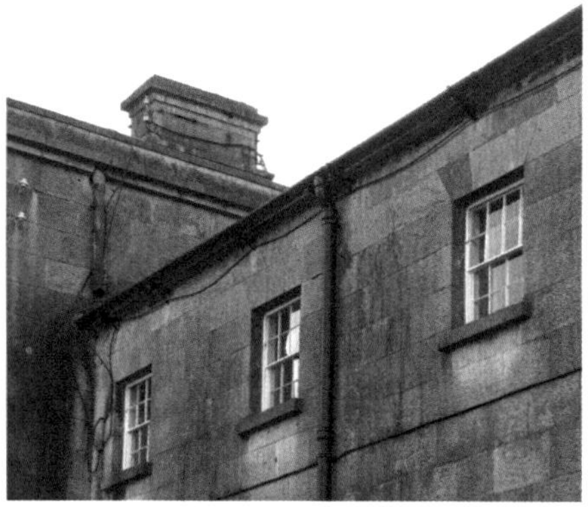
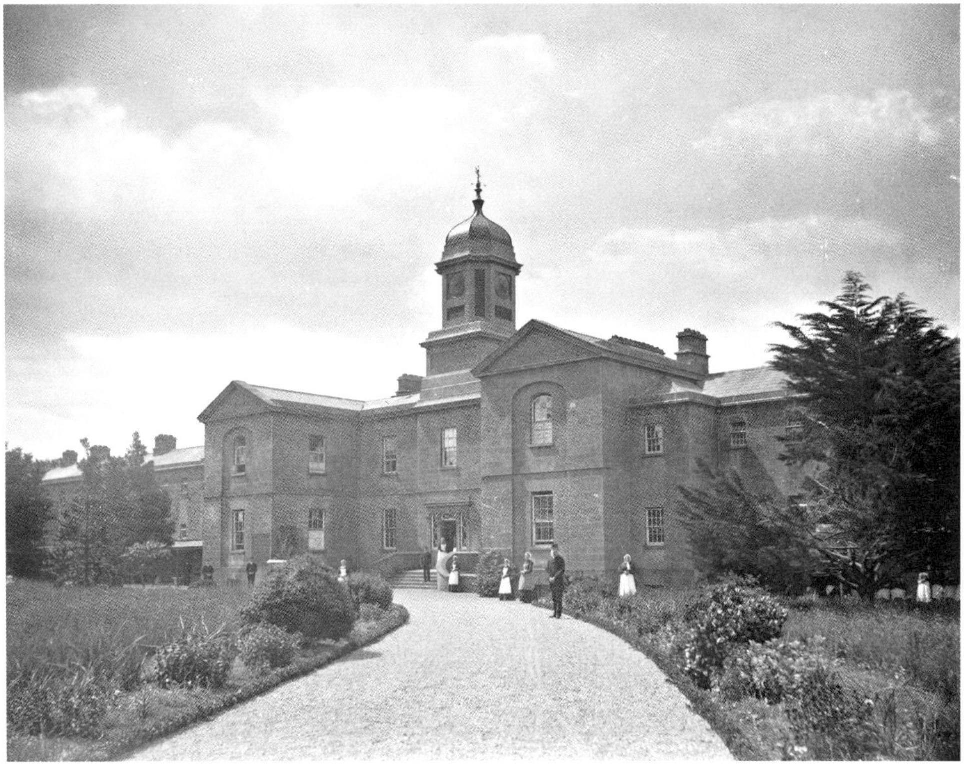
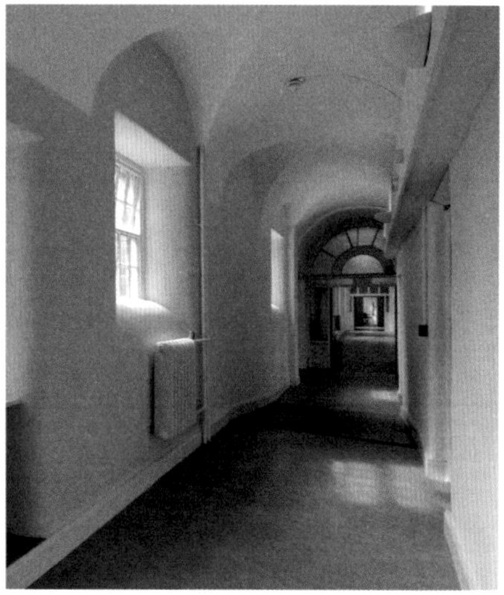

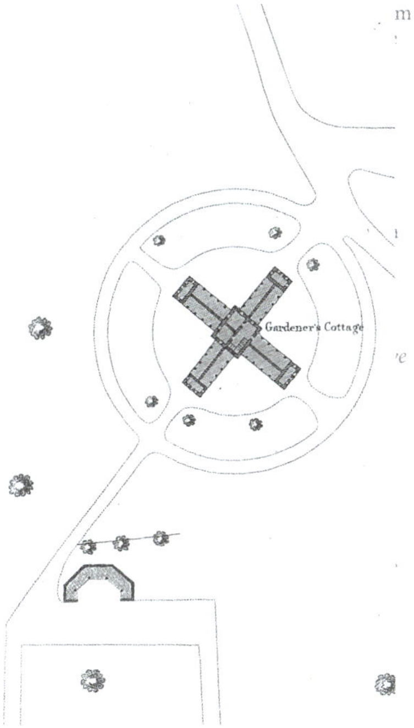

2.12 Ballinasloe: Landscaped forecourt c. 1910. Note more elaborate cupola with engaged Corinthian columns, and the unmodified cell windows, *Image courtesy of the National Library of Ireland (EAS_2159).*

2.13 Maryborough / Portlaoise: Rare example of cell unaltered cell windows, albeit cill level internally has been lowered, *Photograph by David Killeen, 2019.*

2.14 Waterford: Asylum staff posing as if outside a country house c. 1900. Patients are more discreetly placed, *Image courtesy of the National Library of Ireland (POOLEWP 0131).*

2.15 Carlow: The ground floor cells and corridors of all asylums of this era were vaulted throughout in solid masonry - principally as a defence against fire, *Photograph by David Killeen, 2019.*

2.16 Richmond Asylum, Dublin: Elaborate and unusual garden buildings offer evidence of a landscape of leisure, *Reproduced courtesy Trinity College Dublin (OS-Dublin City-1056-Sheet 7-1866).*

2.17 Maryborough / Portlaoise: Plan and elevation of water pumping house, articulated as classical garden building, *Image courtesy of the Irish Architectural Archive (Workhouse Drawings Collection, 85/138: 218).*

2.18 Clonmel: Landscape design including primary and secondary avenues, formal garden with summer house, orchard, and laundry drying yard, *Reproduced courtesy Trinity College Dublin (OS-Clonmel-500-Sheets 7,13-1876).*

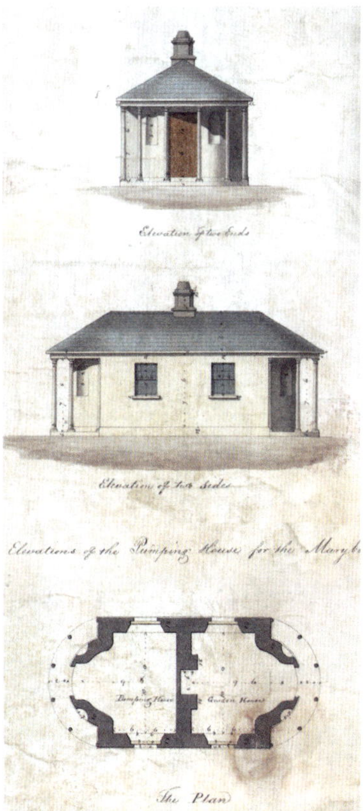

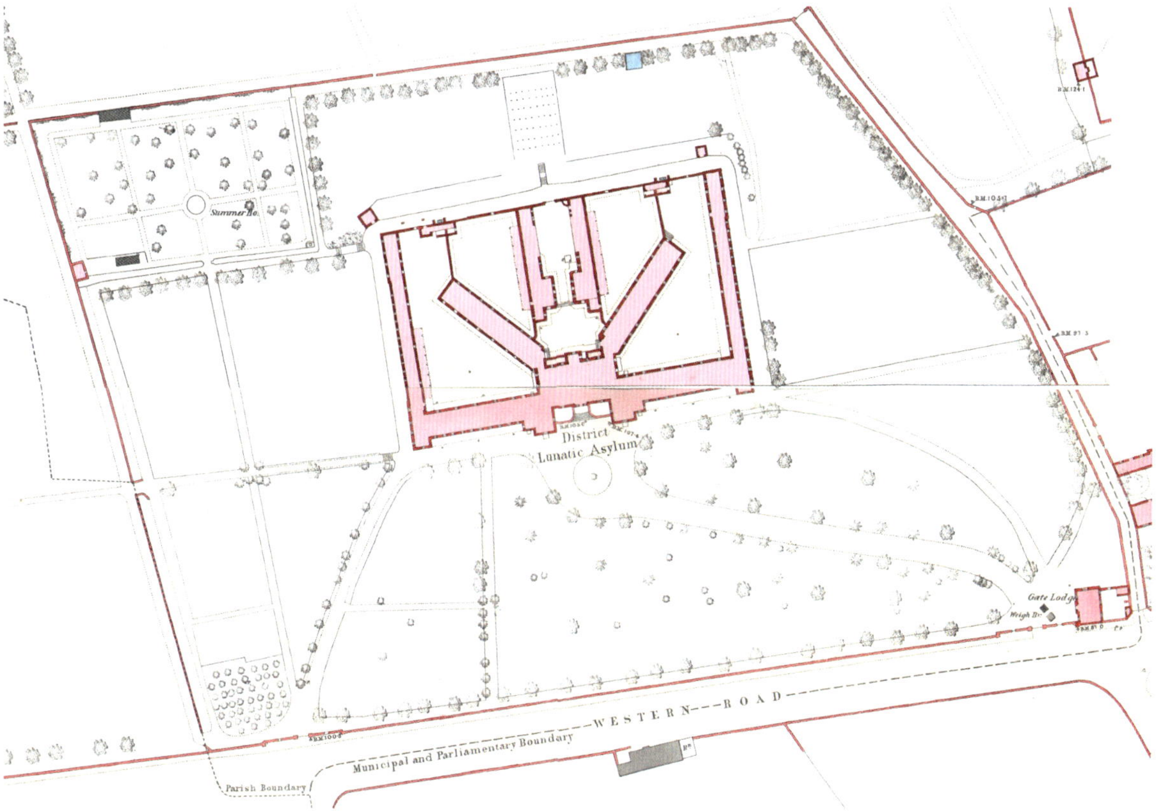

vaulted masonry – a highly effective safeguard against the risk of fire, but also an eye-watering expensive approach copied straight from handbook of 'reformed' prison design.[35] From outside, the cell windows, at three feet and six inches square, would have appeared tolerably generous – better glazed than the cottages in which pauper inmates otherwise resided and far removed from the barred openings of contemporary prisons.[36] Closer examination, however, reveals that the lower half of each window was blocked internally. Combined with differentials in floor level between central block and wing, the result was a meagre opening whose sill was situated some 12 feet above the cell floor. Small, high-cell windows were still common to most asylums of the era – designed to prevent patients' destructive and/or self-destructive impulses; more notable is that Johnston's architectural sleight of hand contrived to convey an outward impression of enlightened benevolence not quite matched by the reality within.[37]

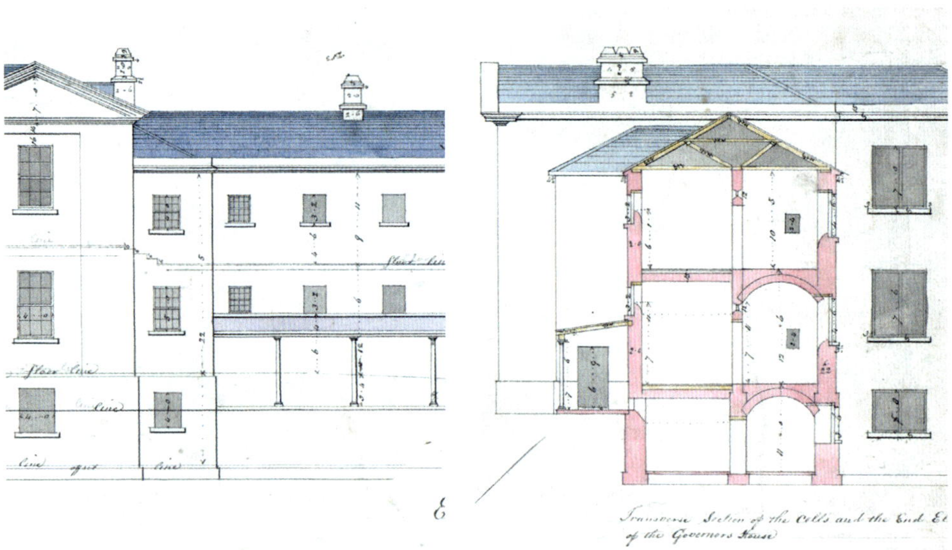

2.19 Belfast: Part elevation and section showing differentials in floor level and partially blocked cell windows, *Image courtesy of the Irish Architectural Archive (RIAI Murray Collection 92/46: 108).*

In a carefully cultivated landscape

Pleasing landscape views and therapeutic outdoor activities featured as part of the curative regime at The Retreat and became a fundamental tenet of moral management, whose value was reiterated in most contemporary writings. It was therefore logical that Ireland's new asylums, guided by a founding commitment to moral management, should have been provided with sufficient grounds to facilitate therapeutic activities – de facto necessitating locations at a slight remove from the urban centre they served. As Philo puts it, the geographical distribution of asylums undergoes a marked shift, from 'an essentially eighteenth-century vision of medical (and hence urban) location [to] an alternative and later vision of moral (and hence rural) location inspired by the York Retreat.'[38] Even in this context, it is still surprising to discover that the first edition Ordnance Survey maps portray the early asylums as miniature demesnes, complete with the ink stipple usually reserved for the 'polite' landscapes that the gentry created around their suburban villas or country seats.[39]

35. Thomas Markus 'The Sad, the Mad and the Bad', in Thomas Markus (ed.), *Order in Space and Society: Architectural Form and its Context in the Scottish Enlightenment* (Edinburgh, 1982), p. 95. Elevations of Bevan's various panoptic proposals were included as appendices in the *1815 Select Committee Report*, HC 1814–15 (296) Plate I and IV. His designs for the Wakefield asylum are of particular interest as the cupolae sit atop the two decentralised inspection nodes, not centrally on the building.
36. A photograph of the demolition of Lifford goal offers a spectacular cut-away view of this construction technique. See Butler, *Building the Irish Courthouse and Prison*, p. 251.
37. It is also worth noting that as late as 1815, the design of New Bethlem left cell windows entirely unglazed. *1815 Committee Report*, p. 32
38. The design of the Retreat pioneered iron casement windows instead of prison-like bars and heavily promoted the value of landscape views from day spaces, but also reverted to high-level windows within individual patient cells. Tuke criticises other designers who engaged in similar architectural deceit to Johnston with respect to partly blanked windows. Tuke, *Practical Hints*, pp 37–8. A similar criticism was made that the lower half of day-room windows at New Bethlem were blanked out. From the discussions it is clear that the prevailing standard was that patients should be afforded a view from day spaces (when it was also possible for staff to guard against breakage) but that high windows (in the case of New Bethlem, still without glass) were indispensable within sleeping quarters when patients were less closely supervised. *1815 Select Committee*, pp 32–3, p. 193. A common architectural solution to the compositional conundrum of small cell windows was to employ lunettes, as at Dance's St Luke's Hospital, Stark's Glasgow and Bevan's several design submissions to the 1815 Committee.
39. Chris Philo, *A Geographical History of Institutional Provision for the Insane from Medieval Times to the 1860's in England and Wales: This Space Reserved for Insanity* (Lewiston, 2004), pp 571–6.

The detail and level of elaboration is suggestive of landscapes whose major features were well established by the time they were mapped, some as little as five years after opening.[40] Fine landscapes would become the default aesthetic setting for 'respectable' educational and enclosed religious institutions of the middle and later nineteenth century, built to serve upper-middle-class cohorts somewhat socially accustomed to such trappings. But what is most remarkable about the asylum landscapes is not their superb quality or relatively early date, but that they were designed for the benefit of inmates drawn from the pauper class.[41]

A visitor approaching one of these asylums is first struck by the boundary wall, similar to those found enclosing countless private suburban villas and country demesnes, only taller. Once admission is granted by the gatekeeper in his lodge, our visitor proceeds along a curved avenue through tree-studded parkland. The main building gradually emerges from its cloak of ornamental planting, revealing itself in a moment of modest drama that echoes the stage-managed approach to a self-respecting country mansion. A late nineteenth-century photo of Waterford plays to this illusion, where formally dressed staff are precisely positioned alongside the raked gravel avenue to portray an image of gentility, as if servants of the 'big house' are awaiting the return of the master. One has to examine this photograph very carefully to even notice the patients in the grounds, and closer yet to discern an inmate peering from behind a barred window – an unwelcome intruder whose presence sabotaged the photographer's idealised image (see Case Study 9).

Surviving drawings for these asylums indicate that the Board of Control's centrally administered construction contracts did not include any landscape works beyond the erection of the gate lodge and boundary walls. Asylum governors – drawn principally from the ranks of the local landed gentry – had no say in the architecture of the asylum buildings, but their influence on the design of the landscape setting is unmistakeable. That the governors saw fit to invest such effort and resources reflects their pride in these new institutions, and offers tangible evidence of the prestige that their involvement projected onto an establishment.[42] While there is a paucity of documentary evidence relating to any landscape matters, it seems certain that the governors took a direct and personal interest, perhaps revelling in this one aspect of the institution where they could actually bring relevant experience to bear: 'The grounds, too, are undergoing the necessary cultivation by direction of the Board of Governors, who have met on several occasions to make contracts'.[43] We can only speculate about how prospective patients perceived this set piece as they were chaperoned up the avenue and into the waiting arms of the asylum. Fear, awe and trepidation were surely present, albeit the most disturbed, depressed or deranged likely remained oblivious. However, the effect would not have been lost on their visitors, who – drawn from the same pauper class – would have been simultaneously reassured by the respectable credentials of the institution and admonished by the aesthetic trappings of their social superiors.[44]

But it would be a mistake to dismiss the landscape ambitions of the early asylums as an exercise in elitist vanity. From the outset, Ireland's asylum landscapes included many of the other features of the private demesne whose primary value was

40. As at Carlow, Maryborough, Clonmel and Waterford. The mapped landscapes at Armagh, Belfast and Londonderry seem relatively spare by comparison, but this is likely due to changes in cartographic conventions as the Ordnance Survey progressed from north to south, as the surviving parkland at Armagh is actually one of the finest in the country and later maps confirm similar parklands (since erased) at Belfast and Londonderry. The urban-scale forecourts enclosed by the larger X-plan asylums at Limerick and Ballinasloe militated against the creation of a more rural parkland aesthetic.
41. The Irish asylum landscapes predated London's New Bethlem, where the ornamental landscaping was not completed until 1837, as recorded on a surviving testamentary plaque on site seen by the author.
42. Newly established Protestant schools such as Wilson's Hospital in Westmeath (1760–1770) were set out in demesne-like parklands. The Ordnance Survey use of stipple to denote 'polite landscapes', while not always consistent, did include the National Seminary at Maynooth and at least some of the earlier Catholic diocesan seminaries and religious-run boarding schools, even if their landscape features were not as yet well developed. For more on these other typologies see Maurice Craig, *The Buildings of Ireland: From Earliest Times to 1880* (Dublin, 1997) pp 303–5; Martin McKeith, 'The Architectural Development of the Irish Diocesan Major Seminary – from 1782 to 1900', (unpublished MUBC Thesis, 2012); McCullough, *A Lost Tradition*, p. 115.
43. All the evidence in Johnston and Murray's surviving drawings and specifications indicate that their responsibilities to landscape matters were limited to the necessities of boundary wall, gate lodge, water supply and disposal arrangements. Surviving site plans are rare but where they do exist, as for Carlow (1831), the building, boundary walls and drainage arrangements are shown, but the remainder of the site is left blank. Landscape matters feature but rarely in the inspector's reports and parliamentary inquiries into the design and procurement of the asylums. A detailed examination of the minute books of individual asylums would be necessary to define what role, if any, was played by professional landscape designers.
44. *Seventh Annual Asylum Report 1855*, HC 1854–55 [1981] xvi, p. 15

45. Especially if we consider that the only circumstance in which the average rural pauper of the era would experience such a landscape setting would be if summoned to their landlord's seat, itself an occasion sufficiently rare as to be a cause of considerable apprehension.

46. In her study of the similarly designed landscapes of England's lunatic asylums, Sarah Rutherford concludes that that the function of such landscapes was predominantly therapeutic, affording less attention to their potential iconographic value.. Sarah Rutherford, 'The Landscapes of Public Lunatic Asylums in England, 1808–1914' (unpublished PhD Thesis, 2003) p. 5, pp 174–8, p. 182; Patrick Quinlan, 'Cure, Care and Containment: The architecture and landscape of Ireland's lunatic asylums, 1814–2014' (unpublished MUBC Thesis, 2014), pp 45–55.

47. By way of comparison, the People's Park in Waterford, which lays claim to being the first municipal park in Ireland, was completed only in 1857, while St Stephen's Green in Dublin would not be re-opened to the general public until 1880. Dermot Power, 'A History of the People's Park', in *The Waterford Archaeological and Historical Society Journal* 52 (1996), pp 113–5.

the leisure and pleasure of its residents rather than the creation of an aesthetic set piece for the benefit of others.[45] Thus we find decoratively planted parterres, ornate summer houses and garden buildings, scenic paths meandering through belted woodland – all unprecedented in institutions designated for the pauper classes. Even if the patients were also necessarily engaged in the less genteel activity of maintaining these grounds, we must recall that in the 1820–30s, such landscapes of leisure otherwise remained the exclusive preserve of the upper classes in their rural demesnes and gated urban squares. The free, universal public urban park would not emerge as a phenomenon in Ireland for at least another generation.[46] The fact that pauper patients were afforded a therapeutic experience of genteel landscape – beyond mere agricultural toil and free from the trappings of surveillance or coercion, which can taint the associated architecture – has barely featured in the debates between bleak and benign interpretations of the asylum. Understanding this aspect of the legacy leads to the view that the Irish asylum system truly did embody benevolent, therapeutic and curative intentions, and, significantly, that this owes at least as much to the local elites who assumed responsibility for their governance as to the central powers that created them.[47] High-quality landscapes would remain a notable feature of the second and third phases of construction and would continue to be maintained and enhanced for a further century, even as the idealism originally underpinning the asylum project crumbled.

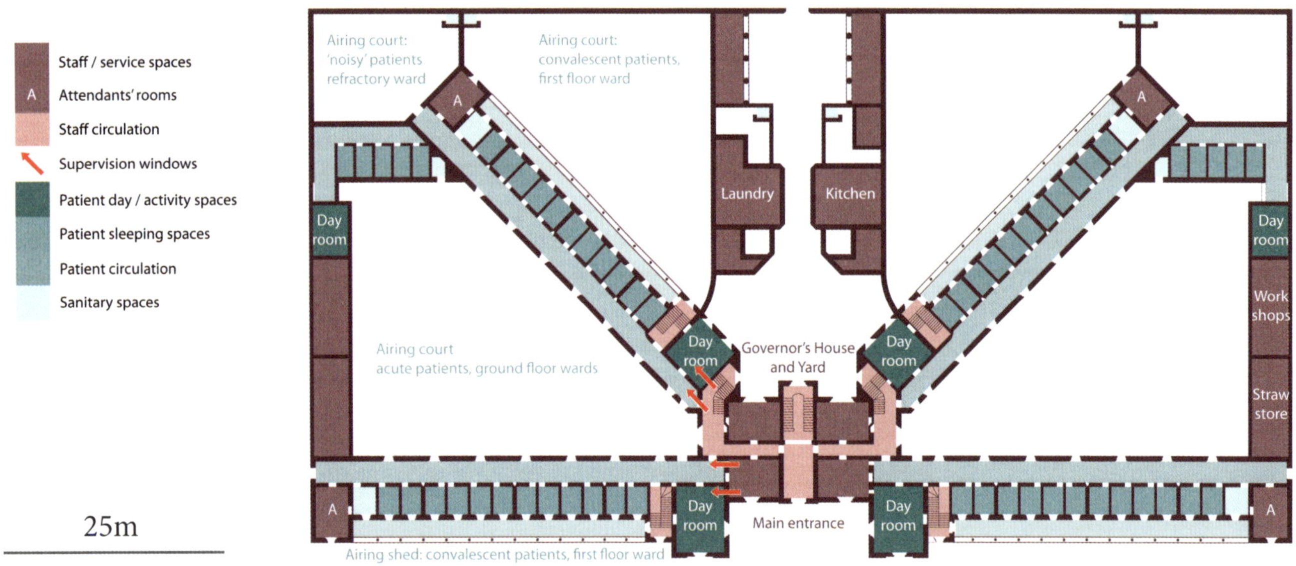

2.20 Plan diagram of Carlow Asylum with key spaces annotated. Note the internal windows which allowed the Governor and Matron to inspect the galleries and dayrooms, *Drawn by the author.*

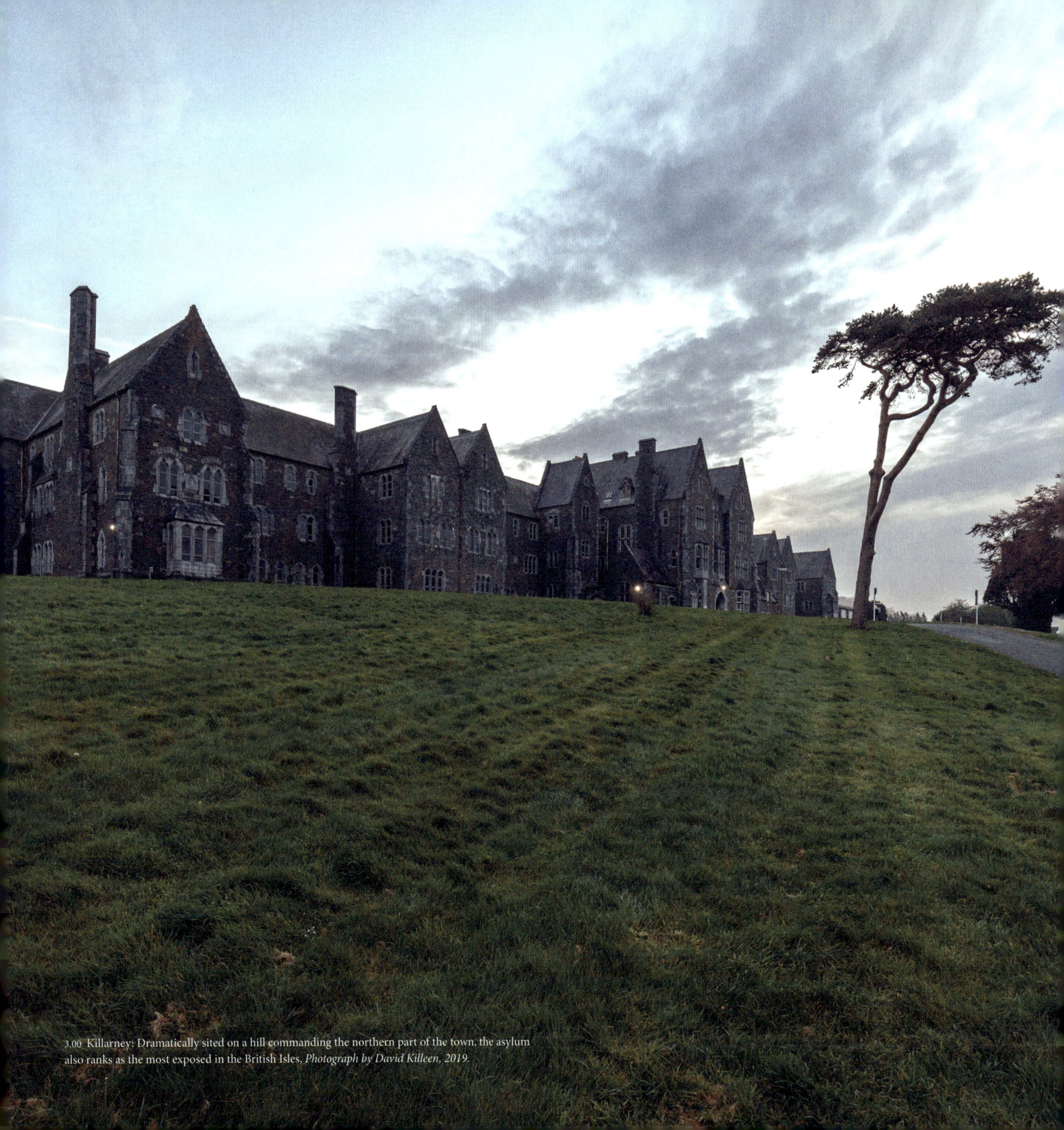

3.00 Killarney: Dramatically sited on a hill commanding the northern part of the town, the asylum also ranks as the most exposed in the British Isles, *Photograph by David Killeen, 2019.*

Architectural Ambitions

giving a splendid waistcoat to a man without a shirt[1]

Upon 'completion' of the district asylum system in 1835, the eight-man Board of Control resigned, their duties passing to the Board of (Public) Works.[2] Yet it must already have been evident that the task of making adequate provision for the insane was far from complete. By 1833 the board of Belfast Asylum was already petitioning for the purchase of additional ground and notwithstanding that this request was initially refused,[3] plans were drawn up the following year to extend Belfast to accommodate '100 incurable patients'.[4]

The use of the term 'incurable' at this juncture is significant, indicating that the optimism that heralded the introduction of moral management was being tempered by the reality that not all patients could be cured.[5] The admission of irredeemably chronic cases from other institutions, a continuing excess of admissions over discharges, and the absence of what today's clinicians would term 'alternative pathways of care' inevitably resulted in an accumulation of patients. The passing of the 1838 Dangerous Lunatics Act[6] exacerbated the situation by creating 'a permissive system of judicial admission', whereby it became relatively easy for families and communities to obtain committal orders for the involuntary commitment of an individual, difficult for asylum management to refuse, and next to impossible for that individual to resist. The admissions process as designed by this legislation and its successor in 1867 operated by default as a one-way valve, with neither time limits nor review mechanisms to check its flow. In becoming the predominant, much abused mode of admission to Ireland's asylums, the dangerous lunatics acts have been identified by many scholars as one of the biggest drivers of the country's inexorable increase in asylum demand.[7]

By 1842, 2,028 patients were housed in accommodation built for 1,220, this on the eve of a famine that would heap further pressure on every aspect of state-funded social provision. A House of Lords Select Committee was convened in 1843 to 'Consider the State of the Lunatic Poor in Ireland.'[8] The blunt title of the legislation that emerged two years later – 'Central Criminal Lunatic Asylum (Ireland) Act'[9] –

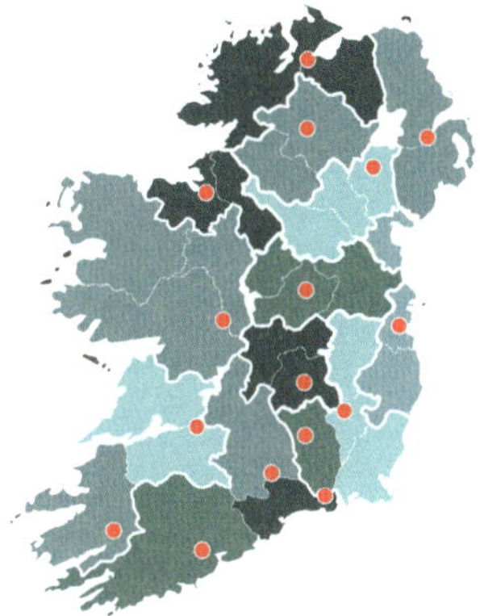

Asylum distribution in Ireland, **1855**, *Drawn by the author.*

1. Henrietta Martineau, *Letters from Ireland* (London, 1852), cited in Frederick O'Dwyer, *The Architecture of Deane and Woodward* (Cork, 1997), p. 104.
2. Predecessor to the modern-day Office of Public Works. Joseph Robins, *Fools and Mad: A History of the Insane in Ireland* (Dublin, 1986), p. 66.
3. National Archives of Ireland, Chief Secretary's Office, 1833, Memorial from five Governors and Directors of the Belfast District Asylum for Lunatic Poor asking authorisation to purchase land, CSO/RP/1833/1072; Ibid., Chief Secretary's Office, 1833, Letters from Joseph Stevenson, [secretary] and chairman and members of the board, Belfast District Lunatic Asylum, [County Antrim], proposing to purchase more land. CSO/RP/1833/1941.

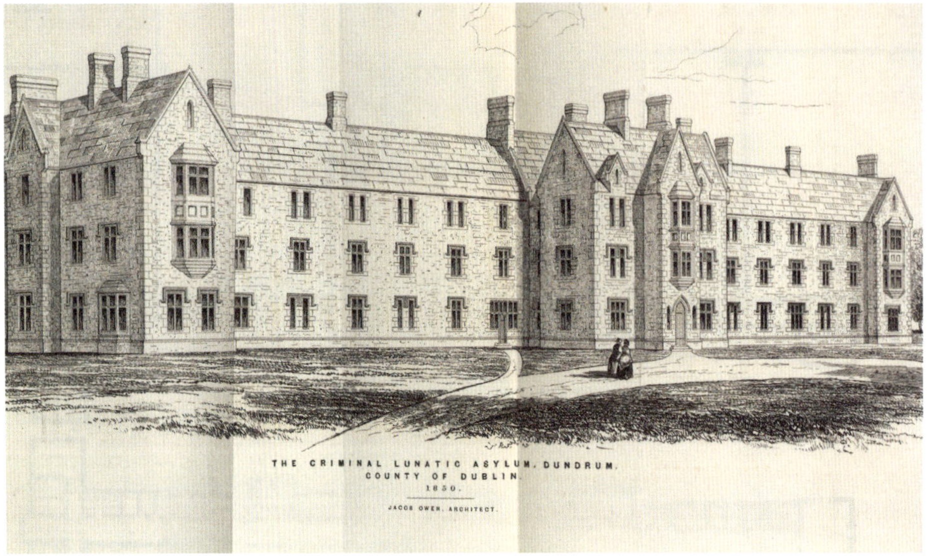

3.01 Dundrum: Jacob Owen's Central Criminal Lunatic Asylum. The main principles established by Owen in this building would be replicated in all of the new asylums of this era, *Civil Engineer and Architect, 1851, Plate 8.*

disguises the breadth of issues addressed by the committee and the exceptional depth of consultation in which they engaged, actively canvassing the views of the board of every District Asylum and many grand juries.[10] Asylum boards generally supported the proposal to establish a specialist criminal asylum – itself a world first – but it was the question of how best to provide for incurable 'cases of epilepsy, idiotcy [*sic*], and chronic disease' that generated most debate. Only one of the ten asylum boards thought it acceptable to return 'harmless cases' to the workhouses; eight supported specialist provision for incurables – gently rebranded as 'Provincial Asylums for the chronic insane classes' – to allow the District Asylums to fulfil their originally intended role as 'Hospitals for the treatment of insanity'. The criminal asylum was built soon afterwards, but the provincial asylums were never realised, dropped in favour of a more conventional approach – expanding existing sites and establishing additional District Asylums to serve smaller districts.[11] The critical operational distinction between acute 'hospital' and long-stay 'asylum' would not fully regain traction until the mid-twentieth century.

The consultation that preceded the 1845 legislation was a moment in time whose significance has been overlooked. This was the first opportunity for various stakeholders to take stock and compare the true performance of an experimental system against the optimistic predictions that had prompted its creation. It was also possibly the last moment at which a dramatic change of direction remained possible: professional structures and power dynamics were still fluid, the local economic impacts of the institutions were not yet significant, the parallel system of Poor Law institutions were in their infancy and the crisis of the famine had yet to come. What is remarkable therefore, is how rapidly institutionalisation in a purpose-built asylum had come to be universally accepted as the only valid solution for insanity in all its forms: not one of the ten asylum boards consulted challenged this fundamental

4. Irish Architectural Archive, Murray Collection, *c.* 1830, A Plan of the Belfast District Lunatic Asylum, shewing [sic] the proposed addition for the accommodation of 100 incurable patients, 92/46, Sheet 0119. Similar plans were prepared for Armagh in 1837, while by 1842 the capacity of Clonmel had been increased from 60 to 100.
5. It is worth noting at this time that the distinction between mental illness – often transitory – and learning disabilities – more often congenital – was not always drawn.
6. An Act for the more effectual provision for the prevention of offences by insane persons in Ireland 1838 (otherwise known as the Dangerous Lunatics (Ireland) Act 1838), 1 & 2 Vic. c.27.
7. Prior and Finnane note that it accounted for over 70 per cent of admissions in the closing decades of the nineteenth century. Pauline M. Prior, 'Dangerous lunacy: The misuse of mental health law in nineteenth-century Ireland', in *The Journal of Forensic Psychiatry & Psychology* 14:3 (2003) p. 531, p. 536; Mark Finnane, *Insanity and the Insane in Post-Famine Ireland* (London, 1981), p. 101. See also Damien Brennan, *Irish Insanity, 1800–2000* (Oxon, 2014), p. 1, pp 83–4; Robins, *Fools and Mad*, p. 77.
8. *Report from the Select Committee of the House of Lords appointed to Consider the State of the Lunatic Poor in Ireland* (hereafter *1843 Select Committee Report*), HC 1843 [625] x, p. v.
9. Central Criminal Lunatic Asylum (Ireland) Act 1845, 8 & 9 Vic. c.107.
10. *Annual Asylum Report 1844*, HC 1845 [645] xxvi, pp 64–81.
11. Reuber suggests that this statutory classification of insanity in the 1845 legislation may have been a world first but, with the exception of the criminal asylum, the institutional infrastructure did not match the intention. Markus Reuber, 'Moral management and the "Unseen Eye": Public lunatic asylums, 1800–1845', in Elizabeth Malcolm and Greta Jones (eds), *Medicine, Disease and the State in Ireland, 1650–1940* (Cork, 1999), p. 226.

presumption.[12] Rising patient numbers were interpreted as justification to expand the system further; potential shortcomings would be resolved through a more rigorous system of classification. The die was cast for the century to come. A progressive feature of the 1845 legislation that did become reality was the establishment of a new Lunacy Inspectorate – separate from the Inspectors General of Prisons who had fulfilled the role since 1787 – breaking another link between the prison and asylum systems. The first Inspectors of Lunacy, Francis White and John Nugent, were both doctors whose increasing influence and conceptual commitment to the asylum project would shape the system over the following decades.[13]

Effective for all the purposes of such institutions

Given the extraordinary confluence of architectural and curative theories embodied in the design of the Phase 1 asylums, and the acclaim with which they were greeted, it is remarkable how opinions of these buildings changed so dramatically during the first decades of their operation – albeit this was probably also reflective of rising expectations in matters of comfort and sanitation:

> *with regard to the interior arrangement of the building, for the purposes of ventilation, light, inspection, and every other particular necessary for the accommodation of patients, I consider it perfectly adapted to the end proposed in its erection.*[14]

> *These buildings were not provided with any modern improvements: no water was laid on – the patients, as in Carlow, being left to wash in the open courts under shelter of a shed… The kitchens were usually small and inconvenient… No places of worship or recreation halls were provided, nor any artificial means of ventilating the cells and galleries…*[15]

This sharp shift in opinion went beyond merely pragmatic matters. A close personal relationship between the patient and their 'moral governor' had been a core tenet of moral management, a feature that led the original legislation to include an upper limit of 150 beds per asylum. Contrary to the balance of views expressed by the ten asylum boards, the 1845 Act lifted this limit. The influential John Connolly reckoned that asylums could safely be scaled up to 400 beds – 'beyond which almost every desirable quality, both in the construction and government of an asylum, becomes more difficult to be obtained or preserved'[16] – but this pragmatic decision can only be read as a blow to their original curative intent.[17]

But the most significant philosophical shift from the earlier generation of asylums was the quiet retirement of the 'all-seeing eye': there were no clever contrivances to convey a sense of constant surveillance, and centralised visual oversight of the extremities of such long buildings would in any case have been impossible. Instead, the emphasis would shift to prioritise large windows and buildings of southerly aspect, on elevated sites selected for their healthy air and commanding views. Therapeutic priorities were clearly changing. Where the curative power of moral management

12. A review of the responses from the ten asylum boards also give the lie to any accusation of 'empire building' on their part – while most concurred that lunatics were better in an asylum than poorhouse or gaol, they were not specifically enthused at the prospect of expanding their own institutions further. *Annual Asylum Report 1844*, HC 1845 [645] xxvi, pp 64–81.
13. Catherine Cox, *Negotiating Insanity in the Southeast of Ireland, 1820–1900* (Manchester, 2012), pp 34–5.
14. John Jackson, 'First manager of Limerick District Lunatic Asylum (opened 1827)', cited in Reuber, 'Moral management and the "Unseen Eye"', p. 223.
15. *Report of the Commissioners of Inquiry into the state of the Lunatic Asylums… in Ireland 1858* (hereafter *1858 Commissioners Report*), HC 1857–58 [2436-I], p. 13.
16. The committee had regard to evidence from John Connolly, a few years prior to the publication of his influential book. John Connolly, *The Construction and Government of Lunatic Asylums* (London, 1847), p. 10.
17. Curiously, nobody seems to have considered the possibility of increasing the number of moral governors pro rata within a single larger asylum, which would have preserved the supposed therapeutic benefits of the former while enjoying most of the cost economies of the latter. The size cap was also lifted for England during the same parliamentary session: *County Asylums Act (England) 1845*, 8 & 9 Vict. c.126.

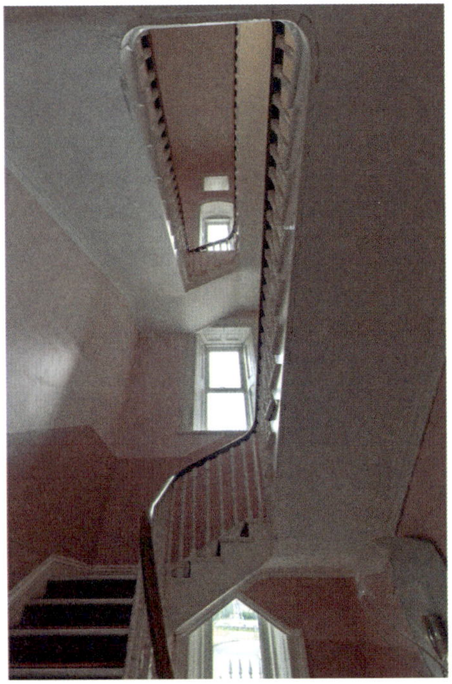

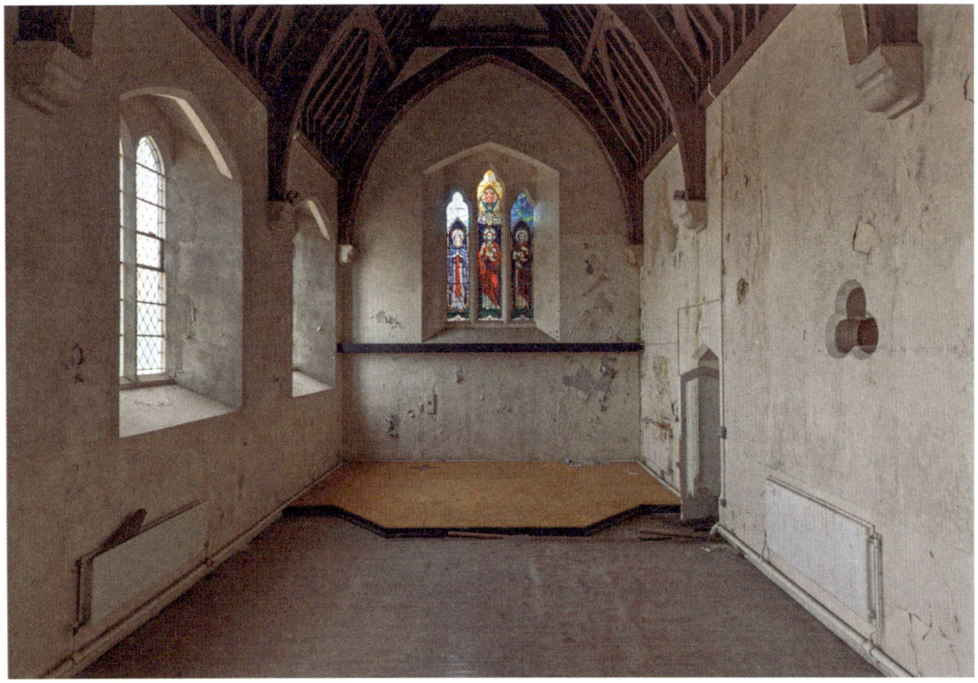

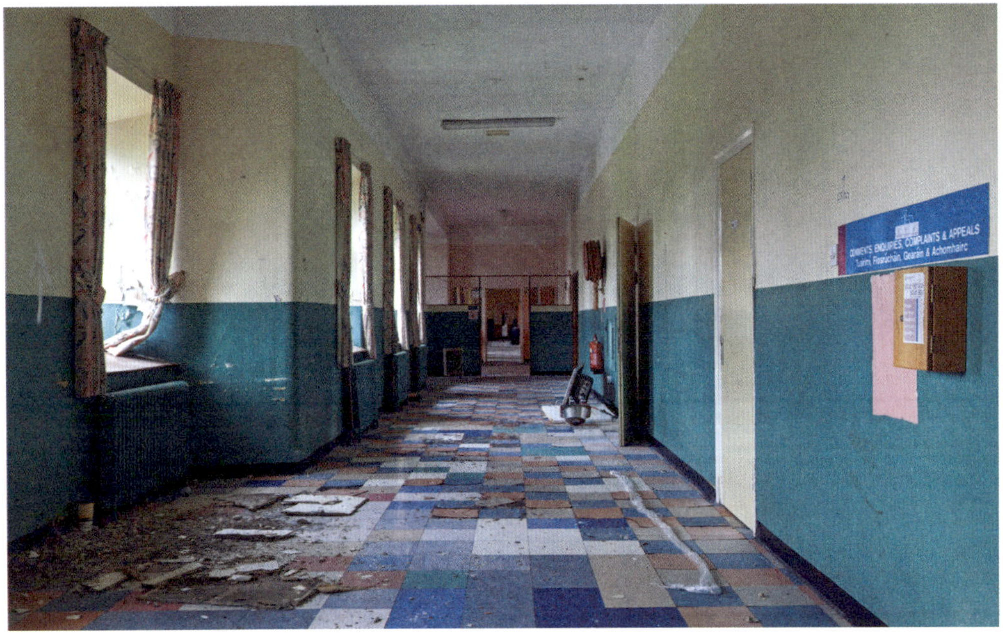
COMMENTS, ENQUIRIES, COMPLAINTS & APPEALS
Tuairimí, Fiosrúcháin, Gearáin & Achomhairc

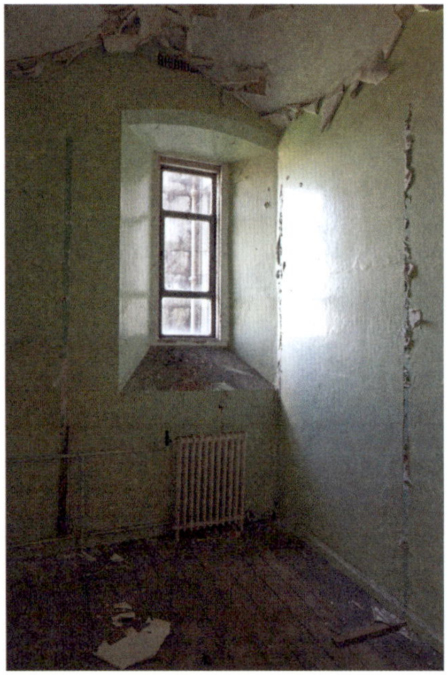

3.02 Mullingar: High quality joinery in the central block would not have looked out of place in a contemporary gentleman's residence, *Photograph by David Killeen, 2019.*

3.03 Killarney: Asylums of the second phase generally included chapels on the upper floors to the rear of the central block. This example at Killarney is a rare, unaltered example, *Photograph by David Killeen, 2019.*

3.04 Mullingar: Interior view of south-facing 'galleries' which doubled as patient day-spaces, *Photograph by David Killeen, 2019.*

3.05 Mullingar: Typical cell interior, *Photograph by David Killeen, 2019.*

3.06 Dundrum: The more generous fenestration and exuberant detailing of the later asylums would make Owen's Central Asylum seem restrained by comparison, *Photograph by David Killeen, 2019.*

3.07 Killarney: Architects working in the Gothic style deployed gables, buttresses, bay and oriel windows and chimney stacks to picturesque effect, *Photograph by David Killeen, 2019.*

3.08 Eglinton Asylum, Cork: Atkins uses the same devices at Cork, albeit his brick water-towers feel like an incongruous addition, *Photograph by David Killeen, 2019.*

3.09 Kilkenny: Its relatively small size and robust Tudor detailing make Kilkenny one of the more successful compositions of the era, *Photograph by David Killeen, 2019.*

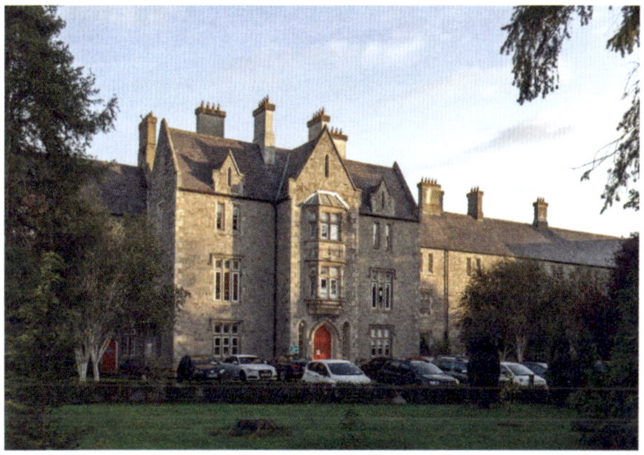

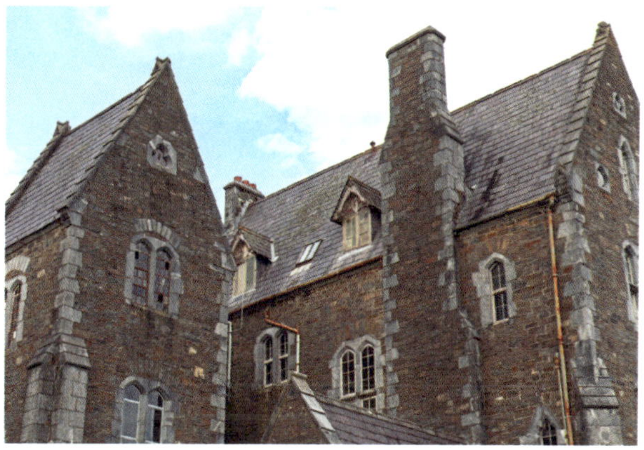

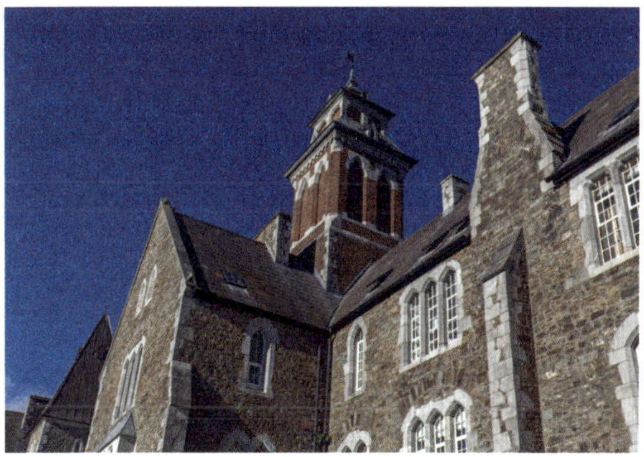

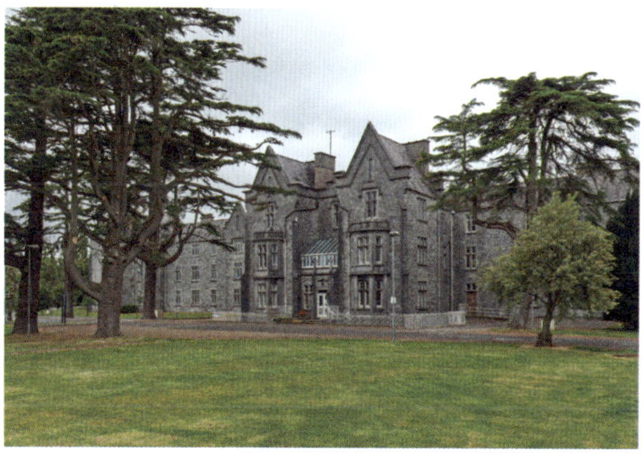

had once depended on patients being subject to the ever-watchful eye of the moral governor within the spaces of the asylum, patients' own eyes were now encouraged to partake of the therapeutic benefits of the view from their windows.

In addition to the specialist Central Criminal Lunatic Asylum (opened 1850) enabled by the new legislation, five conventionally constituted District Asylums were sanctioned for Kilkenny (1852), Killarney (1852), Omagh (1853), Sligo (1855) and Mullingar (1855), as well as major new buildings for the existing asylums at Cork (1852) and The Richmond (1854). The differing capacities of each new asylum militated against a standard design, and with the Board of Works already struggling under a heavy workload (which included commissioning new 'Godless' colleges at Cork, Galway and Belfast and a godlier one at Maynooth), it was necessary to outsource to private practitioners: 'The great increase of business connected with the erection of various public buildings, has rendered the employment of private architects indispensable, to enable us to carry them out satisfactorily.'[18] The architectural profession was, needless to say, delighted by this turn of events. The editor of *The Dublin Builder* commended the Board of Works for acting on a 'truly liberal and art-encouraging principle… their patronage has been judiciously bestowed… [giving] the young and ardent members of the profession… encouragement and hope.'[19] Such 'liberal patronage' would ultimately become a matter of controversy and regret for the Board, as soon we shall see.

Given that every public asylum to date had been delivered by the incumbent partnership of Francis Johnston and William Murray, prior experience of asylum design could not be a pre-requisite for these prestigious appointments. Membership of the council of the recently established Royal Institute of Architects of Ireland seems to have been a more influential factor: all but two of the appointees were well established practitioners who served on the council alongside Board of Works Architect and RIAI elder statesman Jacob Owen during the 1840s. In January 1848 the Board of Works issued all architects with a set of *Instructions to Architects* outlining their preferred design approach. By contrast with the relative freedom that Francis Johnston enjoyed when conceiving the first asylum typology 30 years earlier, the *Instructions* were extraordinarily prescriptive, drawing upon the practical experience of the likes of Eyre E. C. Kenny in operating such institutions over several years, as well as contemporary best practice gleaned from a tour of the most modern English corridor asylums, including Surrey, Hanwell and Maidstone.[20] O'Dwyer notes that most of the architects were either already appointed prior to the issuance of the *Instructions* or were working in anticipation that they soon would be, so that it is not inconceivable that their early design work and correspondence actually helped the Board of Works to refine their own brief.[21]

All eight architects ultimately produced designs in strict accordance with the operational orthodoxy of the Instructions. At the centre every new asylum was an entrance block of three (occasionally four) storeys containing administration, board and reception rooms, private quarters for the Manager (later RMS) and Matron; all were well appointed with high-quality joinery, plasterwork and chimneypieces that would not be out of place in a contemporary mansion. Despite the chapel forming the

18. *Sixteenth Report from the Board of Public Works, Ireland, with Appendices* (hereafter *Sixteenth Board of Works Report*), HC 1848 [983] xxxvii, p. 14.
19. This approach sat in stark contrast with the 'stereotyped edition… the same style, the same plan, the same arrangement, repeated in every one, no matter what the site' that had characterised Wilkinson's workhouses. *The Dublin Builder*, 17 Aug. 1850, p. 387.
20. Eyre E. C. Kenny, superintendent of the auxiliary asylum at Islandbridge, Dublin, simultaneously published his *Short Hints and Observations on the Arrangement and Management of Lunatic Asylums* (Dublin, 1848).
21. The new brief seems to have become retrospectively binding on those already appointed; compositionally outstanding early designs for the Killarney asylum prepared by Benjamin Woodward in 1847 were superseded by a more mundane design that adhered strictly to the requirements of the 'Instructions'. Frederick O'Dwyer, *The Architecture of Deane and Woodward* (Cork, 1997), pp 90–2. Una Sugrue also suggests that Murray sought the views of Kenny at Islandbridge to inform his design of the New Richmond.

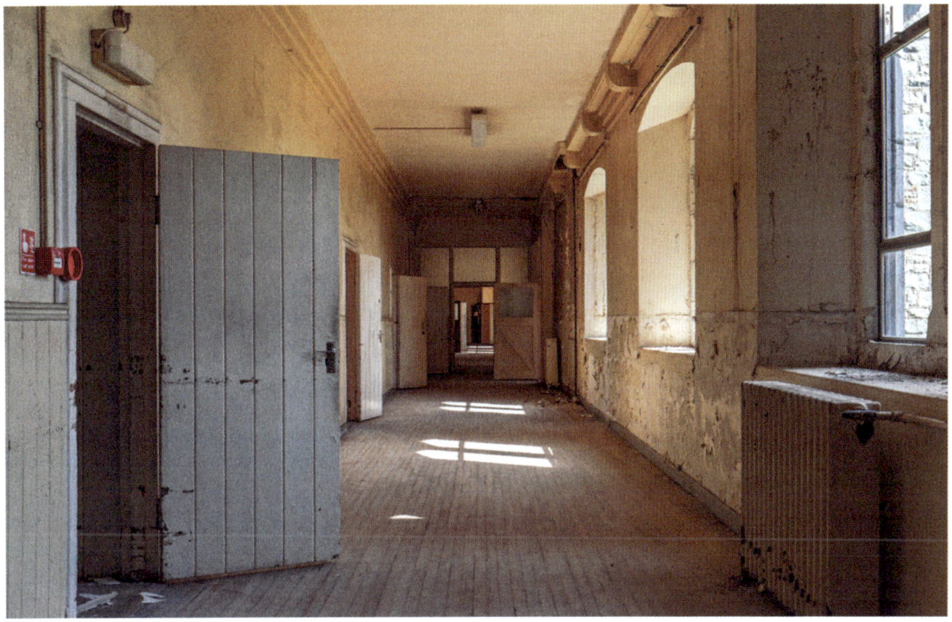

3.10 Killarney: Interior view of south-facing 'galleries' which doubled as patient day-spaces, *Photograph by David Killeen, 2019.*

22. This is a potentially fruitful area for further research. Did the (Anglican) political establishment wish to avoid a situation whereby the external expression of these new civic institutions would be defined by a feature that would potentially be contested between the creeds, or indeed risk being dominated by adherents of the (Catholic) majority?

architectural centrepiece of many contemporary English asylums, it was conspicuous by its absence in these Irish buildings, being generally located on the upper floors within the rear part of the main block. In architectural terms, this can only be seen as opportunity lost, particularly when we consider the rich potential of an externally expressed chapel as in Benjamin Woodward's abortive designs for Killarney (see Case Study 14).[22]

Gender-segregated patient accommodation was located in long, three-storey wings extending to the east and west, with 20–50 patients per floor on each side. Sleeping spaces were placed on the north facade, laid out in varying proportions of single cells and dormitories depending on the category of patient – from single cells for the 'refractory' or disturbed on the ground floor to dormitories of 10 to 14 beds for the 'quiet and harmless' on the top floor. Sleeping accommodation was accessed directly from wide, bright, south-facing corridors or 'galleries' that doubled as day spaces, broadening out locally into more usefully proportioned day rooms. Separate single-storey blocks to the rear accommodated a laundry department with a wash house and drying room, a kitchen including a bakery and dairy, assorted workshops, and out-offices. To isolate these potential sources of fire, all were generally detached from the main building and linked back to it via a pair of communicating corridors. Acknowledging the shortcomings of the earlier asylum designs, considerable effort was invested in the technical specification of these spaces, with surviving drawings for Mullingar showing the fascinating means by which hot water and steam were generated and distributed through kitchen and laundry spaces in an era before factory-produced equipment.

Fireplaces in patient spaces were too small and few in number to adequately heat them in winter; the handful of senior officers privileged to lodge in the central block typically enjoyed the warmth of as many hearths as the rest of the building combined. Each ward was provided with at least one water closet, wash room and bath for 20–30 patients – an improvement on the earlier asylums, which had indoor baths but not initially water closets, and generations before the pauper class would see the benefit of indoor sanitation in their own homes.[23] The medically unwell or potentially infectious were physically isolated in infirmaries, provided either as detached buildings, or in smaller wings at each extremity of the building. This layout readily lent itself to both parallel and perpendicular extension, ultimately resulting in impractically long buildings whose distant wards could only be accessed by passing through other wards – an arrangement that John Connolly advised against as early as 1847 but which became a feature of almost all asylums, in both Ireland and Britain.[24]

And not devoid of architectural character

Just as the spatial planning of the earlier panoptic asylums became too closely associated with emerging prison architecture, so the Board of Works also sought to clearly distance the outward appearance of the new asylums from those that went before. The opening lines of the *Instructions* reminded architects that they were 'designing an hospital, not a prison', and that 'the *appearance* of restraint and confinement may be as much as possible avoided.'[25] Nowhere was this more pertinent than in Jacob Owen's own design for the world's first specialist asylum for criminal lunatics at Dundrum, south Dublin – a brief that explicitly combined the curative aspirations of the asylum with the security imperatives of the prison, and a topic worthy of a book in its own right. It is clear that many of the principles adopted by Owen in designing this asylum would go on to be included in the *Instructions*, which is another way of observing that the design of the central criminal asylum is actually far closer to that of a conventional district asylum than might have been expected.

The *Instructions* went on to state that 'the style of architecture best suited to the general quality of the building materials in this country, and admitting also of additions being easily made to the asylums hereafter, is the "Gothic".' The Board emphasised that the new asylums should be of architectural merit, and clearly distinguished from the Union Workhouses that were then rising all around the country:

> *It is hoped that the buildings will be found effective for all the purposes of such institutions, and, at the same time, not devoid of architectural character… the cost of lunatic asylums must necessarily be great, and should not be compared with that of workhouses and ordinary charitable institutions, which is the comparison generally made by inexperienced persons.*[26]

Architects were permitted to propose styles other than Gothic, but it seems to have been universally understood that this licence did not extend to any repetition of the classical style employed in the earlier asylums. The resultant buildings occupied various points along a spectrum of historical-revival styles, from Early-English Gothic via watered-down Tudor to full-blown Elizabethan. Architects in both camps employed a similar array of devices including bay- and oriel-windows, decorative

23. By way of further contrast: the contemporaneous new model prisons designed on the 'separate system', such as Pentonville in London (1842) or Mountjoy in Dublin (1850), were provided with individual in-cell sanitation for every prisoner.
24. Connolly, *The Construction and Government of Lunatic Asylums*, p. 19.
25. Emphasis added by author. 'Instructions for the guidance of Architects when furnishing Designs for Lunatic Asylums', appendix to *Sixteenth Board of Works Report*, HC 1848 [983] xxxvii, p. 236. Architects also likely referred to Connolly's contemporary book, *The Construction and Government of Lunatic Asylums*, which the Instructions broadly paralleled.
26. *Sixteenth Board of Works Report*, HC 1848 [983] xxxvii, p. 16. It is also notable that the preference for the Gothic style for these asylums is pitched in such bluntly pragmatic terms – the fundamentalist and moralistic justifications for the Gothic Revival as espoused by Pugin, amongst others, are notable for their absence.

buttresses, vertiginous chimney stacks and a multiplicity of steep gables to enhance the picturesque effect of what otherwise threatened to be domineering institutional buildings. Those who chose the Gothic idiom – including Sir Thomas Deane at Killarney and William Atkins at Cork – attempted to introduce variety with their studiously irregular disposition of single, bi- and tri-partite openings and bay- and oriel-windows. William Murray[27] went one better at the New Richmond by alternating shallow and deeply projecting day rooms. Surviving images of this now demolished building suggest that it come closest to submerging the tyranny of symmetry dictated by the building's brief beneath a picturesque architectural veneer.

In decorative terms William Deane Butler at Sligo surpassed his peers, employing an elaborate Elizabethan-Revival style that strikes an exotic note in a country where Elizabethan architecture in its original conception is all but unknown. The massing and roofscape of the building was simpler than most of its peers, but Butler compensated with a panoply of decorative stonework including curvilinear

27. Or more likely, his son William G. Murray, who took over the project after William Senior's death in 1849.

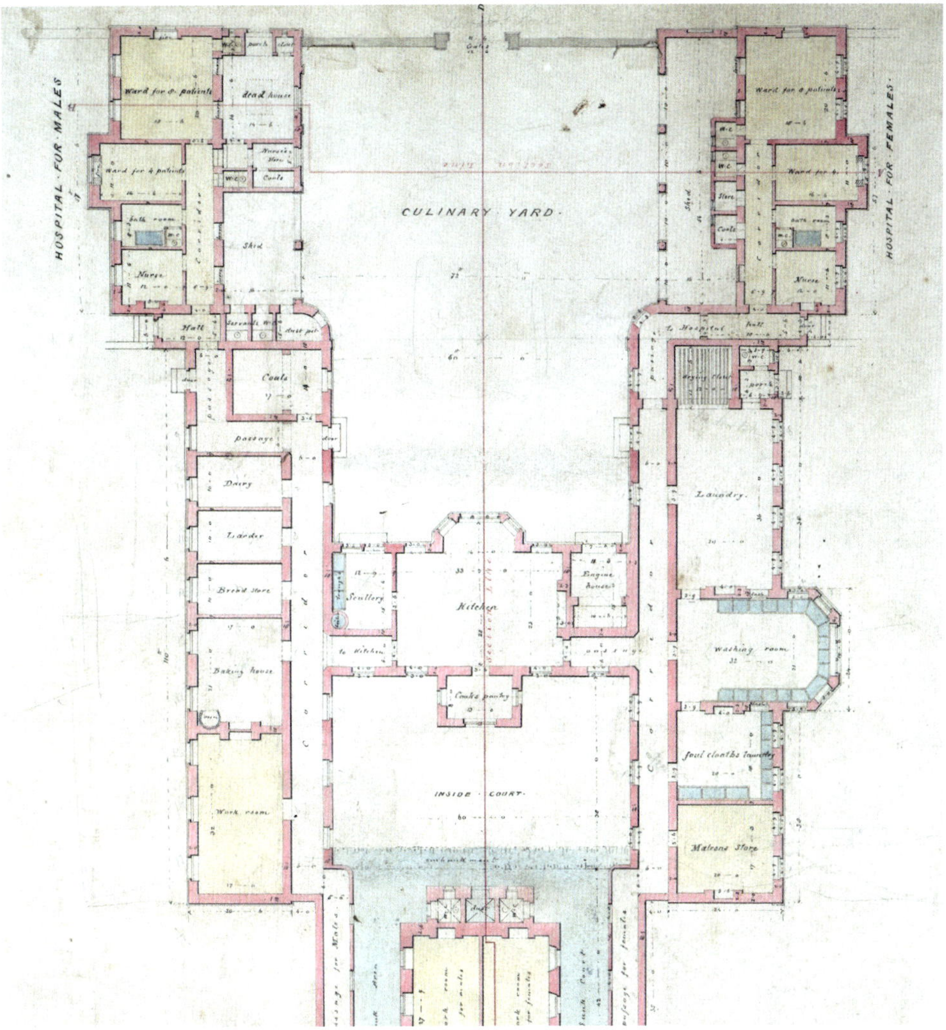

3.11 Sligo: Plan of service quarters, showing extensive kitchen and laundry departments, with infirmaries in an unusual location beyond, *Image courtesy of the Irish Architectural Archive (Sligo Lunatic Asylum Collection, 89/11: 2)*

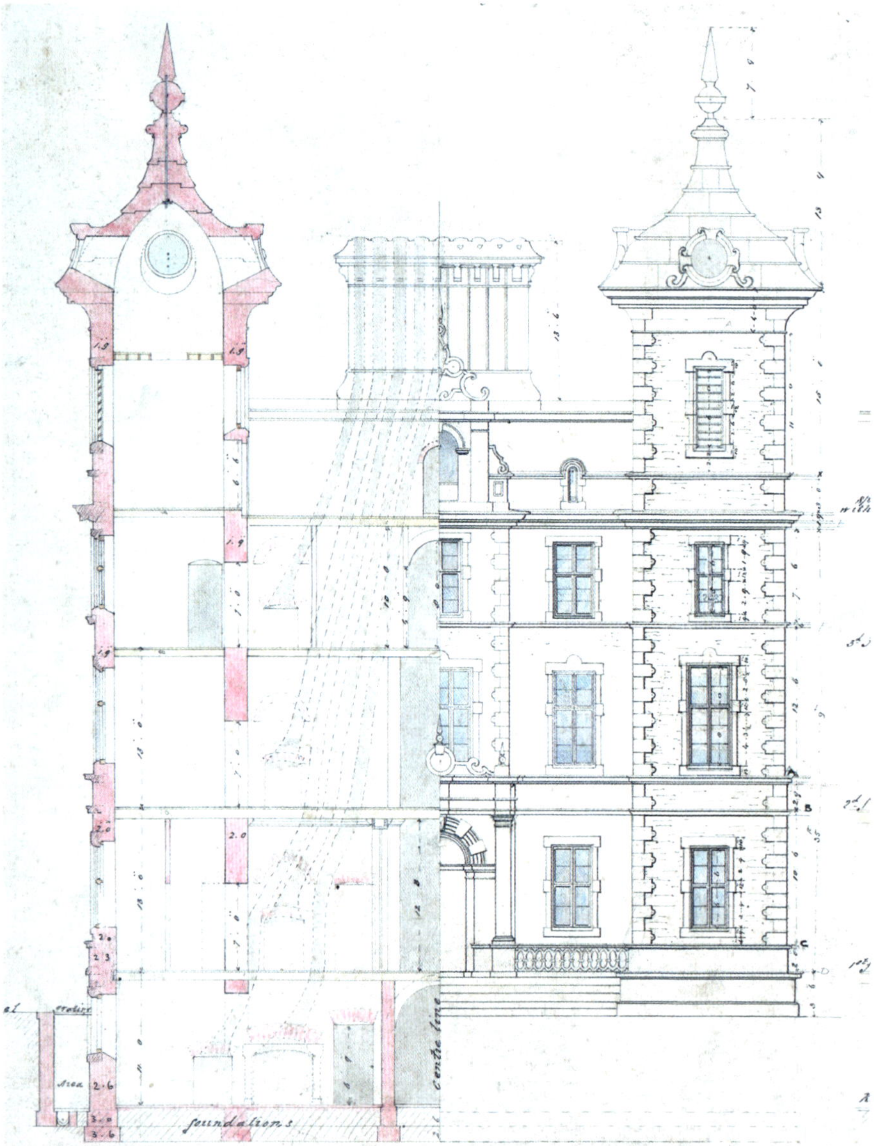
foundations
Centre line

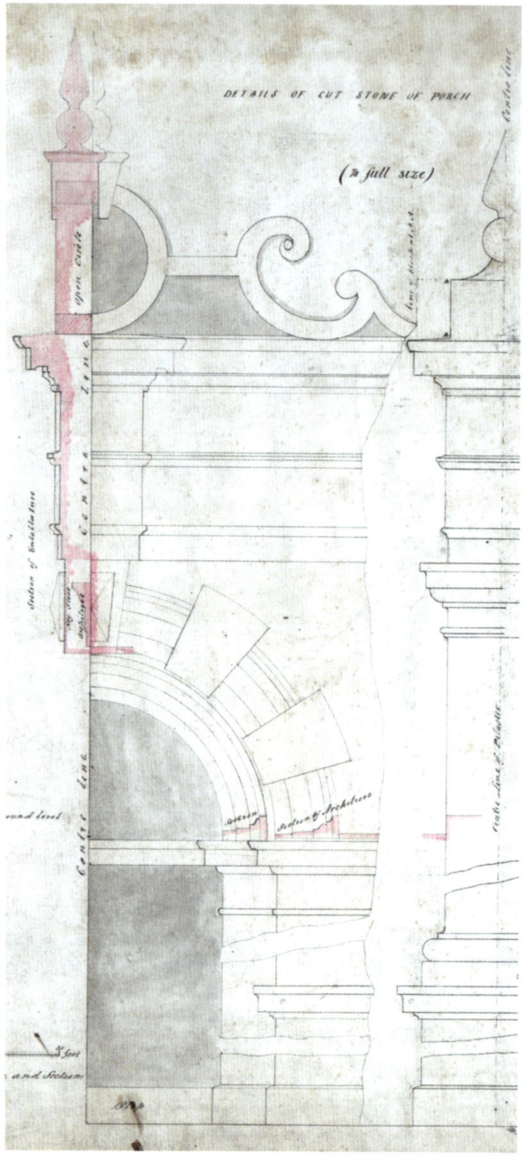
DETAILS OF CUT STONE OF PORCH
(½ full size)

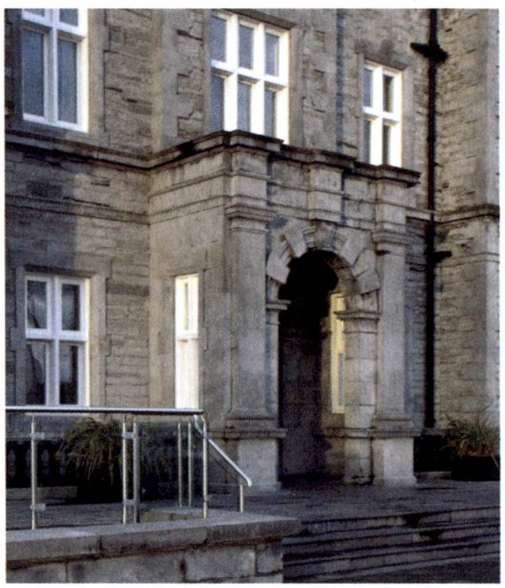

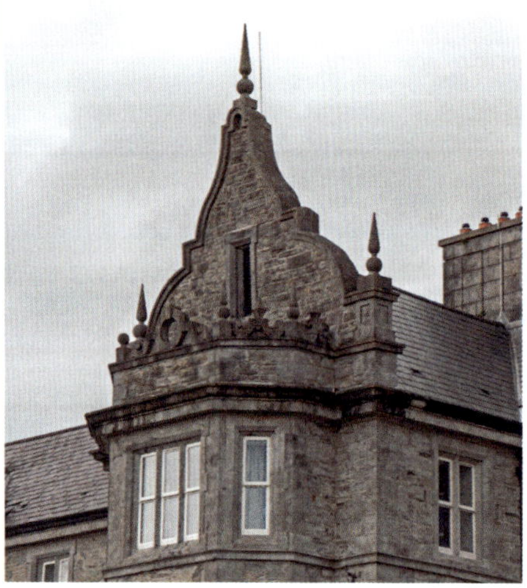

3.12 Sligo: Part elevation, part section of central block. Note elaborate decorative detailing, including cut stone spires not executed, *Image courtesy of the Irish Architectural Archive (Sligo Lunatic Asylum Collection, 89/11: 11).*

3.13 Sligo: Detail of cut stone to entrance porch, Image courtesy of the Irish *Architectural Archive (Sligo Lunatic Asylum Collection, 89/11: 11)*

3.14 Sligo: Cut stone detailing of exceptional quality and controversial cost, *Photograph by author, 2013.*

3.15 Sligo: The florid Elizabethan-revival style strikes an exotic note in a country where Elizabethan in its original conception was all but unknown, *Photograph by David Killeen, 2019.*

3.16 Dundrum: Twentieth-century modifications rendered the airing yards definitively 'prison-like', *Photograph by David Killeen, 2019.*

3.17 Mullingar: Walled gardens offered therapeutic and practical benefits within (another) secure boundary, *Photograph by David Killeen, 2019.*

3.18 Eglinton Asylum, Cork: Dramatic silhouette of Atkin's 285 metre long façade which dominates the Lee valley west of the city, *Photograph by David Killeen, 2019.*

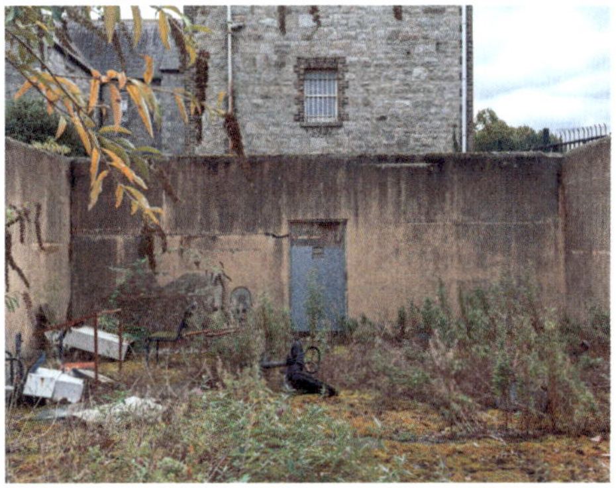

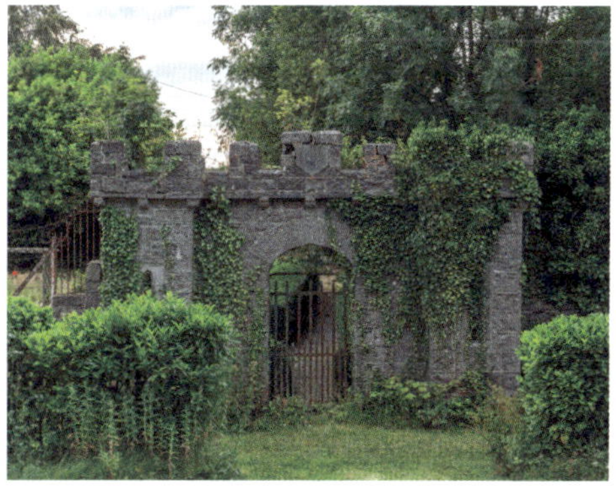

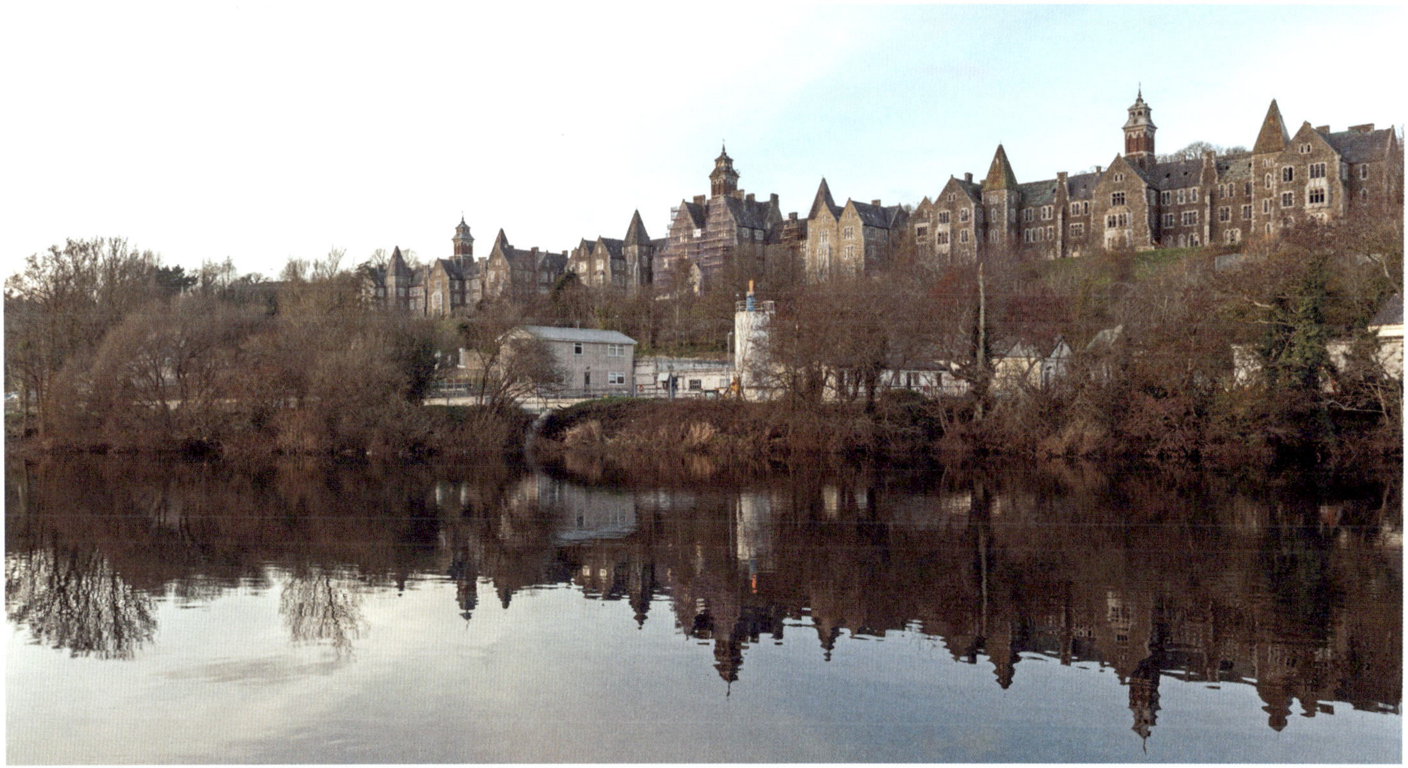

28. Reuber regards Atkin's disaggregation of three detached blocks in Cork as the first 'pavilion' asylum, an interpretation the author struggles to share. It is a distinguishing feature of the pavilion model that the circulation routes are entirely separate from the patient blocks, whereas at Cork the ground floor wards remain principal thoroughfares. Markus Reuber, 'The architecture of psychological management: the Irish Asylums, 1801–1922', in *Psychological Medicine*, no. 26 (1996), p. 1185.

29. Interesting to observe that, although wrapped in superficially similar architectural clothing, the internal programmes of the asylums and the colleges were utterly different, and the quality of their internal finishing likewise a world apart.

gables, pinnacles and open fretwork parapets. Butler's ambitious plans for curvaceous cut stone roofs to the pair of central water towers proved to be a bridge too far and were greatly simplified in execution, explaining their slightly discordant appearance today. The designers of the smaller buildings – most obviously George Papworth at Kilkenny – succeeded in creating an attractive character which, if not convincingly domestic, was at least less overtly institutional. But disguising the sheer scale of the largest asylums of the period – Omagh, Mullingar and Cork – would prove a much greater challenge to their respective architects.

The Omagh commission was the swansong of a long and fruitful career for architect William Farrell, but is also the most disappointing building of the period. A late decision to completely reverse the orientation of the building after contracts had been signed left little time to redesign a façade of barrack-like grimness. We might also speculate that additional costs arising from this late change may have obliged Farrell to achieve savings by omitting other architectural features, and the effect is not improved with the more recent removal of most of the original chimneystacks. But of the three largest and most lucrative commissions, two were entrusted to architects still aged in their 30s, neither of whom were (yet) members of Owen's RIAI inner circle. Of the two, John Skipton Mulvany was already accomplished beyond his years with a variety of high-profile commissions to his name, but even he struggled to overcome the compositional challenges presented by the sheer scale of the building. In truth no amount of architectural wallpaper could disguise the underlying monotony of Mullingar's 200-metre, three-storey frontage; Mulvany might have done better to reconfigure the overall massing by staggering the layout in plan and introducing taller elements in elevation.

Maybe it is no coincidence that the 'youngest and most ardent' architect proved the most willing to innovate. William Atkins faced the biggest challenge of all in designing the Cork asylum – at 500 patients it was the largest yet conceived in Ireland – and he had the least professional experience to draw upon. But his approach represented a rare example of programmatic innovation in this era: splitting the building into three free-standing pavilions, connected by corridors, with a clear visual break between each. These blocks were reasonably successful compositions in their own right, but not long afterwards the overall effect was lost with the construction of full-height links, creating the impossibly long 285-metre building that dominates the Lee valley to this day.[28]

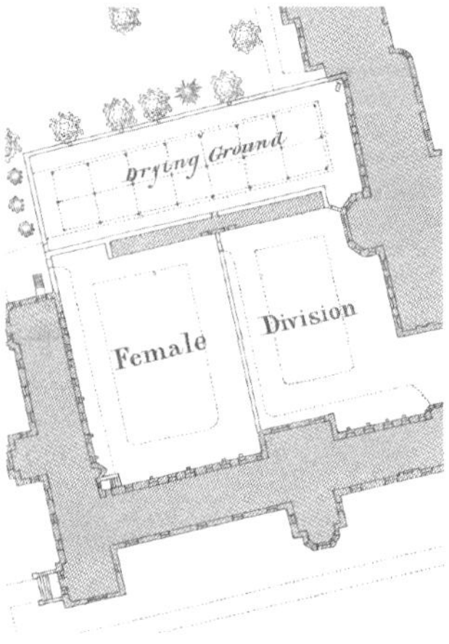

3.19 Sligo: Behind the ornate façade, the airing yards lay in a state of perpetual gloom. *Reproduced courtesy of Trinity College Dublin (OS-Sligo-500-Sheet 2-1877).*

Individual critiques notwithstanding, the aesthetic quality of these buildings as a collective was on a par with the prestigious third-level colleges on which the Board of Works were simultaneously engaged, and a world removed from the overt architectural poverty of the Union Workhouses.[29] All were approached via sweeping avenues that arrive obliquely at the central block through attractive landscapes that would be planted with boundary woodlands and specimen trees, further reinforcing their presentation as high-status buildings. Indeed the contrast between the new asylums and the general living conditions of the class for whom they were built could not have been more stark, as observed by a visitor to Killarney in 1852: 'Looking from it to the styes in the outskirts of the town, where human families are huddled like swine, we could not but feel that to build such an establishment in such a place was like giving a splendid waistcoat to a man without a shirt…'[30]

Life within the walls

Architecturally impressive from afar they may have been, but life within the walls was far from luxurious. Historic photographs of patient living spaces are exceedingly rare, so we have little to contradict our current perception of these as relatively stark, comfortless places. Timber wainscoting and ceiling linings in patient spaces at Killarney and decorative plaster cornices at Mullingar are rare exceptions to the rule of Spartan interiors, while the lighter touches that could have lifted the spirits appear to have been entirely absent in these early years:

> *In corridor or day room, the lunatic sees nothing but the one undiversified white wall – giving to these hospitals, intended for the restoration of the alienated mind, an air of blankness and desolation more calculated to fix than to remove the awful disease under which it labours.*[31]

Patients would doubtless have appreciated it if their designers had paid more heed to curtains – or even internal plaster – than cut stone, as recommended by Samuel Tuke's thirty years earlier:

> *The internal comforts of public Institutions are obtained at much less expense than external ornament… in determining to prefer internal convenience to external decoration: the comfort of the inmate, to the gratification of the passing traveller.*[32]

The smooth operation of the institution demanded a highly regimented routine that severely curtailed individual freedom. Standardised rules were adopted by the Lord Lieutenant in 1843 for use across all asylums. In summer, patients were woken at 6 a.m. and locked out of their sleeping quarters until 8.30 p.m., at which time they were locked back in until the following morning. From October to March, the respective times were 7 a.m. until 7 p.m., so that averaged across the full year, patients spent 45 percent of their time confined within their cells or dormitories – and this in an era before artificial lighting.[33] Breakfast, dinner and supper were served at set times and partaken of in the day rooms until the advent of centralised dining halls. Sligo's governors were the first to propose the addition of a dining hall before their building was even finished; most other asylums would eventually follow suit. The original design for Sligo was also unique in featuring a separate recreation hall – distinct from both chapel and dining hall – functions that on other sites were more commonly combined.

The designed landscapes described in the previous chapter offered therapeutic relief from this regimented indoor existence, but not all patients were free to roam. Difficult, 'refractory' and dangerous patients were typically confined indoors with access only to walled 'airing courts' – swathes of featureless paving depressingly reminiscent of prison yards. Despite instructions that airing courts should be located

30. Henrietta Martineau, *Letters from Ireland* (London, 1852), cited in O'Dwyer, *The Architecture of Deane and Woodward*, p. 104.
31. *1858 Commission Report*, HC 1857–58 [2436-I] p. 14.
32. Samuel Tuke, *Practical Hints on the Construction and Economy of Pauper Lunatic Asylums* (London, 1815), p. 50.
33. *Annual Asylum Report 1843*, HC 1844 [567] xxx, p. 44.

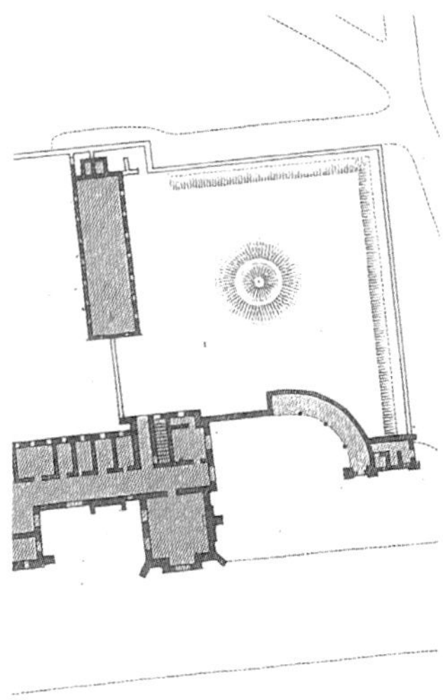

3.20 Richmond Asylum, Dublin: Viewing mound and sunk-fence to allow patient views out of airing yard, *Reproduced courtesy of Trinity College Dublin (OS-Dublin City-1056-Sheet 7-1866).*

to the south of the buildings to maximise exposure to fresh air and sunlight, this guidance was almost universally ignored:

> *in no instance have the airing-yards been placed in the front. The consequence is that they are generally too much enclosed… and surrounded by buildings and high enclosure walls, which exclude the view of the country [and]… the genial influence of the sun's heat.*[34]

34. *1858 Commission Report*, HC 1857–58 [2436-I], p. 6.

Even though sunk-fences and ha-has were commonly employed to diminish the apparent height of the airing yard walls, and viewing mounds were occasionally formed to enable views over them, airing courts remained for the most part joyless. The imperative to compose a set piece of an architecturally distinguished façade within a genteel parkland setting clearly took precedence over the daily experience of patients, particularly disadvantaging the more acutely disturbed for whom the airing court offered their only release from the indoor regimen. It was an unfortunate shortcoming in a building programme whose commissioners and designers otherwise demonstrated a laudable commitment to best practice as it was then perceived, who had gone to great lengths to learn from the lessons of the first generation of asylums, and who took such obvious pride in their creations. But this would prove to be far from the only major failing of these ambitious buildings, as we shall soon see.

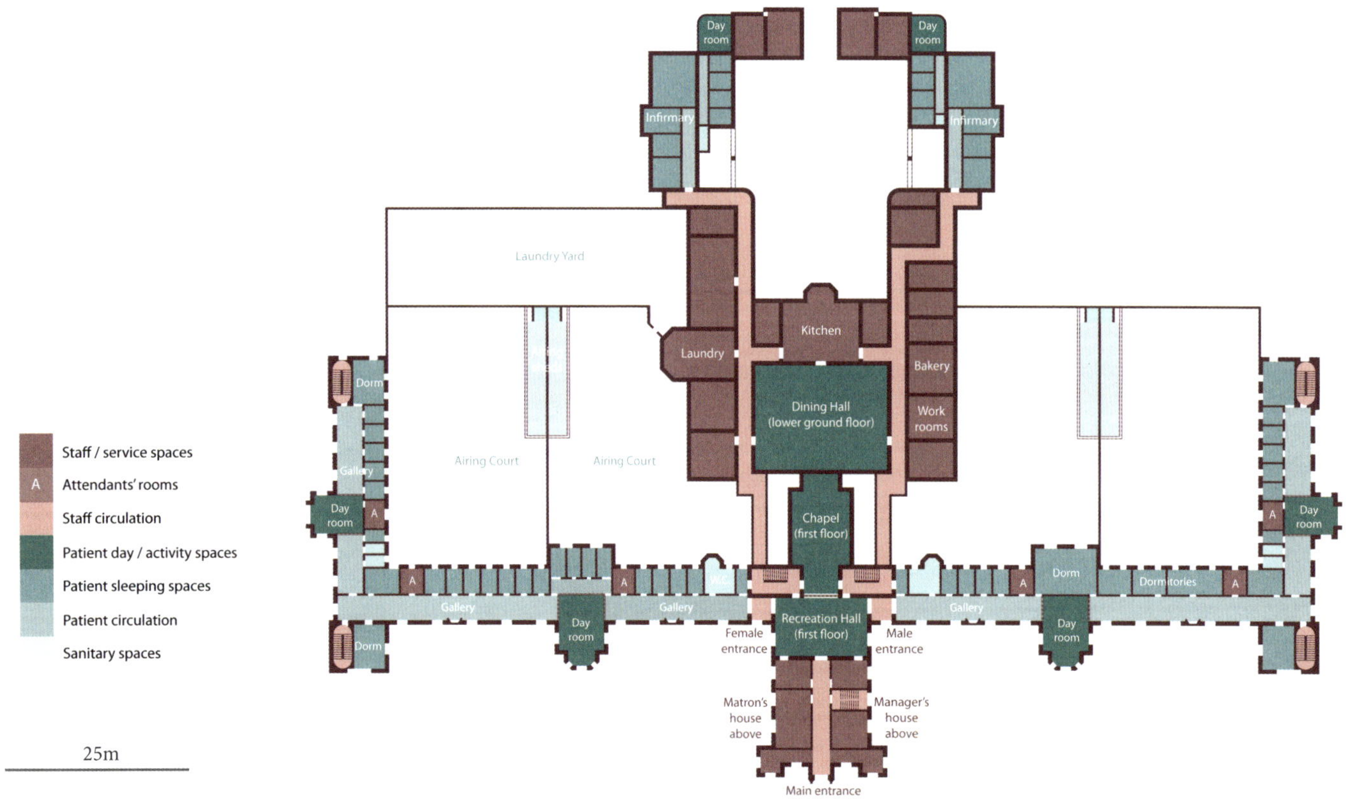

3.21 Plan of Sligo Asylum with key uses annotated. Note how the wider galleries double as day rooms and the growth of communal and ancillary spaces, *Drawn by the author.*

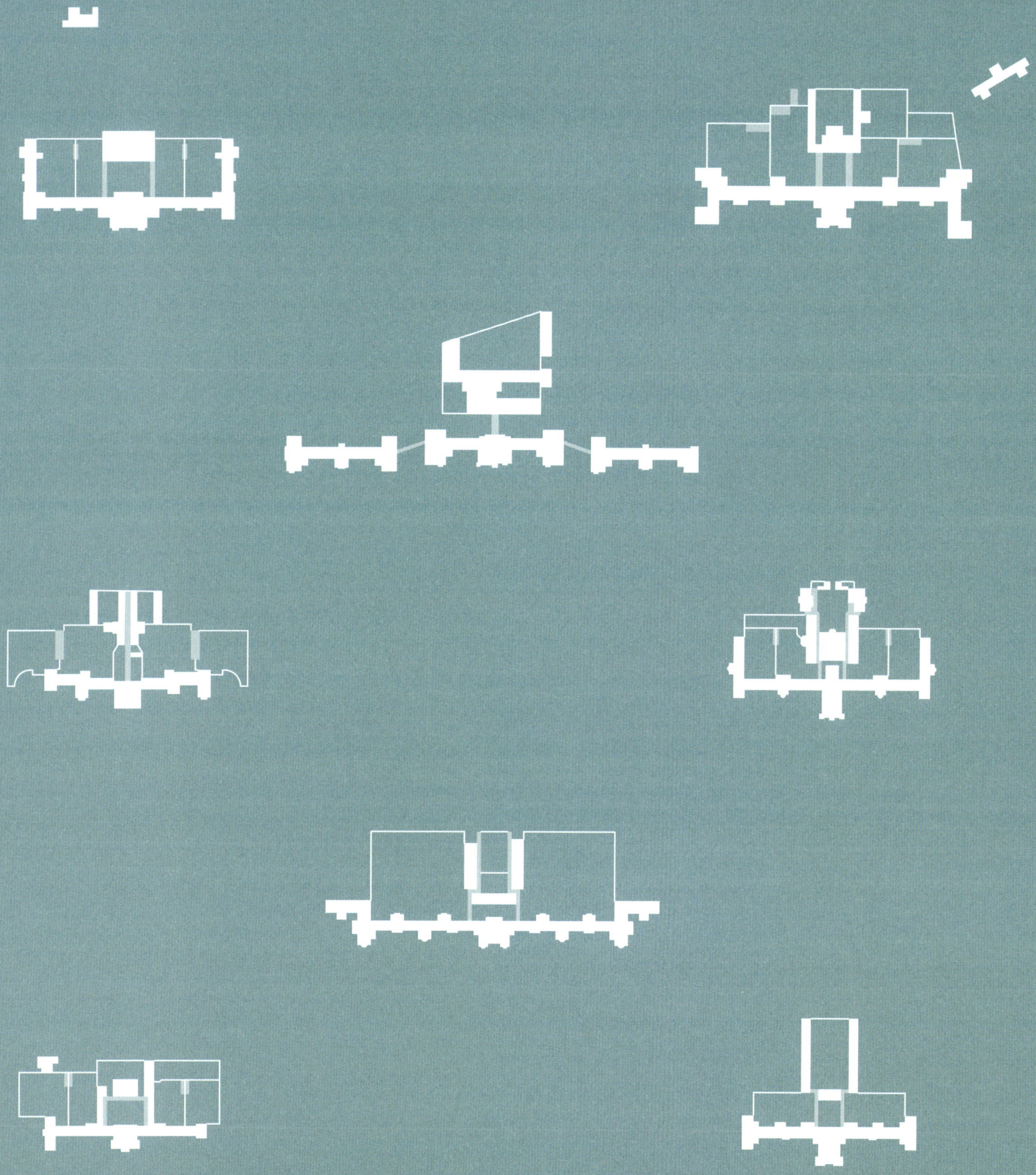

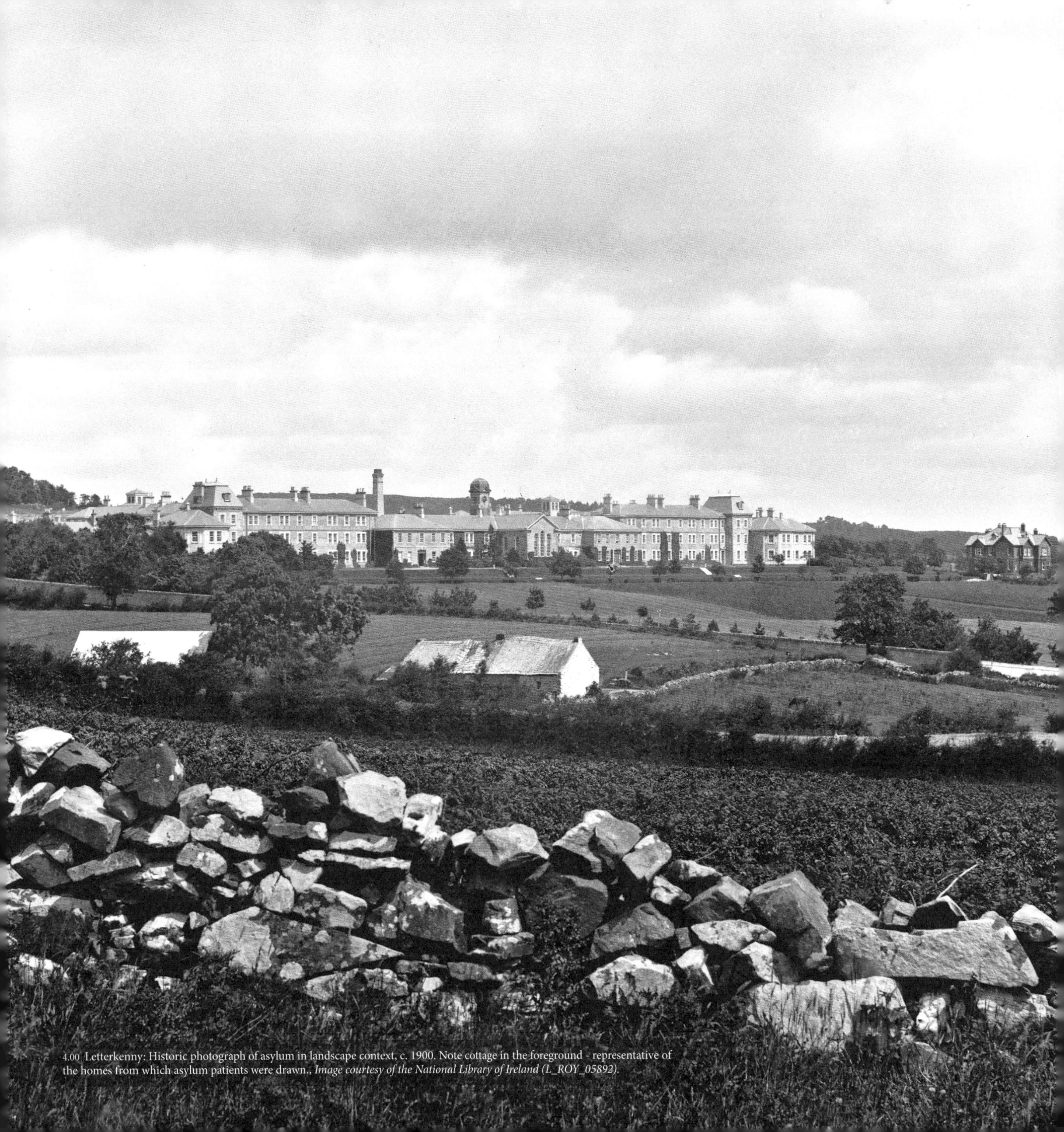

4.00 Letterkenny: Historic photograph of asylum in landscape context, c. 1900. Note cottage in the foreground - representative of the homes from which asylum patients were drawn., *Image courtesy of the National Library of Ireland (L_ROY_05892).*

1855 - 1885

Demise of Innocence

fully calculated to meet the wants of the country[1]

Between 1844 and 1854 the Board of Works and their private architects succeeded in the impressive feat of doubling Ireland's asylum accommodation during one of the most traumatic periods in Irish history. The new network of asylums was undoubtedly impressive to behold, but almost immediately proved controversial amongst local communities who were obliged to repay the loans issued to cover their capital costs, as well as meeting their ongoing operating expenses. Regardless of the actual merits of the complaints that follow, it is worth recalling that these new asylums opened their doors into a completely different world from that in which they were planned, barely a decade earlier. A constituent nation of the world's most powerful empire had witnessed a catastrophe of starvation and mass emigration that local government had proven wholly unable – and national government, grimly unwilling – to mitigate. Beyond the immeasurable humanitarian toll, the economy locally and nationally was still reeling, and costs that may have seemed reasonable and proportionate in the pre-Famine world would now be seen in an entirely different light.

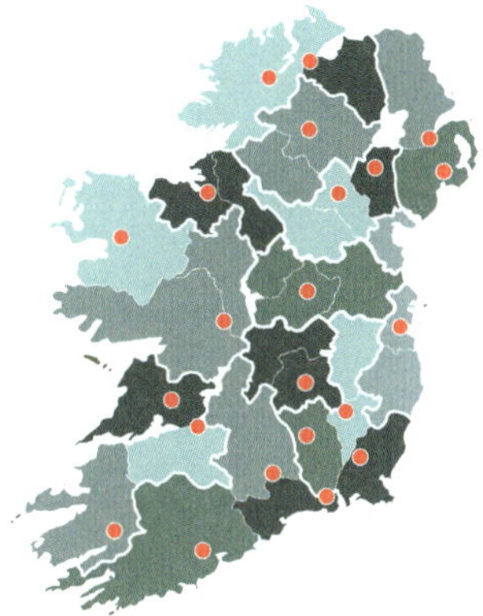

Asylum distribution in Ireland, **1885.** *Drawn by the author.*

By failing to issue clear cost guidance to their architects at the outset, the central authority of the Board of Works in effect wrote blank cheques that would fall to individual counties to honour. It was bad enough that the counties found themselves burdened with paying for expensive, architecturally elaborate buildings in whose design they were not consulted, but to add insult to injury, the structures themselves soon proved to be highly defective. Local grand juries accused the Board of Works of mal-administration, citing the 'useless expense of [cut stone] decoration' and substandard workmanship that resulted in widespread dampness and dry-rot in newly completed buildings, the latter especially prevalent at Killarney and Cork:

> *The building, when given up, was really not habitable by the patients. The water streaked off the walls in buckets full; mops were used every day soaking it up, and this was so for the first year here. The asylum was obliged to be pointed every winter to try and exclude damp. So great was the damp, that every joist running across the corridors became rotten as a pear. The Board of Works found it necessary to make additions in order to*

1. *1858 Commission Report*, HC 1857–58 [2436-I], pp 22–4.

correct the evils, and they sought to throw it upon the Board of Governors after they got the responsibility off their own shoulders.[2]

A parliamentary commission of enquiry was established in 1855 and having gathered exhaustive evidence, substantiated many of these claims. The commission authorised financial rebates from central funds to local grand juries to cover the costs both of remedying defective workmanship and instances where architectural ornamentation exceeded what was deemed reasonable for buildings of public charity. The Board of Works were criticised for their lax oversight and relieved of any further duties with respect to lunatic asylums. A new Board of Control – similar to that which existed prior to 1835 – would henceforth be responsible for 'superintending and directing the Erection, Establishment and Regulation of Pauper Lunatic Asylums'.[3] In the Board of Works' defence, the commission concluded that the second-phase asylum buildings were, in toto, actually one-third cheaper than those erected by the first Board of Control to the designs of Johnston and Murray, and one-quarter cheaper per patient than their English counterparts.[4]

Fully calculated to meet the wants of the country

At this point it is worth recalling that the asylum was far from the only institution where Ireland's insane paupers could be found. The continued detention of lunatics in county goals was a cause for humanitarian concern, while thousands of insane persons – often but not exclusively congenital idiots and imbeciles – were still lodged in union workhouses. The relative fluidity that was still evident in the movement of insane persons between the community and the three main institutional settings is a complex topic outside the scope of this book, but suffice to observe that beyond the question of defective law, the territorial interests of the different institutions and their administrators played no small role. Gaol governors and workhouse masters were eager to divest their most troublesome cases to the asylum, while Poor Law Guardians, being slightly more answerable to their rate-paying electorate than grand jury elites, were keenly incentivised to minimise the burden on their rates by exporting

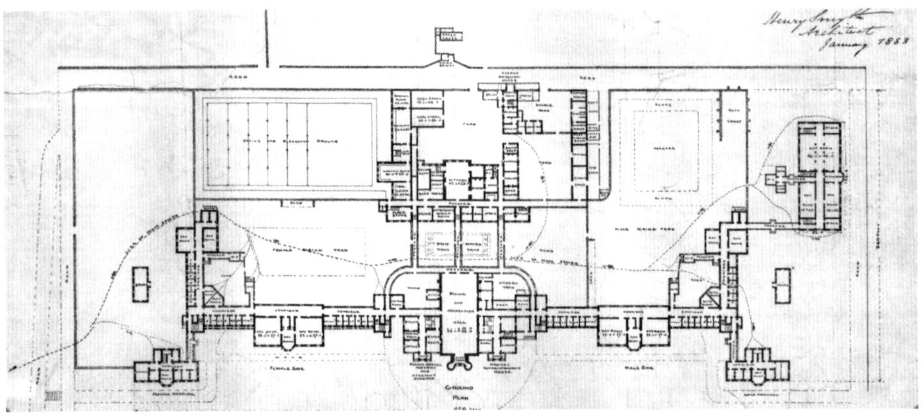

4.01 Downpatrick: The increasing scale and complexity of asylums of this era is evident from the layout of the new Downpatrick Asylum, *Image courtesy of the National Archives of Ireland (Office of Public Works Collection, OPW/5HC/4/944).*

2. *Report of a Commission Inquiring into the Erection of District Lunatic Asylums in Ireland* (hereafter *1856 Commission Report*), HC 1856 [9] liii, pp 493–4. Considering both average annual rainfall and average wind speed, Killarney ranks as the most climatically exposed asylum in the British Isles. The deleterious effect of wind-driven rain off the Atlantic is as evident now as in the 1850s: vandalism and arson aside, no building has displayed a more dramatic or rapid deterioration since being vacated than Killarney.
3. Ibid., p. 1. See also *Lunatic Asylums Repayment of Advances (Irl) Act 1855*, 18 & 19 Vic. c.109.
4. *1856 Commission Report*. The Commission revealed that the Board abandoned its preconceived cost of £100–120 per bed, issued no instructions to architects regarding construction budget, did not seek cost estimates from architects during design development, and thus had no idea of the likely cost of the plans before proceeding to tender. Final construction cost of phase-two Irish asylums averaged £148/bed, compared to £222/bed for the phase one asylums and £201/bed for contemporary English asylums.

the costs of maintaining such patients to the asylum budget – even though the per-capita cost of an asylum place was far higher than the workhouse.[5]

It was in this context that yet another commission was appointed to examine every aspect of the provision for the insane in Ireland, including district asylums, workhouses and gaols. The commission's 1858 report calculated the number of lunatics either poorly accommodated or 'at large' to inform forecasts for future asylum demand. Implicit in their outlook was the premise that the only appropriate place for poor, mentally ill or intellectually disabled people was the asylum, helping to drive the demand that would make their forecasts self-fulfilling. The commission were also supportive of the conceptually attractive prospect of a district asylum system organised along county lines:

> *We think it very desirable that where a county is large enough to require an asylum, say for 250 patients, it should… possess an asylum for itself… [and so] complete the distribution of Ireland into Lunatic Asylum Districts, in a manner fully calculated to meet the wants of the country, so far as we can anticipate they will arise for some time to come.*[6]

After the usual politicking about districts and locations, new asylums would ultimately be constructed for Counties Donegal (Letterkenny, opened 1865), Down (Downpatrick, 1865), Mayo (Castlebar, 1866), Clare (Ennis, 1868), Wexford (Enniscorthy, 1868) and Cavan–Monaghan (Monaghan, 1869). No doubt prompted by the controversies around the cost of the last phase of construction, the Inspectors predicted – with optimism that verged on the delusional – that the new asylums could be constructed at a total cost of £70 per bed including land, buildings and fittings.[7] The buildings of this phase would indeed prove to be cheaper on a per-bed basis than their predecessors, but with final costs in the range of £126 – £202 per bed.

As this phase of building drew to a close, parliament took the opportunity to reform the 1837 Dangerous Lunatics Act, outlawing the objectionable practice of committing dangerous lunatics to prisons while they awaited transfer to asylums. However, this seemingly benign motive helped to reinforce a system of involuntary detention in asylums that was 'poorly controlled, had limited safeguards and no in-built system of review'.[8] Admissions under the 1867 Dangerous Lunatics Act[9] would become a prevalent and much abused mode of entry to Irish asylums, used in respect of individuals who posed little or no danger. Being a judicial process that the medical men running the asylums had no authority to overrule, asylums were effectively obliged to accept detainees regardless of the potential of cure or the limitations of the available space.

Trust and obey

From the siting of the six buildings in this period we can see that while elevated sites with fine views remained essential, a southerly aspect was negotiable. Landholdings of 40–50 acres were now typical, as required to fulfil the pragmatic, therapeutic and programmatic needs of the institution. And while Foucault and others have described

5. At this time the maintenance of gaols and asylums was the responsibility of the grand jury, funded by the county cess, which was levied on landowners and larger occupiers. Workhouses established under the Poor Law were administered by elected Poor Law Guardians, who struck a rate payable on all property. However, landlords paid half the poor rates burden on tenanted land, and the entire rate on tenancies valued below £4. An exploration of the political dimensions of the different political and funding structures is beyond the scope of this study, but for further reading about how patients circulated between all three institutions, see Oonagh Walsh, 'Lunatic and criminal alliances in nineteenth -century Ireland', in Peter Bartlett and David Wright (eds), *Outside the Walls of the Asylum: The History of Care and Community 1750–2000* (London, 1999), pp 132–52.
6. *1858 Commission Report*, HC 1857–58 [2436-I], pp 22–4.
7. *Ninth Annual Asylum Report 1859*, HC 1859 session 2 [2582] x, pp 7–8.
8. Brennan, *Irish Insanity*, pp 83–4.
9. Lunacy (Ireland) Act 1867, 30 & 31 Vict., c.118, s.10.

the trend towards increasingly rural and remote asylum sites as evidence of an exclusionary impulse, in the Irish context at least, the modest increase in distance between town and asylum through the nineteenth century probably owes as much to the pragmatics of purchasing suitably large land holdings on reasonable terms.[10] In architectural terms the corridor model remained dominant, but with certain modifications compared to the second phase of buildings, and a higher priority afforded to economy and efficiency in accommodating ever greater numbers of patients within a single institution. The number of single cells was reduced in favour of larger dormitories, while wholly separate day rooms were re-introduced in response to the criticisms that attended the use of draughty and uncomfortable galleries as day spaces. Day rooms would more commonly be found on the ground floor with sleeping spaces on the floors above, an arrangement seen as 'assimilating their circumstances [more closely] to those of ordinary life'.[11] But that modest adjustment could not disguise the realities of institutional life where patients found themselves herded into ever larger groups by both day and night, with obvious implications for privacy and individual dignity. The universal inclusion of large dining and recreation halls may have been small compensation, offering patients a new range of possibilities for indoor recreation and leisure. Behind the scenes a growing array of ancillary structures of increasing technical complexity was needed to service the institution – a point vividly illustrated in the fascinating and near-complete set of contract drawings that survive for Ennis.

The 1855 Commission had criticised the second-phase asylums for their 'excess of embellishments… beyond what is suitable for such an institution', effectively vetoing a recurrence of the fine mullioned windows, buttresses and gables that characterised those buildings. Nevertheless a certain level of architectural aspiration

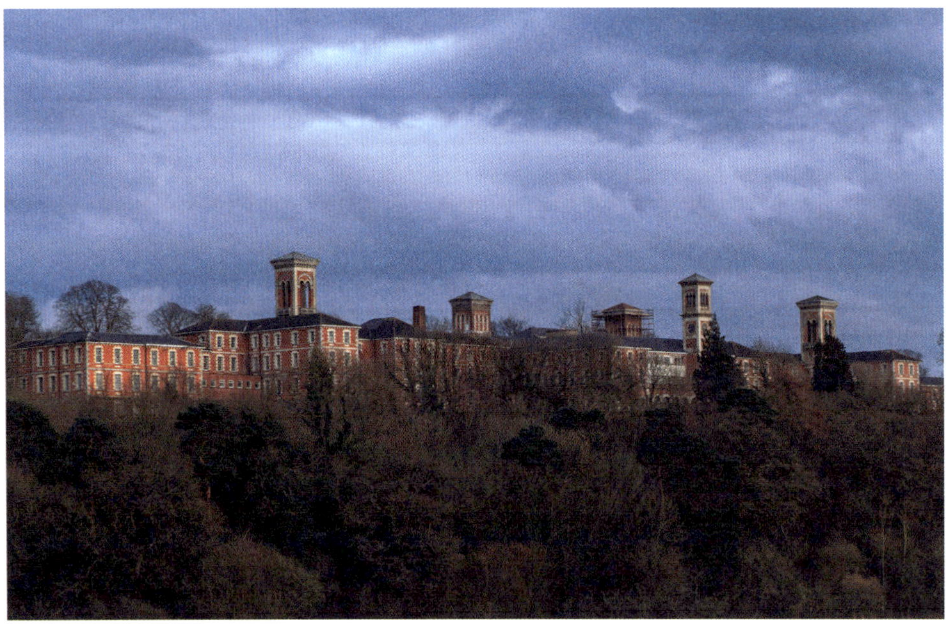

4.02 Enniscorthy: No less than five Italianate campanile make for a superb composition along the steep wooded banks of the Slaney, *Photograph by David Killeen, 2019.*

10. Philo's research in the English and Welsh context concurs, citing multiple references to the positive 'pull' factors of the countryside, and very few to support the 'push' factors implied by Foucault's 'contaminationist' argument. Chris Philo, *A Geographical History of Institutional Provision for the Insane from Medieval Times to the 1860's in England and Wales: This Space Reserved for Insanity* (Lewiston, 2004), pp 580–1; Patrick Quinlan, 'Cure, Care and Containment: The architecture and landscape of Ireland's lunatic asylums, 1814–2014' (unpublished MUBC Thesis, 2014), pp 40–5.

11. Clare County Lunatic Asylum,' *The Irish Builder*, 15 Mar 1866, p. 71. One might also challenge the middle-class assumption that the experience of 'going upstairs to bed' would be shared by the pauper class who populated these buildings, a plurality of whom would still have occupied single-storey cabins in the 1860s.

was still expected, and high-quality-cut stone detailing would still feature at Ennis and Castlebar to enliven otherwise lacklustre elevations:

> *the public institutions of the country should not reflect too much its poverty, its crime, or its misfortune, and … the lunatic asylums, at the same time that they receive a sober architectural treatment, should not be mere repetitions of the character of an union workhouse or prison, and thus give an unhappy aspect to a locality.*[12]

In the context of such pointed advice it is surprising that the newly reconstituted Board of Control would retain none other than the architect of Ireland's workhouse system, George Wilkinson, whose services local grand juries could directly engage for a highly competitive fee.[13] Wilkinson could claim to have delivered a greater quantum of accommodation in Ireland than any architect before (or, likely, since) within the strictest of budgets,[14] but was therefore also the individual most directly responsible for introducing that 'unhappy aspect' to some 160 localities. Wilkinson's unrivalled expertise in the design of pauper institutions equipped him to develop an operationally effective layout for his two almost identical asylums at Castlebar and Letterkenny. His main innovation was the provision of a pair of smaller, off-centre administration blocks for the male and female sides of the house, creating a less intimidating admissions experience for prospective patients. However, his workhouse career inevitably blunted his aesthetic judgement. Wilkinson followed English precedent in promoting the chapel to form the centrepiece of the composition, but even with the addition of a modest cupola, it proved too weak and undistinguished to anchor a wide building rendered incoherent by the presence of two front doors and strangely inverted massing – two stories at the centre rising to three at the extremities. Later extensions to both buildings have only compounded the confusion.

Ireland's architectural landscape is certainly richer for the fact that most counties instead engaged their own architect, even if the resulting buildings were a decidedly mixed bunch. With costs now firmly in focus, Wilkinson's razor-thin fees as a benchmark and the obligation in many cases to collaborate with the County Surveyor, few of the appointees in this era would be drawn from the top tier of contemporary architectural talent. A case in point is Henry Smyth's Down District Asylum at Downpatrick, whose nondescript ward blocks flank a dashing and flamboyant clocktower with a nine-metre-high arched window, flanked by circular turrets, surmounted by with a heavily sprocketed roof and crowned with an orgy of High-Victorian decorative ironwork. The visual effect is as compelling as it is bizarre; its impact heightened further by being approached on-axis.[15] From an aesthetic point of view the pick of the period is Enniscorthy, designed by county surveyor and architect pairing of James Bell and James Barry Farrell. Dramatically situated on a steep, wooded hillside overlooking the River Slaney, the skilful handling of massing, punctuated with no fewer than five Italianate towers of varying heights, makes for a sublimely picturesque vista, achieved using economic brick construction enlivened by the use of red and yellow polychromy rather than expensive dressed stone.

12. *1856 Commission Report*, HC 1856 [9] liii. See also *Lunatic Asylums Repayment of Advances (Irl) Act 1855*, 18 & 19 Vict., c.109 s.5.
13. Frederick O'Dwyer, *Irish Hospital Architecture: A Pictorial History* (Dublin, 1997), p. 12.
14. With 160 workhouses each accommodating between 200 and 2000 inmates to his name, Wilkinson is one of the most prolific architects in terms of sheer output ever to have worked in Ireland – albeit not in terms of design quality or variety. Denis Cogan, 'The Irish Workhouses: a study of their architectural legacy' (unpublished MUBC thesis, 1998).
15. With the exception of the formal urban forecourts of Limerick and Ballinasloe, asylums of every era were approached obliquely rather than head-on, reflecting the prevailing convention in country house landscape design in the period.

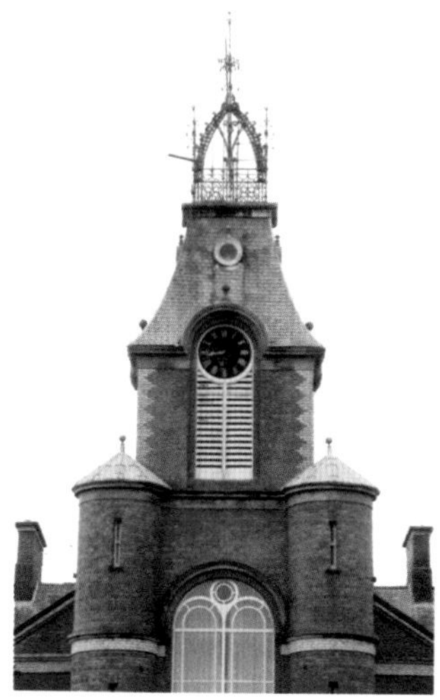

4.03 Downpatrick: A flamboyant central tower marks the great hall at the centre of an otherwise mundane and economic brick façade, *Photograph by the author, 2020.*

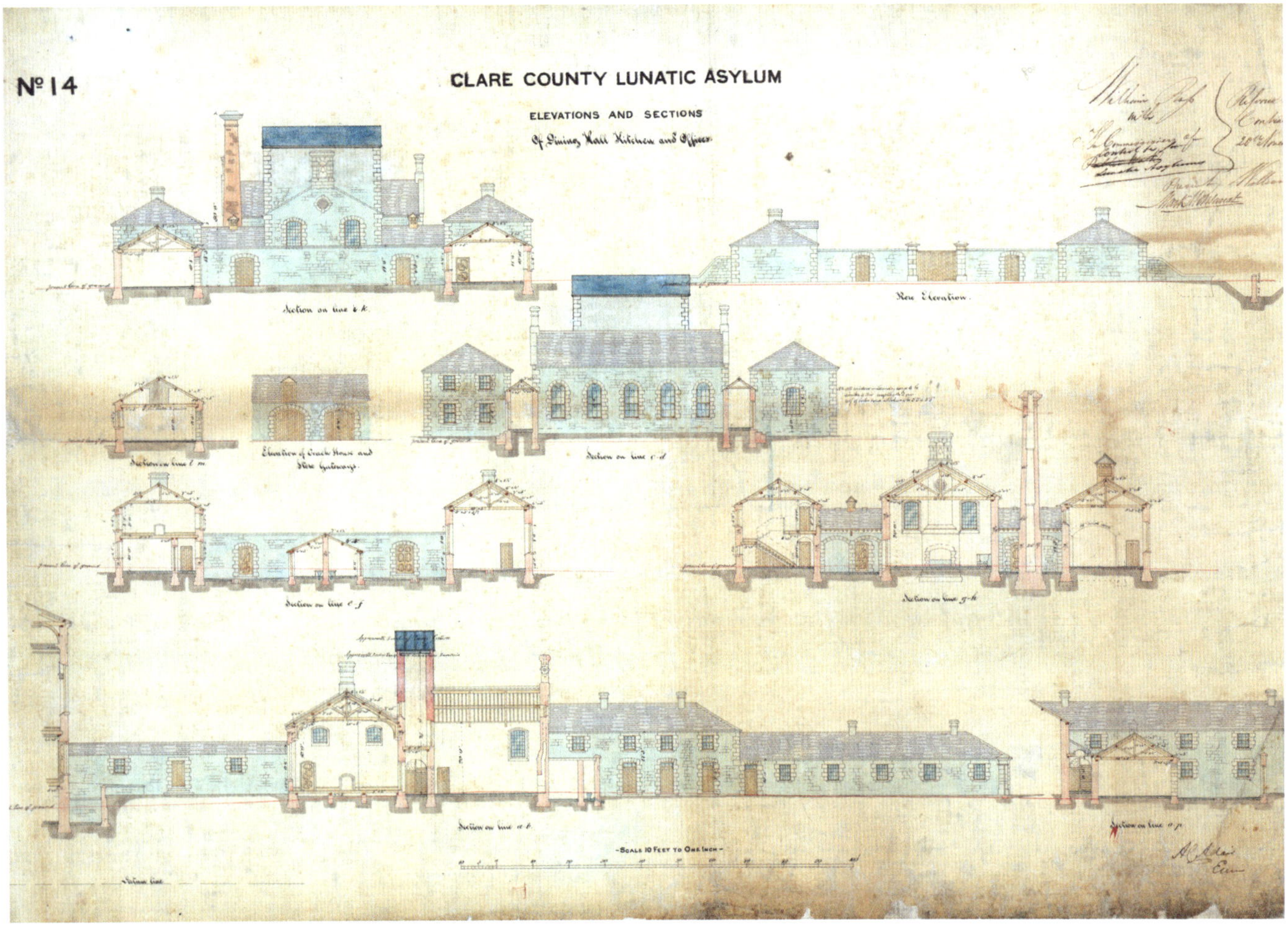
Nº 14
CLARE COUNTY LUNATIC ASYLUM
ELEVATIONS AND SECTIONS
Of Dining Hall Kitchen and Offices
SCALE 10 FEET TO ONE INCH

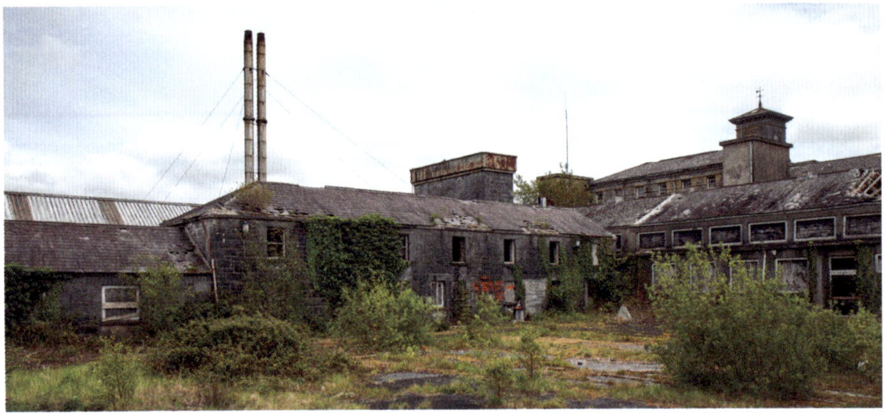

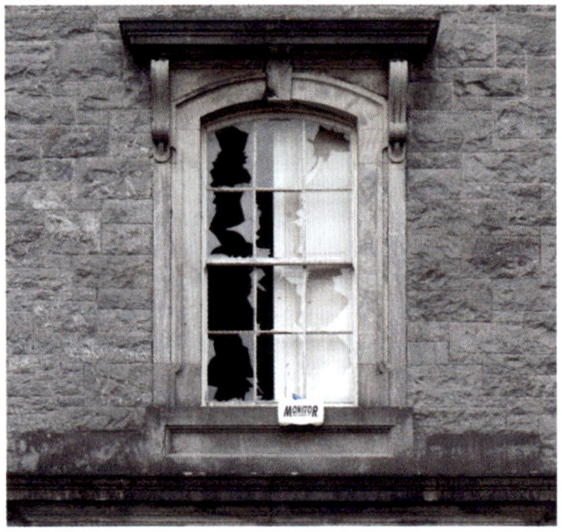
MONITOR

4.04 Ennis: Sections and elevations of ancillary structures, *c.* 1864, *Image courtesy of the National Archives of Ireland (Office of Public Works Collection, OPW/5/HC/4/800, 14).*

4.05 Ennis: The complex back-of-house area encountered in the contract drawing as it stands today, *Photograph by David Killeen, 2019.*

4.06 Ennis: High quality dressed stone enlivens the central block of an otherwise undistinguished building, *Photograph by David Killeen, 2019.*

4.07 Monaghan: Dayrooms tend to be large and bright, but by now far removed from any sense of 'homeliness', *Photograph by David Killeen, 2019.*

4.08 Enniscorthy: The third phase of asylums accelerated the trend towards larger internal dayrooms and dormitories, *Photograph by David Killeen, 2019.*

4.09 Letterkenny: Rendered walls with brick dressings made for a most utilitarian apperance, *Photograph by David Killeen, 2019.*

4.10 Castlebar: Modest central chapel flanked by separate admissions blocks for male and female sides, *Photograph by David Killeen, 2019.*

4 5 6 7 8 9 10

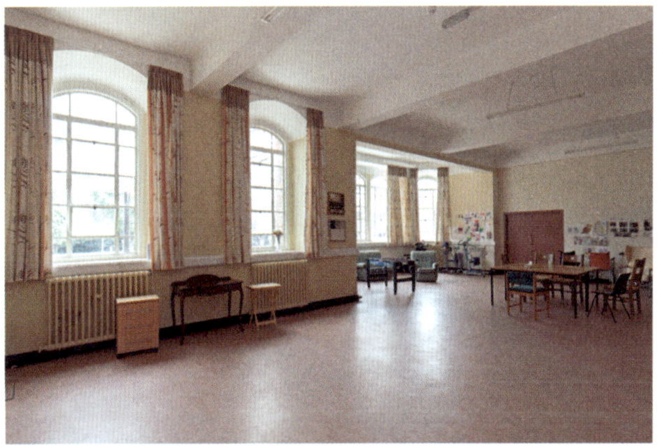

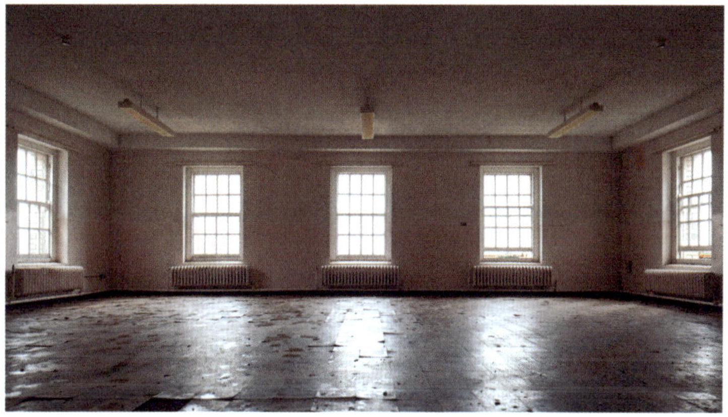

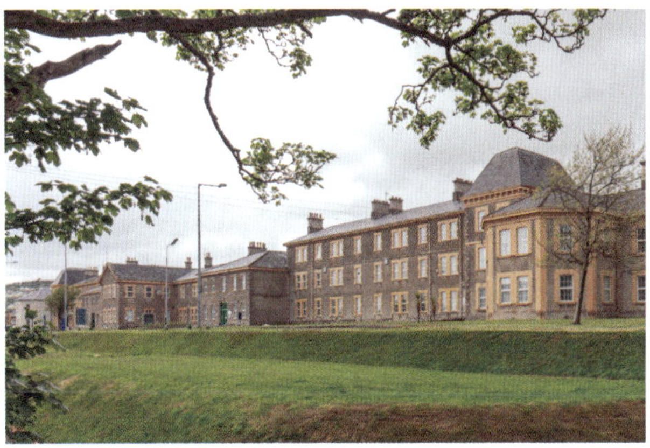

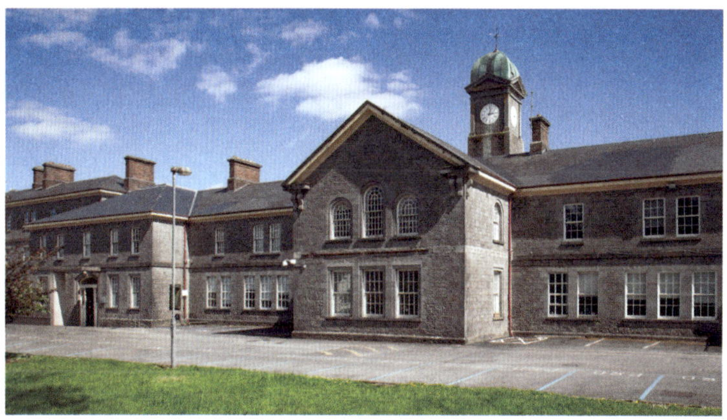

The external appearance of the lunatic asylum had evolved far from the visual imagery of a prison which had tainted Johnston's earliest buildings, becoming a distinctly recognisable typology in its own right. It had moved even further from the precepts of moral management, which regarded asylum patients as a 'family' in a home environment – nobody could discern the slightest hint of domesticity in these domineering buildings. The enormous institutional facades of the era may have been less architecturally ambitious than their immediate predecessors, but it remained universally understood that the asylum building should project an image of sobriety, stability and authority. The stage-managed approach, the dominant tower, the monumental scale and seldom relieved symmetry combined to warn the prospective patient that they were submitting to a regime more powerful than themselves. The buildings needed no carved inscriptions to convey their implicit admonishment: Trust and Obey.

An exemplary client

Regardless of the various facade treatments employed, the foregoing are all versions of the traditional corridor asylum. Only one building in this era broke convention to pursue a path of programmatic innovation, and that building was at Monaghan. Inspired by an asylum committee who crafted a comprehensive brief informed by the careful research of international precedents, architect John McCurdy's competition-winning entry ventured further with a design that anticipated later international developments in asylum design, and which would still be highly regarded nearly three decades after opening: 'unlike the other Irish asylums built at this time, the original plan would appear to have been an excellent one – answering in many of its details the requirements of modern asylum architecture.'[16]

Locating the entrance and administration block (now demolished) of genuinely domestic scale to the north allowed the entire southerly aspect of the asylum to be given over to patient spaces, with bay windows and verandas opening directly onto pleasant south-facing airing grounds discreetly enclosed by ha-has. This logical and eminently desirable arrangement was already mainstream across Britain, but strangely had not been employed in Ireland to date.[17] However, it was McCurdy's disaggregation of the monolithic asylum into a series of freestanding pavilions, laid out around a grand central dining hall and linked by communication corridors (also demolished), that placed McCurdy in the vanguard of an approach that would come to define asylum design through to the dawn of the twentieth century.

The disjointed arrangement of architecturally indifferent rubble-stone buildings that survive on site today offer few clues as to the ground-breaking nature of McCurdy's original concept, but his innovative layout merits a place in the story of international asylum design. Monaghan predated England's first 'pavilion-echelon' asylum at Gloucester by over a decade, but McCurdy and his far-sighted client body fell short in one crucial respect – they missed the opportunity to promote and publicise their innovation. Thus a building that had the potential to influence asylum architecture across Britain and Ireland for a generation has seldom commanded as much as a footnote in history.[18]

16. *Forty-Fifth Annual Asylum Report 1895*, HC 1896 [8251] xxxix Pt.II.1, p.18.
17. If we accept that the eleventh-hour decision to invert the layout at Omagh was more accident than design.
18. The design for Monaghan predates the first major English pavilion asylums (Leavesden and Caterham, competition design 1868), the first corridor-pavilion asylum (Lancashire 1873) and the first pavilion-echelon asylum (Gloucester 1881); Jeremy Taylor, *Hospital and Asylum Architecture in England 1840–1914, Building for Health Care* (London, 1991), pp 142–9. NicGhabhann explores many of Monaghan's innovative design features, but does not contextualise the building's wider significance. Anne McLellan, Niamh Nic Ghabhann and Fiona Byrne (eds), *World Within Walls: From Asylum to Contemporary Mental Health Services* (Monaghan, 2015), pp 159–72.

The demise of moral management

In both new and existing asylums we can see a clear shift from an architecture that sought to contribute directly to the cure of patients, to designs that prioritised the efficient and economic provision of care, albeit with undeniably improved levels of material comfort for those compelled to dwell there. The softer touches – pictures, soft furnishings, potted plants and the like – remained largely absent, by contrast with English asylums where:

> *there is more appearance of comfort and more social enjoyment… which the inmates had been familiar with to a much greater extent in their own homes than are the insane of… this country; for it would be idle to deny the difference which exists in the domestic habits and surroundings which exists between the humbler classes in the two countries.*[19]

More pressing than plants and pictures, pragmatic concerns around the adequacy of water supply, indoor sanitation, forced ventilation, hot water and steam for kitchens and laundries came to the fore. Driven more by the input of the county surveyors than the architects, the new asylums frequently harnessed the latest available technology to service back-of-house areas of increasing complexity. The ever-taller water towers and chimney stacks that resulted were a response to practical need, but would also become part of the visual language of asylumdom. Overloaded and defective drainage systems demanded continuous improvement, but all too often it took one or more fatal outbreaks of dysentery to spur the necessary investment.

The large central dining halls of the new asylums gradually inspired the governors of existing asylums to add their own, though many first had to overcome the moral terror inspired by the prospect of co-mingling of the sexes. The governors at Mullingar

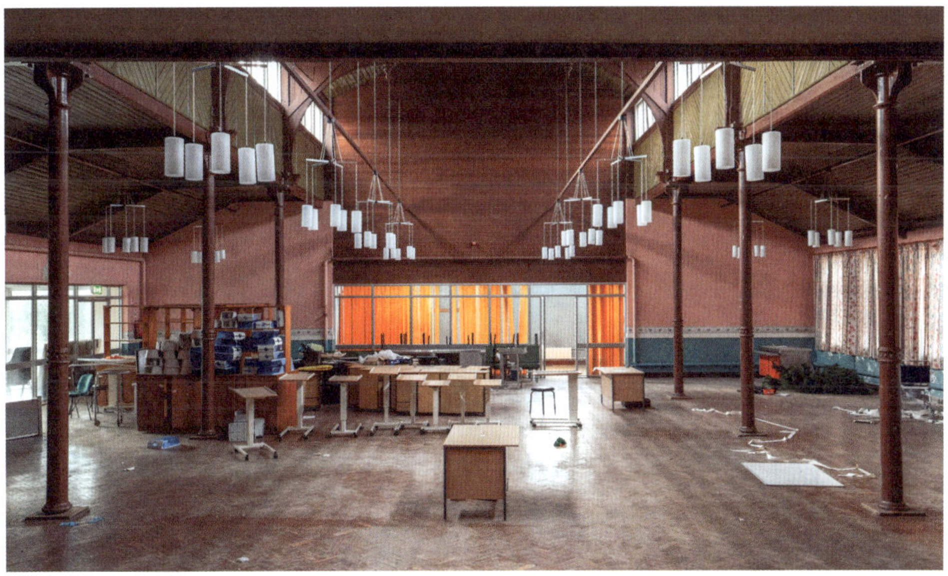

4.11 Mullingar: Central dining hall added once the governors overcame their terror of the sexes mingling, *Photograph by David Killeen, 2019.*

19. *Fifteenth Annual Asylum Report* 1866, HC 1866 [3721] xxxii, p. 9.

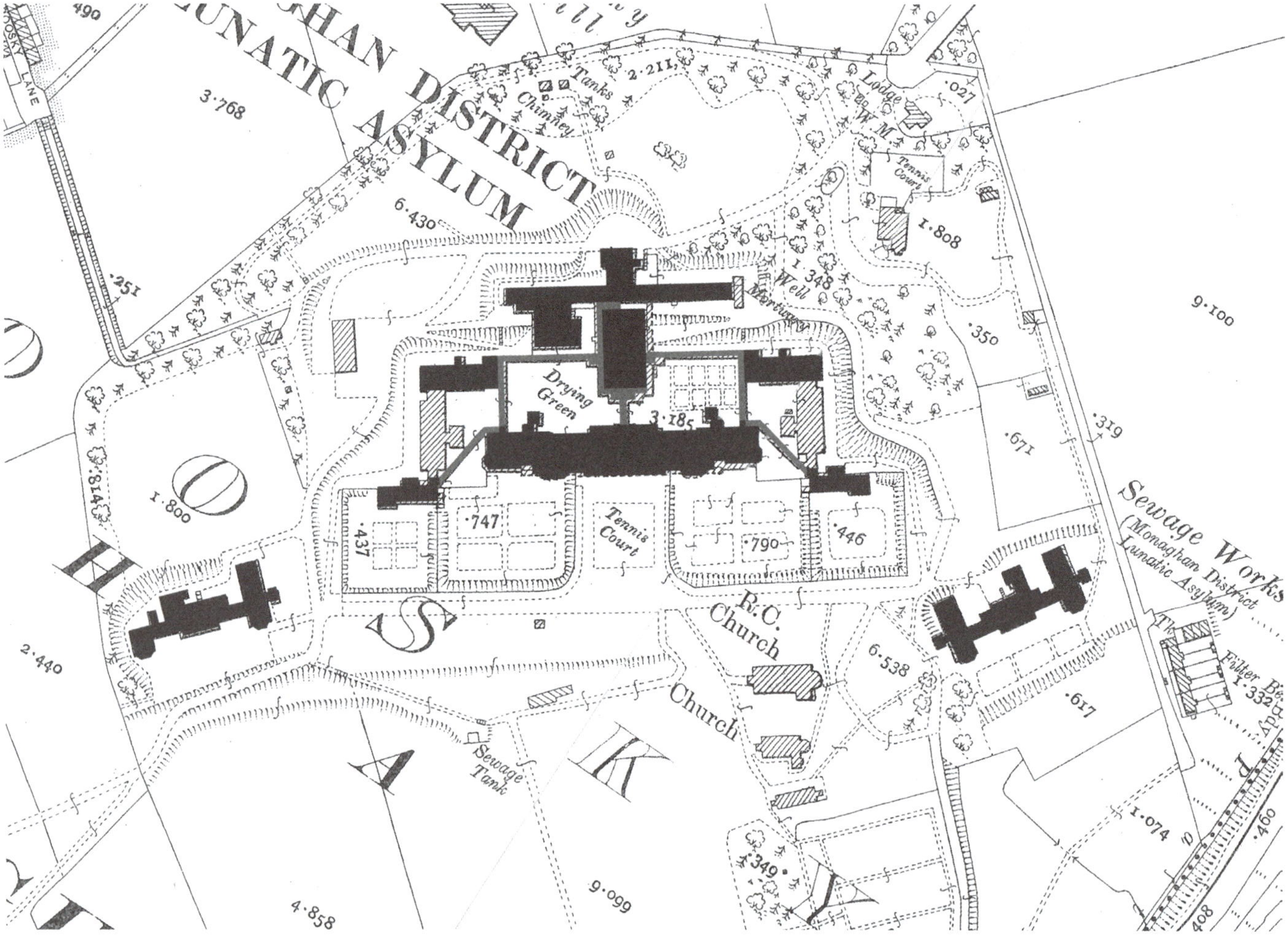

HAN DISTRICT
LUNATIC ASYLUM
Tanks
Chimney
Lodge
W.M.
Tennis Court
Well
Drying Green
Tennis Court
R.C. Church
Church
Sewage Tank
Sewage Works (Monaghan District Lunatic Asylum)
Filter Bs

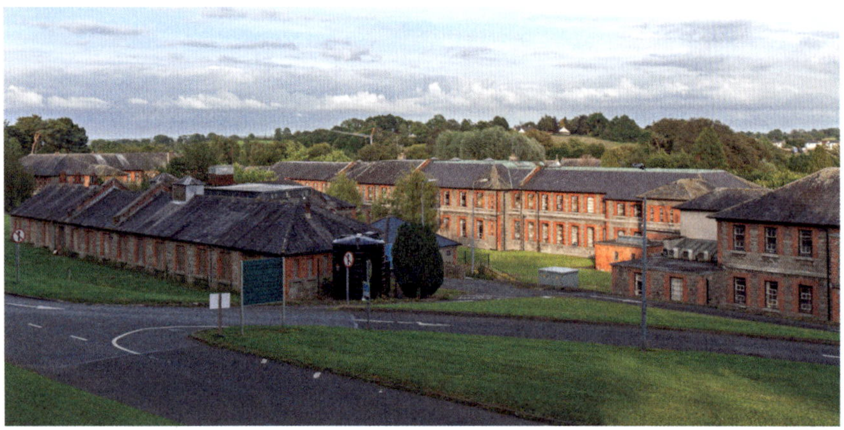

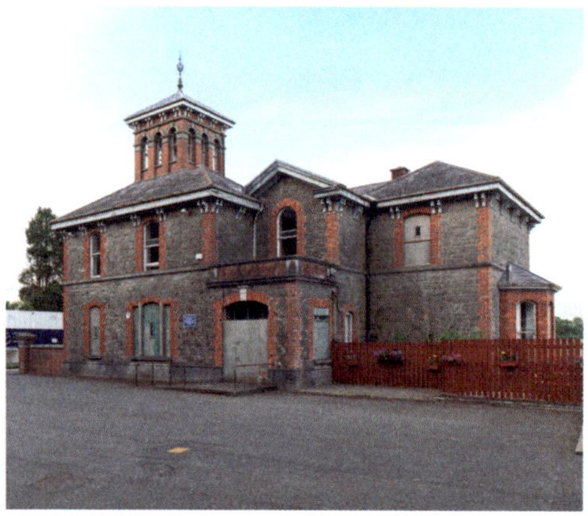

4.12 Monaghan: McCurdy's original layout of individual pavilions linked by a network of corridors - the first pavilion-echelon asylum, *Author's markup of OS map. Reproduced courtesy of Trinity College Dublin (OS-2500-1908, Sheet 9-11).*

4.13 Monaghan: The disjointed arrangement of architecturally indifferent rubble-stone buildings offer few clues as to the ground-breaking nature of McCurdy's original concept, *Photograph by David Killeen, 2019.*

4.14 Monaghan: The fine detached house built in the hope of attracting a 'more than ordinarily efficient' candidate for the role of Resident Medical Superindendent, *Photograph by David Killeen, 2019.*

4.15 Waterford: Central dining hall, c. 1900, enlivened by murals, stencilled decoration and lit by gaslight, *Image courtesy of the National Library of Ireland (POOLEWP_0131).*

4.16 Downpatrick: The Great Hall has been refurbished as an intensively used cultural venue, *Photograph by the author, 2020.*

4.17 Eglinton Asylum, Cork: Secondary dining / recreation hall complete with organ gallery, *Image courtesy of the Irish Architectural Archive (Photographic Collection, 075_088_CS_13_007).*

4.18 Eglinton Asylum, Cork: Main dining hall, *Image courtesy of the Irish Architectural Archive (Photographic Collection, 075_088_CS_13_008).*

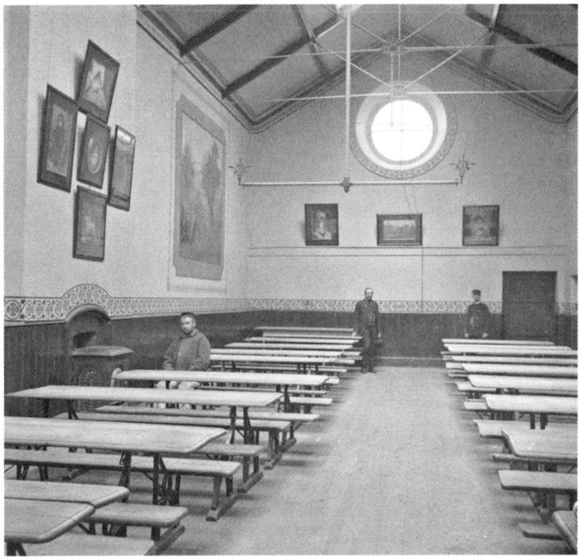

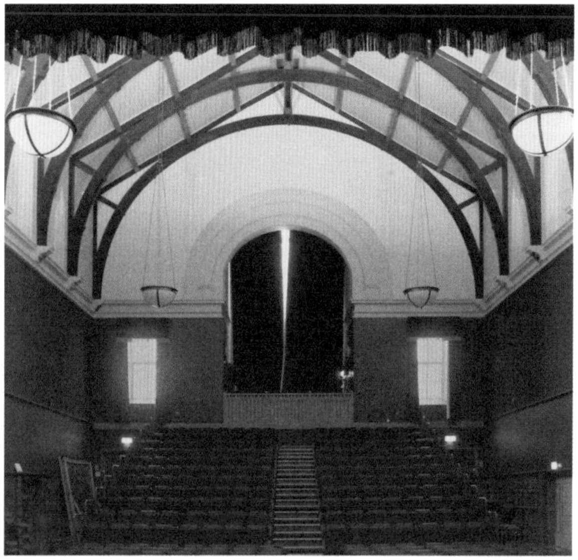

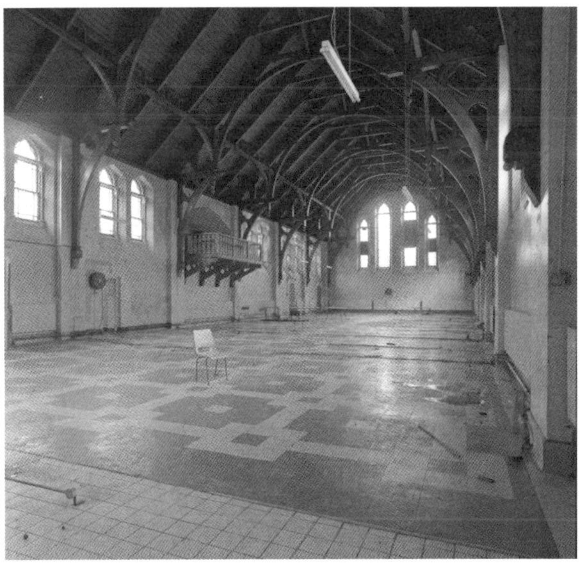

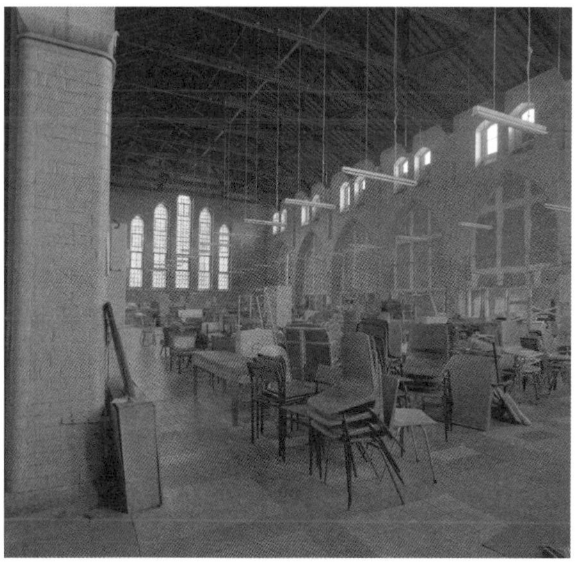

initially compromised by building two separate dining halls before later conceding to the construction of a cavernous central hall. These developments often necessitated the demolition and renewal of earlier ancillary structures - which explains their low survival rate - but in their place created large, architecturally impressive spaces where the entire asylum community could gather for a range of recreational activities. The dances, shows and indoor sports that these spaces accommodated would become an important way to mitigate the monotony of institutional life, especially for the ever increasing number of patients condemned by the Dangerous Lunatics Act and proto-eugenicists to live out the rest of their days within the walls of the asylum.

As the accumulation of 'incurable' cases extinguished any remaining faith in the doctrine of moral management, the Inspectors referred more frequently to external factors beyond their control, citing especially 'hereditary disposition and intemperance' as the 'two great feeders' of asylums. Theories around mental illness as a genetic defect evolved neatly into a narrative that justified lifelong incarceration of those afflicted as a means of preventing the 'germs of disease [from] develop[ing] at a future period'.[20] Containment had displaced cure as the modus operandi of the asylum system. The asylum as an *idea* was dead and buried, but as we shall see, the asylum as an *institution* had developed a life and momentum of its own, no longer truly under the control of its creators.

20. *Eighth Annual Asylum Report 1857*, HC 1857 session 2 [2253], p. 13.

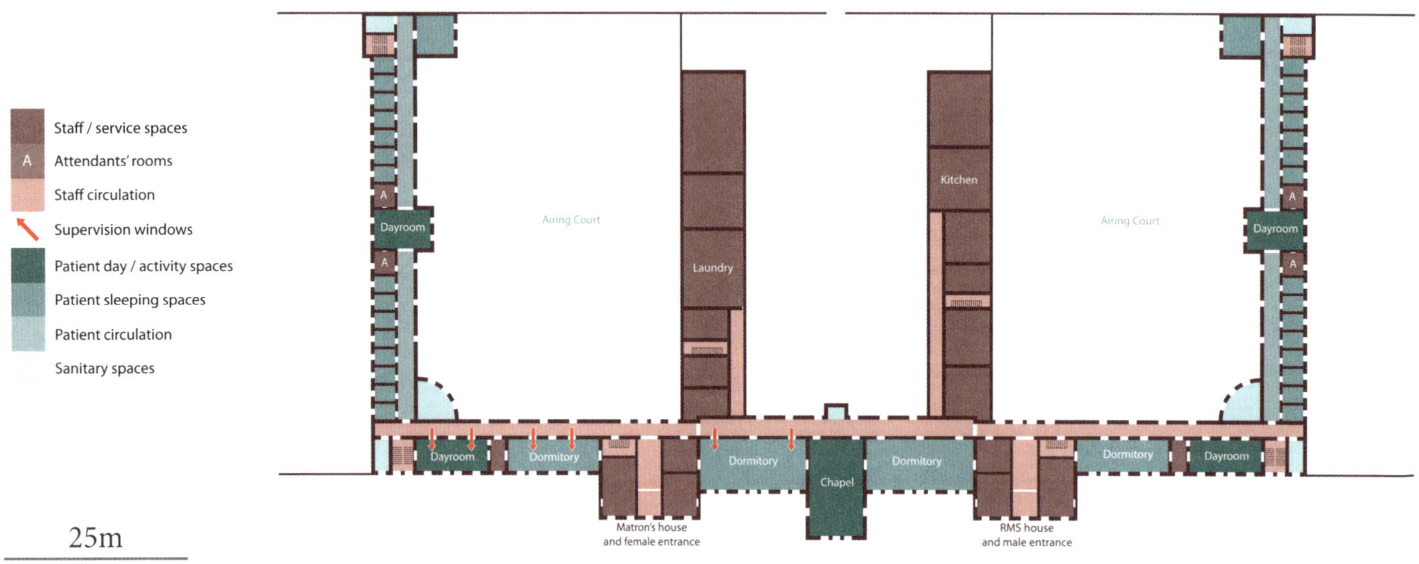

4.19 Plan diagram of Castlebar Asylum with key uses annotated. Note the pair of entrance blocks, the reintroduction of separate dayrooms, and the trend towards larger dormitories. *Drawn by the author.*

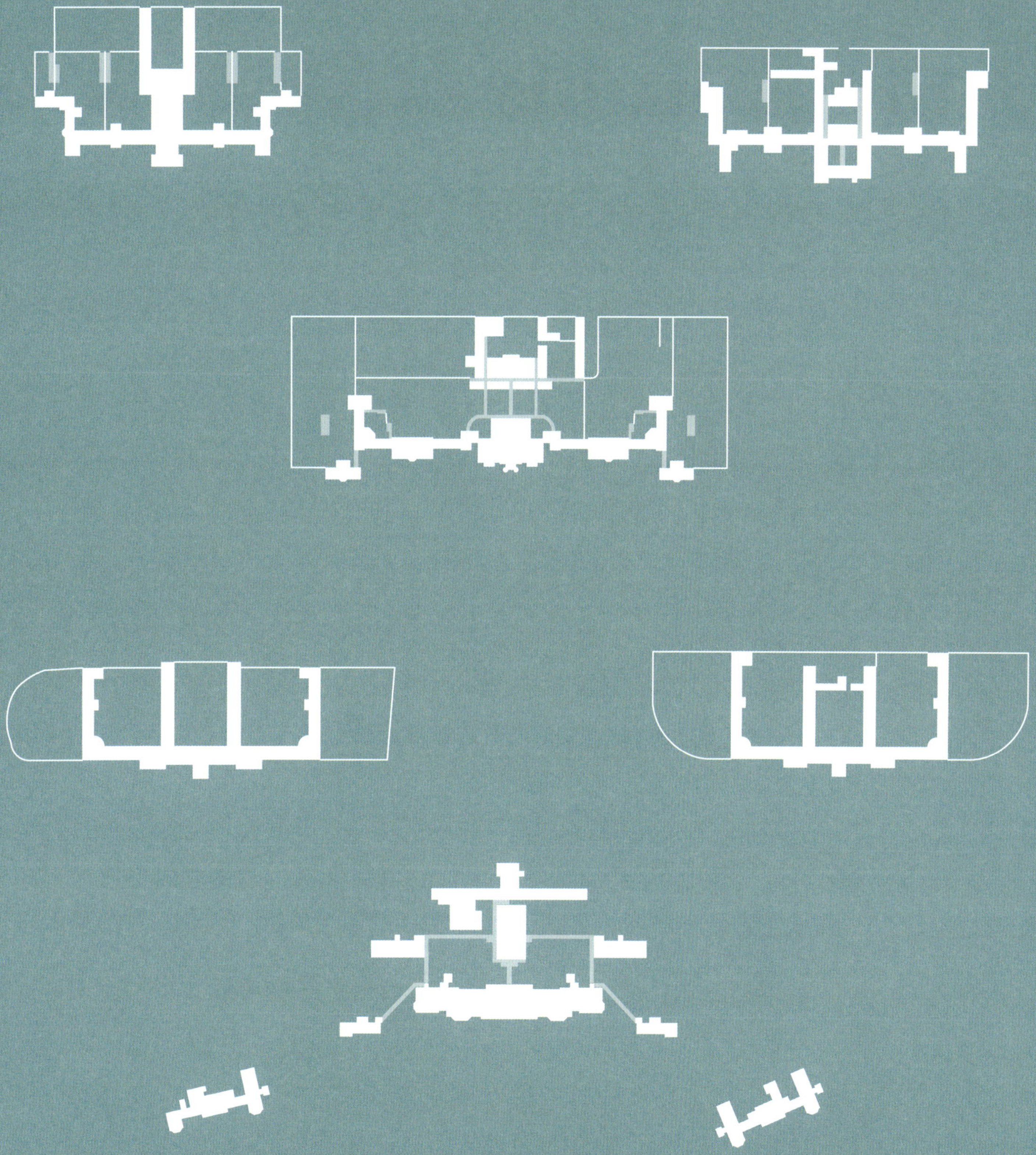

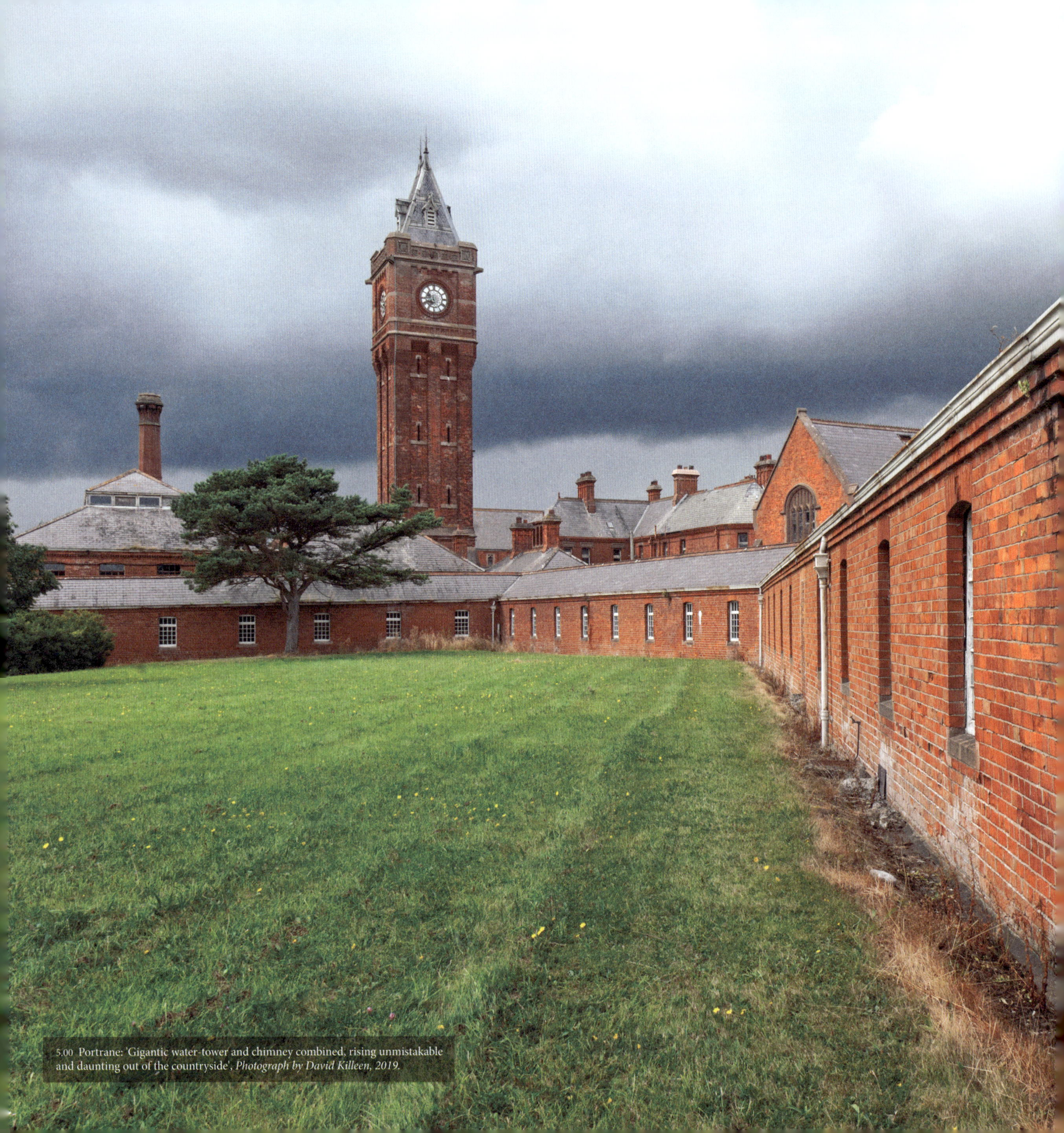

5.00 Portrane: 'Gigantic water-tower and chimney combined, rising unmistakable and daunting out of the countryside', *Photograph by David Killeen, 2019.*

1885-1922

A Definition of Insanity

the Irish branch of the Celtic race is… specially predisposed to mental breakdown [1]

Far from solving the issue of overcrowding, the increased supply of asylum beds during the second and third phases of asylum construction would again be outstripped by demand. The asylums of many western nations experienced rapid growth throughout the second half of the nineteenth century as societies grappled with urbanisation, industrialisation and population growth. Yet patient numbers in poor, agricultural Ireland burgeoned faster than most even as the national population went in the opposite direction,[2] challenging theories that asylum expansion was a side-effect of the rise of industrial capitalism, or was positively created by it as a means of exerting social control.[3]

By the end of the nineteenth century the annual reports of the Inspectors of Lunacy invariably exceeded 200 pages of dense content, which arguably did more to obfuscate than illuminate. A lay person or politician who might be minded to take an interest in the workings of asylumdom would be given the reassuring impression of a highly effective and trustworthy bureaucracy at work, and easily fail to notice that the underlying trend was of a system that changed its own definitions of success to mask its continued failure to deliver against its original curative goals, which often conflated the increase in admissions with the actual incidence of insanity, and yet remained blind to its own contribution to the problems it sought to remedy. Seemingly helpless against a relentless tide of insanity, medical men felt obliged to offer pseudo-scientific rationalisations to justify their continued existence. The Inspectors' reports became an echo chamber for theories as diverse as political agitation, religious fervour, hereditary disposition, use or abuse of substances from tea to alcohol, but seldom challenged the basic assumptions and legislative provisions on which the entire edifice of asylumdom was founded.[4]

The irony of professionals in the field of insanity 'doing the same thing over and over again and expecting different results' will not be lost on modern readers, but the Inspectors seemed largely oblivious to their own role in what Brennan has described as:

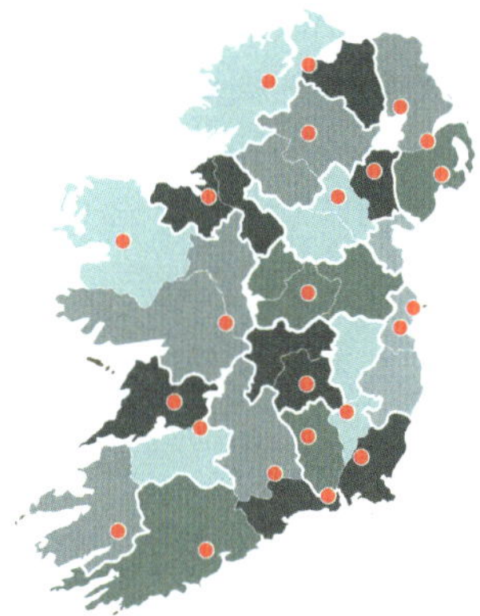

Asylum distribution in Ireland, **1922**, *Drawn by author.*

1. *Supplement to the Fifty-Fourth Report of the Inspector of Lunatics… being a special report on the alleged increase in insanity*, (hereafter *Supplement to the Fifty-Fourth Report*) HC 1906 [3126] xxxix, p. xxvii.
2. Between 1841 and 1911, the asylum population increased seven-fold from 3,498 to 24,655, even as the general population halved from 8,175,124 to 4,390,319.
3. Damien Brennan, *Irish Insanity, 1800–2000* (Oxon, 2014) p. 65, in Andrew Scull, *The Most Solitary of Afflictions: Madness and Society in Britain, 1700–1900* (New Haven and London, 1993).
4. Catherine Cox, *Negotiating Insanity in the Southeast of Ireland, 1820–1900* (Manchester, 2012), pp 57–60 ; Joseph Robins, *Fools and Mad: A History of the Insane in Ireland* (Dublin, 1986), pp 109–27.

5. Brennan, *Irish Insanity*, pp 63–4.

6. Amongst other assertions that the excessive consumption or over-brewing of tea led to melancholia, dyspepsia and nervous irritability. To the relief of the tea-guzzling author, empirical population-based data was brought to bear on this important question: 'the fact that whole nations, such as the Chinese and Japanese, consume it on a much larger scale than the people of this country, and with apparently little, if any, injurious effect, goes far to negative this hypothesis, which, at best, is merely a surmise, unsupported by any adducible facts or statistics.' *Supplement to the Fifty-Fourth Report*, , HC 1906 [3126] xxxix, p. 4, p. 8, p. 15, p. 30, pp 40-4. For the curious, Mrs Sairey Gamp was a habitually drunken nurse and popular comic character in Charles Dickens' *Martin Chuzzlewit*.

> *a circular pattern of policy planning which entailed a number of characteristics: a perception of the existence of an unusually high rate of insanity in Ireland; the need to relieve communities of the burden of insanity… chronic overcrowding... spiralling cost… and further plans for expansion in the form of extensions, annexes and new building projects, which started the cycle once again.*[5]

In 1905, the Inspectors took it upon themselves to formally invite every asylum Resident Medical Superintendent (RMS) to share their views on the perceived epidemic of insanity. Even allowing for the strides in scientific knowledge in the intervening time, some individual contributions to our eyes might seem comical were they not the sincere professional views of men who were each responsible for the fate of a thousand or more vulnerable human beings:

> *To make matters worse, the tea that is consumed so abundantly is stewed, kept on the stove, or near the fire, and, like Mrs Sairey Gamp's brandy bottle, resorted to 'whenever they feel disposed'. No wonder that children reared on this beverage, supplemented by innutritious white bread, should develop all kinds of neurotic affections, which lay the foundation for the pathological evil we are trying to extirpate.*[6]

Yet the Inspectors' synthesis of the responses of multiple doctors were more rigorous than some recent scholars have given them credit for. Amidst some dubious conclusions around the role of emigration and the 'fact that the Celtic race, notwithstanding their undoubted intellectual gifts, are peculiarly prone to mental disease', they correctly cited the effects of increased life expectancy, accumulation

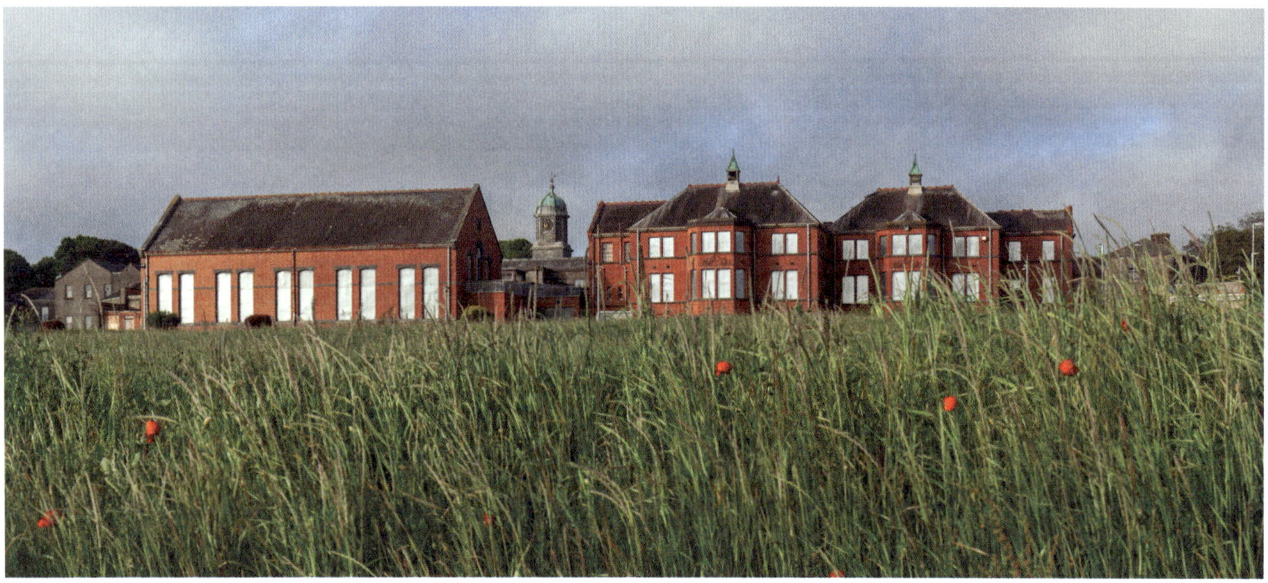

5.01 Waterford: With only three 'green-field' asylums built in a period when the patient population more than doubled, the majority of growth would be accommodated by extending existing asylums, *Photograph by David Killeen, 2019.*

due to low discharge and death rates, the gradual absorption into the asylum of cases previously cared for in unregulated settings (i.e. in the community) and, importantly, the 'widening of medical opinion as to the degree of insanity which justifies certification'.[7] Readers will doubtless be relieved to learn that the case against the nation's favourite brew was dismissed for want of sufficient evidence.

The Inspectors also concluded that the increase in the number of asylums and their greater accessibility (via an expanding rail network) fed into a 'greater confidence on the part of the poorer classes to… send their insane relatives to such institutions instead of keeping them at home'.[8] As Cox reminds us, demand for asylum places was ultimately driven by families on whom the burden of insanity falls first, and who, often having exhausted their own social and economic capacities, proved increasingly willing and able to navigate, use and even at times abuse the institutional system to their own ends.[9] To challenge conventional perceptions of free will one step further, Walsh has even identified individual patients who, when deemed recovered and eligible for discharge, refused to leave the institution, voluntarily deciding to live out their days within the walls.[10]

However, the most popular theme amongst the doctors who responded to the Inspectors' 1905 survey was the observation that many mental illnesses appeared to run in families.[11] From there it was but a short leap to the emerging field of eugenics – the promotion or suppression of certain heritable traits by encouraging or discouraging human reproduction. Twentieth-century history reveals such thinking as a step along the road to the gas chambers of the Third Reich.[12] However, for professionals and policy makers at the dawn of the century who had few effective tools with which to battle a seemingly inexorable epidemic of insanity, eugenics appeared to offer much needed scientific credibility. The eugenics movement enjoyed greater popular appeal and political influence in Britain than Ireland, but amongst Ireland's asylum doctors, the slow disaster of hereditary insanity and population degeneracy justified – even demanded – the containment of the insane and their supposedly defective traits in safe and celibate seclusion.[13] Such reasoning could only have thwarted initiatives that ran contrary to the prevailing wisdom of institutionalisation, even when made by a figure as eminent as Dr Connolly Norman, RMS of The Richmond. Norman's proposal in 1890 to introduce community care or 'boarding out', proven in practice in nearby Scotland, in Ireland fell on deaf ears.[14] While earlier chapters may have identified benign and benevolent evidence in opposition to Foucault's conception of a 'gigantic moral imprisonment', this period of Ireland's asylum history comes closest to matching that dark worldview.[15]

For many of the thousands of patients thus incarcerated, the asylum would retain its hold in death as in life. If the landscape to the front of the asylum played to an image of genteel respectability, the rear concealed a feature that firmly marked it as a pauper institution – the burial ground containing the unmarked graves of those patients whose mortal remains families either could not or would not reclaim. While entirely unremarkable in the nineteenth-century context, the unmarked grave offends modern sensibilities as the final indignity inflicted upon the vulnerable by an uncaring institution, such that new memorials have latterly been erected in almost

7. An interesting aside is the observation that General Paralysis of the Insane (late-stage syphilis), although endemic in England and growing in Ireland's larger cities, remained almost non-existent in rural areas due to the 'high standard of sexual morality which obtains'. *Supplement to the Fifty-Fourth Report*, HC 1906 [3126] xxxix, pp xxx–xxxii.
8. Ibid.
9. As elaborated in her detailed exploration of the admission records of Carlow Asylum: Cox, *Negotiating Insanity*, pp 133–68.
10. Oonagh Walsh, 'Lunatic and criminal alliances in nineteenth-century Ireland', in Peter Bartlett and David Wright (eds), *Outside the Walls of the Asylum: The History of Care and Community 1750–2000* (London, 1999) pp 143–52. A more recent parallel might be drawn with some of the women admitted to Magdalen Asylums who freely elected (and in some cases continue) to live on within the institution as 'Consecrates', a choice that seems incomprehensible to many contemporary commentators. Such decisions cannot be entirely divorced from the confidence-sapping experience of institutionalisation and the perceived dangers of the outside world, but extreme caution is warranted by those who would presume to critique the life decisions of others.
11. *Supplement to the Fifty-Fourth Report*, HC 1906 [3126] xxxix, p. 15.
12. Not forgetting that even supposedly free democracies imposed forced sterilisation on marginalised members of society.
13. Amongst the RMSs who contributed to a special report on insanity in 1905, only the question of emigration as a cause of insanity generated as much discussion as questions of hereditary insanity and congenital idiocy. *Supplement to the Fifty-Fourth Report*, HC 1906 [3126] xxxix, p. xxxix.
14. Joseph Reynolds, *Grangegorman: Psychiatric Care in Dublin since 1815* (Dublin, 1992), p. 159, p. 166. Boarding-out accounted for up to 25 per cent of Scottish patients during the period. Harriet Sturdy and William Parry-Jones, 'Boarding-out insane patients: The significance of the Scottish system 1857–1913', in Bartlett and Wright, *Outside the Walls of the Asylum*, pp 86–114.
15. Michel Foucault, *Madness and Civilisation* (tr. Richard Howard; New York, 1965) p. 278.

every burial ground to commemorate the countless unnamed patients who repose there. A headstone at the twentieth-century mental hospital at Ardee is unique in (retrospectively) naming 88 patients interred between 1946 and 1995, from which it is reasonable to estimate that up to 100 times that number in total may repose across the island's 12 known asylum burial grounds.[16] The other unsettling implication of Ardee's memorial is that, far from being the practice of a dim and distant past, unmarked internments continued right into the 1990s.

Victims of democratic progress

The most significant legislative reform of this era was not actually in the area of insanity, but local government. The 1898 Local Government Act, which established County Councils in their modern form, also reformed the governance of the District Lunatic Asylums. Gentry-dominated boards of governors were replaced with committees of management, largely populated by elected representatives.[17] Such administrative reform would have seemed irrelevant to those behind the walls had it not resulted in an even more parsimonious approach to their care. Changes to the funding model tilted the burden of cost further towards local communities, especially after 1909 when central government grants were capped and all further increases fell on the local rate payers. With elected representatives now directly accountable to a newly enfranchised electorate (which naturally did not include those behind the walls), the political imperative to contain the costs of the system would come to dominate all other considerations:[18]

> *Those in the institutions were receiving care rather than treatment. Isolation and safe custody had taken over from moral treatment… There was… a ready public acquiescence in the policy of confining the problem of insanity behind high walls both in the literal and the figurative sense and no great inclination on the part of anyone to spend more money on improving the quality of care.*[19]

Between 1890 and 1910, asylum populations expanded more in real terms than in any other period, adding almost 8,000 patients to a previous total of 9,000.[20] With only three new 'greenfield' asylums completed in the period, most of this growth had to be absorbed by the existing institutions. Committees of management demanded low-cost and high-capacity architectural solutions in response to the crisis. With the sole exception of Armagh's flamboyant neo-Elizabethan 'Hill Building' of 1898 (see Case Study 2), economy of means had firmly superseded any desire to propagate a particular self-image of the institution. The best buildings of the era may be seen as competent essays in the 'institutional vernacular' of the late Victorian era; the worst were generic mediocrities.

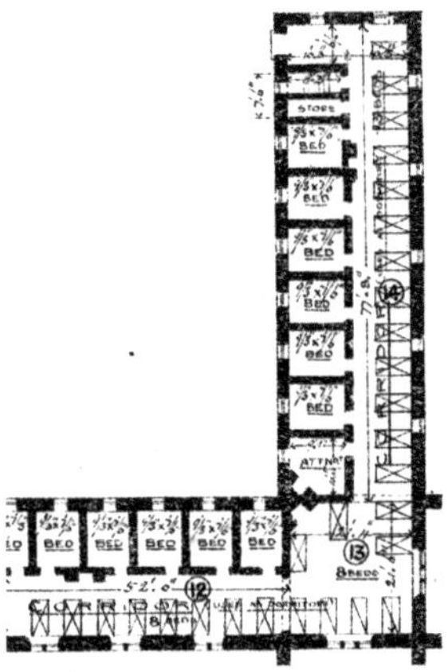

5.02 Richmond Asylum, Dublin: As the institution filled beyond bursing point, beds would fill every available space. *Image courtesy of the National Archives of Ireland (Office of Public Works Collection, OPW/5HC/4/799, 3).*

Beds in corridors – and everywhere else

The extensions to Irish asylums built during this era reflect these priorities. The most common model comprised enormous warehouse-like wards, each accommodating

16. The author has identified at least 12 on-site asylum burial grounds. With the exception of short-lived Castlerea, the remaining ten served institutions accommodating three to five times as many patients as Ardee, and remained in operation for two to three times longer. (88*10*4*2.5 = 8,800) Even this estimate could be conservative, if we allow that the percentage of asylum internments was probably higher in the nineteenth century than the twentieth.
17. Local Government (Ireland) Act 1898, 61 & 62 Vict., c.37.
18. Under the third electoral reform act (Representation of the People Act 1884, 48 & 49 Vict. c.3, the franchise was extended to men paying rent or holding land valued over £10/annum. The mandate was expanded further in 1918 and became universal after independence.
19. Robins, *Fools and Mad*, p. 171, p. 174
20. Patient population in 1890: 9,075. Patient population in 1910: 17,032.

40–50 beds in 4 or 5 rows around a central chimneybreast. Large 'nightingale' style wards had by now become a familiar feature of medical hospitals, but lengths of stay for medical patients tended to be measured in weeks or months. The prospect of living 40 or more years in such a setting affronts modern sensibilities around personal dignity and privacy, but even in a time before the prevalence of such concepts, there was an awareness in some quarters that the pursuit of economy could be taken too far: 'it may be said generally that the building is well arranged for the *storage* – we use the word advisedly – of imbeciles.'[21]

Some of the extensions erected to the rear of the institution would morph into the dark 'back wards' of infamy, the repository of the hopeless, physically and psychologically isolated from the core of the establishment. But on balance, it must be observed that the majority of these wards were high-ceilinged, south-facing or dual-aspect spaces, bathed in light from tall windows. Thus Scull's description of asylum architecture towards the end of the nineteenth century as 'increasingly monotonous, drearily functional, prison-like', is correct on only two counts – objectively, even the worst buildings of this era could not have passed for prisons.[22]

But building projects, however flawed, always lagged behind demand. In the meantime asylum superintendents were obliged to pack more and more patients into already cramped quarters. The Inspectors' mot du jour was 'overcrowding', but this term seems hopelessly inadequate to describe Dublin's Richmond Asylum in 1901. An extraordinary series of drawings by architect W. H. Byrne show rows of beds, not two feet apart, lining the galleries and corridors, in dining rooms and day rooms, repurposed workshops and staff spaces. In the largest male dormitory, restful sleep would have been an impossible dream in a space whose air was vitiated with the smells and sounds of 77 coughing, snoring or moaning patients, all served by only two water closets.[23]

From pavilion-echelon to villa colony

For the Richmond, the remedy for these ills seemed imminent. Even as Byrne's draughtsmen were eking out every last bedspace from the old asylum, an enormous new building was rising from the healthy soil of north county Dublin, to which almost one half of the Richmond's patients would soon depart. The Portrane Auxiliary Lunatic Asylum (1896–1903) was a building of scale and complexity unprecedented in Ireland and seldom exceeded since.[24] George Ashlin's competition-winning design for 1,200 patients was equivalent in scale to a new town, sited on a remote coastal peninsula 13 miles north of the capital and aired by fresh breezes off the Irish Sea. Portrane represents a literal application of the 'broad arrow' or 'pavilion-echelon' layout that had become the standard approach in the design of larger English asylums,[25] but whose application in Ireland was limited to Portrane and its smaller, if older cousin, Antrim's Holywell Asylum (1890–8).

The classic echelon layout comprises a series of individual ward blocks symmetrically arrayed to maximise southerly exposure, each of which accommodated patients classified by gender and degree of insanity (four at Holywell, eight at Portrane). All were connected via a web of corridors to central facilities including a

21. Emphasis in original. Burdett's caustic comments were specifically aimed at the London Metropolitan Asylums Board 'economic' asylum design for incurables at Caterham and Leavesden, which comprised a dozen identical blocks similar to those described above, each containing four forty-bed dormitories and associated dayrooms, but the criticism is no less applicable to some of the spaces considered here. Henry C. Burdett, *Hospitals and Asylums of the World: Volume 2: Asylum Construction, Plans and Bibliography* (London, 1891), p. 103. See also Jeremy Taylor, *Hospital and Asylum Architecture in England 1840–1914, Building for Health Care* (London, 1991), p. 142.
22. Andrew Scull, *The Most Solitary of Afflictions: Madness and Society in Britain, 1700–1900* (New Haven and London, 1993), p. 167.
23. The staff fared little better – a tiny room containing 3 attendant beds opened off the 77-bed dormitory; elsewhere in the institution 17 male attendants shared a single dormitory. National Archives of Ireland (hereafter NAI): Office of Public Works, 1899, *Richmond Lunatic Asylum Drawings*, OPW/5HC/4/799.
24. Only the very largest workhouses and army barracks would have accommodated similar numbers at such close quarters, and neither of these typologies approached the programmatic complexity of the asylum.
25. All three shortlisted designs were of the pavilion-echelon design; the two runner-up designs were by Carroll & Bachelor and William Kaye-Parry. The latter was deeply unhappy with the conduct of the competition, arguing, *inter alia*, that the integrity of the process had been compromised by holding a public exhibition before announcing the chosen design from the three shortlisted schemes. 'The Portrane Asylum Competition', *The Irish Builder*, 15 Apr. 1895, p. 99, and *The Irish Times*, 24 Jan. 1895.

26. Erving Goffman, *Asylums: Essays on the Social Situation of Mental Patients and Other Inmates* (Chicago, 1962), p. 74.

27. Leslie Topp, *Freedom and the Cage: Modern Architecture and Psychiatry in Central Europe, 1890–1914* (Pennsylvania, 2017), pp 32–3, p. 201.

28. 'The latest development in asylum planning: The villa colony system', in *The Irish Builder*, 10 Apr. 1901, pp 689–90.

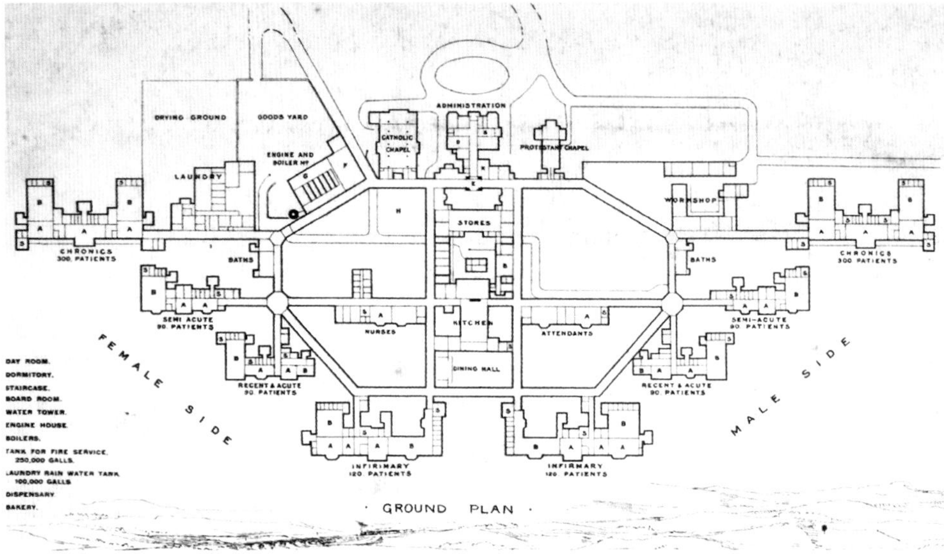

5.03 Portrane: The classic pavilion-echelon layout with south facing pavilions around a central core of ancillary spaces, *Image courtesy of the Irish Architectural Archive (Ashlin and Coleman Collection, 76/1:144)*

dining/recreation hall, chapels, a kitchen, stores, staff quarters, offices, laundry and a boiler house. The design allowed for efficient circulation of staff and supplies without passing through individual wards – a deficiency of older corridor asylums which had only worsened with each successive extension. The echelon layout represents the climax of traditional asylum design – an immense, finely tuned machine optimised to deliver the basic necessities of life for over a thousand patients in the most economic and efficient manner. Patients undoubtedly enjoyed a higher standard of material comfort and a wider range of amenities than in the earlier asylums, but such modest advantages were paid for by the complete subjugation of their individuality to the power and operational demands of the institution. The echelon asylum could be seen as the physical manifestation of the paradox identified by Erving Goffman in his seminal work on 'total institutions' over 50 years later: 'Many total institutions… seem to function merely as storage dumps for inmates, but… present themselves to the public as rational organisations designed consciously, through and through, as effective machines for producing a few officially avowed and officially approved ends.'[26]

On mainland Europe a new type of asylum had emerged to break the dominance of the monolithic institution and the antiquated practices of control and coercion that it appeared to represent. Inspired by the renowned German asylum at Alt Scherbitz, advocates of the villa colony system deconstructed the asylum into a series of domestic scale buildings dispersed across the landscape to convey the impression, if not always the reality, of freedom.[27] First promoted in the Irish construction industry press as a model worthy of emulation in 1901,[28] it was the asylum committee in Belfast – a city flush with the fruits of a booming industrial base – that took the initiative. Belfast's board of governors had purchased the 'extensive and beautiful' 295-acre estate at Purdysburn in 1894 as the site for a new asylum to replace the original 1829 facility, which had since been hemmed in

5.04 Purdysburn: Aerial photgraph, c.1940s, showing the key elements of a centrally located hospital, recreation hall, administration building and laundry amidst a wider landscape of freestanding villas, are all evident, *Image courtesy of National Museums Northern Ireland (Belfast Telegraph, HOYFM.BT.22).*

5.05 Purdysburn: Early design for 'Proposed Villa Colony at Purdysburn' by G.T. Hine, after the first four villas had been constructed, *Image courtesy of the Irish Architectural Archive (Workhouse Drawings Collection, 85/138: 086).*

5.06 Portrane: Competition winning entry by George Ashlin, published in the Irish Builder, 1900, *Image courtesy of the Irish Architectural Archive (Ashlin and Coleman Collection, 76/1:144).*

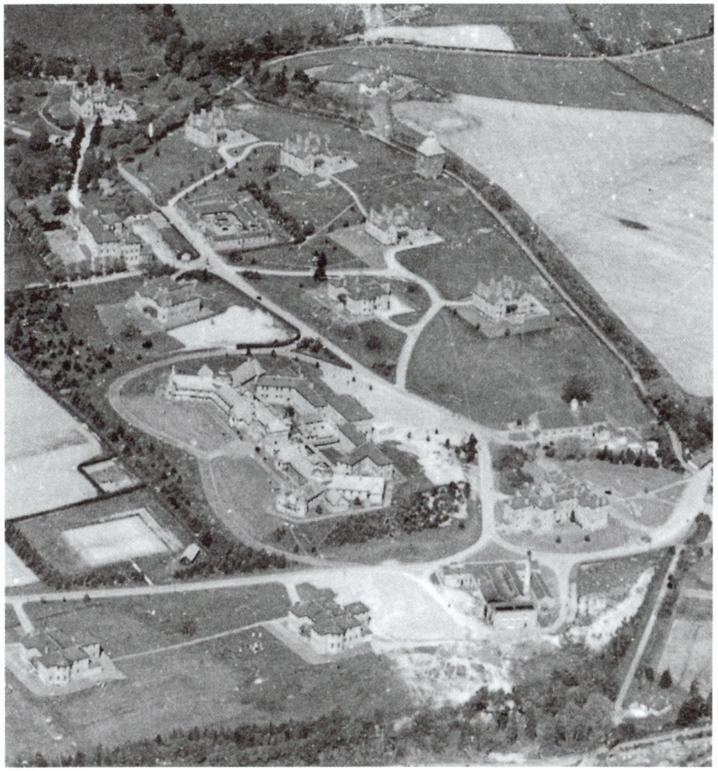

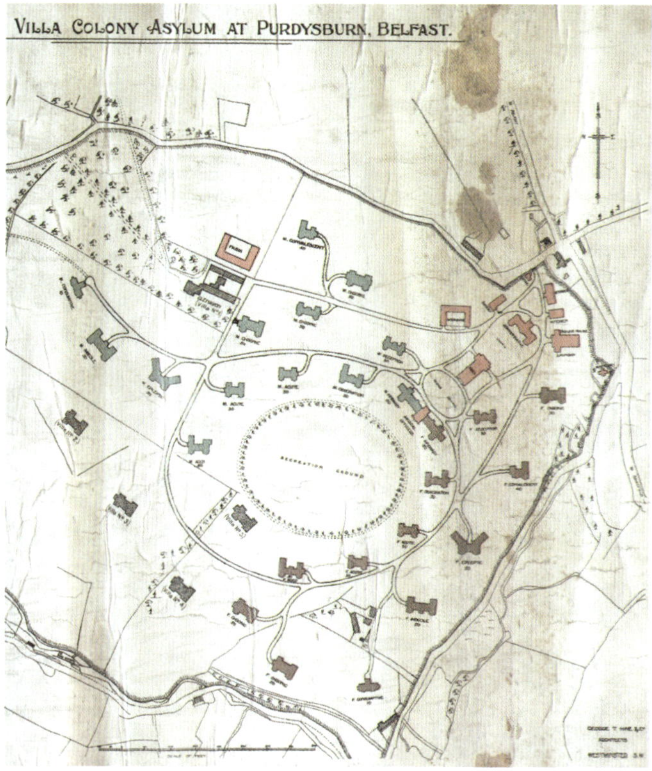

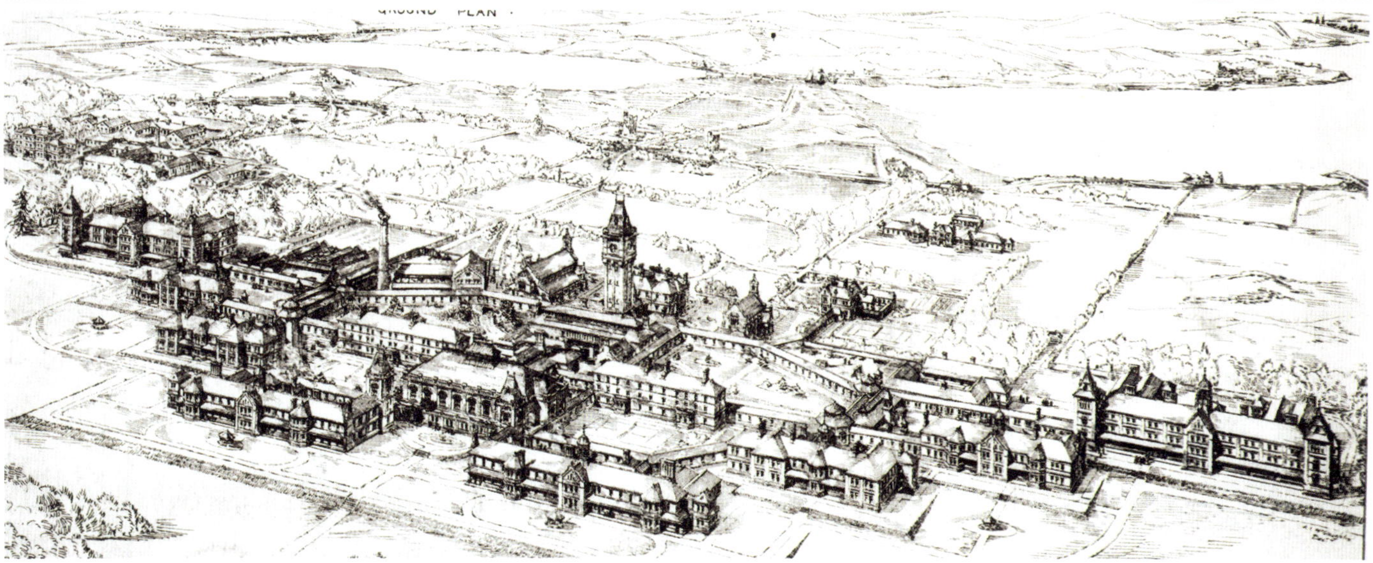

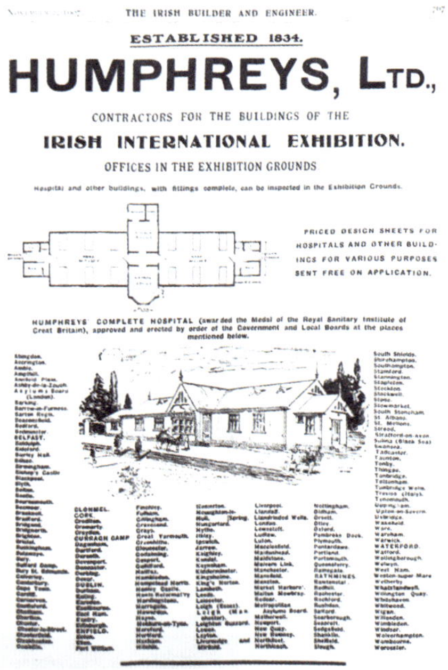
THE IRISH BUILDER AND ENGINEER.
ESTABLISHED 1834.
HUMPHREYS, LTD.,
CONTRACTORS FOR THE BUILDINGS OF THE
IRISH INTERNATIONAL EXHIBITION.
OFFICES IN THE EXHIBITION GROUNDS
Hospitals and other buildings, with fittings complete, can be inspected in the Exhibition Grounds.
PRICED DESIGN SHEETS FOR HOSPITALS AND OTHER BUILDINGS FOR VARIOUS PURPOSES SENT FREE ON APPLICATION.
HUMPHREYS COMPLETE HOSPITAL (awarded the Medal of the Royal Sanitary Institute of Great Britain), approved and erected by order of the Government and Local Boards at the places mentioned below.

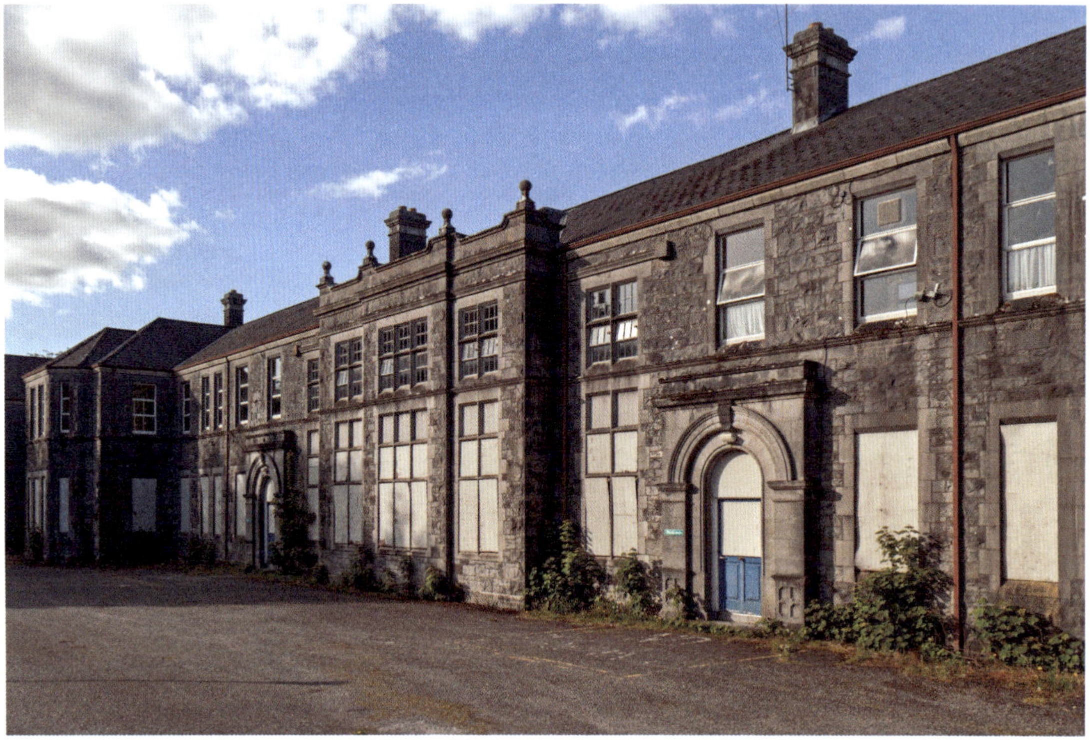

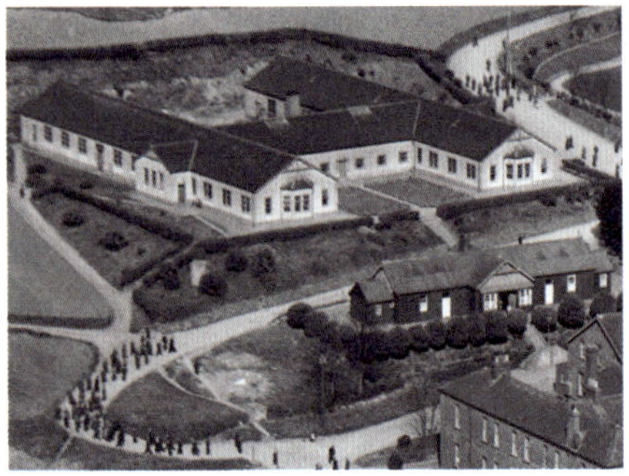

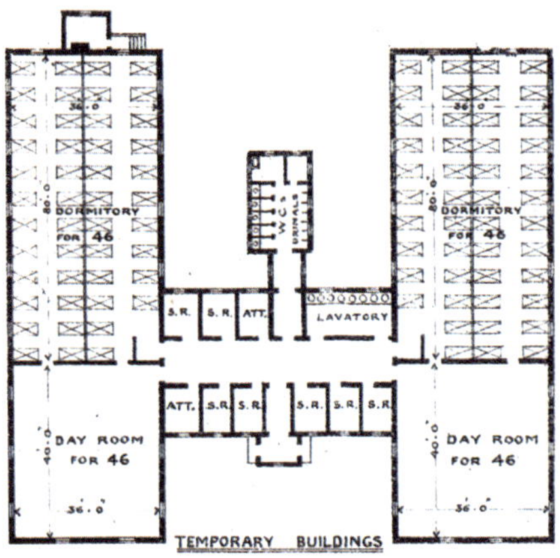
DORMITORY FOR 46
DORMITORY FOR 46
W.C.
URINALS
S.R.
S.R.
ATT.
LAVATORY
ATT.
S.R.
S.R.
S.R.
S.R.
S.R.
DAY ROOM FOR 46
DAY ROOM FOR 46
36.0
40.0
TEMPORARY BUILDINGS

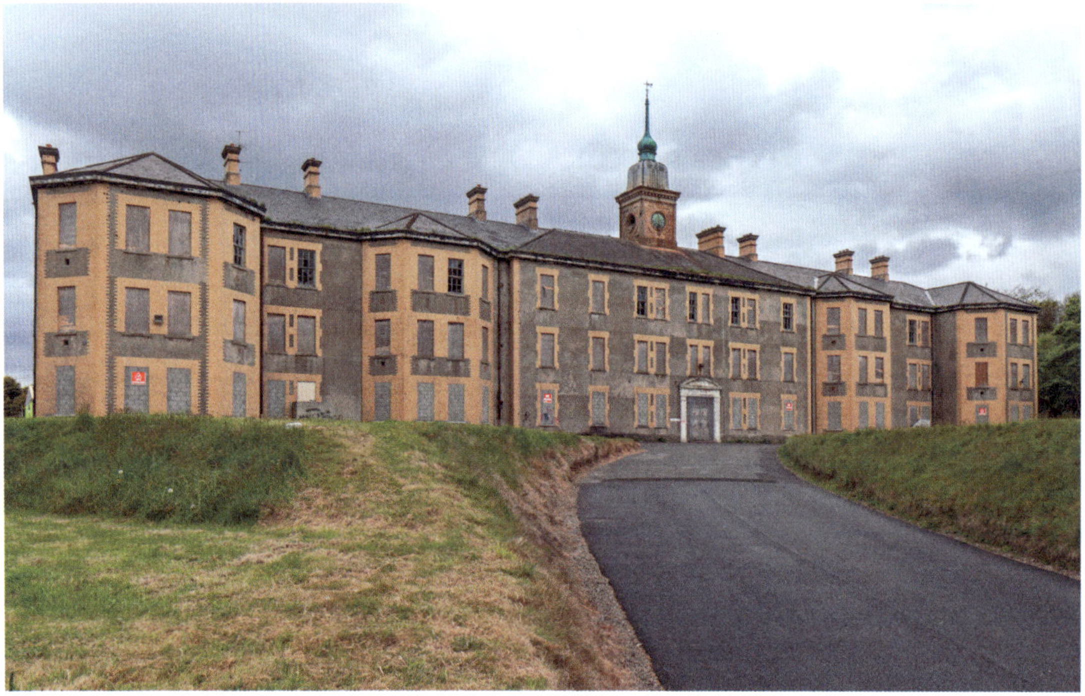

5.07 Historic advertisement for Humphrey's Ltd; the supply of temporary buildings to overcrowded hospitals was clearly a successful business model, *Irish Builder, 1907*, p. 767.

5.08 Ballinasloe: Detached pavilion for 260 patients, completed 1901, *Photograph by David Killeen, 2019.*

5.09 Eglinton Asylum, Cork: Rare image of the 'temporary' buildings once found on many asylum sites but now in all cases demolished, *Image courtesy of the National Library of Ireland (NPA MOR980).*

5.10 Richmond Asylum, Dublin: Typical layout of 'temporary' ward, *Image courtesy of the National Archives of Ireland (Office of Public Works Collection, OPW/5HC/4/799, 3).*

5.11 Letterkenny: Detached pavilion for 200 patients, completed 1906. The cupola was relocated here from the main building for reasons that are not entirely clear, *Photograph by David Killeen, 2019.*

5.12 Portrane: Open plan dayrooms and dormitories commonly contained 40, 60, or even 80 patients in a single space, *Photograph by David Killeen, 2019.*

5.13 Portrane: Single rooms were now much fewer in number, though whether seen by patients as a privilege or punishment is moot, *Photograph by David Killeen, 2019.*

5.14 Purdysburn: Interior photograph, 1935. The individual villas featured living spaces of more domestic scale, *Image courtesy of National Museums Northern Ireland (A. R. Hogg, BELUM.Y910).*

5.15 Purdysburn: Interior photograph, 1935. Multi-bed dormitories remained, but seldom exceeding 12 beds, *Image courtesy of National Museums Northern Ireland (A. R. Hogg, BELUM.Y913).*

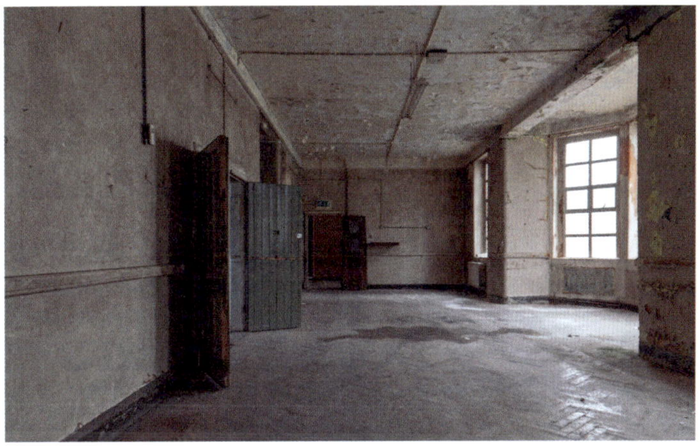

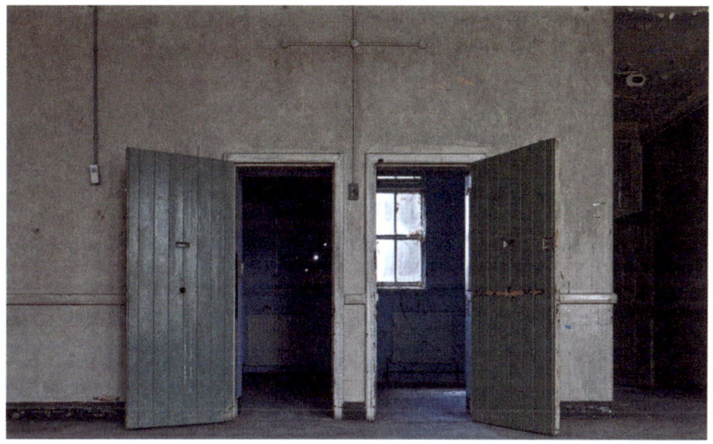

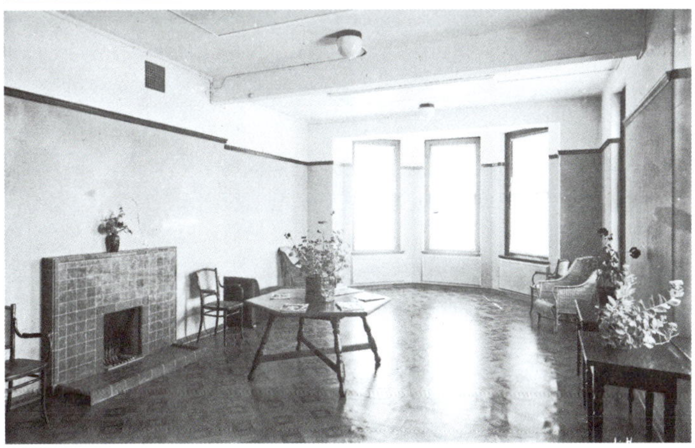

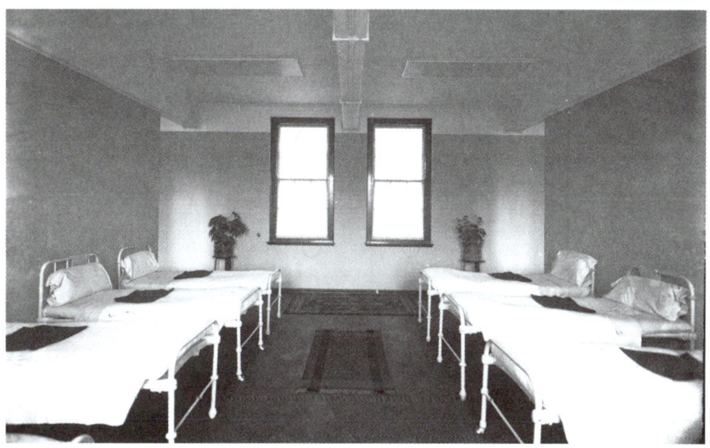

on all sides by urban growth. An architectural competition was held and plans for a conventional asylum were prepared by the winning Belfast firm of Jackson, Ferguson and Tilley.[29] But following the changes wrought by the 1898 Local Government Act, the newly constituted asylum committee decided to reappraise the project, and in 1901 determined that their new institution would be the first 'villa colony' asylum in Ireland.[30] The first two phases, built between 1902 and 1912, comprised ten domestic style villas, a 100-bed hospital (for the medically unwell), an administration block, recreation hall, laundry, two chapels and a variety of ancillary structures. Eminently flexible as a model, further villas would be added through the 1920s and 30s. All were constructed as detached buildings scattered informally across the gently undulating landscape, a vision of freedom when compared to the spider's web of buildings and corridors of the recently completed pavilion-echelon asylums at Holywell and Portrane.[31]

The two biggest cities on the island at the turn of the century thus faced similar challenges of congested asylums that had long outgrown their urban sites. The solutions adopted by their respective authorities may imply something about their differing senses of municipal identity. Dublin – a large but staid metropolis whose best days had departed along with its resident parliament and seasonal aristocracy a century earlier – blindly followed English convention for its new overflow facility at Portrane and shunned any more radical proposals to either improve or replace its discredited Grangegorman complex.[32] Belfast – a booming, self-confident, self-made city, home to world-beating industries – looked to mainland Europe in the belief that it could do better. In replacing their old asylum with an entirely new 'villa colony' at Purdysburn, they demonstrated renewed faith in the potential of better architecture to achieve better outcomes, while also consciously positioning themselves as one of the most progressive municipalities in the kingdom.[33]

Pavilions, sheds and chapels

As a purpose-built villa colony, Purdysburn would remain exceptional in the Irish context. However, as other asylums grew in scale and complexity, some would come to superficially resemble mini-colonies, as a multiplicity of new buildings were erected to accommodate uses formerly housed in the main building, or not previously provided for at all. We have already seen how McCurdy's innovative design for Monaghan preceded the echelon layout by several decades, but he also pioneered the construction of free-standing 'pavilion' blocks, entirely detached from the main edifice.[34] The pavilion approach would prove attractive as a practical means of providing additional accommodation in asylums where principal buildings had been extended past the point of absurdity.

At one end of the spectrum, single-storey villas would mushroom across the landscape at Waterford and Clonmel; the architect of the latter under strict instructions from the indomitable local priest and committee member Fr Scanlon, who insisted: 'the Committee want a plain building, and not an ornamental one… we don't want any baby houses, or houses for show… we should only have the best rubble masonry, and it will be done for less than £13,000.'[35] Whether down to Fr

29. *Forty-Eighth Annual Asylum Report 1898*, HC 1899 [9479] xl, p. 27.
30. The article references the application of the villa colony concept in Scotland, but strangely makes no mention of concurrent developments in Belfast. Yet the timing of this publication and the Belfast decision is no mere co-incidence, as the article's author acknowledges the *Belfast Weekly Telegraph* as a source. *The Irish Builder*, 10 Apr.1901, p. 690.
31. Gillian Allmond, 'Light and darkness in an Edwardian institution for the insane poor: Illuminating the material practices of the asylum age', in *International Journal of Historical Archaeology* 20:1 (2016), p. 4.
32. House of Lords (HL) Debate, 16 May 1895, vol. 33, cc. 1299–1306.
33. Alongside their overt propaganda value, Topp reveals that the villa-colony asylums of Habsburg lands were highly political projects through which individual municipalities defined themselves in a wider empire – Belfast's Purdysburn is open to similar readings. Leslie Topp, *Freedom and the Cage: Modern Architecture and Psychiatry in Central Europe, 1890–1914* (Pennsylvania, 2017), pp 39–41. English pavilion-echelon asylums of the period were beginning to introduce detached villas alongside the dominant main asylum building, but the only true villa colony of the period in England was the Ewell Epileptic Colony (1903). The model was adopted more enthusiastically in Scotland at Kingseat (1904), Bangour Village (1908) and Dykebar (1909). Taylor, *Hospital and Asylum Architecture in England*, p. 152; Gillian Allmond, 'Liberty and the individual: The colony asylum in Scotland and England', in *History of Psychiatry*, 28:1 (Mar. 2017), p. 31.
34. Looking further afield to the United States, Yanni notes that the merits of 'cottage' blocks only gained traction there after 1869. Coincidentally, an Irish-born architect designed the first new-build asylum to incorporate cottage wards alongside a corridor hospital in 1878. However, Willett emigrated decades before Monaghan was built and sadly is unlikely to have known of it. Carla Yanni, *Architecture of Madness: Insane Asylums in the United States* (Minneapolis, 2007), p. 91.
35. *The Irish Builder*, 18 Jul. 1901, p. 799.

Scanlon's intervention or otherwise, the domestic scale and simple character of architect James F. Fuller's resulting buildings has allowed them to remain in use to this day, discreetly evading the contemporary campaign seemingly fixated on decommissioning any building that predates the Emergency. Larger examples, as at Cork (1894), Ballinasloe (1901) and Letterkenny (1906) were more akin to standalone asylums, each accommodating several hundred patients and several featuring their own dining halls. A new 'farm colony' at Mullingar (1902) provided accommodation for 146 'working male patients' overlooking the asylum farmyard.[36] All were buildings of solid construction and minimal architectural pretension, with generic institutional facades and generally bright interiors characterised by enormous, open-plan dormitories and day rooms similar to the extensions already discussed.

All proved insufficient to deal with a patient population that grew by an average of 400 patients a year, every year, for two decades around the turn of the century. *In extremis,* committees resorted to temporary buildings – timber and corrugated iron wards such as those sold by Humphreys Ltd. Initially devised to meet military demand for rapid-erection field hospitals, these flat-pack, mail-order buildings were embraced by committees at Clonmel, Cork, Limerick, Mullingar and the Richmond. In the best tradition of temporary buildings everywhere, most continued in use for a lifetime.[37] Even the enormous new asylum at Portrane was overcrowded within a few years of its opening, such that in 1907, six temporary timber huts that had been erected to house construction workers were 'being fitted up for the reception of some of the lunatic inmates of the workhouse of the district'. Two hundred unfortunate patients still called them home in 1978.[38]

Asylum chapels offer a more encouraging example of the trend towards disaggregation. Even though chapels were not uncommon in contemporary prisons and houses of industry, they were notable by their absence from Johnston and Murray's early asylums. Criticisms soon emerged around the unsuitability of the spaces later commandeered for worship, such as at Clonmel, where 'a room occupied as a day-room, breakfast, dining and supper-room, and moreover, too limited in size, is used for the purpose.'[39] Even in the second phase of asylums, where chapels had been provided, the 1858 Commission of Inquiry highlighted 'objectionable arrangements' around religious observance, including the ecumenical horror of Anglicans and Catholics using the same space for worship. The Commission's report recommended the provision of dedicated, separate chapels for the two main denominations, leading to the gradual construction of freestanding chapels at almost every asylum between the 1860s and 1930s.[40] The majority were built for use by Roman Catholic patients, but on around half of sites, a second (smaller) chapel for Church of Ireland patients would also be added, often constructed at the same time, by the same architect and in a similar idiom, making for some pleasingly quirky couples. The central partitions that had divided males from females in the earlier chapels were dispensed with,[41] but the new chapels usually retained separate doors for male and female patients. Stricter denominational division was no excuse to relax gender separation.

36. *Fifty-Second Annual Asylum Report 1902*, HC 1903 [1762] xxvii, p. 38.
37. The 'Red Building' at Clonmel was built in 1898 and was still in occupation in 1984. Eamon Lonergan, *St Luke's Hospital Clonmel 1834–1984* (Thurles, 1984), pp 37–8.
38. *Fifty-Seventh Annual Asylum Report 1907*, HC 1908 [4302] xxxiii, pp 136–7; Annie Ryan, *Walls of Silence* (Callan, 1999), p. 17.
39. *Sixteenth Annual Asylum Report 1867*, HC 1867 [3894] xviii, p. 17. Despite these complaints, the new chapel at Clonmel would not be completed until 1890. Lonergan, *St Luke's Hospital Clonmel*, pp 34–5.
40. The exceptions being Killarney, Downpatrick and Enniscorthy.
41. As seen in contract drawings for Dundrum (NAI: Office of Public Works, 1845, Central Criminal Lunatic Asylum, OPW/5/HC/4/779, Sheet 7), Sligo (Irish Architectural Archive: Sligo Lunatic Asylum Collection, ca. 1850, Sligo District Lunatic Asylum, 89/11 Sheets 4, 13) and Ennis (NAI: Office of Public Works, 1864, Clare District Lunatic Asylum, NAI OPW/5/HC/4/800, Sheet 10).

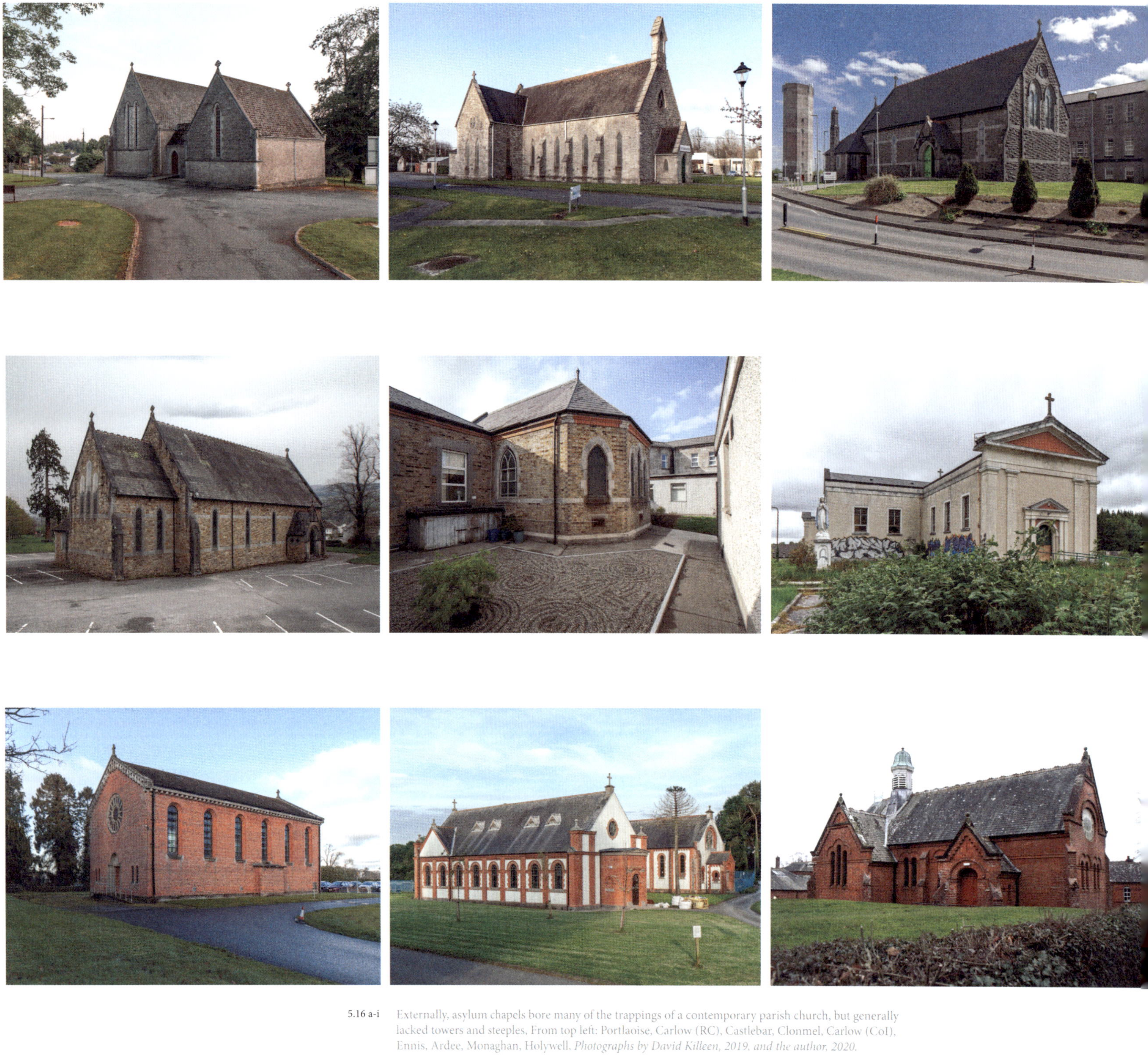

5.16 a-i Externally, asylum chapels bore many of the trappings of a contemporary parish church, but generally lacked towers and steeples, From top left: Portlaoise, Carlow (RC), Castlebar, Clonmel, Carlow (CoI), Ennis, Ardee, Monaghan, Holywell. *Photographs by David Killeen, 2019. and the author, 2020.*

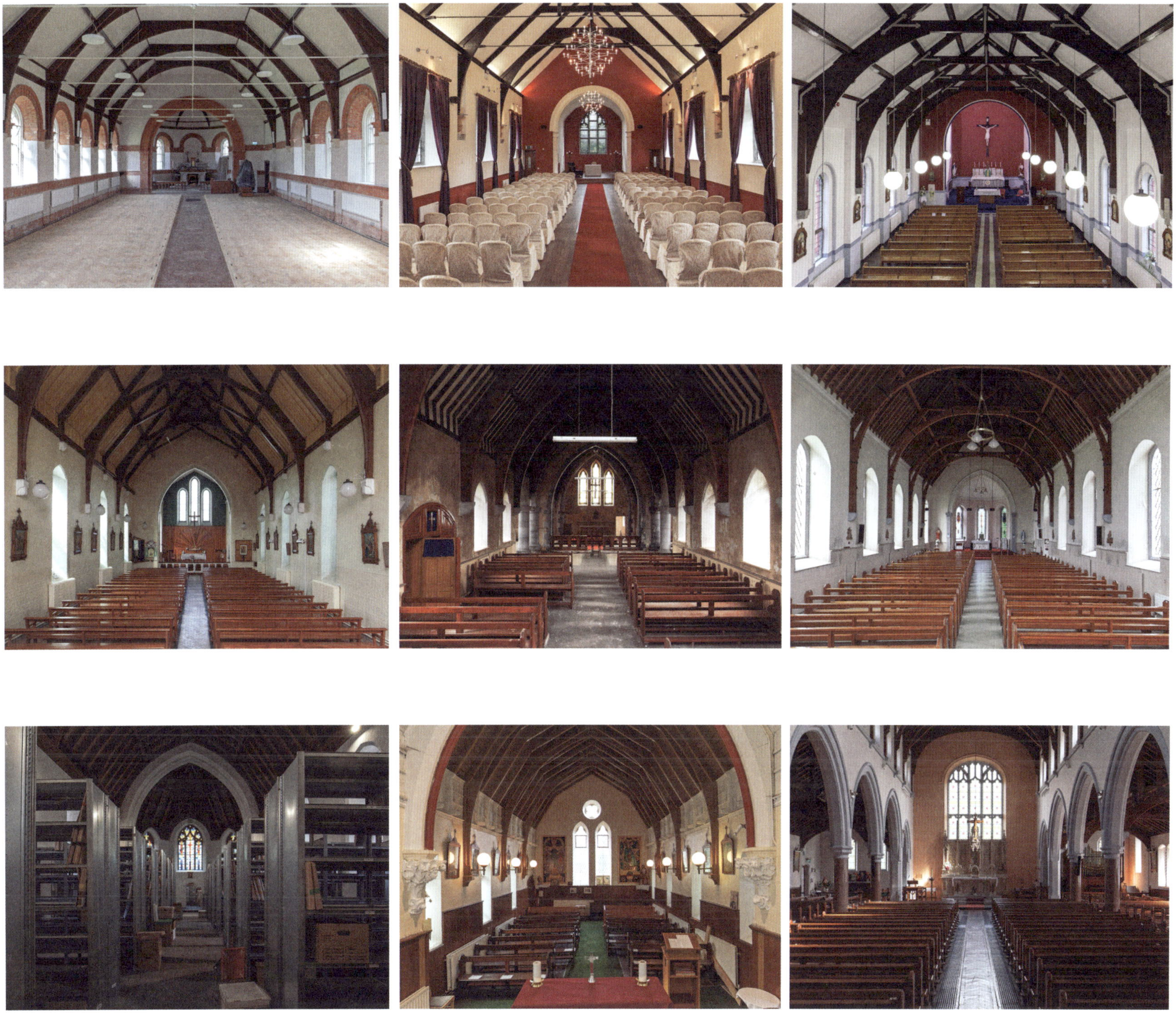

5.17 a-i Chapel interiors were generally spare, and seldom gained the trappings of stained glass and marble with which most ordinary churches would be embellished over time. From top left: Monaghan, Sligo, Castlerea, Clonmel, Limerick, Mullingar, Kilkenny, Dundrum, Portrane, *Photographs by David Killeen, 2019.*

So even as the architectural quality of new wards declined, asylum governors and committees still proved willing to pay for the outward architectural trappings of a dignified place of worship. Externally, most would have been indistinguishable from the simpler parish churches of the day but for the absence of belfries and steeples – neither visual cues nor audible calls to prayer were needed by a congregation whose days were already governed by the asylum bell. The new chapels were proudly sited in visually prominent positions but paid little heed to the established structure of the designed landscape; by the late nineteenth century, asylum governors seem to have lost interest in curating the visual set piece of building-and-landscape that had so exercised their fore-fathers.[42] Internally, the chapels today are striking for their spareness: a congregation without financial means militated against the addition of stained glass windows and marble altars with which generations of the faithful have embellished even the most humble parish churches.

Flying the cuckoo's nest

The curative aspirations of the first asylums demanded that their senior officers, as parents of the 'moral family', should be quartered within the building. This approach was mostly continued in the second and third phases of building – the principal rooms of the main block were divided between the (no longer matrimonially bonded) Governor and Matron, whose personal comfort was attended by servants operating from separate basement kitchens. As the perceived effectiveness of 'moral management' diminished and asylum populations grew, the era of the Moral Governor succumbed to the dominance of the Resident Medical Superintendent, and any sense of the asylum as a 'family' environment watched over by a benign, paternal, if not omni-present figure, was lost. Thus, barely fifteen years after Dr John Connolly observed that the resident physician 'will almost regard his patients as his children',[43] the medical profession was demonstrating a distinct eagerness to escape the tumult of the asylum 'family':

> *Another glaring want in this institution… [is the fact that] no suitable accommodation [is] provided for that officer [RMS] who, like others similarly placed, is 'cabin'd, cribb'd, confined in such a manner as to be both injurious to health, and highly derogatory to him as the head of an important public establishment…, who has to bear the burden and heat of the day, and who should, after his day's toil and ever-anxious duties, have his own house to retire into from the carking cares and annoyances by which he is continually surrounded.*[44]

Such supposed affronts to their professional dignity went unresolved for many more decades. The RMS continued to be 'cribb'd' in the central administration block, with Monaghan providing the rare early exception. There, the local asylum committee in 1863 considered that a superior detached dwelling would allow them to attract a 'more than ordinarily efficient' candidate to manage their institution, and successfully defended their decision against the conservative bureaucracy of the Board of Control

42. The author had considered the elegantly sectarian theory that chapel construction was a way for the new (middle-class and Catholic) asylum committees to parade their religious values at the expense of a demesne-style landscape inherited from the gentry-dominated boards of old, but no distinction is obvious in the siting of chapels that pre- and post-date the 1898 Local Government Act. Asylum committees in Northern Ireland, which were not Catholic-dominated, showed similar disregard for the nuances of designed landscapes, albeit it is hard not to infer motive in decisions at both Armagh and Omagh to position Anglican chapels prominently to the front, while their larger Catholic counterparts were discreetly tucked away to the rear. At Purdysburn, both chapels were discreetly located on a wooded knoll.
43. John Connolly, *The Construction and Government of Lunatic Asylums* (London, 1847), p. 144.
44. Anon, *Dublin Journal of Medical Science*, 32 (1861), p. 379, cited in Markus Reuber, 'Moral management and the "Unseen Eye": Public lunatic asylums, 1800–1845', in Elizabeth Malcolm and Greta Jones (eds), *Medicine, Disease and the State in Ireland, 1650–1940* (Cork, 1999), p. 228.

in Dublin Castle.[45] Even Henry Burdett, an international expert on asylum and hospital design whose monumental publication of 1891 firmly endorsed the connection of every function by a web of corridors, made an exception for the RMS. His advice made clear the high social status of the late nineteenth-century RMS by the scale of detached dwelling to be provided: 'His residence should be a comfortable house, containing not fewer than three public rooms and eight bedrooms.'[46] Whether Burdett's bedroom tally represented expectations of hospitality or fecundity remains moot.

Monaghan's competitive advantage in the employment market would remain intact for almost 20 years. The majority of RMS houses were built in the period between 1890 and 1910 – perhaps reflecting the point at which overcrowding finally rendered life in the main building intolerable, and in several instances allowing the vacated quarters to be repurposed for patients. Most are solid, conventional specimens of late Victorian or Edwardian middle-class residential architecture, with those at Letterkenny and Limerick improved by attractive arts and crafts detailing. The largest of all is naturally found at The Richmond, a sombre red-brick pile that finally rescued Ireland's busiest RMS from his 'carking cares'. A late flurry of utilitarian doctor's houses in the 1950s implies that a significant number of RMSs (and many of their deputies) up to that point had still been obliged to lodge under the same roof as their charges almost a century after first agitating for change. If the medical profession's increasing influence and ultimate monopolisation of the asylum system was a self-serving exercise designed to boost their power and prestige as is argued by Scull and others, then the nature of their living quarters implies that in Ireland, at least, that project was far from an unqualified success.[47]

War and revolution

At the outbreak of war in Europe in 1914, Ireland's asylums were home to 21,480 patients and on the basis of prevailing admission and discharge rates, that number could have been expected to increase to around 22,350 by 1918. Instead, the war years saw the first ever sustained drop in patient numbers, to 19,907 in 1918. Surprisingly, the number of (civilian) admissions for which the war was given as a primary or contributory cause of insanity never exceeded 2%, while the overall admissions rate actually dropped during the war.[48] Unfortunately, the more significant cause of falling patient numbers was a spike in mortality, caused by general shortages of food, fuel and medicine, unusually cold winters and a staff cohort much depleted by the call of 'King and Country'.[49] The misery was compounded in 1917 and 1918, as the influenza pandemic ripped through cold and undernourished populations packed into poorly ventilated and overcrowded spaces. In a strange irony it was Belfast – whose asylum comprised modern, spacious villas in the 'admirable surroundings' of a healthy rural site – that suffered the highest mortality rate of all, losing one third of its inpatient population in just two years.[50] Then, as now, residential institutions are inherently vulnerable to the silent scourge of contagious disease.

As the war progressed, sections of Dublin's Richmond Asylum and Belfast's old city asylum were requisitioned to serve as War Hospitals, necessitating the redistribution of patients across the remaining accommodation. Upon closure of

45. Anne McLellan, Niamh Nic Ghabhann and Fiona Byrne, *World Within Walls: From Asylum to Contemporary Mental Health Services*. (Monaghan, 2015) p. 4.
46. Burdett, *Hospitals and Asylums of the World*, p. 18.
47. Of the 20 asylums built prior to 1869 where RMS lodgings were originally within the main building, new detached houses were built at approximately one third of these sites prior to 1900, and at least another third between 1900 and 1960. Purpose-built houses were provided in all new asylums after Monaghan.
48. *Sixty-Seventh Annual Asylum Report 1917*, HC 1919 [32] xxv, p. vii. Research in other quarters has identified that national solidarity in times of adversity seems to contribute to a reduction in admission rates – it is too soon to see how this finding weathers the pandemic of 2020–21.
49. Volunteers were drawn from all grades, including at least three Resident Medical Superintendents (RMSs) and seven Assistant Medical Officers.
50. Mortality rates were 15.4 per cent in 1917 and 19.7 per cent in 1918. *Sixty-Seventh Annual Asylum Report 1917*, HC 1919 [32] xxv, p. xix, and *Sixty-Eighth Annual Asylum Report 1918*, HC 1920 [579] p. xxi, p. xix. The necessity of moving 400 patients from the old city asylum, via temporary lodgings in workhouses before arriving at Purdysburn, may have helped to seed and spread the virus in each new setting.

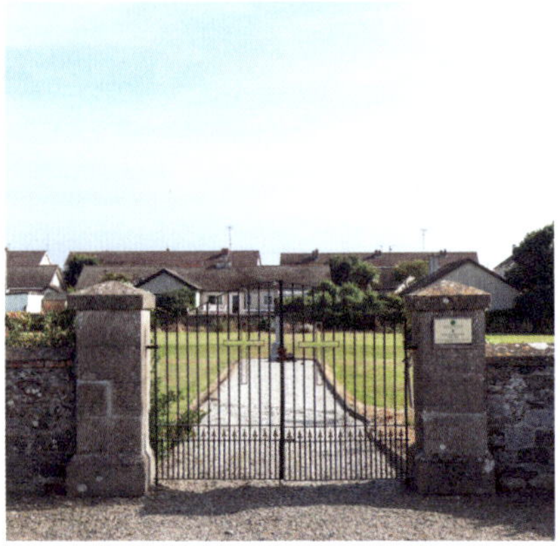

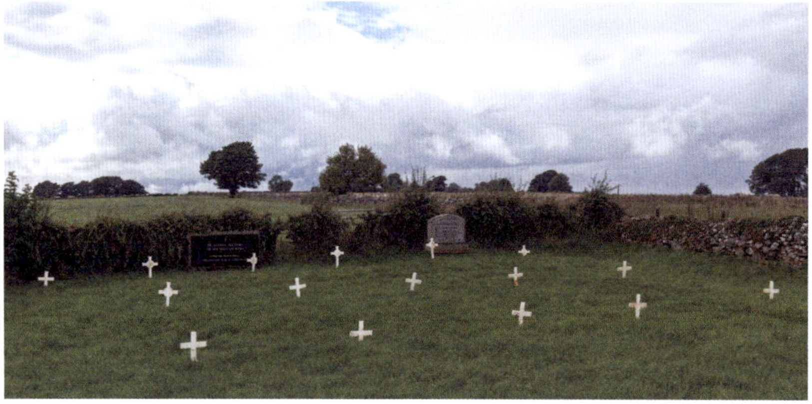

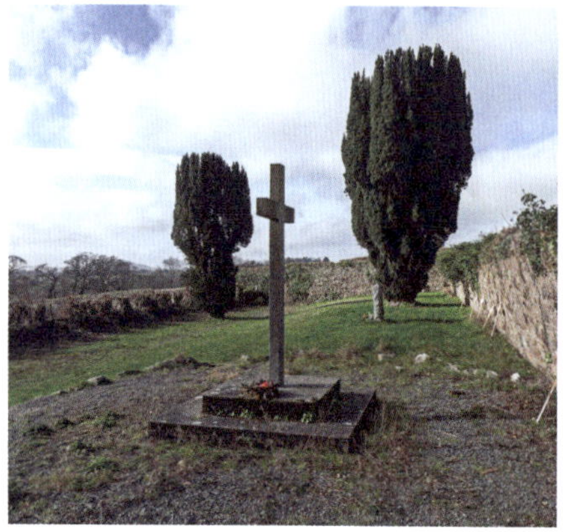

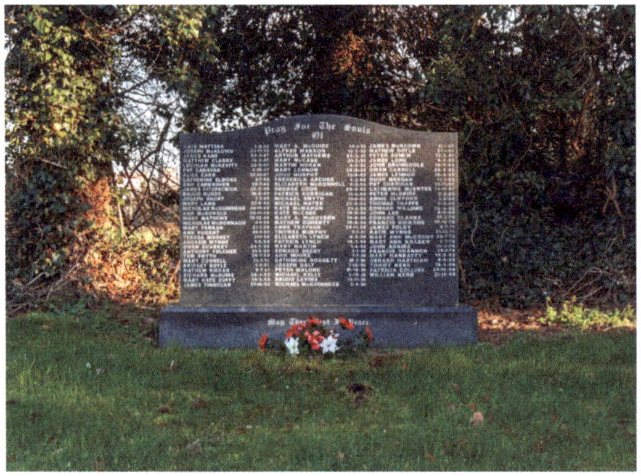
Pray For The Souls
Of

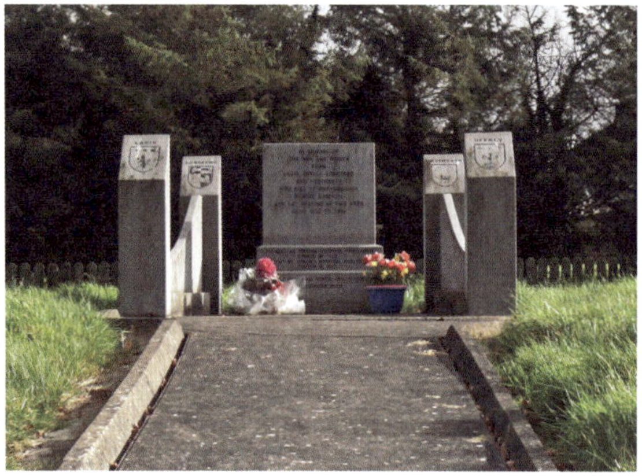

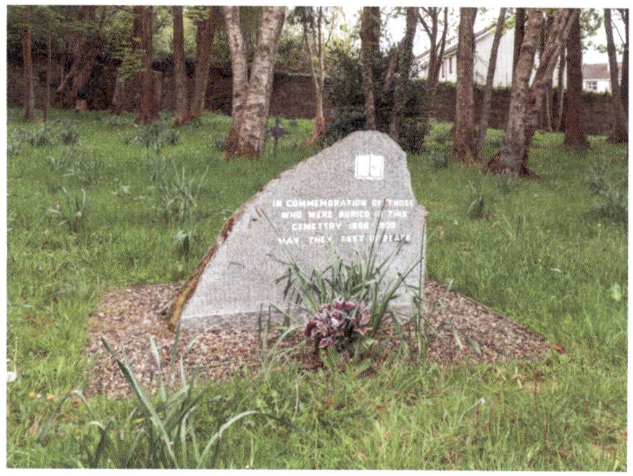
IN COMMEMORATION OF THOSE

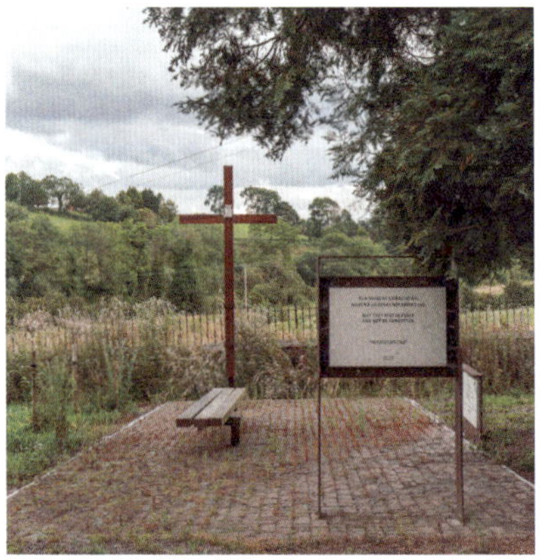

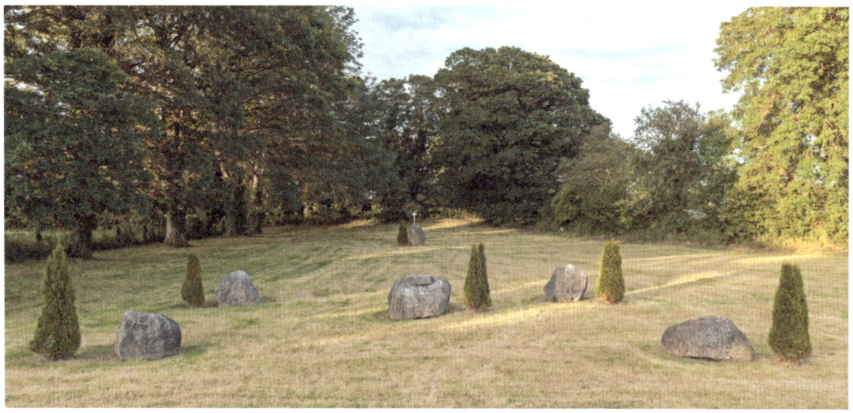

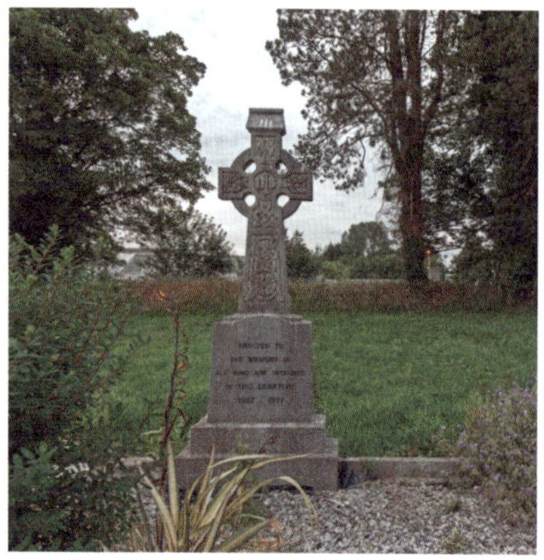

18 19

5.18 a-i Final resting place for up to 10,000 anonymous former patients, most asylum burial grounds have been provided with later memorials. From top left: Portrane, Castlerea, Enniscorthy, Ardee, Portlaoise, Letterkenny, Monaghan, Ballinasloe, Mullingar. *Photographs by David Killeen, 2019.*

5.19 a-f Resident Medical Superintendents gradually gained substantial detached dwellings commensurate with their social standing. From top left: Monaghan, Waterford, Castlebar, Letterkenny, Limerick, Portrane. *Photographs by David Killeen, 2019.*

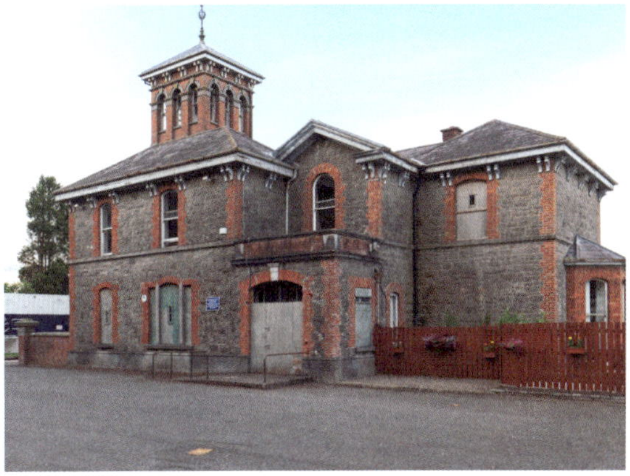
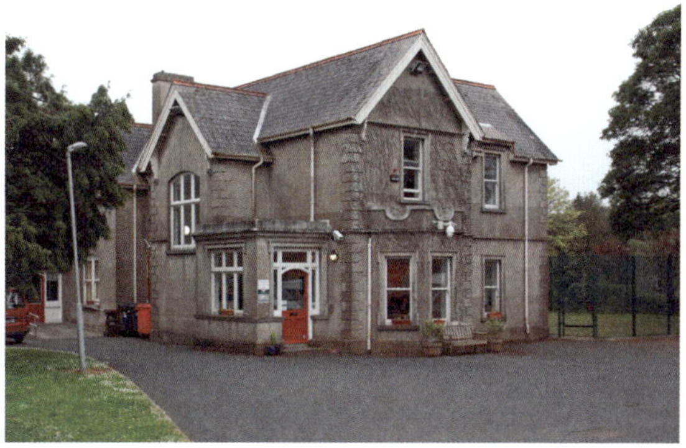
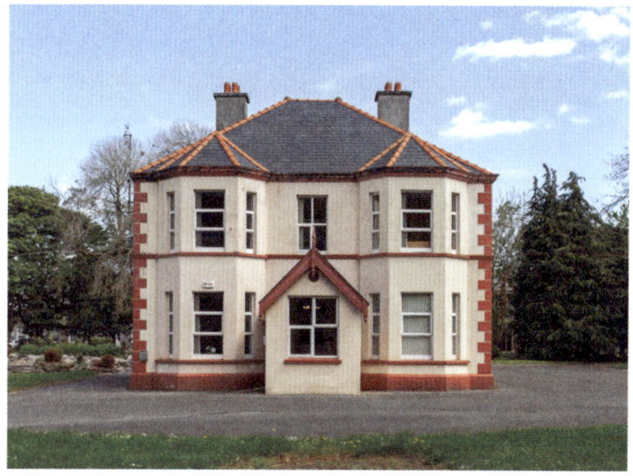
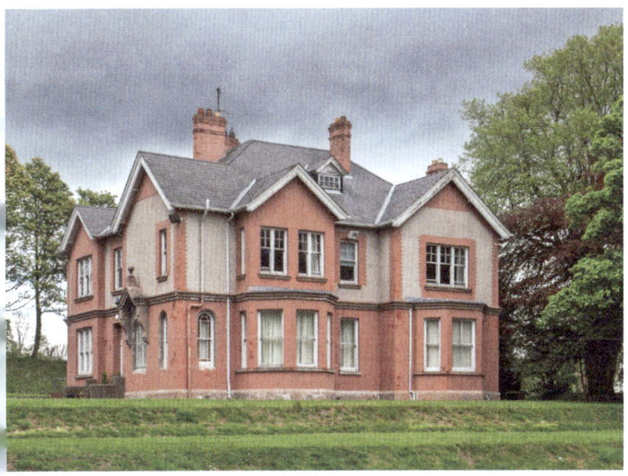
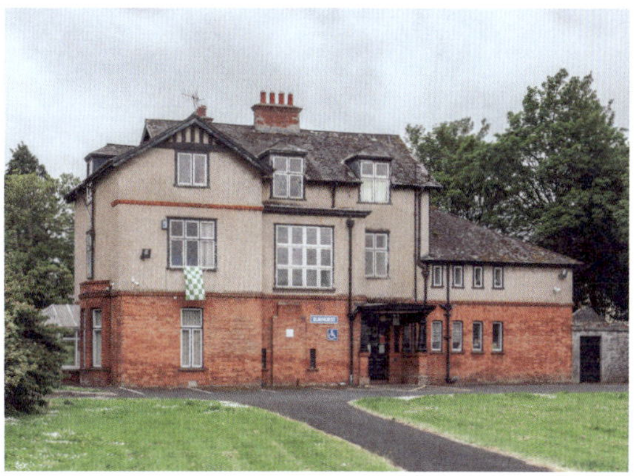
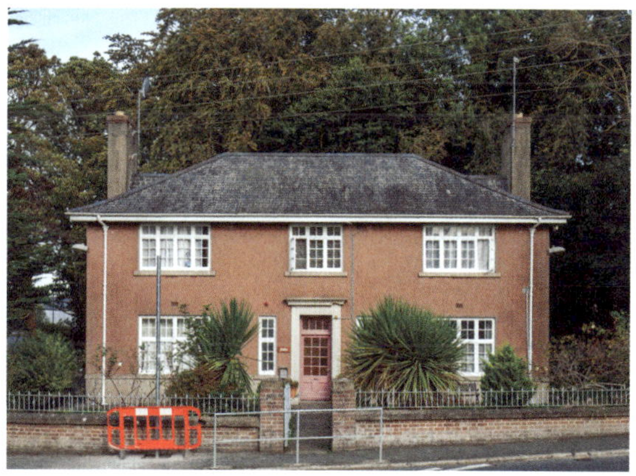

51. The public expenditure estimates for 1921–2 included an allowance of £6,136 for the salaries and expenses of the two inspectors and their four support staff (or enough to maintain approximately 140 patients for a year), but their report was never published. *1921–22 Estimates for civil services for the year ending 31 March 1922*, HC 1921 [41] xxii, p. 190, p. 194.

52. *Sixty-Eighth Annual Asylum Report 1918*, HC 1920 [579] xxi; *Report of the Inspector of Mental Hospitals, 1923*.

53. Research into the individual institutional records would doubtless reveal a much richer story of these times. It seems certain that some asylum staff would have participated in the conflicts, perhaps finding themselves in opposition to an officer class whose loyalties more likely rested with the Union.

these hospitals in 1919, the District Asylums received some 400 chronic mental cases from these hospitals – shattered sailors and shell-shocked soldiers, many of whom would spend the rest of their lives in institutional care, paid for by the British Ministry of Pensions as 'Service Patients'. Of course, conflict was soon to erupt much closer to home, but beyond a gap in annual reporting between 1920 and 1922, revolutionary war, civil war and an end to '800 years of British rule' failed to register on the bureaucratic radar.[51] There is an almost eerie degree of continuity between the last reports of the outgoing Inspectors of Lunacy and the early reports of the Saorstát's new Inspector of Mental Hospitals. Both studiously avoided any mention of the disturbed state of the country or its effect on the institutions, focusing determinedly on the inadequacy of fire drills, the desirability of better bedding and the commendable utility of hair-teasing machines in upholstery workshops.[52] But then, for those living within the walls, the small comfort of a better pillow was probably of greater consequence than whether it came wrapped in a Union Jack or a tricolour.[53]

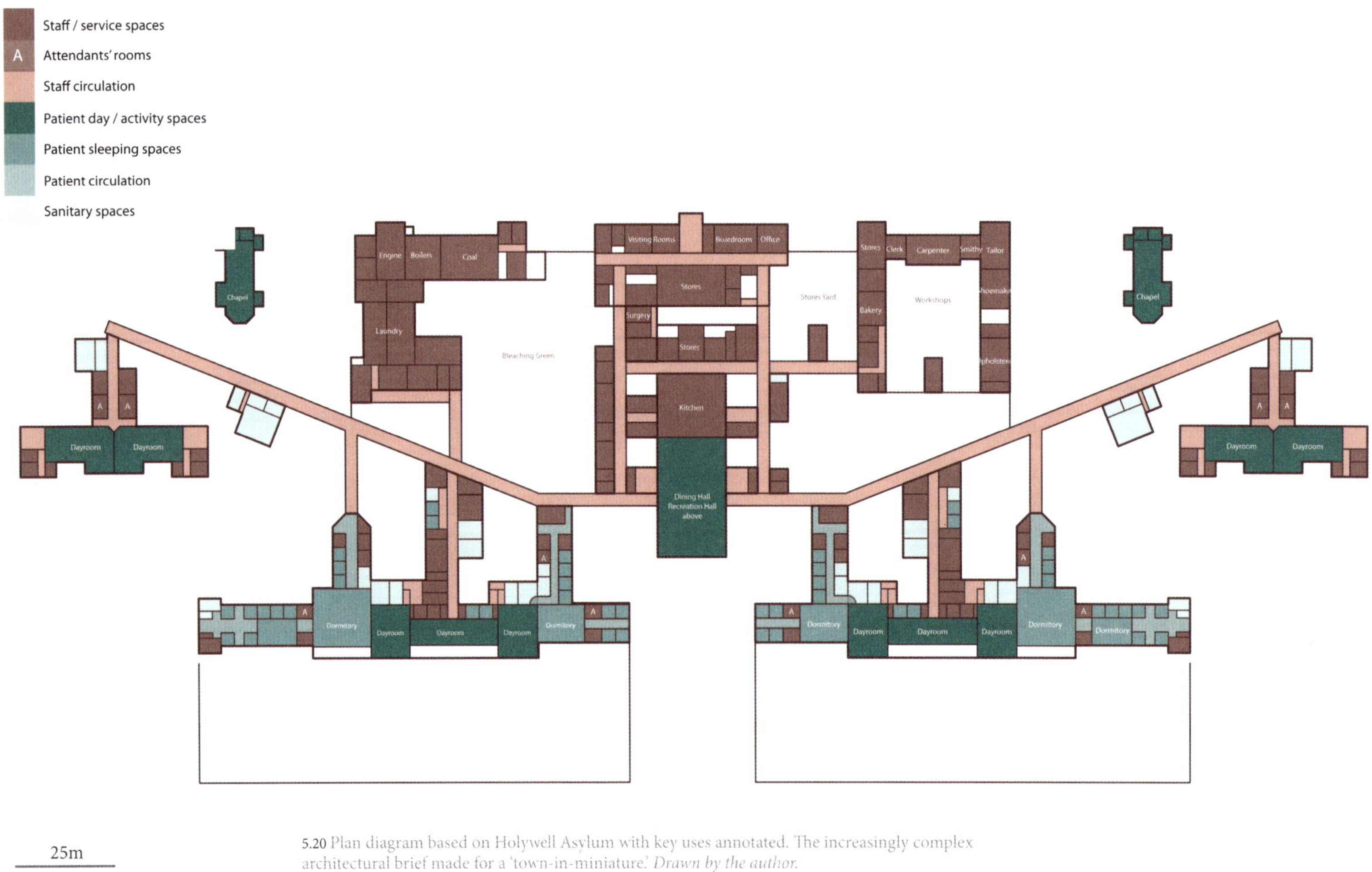

5.20 Plan diagram based on Holywell Asylum with key uses annotated. The increasingly complex architectural brief made for a 'town-in-miniature.' *Drawn by the author.*

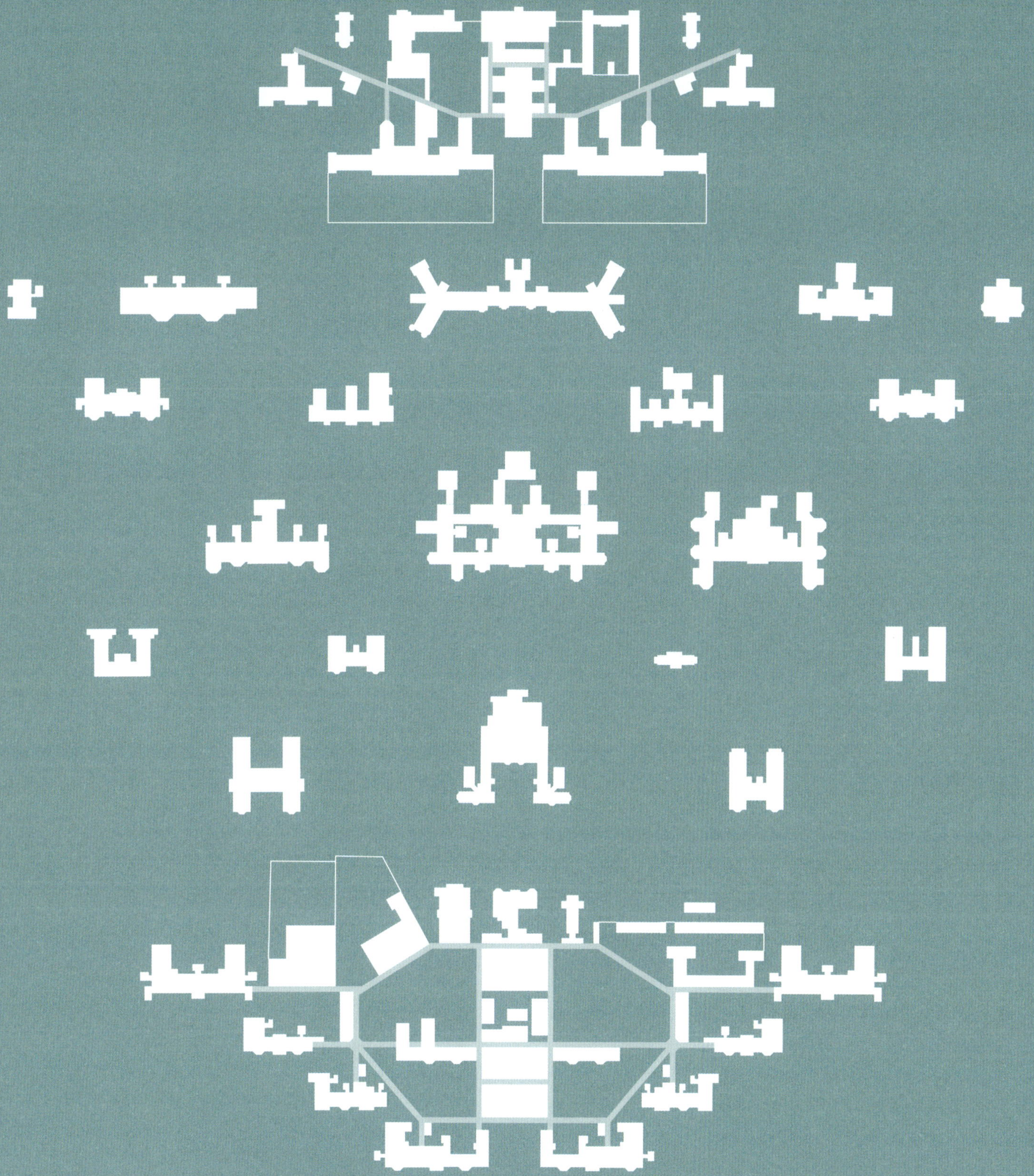

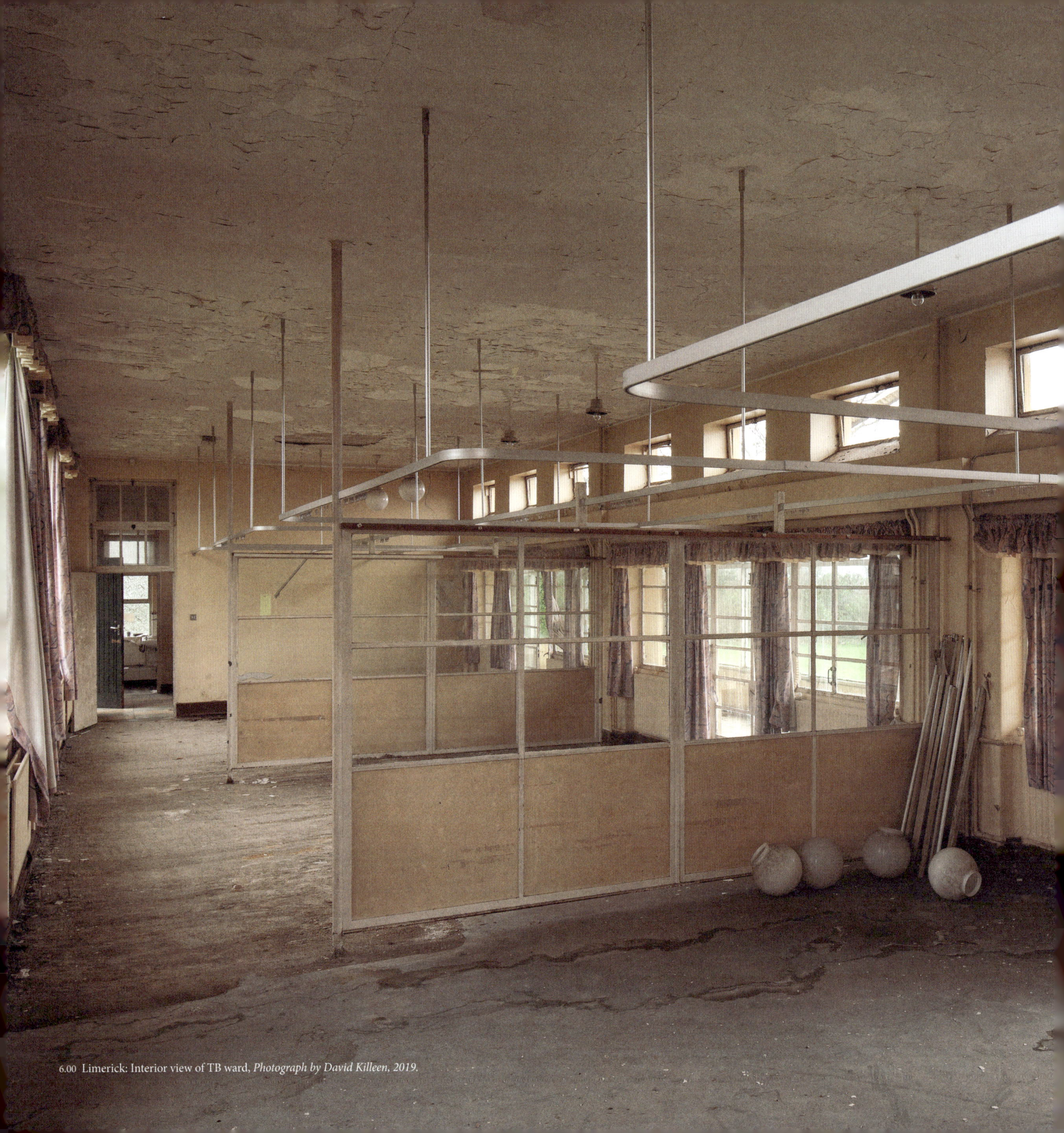

6.00 Limerick: Interior view of TB ward, *Photograph by David Killeen, 2019.*

New Name, New Nation, Old Problems

these farms offer a most suitable form of occupational therapy [1]

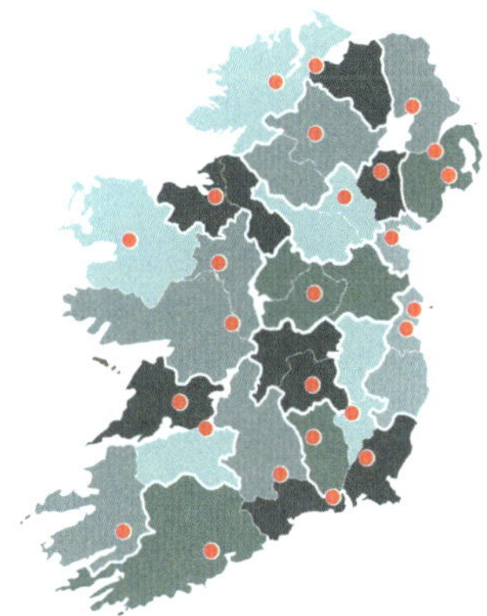

Mental hospital distribution in Ireland, 1945, *Drawn by the author.*

The first sitting of an independent Irish Dáil in January 1919 set out its intention of 'abolishing the present odious, degrading, and foreign Poor Law system, substituting therefor [*sic*] a sympathetic native scheme for the care of the Nation's aged and infirm, who shall not be regarded as a burden, but rather entitled to the Nation's gratitude and consideration.'[2] By the time the new Free State government established a formal 'Commission on the Relief of the Sick and Destitute Poor Including the Insane Poor' in 1925, Ireland's institutional landscape had already been transformed by a series of 'County Schemes' that saw most former workhouses closed or converted into County or District Hospitals or County Homes caring principally – though not exclusively – for the destitute elderly.[3] This was also the period that saw the establishment of specialist Mother and Baby Homes designed to keep 'unmarried mothers in the pre-natal period out of… the County Homes',[4] joining a network of religious-run Industrial Schools, Reformatories and Magdalen Asylums whose number had multiplied through the later nineteenth century. The Free State may have succeeded in its goal of deconstructing a Westminster-designed regime that reflected Victorian England's economically conservative terror of incentivising the 'undeserving poor', but in its place it facilitated an even more formidable institutional infrastructure that policed the moral order of socially conservative Irish Catholic values – itself now in turn a subject of widespread contemporary opprobrium.[5]

But anyone who hoped that an independent Ireland would begin to remedy the deficiencies of another type of centrally decreed institutional regime would be disappointed. When the Commission published its report in 1927 it included several worthy recommendations around the treatment of acute mental illness in general hospitals and the capping of the size of mental hospitals at 1,000 patients by establishing auxiliary hospitals, and boarding-out patients.[6] The Commission also recommended the consolidation of the complex 'hodgepodge' of lunacy legislation

1. *Report of the Inspector of Mental Hospitals, 1950*, p. 32.
2. Piaras Béalsaí TD, Dáil Éireann, 21 Jan. 1919, F:1.
3. Annie Ryan, *Walls of Silence* (Callan, 1999), p. 142.
4. *Report of the Commission on the Relief of the Sick and Destitute Poor, Including the Insane Poor*, (Dublin, 1928), p. 1623.
5. As evidenced in the reports of several recent investigations, including: *Final Report of the Commission to Inquire into Child Abuse* (Dublin, 2009), *Report of the Inter-Departmental Committee to Establish the Facts of State Involvement with the Magdalen Laundries* (Dublin, 2013) and *Final Report of the Commission of Investigation into Mother and Baby Homes* (Dublin, 2021). See also James M. Smith, 'The politics of sexual knowledge: The origins of Ireland's containment culture and the Carrigan Report (1931)', in *Journal of the History of Sexuality* 13:2 (2004), pp 209–13.
6. Dermot Walsh and Antoinette Daly, *Mental Illness in Ireland 1750–2002: Reflections on the Rise and Fall of Institutional Care* (Dublin, 2004), p. 32.

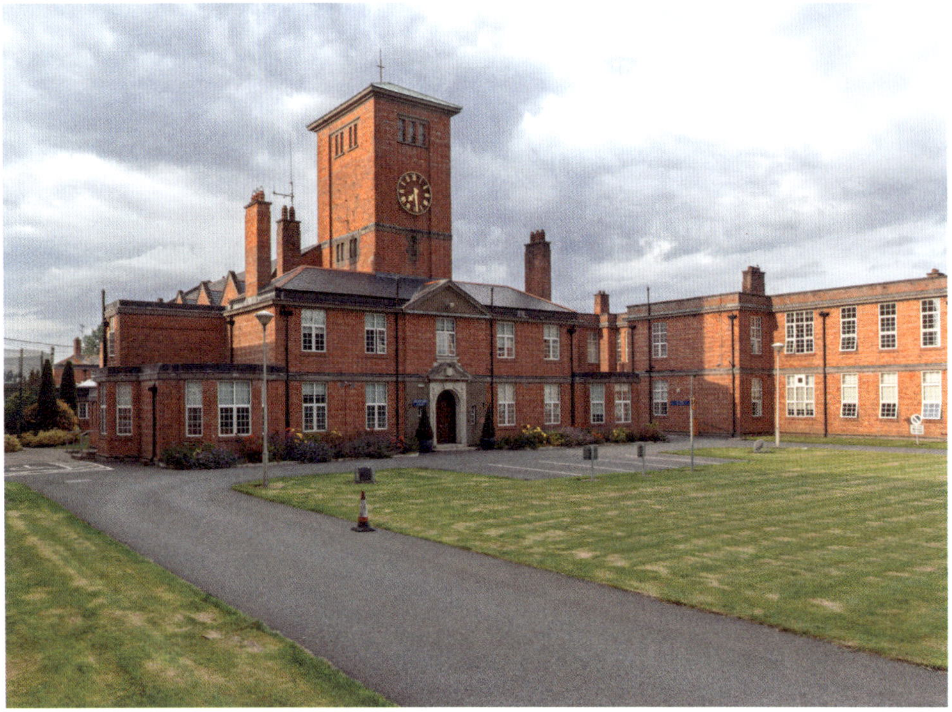

6.01 Ardee: Entrance forecourt dominated by clocktower, *Photograph by David Killeen, 2019.*

that had accreted over the previous century, but such deep reform would have to would wait another 20 years for the Mental Treatment Act of 1945.[7]

Instead, the token legislative initiative of the Free State was to re-style 'District Lunatic Asylums' as 'District Mental Hospitals'; the thousands indefinitely detained therein would remain legally defined as 'dangerous lunatics' under archaic legislation dating from 1867.[8] This empty gesture – the institutional equivalent of applying green paint on a red letterbox – contrasts sharply with the political will invested in the systematic deconstruction of the legacy workhouse system and in the creation of new Mother and Baby Homes. Far from indicating that the asylum system was already well-regarded and in little need of reform, the headline conclusion is that the mentally ill were indeed a 'burden', less deserving of 'native sympathy… and consideration' than the aged and infirm, with the subtext that the existing legislation was already more than effective at neutralising any threat posed by the insane to the social order. Indeed, Scull's contention that 'asylums were now seen as an essential guarantor of the social order, as well as an important symbolic reminder of the awful consequences of non-conformity'[9] becomes much more relevant in the Irish context if we replace the 'capitalist economy' part of his equation with 'conservative theocracy'.[10]

Following partition, the six district asylums of Armagh, Belfast (Purdysburn), Londonderry, Omagh, Down (Downpatrick) and Antrim (Holywell) remained within Northern Ireland and became subject to their own Inspectorate. Reforming legislation introduced in Northern Ireland in 1932 closely mirrored English law introduced two years earlier, modernising the language of lunacy and reforming the categories of admission, but offering little impetus to change the conceptual basis of the service.[11]

7. Ibid. See also Damien Brennan, *Irish Insanity, 1800–2000* (Oxon, 2014), p. 93; Joseph Robins, *Fools and Mad: A History of the Insane in Ireland* (Dublin, 1986), p. 187.
8. Note that the change of name was carried into effect by the 1925 Local Government Act (no. 5 of 1925), and was not a recommendation of the Commission.
9. Andrew Scull, 'A convenient place to get rid of inconvenient people: The Victorian lunatic asylum', in Anthony D. King (ed.), *Buildings and Society: Essays on the Social Development of the Built Environment* (London, 1980), p. 50.
10. And an area eminently worthy of further research. Several unpublished papers presented at the Prisons, Asylums, Workhouses conference at Public Record Office of Northern Ireland (PRONI), Belfast, June 2019, explore the gamut of Irish institutions as part of an infrastructure of social control either directly operated by the Catholic Church, or heavily influenced by its cultural dominance. Even so, the position of the asylum as a state-sponsored, officially secular entity remains nuanced, and much more work is needed to tease out this relationship.
11. Mental Treatment Act (NI) 1932, 22 & 23 Geo.5, c.15. Pauline M. Prior 'Mental health law on the island of Ireland, 1800–2010', in Pauline M. Prior (ed.), *Asylums, Mental Health Care and the Irish 1800–2010* (Dublin, 2012), p. 324.

Arguably, partition had a less immediate impact on the political status of the asylums than the reform of local government 20 years earlier, a reform that had replaced gentry-dominated boards of governors with committees far more representative of their local ratepayers.[12] It was perhaps predictable that mental hospital committees in the new Free State should vote to banish portraits of Queen Victoria from their board rooms; it is more surprising to recall that these same committees had been proud to pass conspicuous motions of sympathy on the death of her son, King Edward VII, little more than a decade before.[13] Unlike the Poor Law Boards of Guardians, whose politicisation by the nationalist cause in the 1880s and 1890s transformed them into hubs of political activism,[14] the middle-class rate-payers who dominated the asylum committees seemed more inclined to follow events than to shape them.

Committees displayed more consistency in representing rate-payer interests through these straitened times, exhorting asylum officers to achieve economies in the management of the institutions, including reduction of patients' 'dietary', and wage cuts for asylum staff. Parsimonious attitudes would persist long after initial fiscal shock of Independence had dissipated, through the Economic War and into the Emergency, with a particularly dramatic example occurring at Killarney in 1940. Over one thousand patients were crowded into a hospital where tuberculosis was endemic, but the prospect of burdening the rates with the wages of a third permanent doctor was sufficient to provoke 100 angry farmers to arrive at the hospital on horseback and storm the meeting of the committee of management.[15]

The Irish Hospitals' Sweepstakes

It is therefore little surprise that new construction projects were a low priority for both local and central government in the early years of the new state, even as the numbers in the mental hospitals resumed their upward trajectory. This only changed with the establishment of the Irish Hospitals' Sweepstakes in 1930 – a lottery established for 'the purpose of helping the sick poor' by funding the construction or improvement of public hospitals – which offered mental hospital committees a potential source of grant aid for capital projects at reduced cost to their local ratepayers.[16] The Sweepstakes funded a dramatic transformation in Ireland's wider healthcare infrastructure, but mental hospital projects accounted for barely 4% of the funds distributed. It is easy to interpret this as further confirmation of the marginalisation of mental health, but it must also be noted that the fledgling state faced a spectacular dearth of buildings for general medicine, in contrast with a relatively large endowment of purpose-built – if sometimes outdated and habitually overcrowded – asylums.

Sweepstakes money would enable the construction of two new district mental hospitals at Ardee and Castlerea – the first purpose-built institutions in 30 years. Ardee opened in 1933 to receive County Louth patients from Portrane, while Castlerea opened in 1940 as an auxiliary branch of Ballinasloe, although it was requisitioned shortly afterwards for use as a tuberculosis sanatorium before being returned to the mental health service in 1955.[17] Both buildings embody a curious mix of tradition and modernity. They were built as modern 'Mental Hospitals' but remained asylums in conception and operation – large self-sufficient institutions set on rural

12. Brennan, *Irish Insanity*, p. 92.
13. As at Killarney and Clonmel. Dermot Dwyer, (ed.), *St. Finan's Hospital Killarney: A Medical, Social & Sporting History 1852–2002* (Killarney, 2002), p. 11, p. 20; Eamon Lonergan, *St Luke's Hospital Clonmel 1834–1984* (Thurles, 1984), p. 56.
14. The governance structures of the asylum system could provide rich material for a separate political study along the lines of Butler's exploration of grand jury patronage in courthouse and prison building or Crossman's study of the Poor Law Boards of Guardians. Richard J. Butler, *Building the Irish Courthouse and Prison: A Political History, 1750–1850* (Cork, 2019); Virginia Crossman, *Politics, Pauperism and Power in Late Nineteenth-Century Ireland* (Manchester, 2006), pp 42–53.
15. Dwyer, *St Finan's Hospital Killarney*, pp 42–5.
16. £1.5 million from a total distribution of £35 million was allocated to mental hospitals between 1931 and 1955. Eamon de Barra and John O'Sheehan (eds), *Oispidéal na hÉireann: Ireland's Hospitals 1933–1950* (Dublin, 1956), p. 8.
17. *Report of the Inspector of Mental Hospitals, 1977–1979*, p. 16.

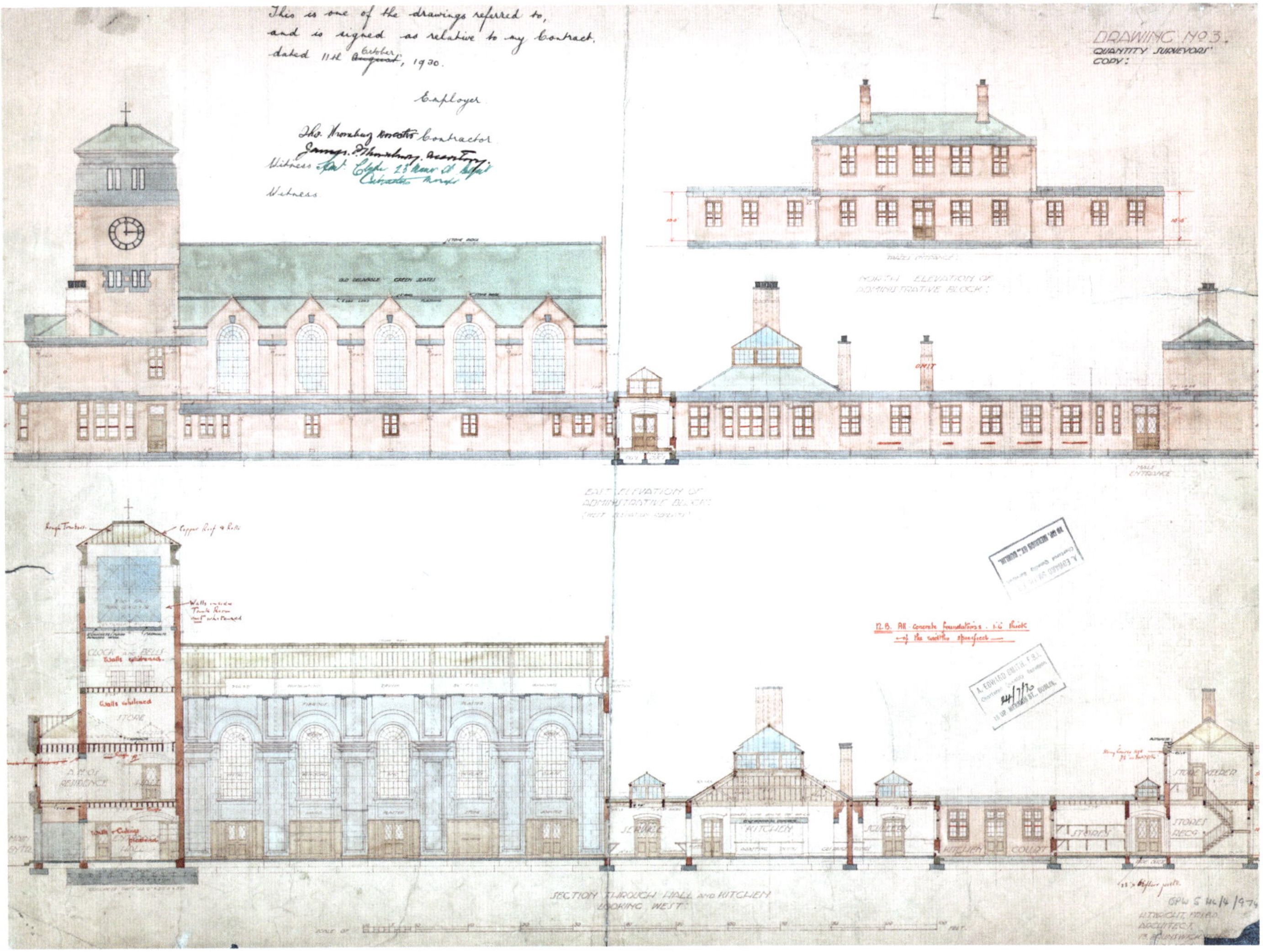

This is one of the drawings referred to, and is signed as relative to my contract. dated 11th October, 1930.
Employer
Contractor
Witness
Witness
DRAWING No 3.
QUANTITY SURVEYORS' COPY.
NORTH ELEVATION OF ADMINISTRATIVE BLOCK.
SECTION THROUGH HALL and KITCHEN LOOKING WEST
KITCHEN
STORES

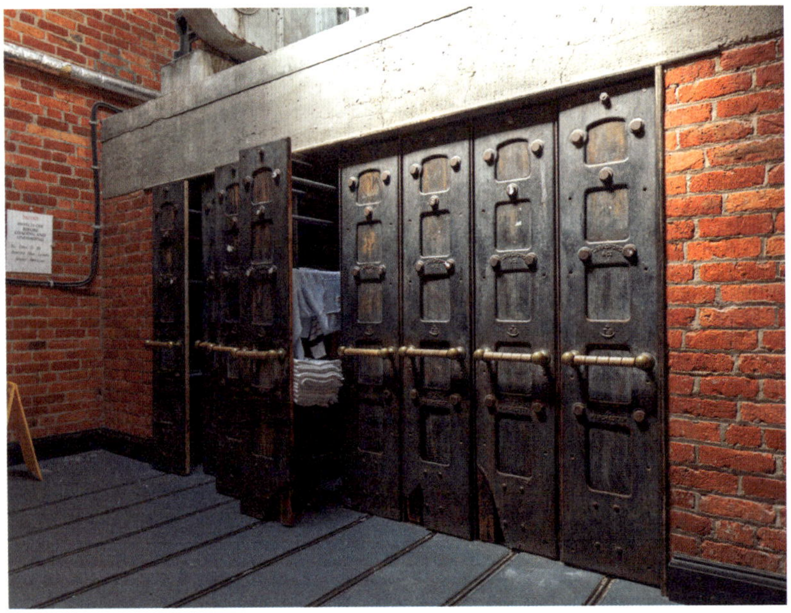

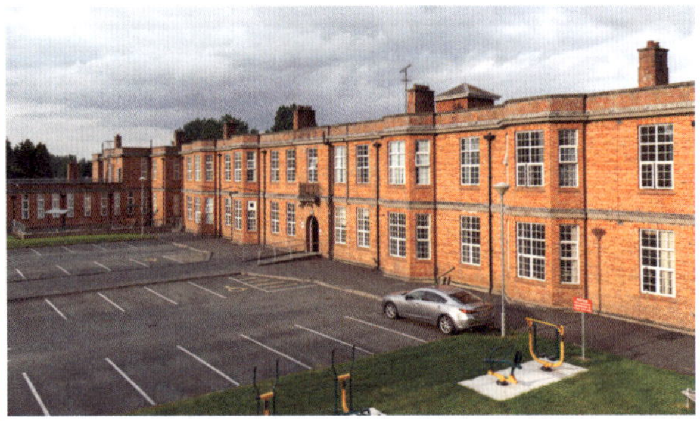

6.02 Ardee: Elevation and sections through administration block and dining / recreation hall, *Image courtesy of the National Archives of Ireland (Office of Public Works Collection, OPW/5HC/4/974,3).*

6.03 Ardee: Hospital laundry equipped with the latest drying equipment, *Photograph by David Killeen, 2019.*

6.04 Ardee: Side entrance to ward block, *Photograph by David Killeen, 2019.*

6.05 Castlerea: High quality terrazzo finishes typical of buildings of this era, *Photograph by David Killeen, 2019.*

6.06 Castlerea: Modest central administration block, with clocktower above and recreation hall behind, *Photograph by David Killeen, 2019.*

6.07 Castlerea: Hospital chapel with squat castellated tower, *Photograph by David Killeen, 2019.*

6.08 Castlerea: Aerial photograph, 1954, with additional buildings added during period of use as TB sanatorium, *Image courtesy of the National Library of Ireland (NPA MOR433).*

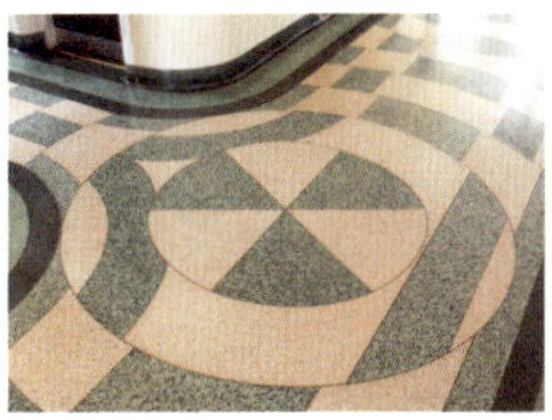

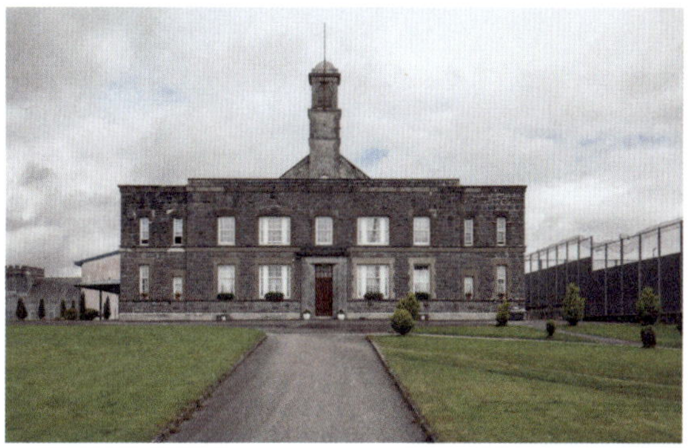

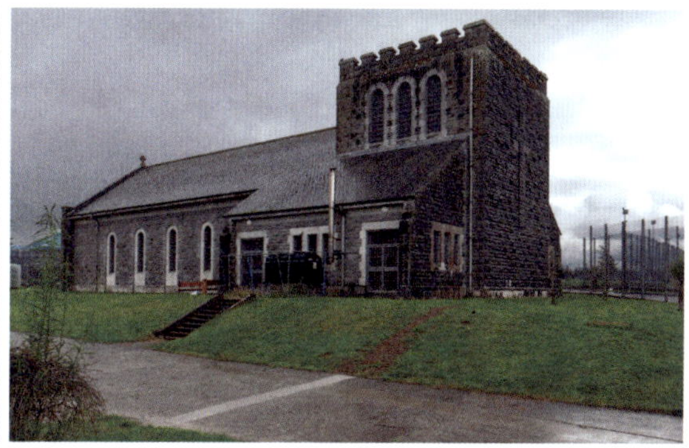

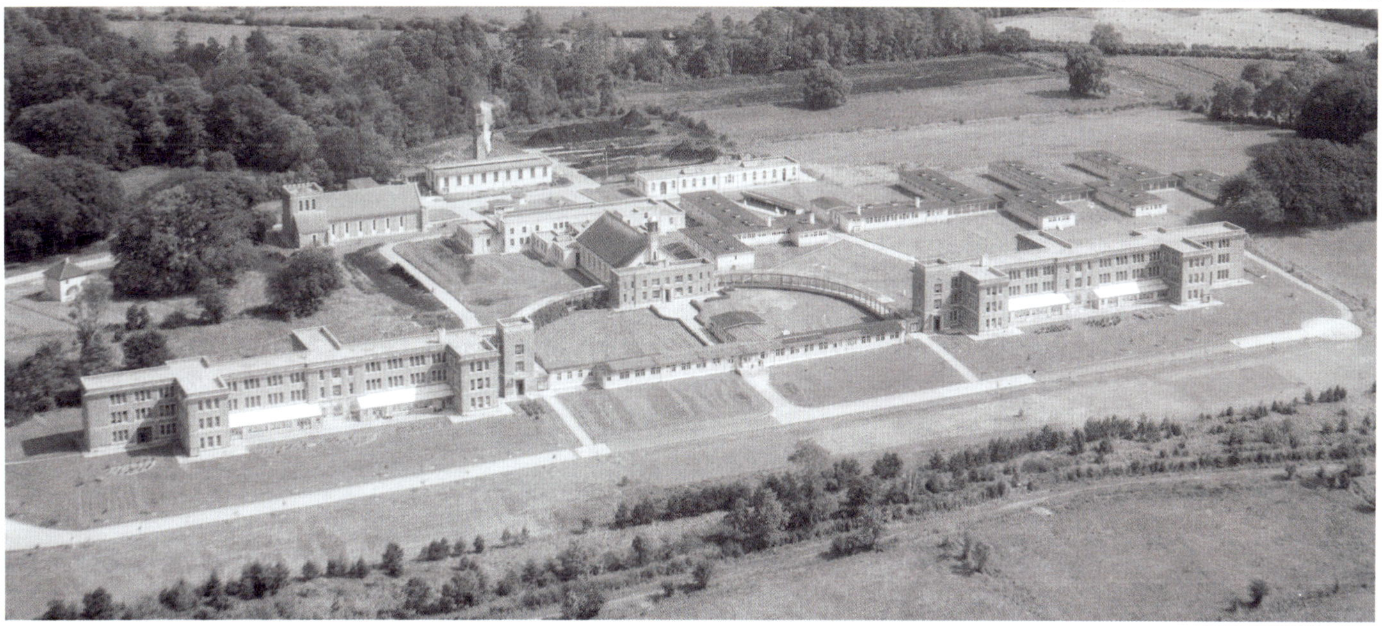

landholdings remote from any general hospital. Their spatial organisation differed little from their Victorian antecedents – symmetrical male and female wards linked to a central administration block, a dining/recreation hall and back-of-house facilities. The architects of both seemed open to the influences of international modernism, yet harked back to traditional motifs, most notably central clocktowers, which had become the obligatory architectural markers of asylumdom.

James Boyd Barrett's design for Castlerea is a curious hybrid of several different architectural impulses. In layout, it feels like a Victorian pavilion-echelon asylum crossed with a Palladian villa; the diagonal link corridors of the former replaced with quadrant-curved, open colonnades of the latter. Boyd Barrett's flat roofed, modernist forms were cloaked in his distinctive conservative attire: rock-faced limestone and enormous sliding-sash windows where one might have expected white render and streamlined metal casements. This was nevertheless a high-quality building whose main architectural shortcoming lay in the diminutive scale of the central block compared to the assertiveness of the projecting ward pavilions. Whereas Boyd Barrett's signature style is evident across numerous mental- and general-healthcare projects of the era, Scottish architect Henry Thomas Wright's design for Ardee is his only known building in either jurisdiction.[18] His was an economic and compact plan, competently executed and detailed in a form that was unmistakably modern, albeit dressed with too many neo-classical details to be considered *modernist*.[19] A muscular clocktower still commands the formal approach, but the overall composition is altogether less domineering than the asylums of old, and a world removed from the legacy buildings of the Richmond and Portrane where Louth patients had heretofore been sent.

Buildings of hope and failure

Wright's Ardee may have outshone Castlerea in both its operational efficiency and its architectural composition, but fell short in the quality of its patient accommodation. The compact plan created few south-facing patient spaces, contrary to the doctrine of maximising sunlight and ventilation that was once again to the fore in an era of rampant tuberculosis. Boyd Barrett, as one of the most prolific healthcare architects of his generation, championed sun-soaked, south-facing patient spaces whether designing for mental health, general health, or tuberculosis, creating buildings that could – and did – migrate between these uses. The 1930s and 40s would see two new building typologies emerge on existing hospital sites, both designed in accordance with the same design principles, but serving radically different purposes, which reflected both the gross failures of the existing system and a continued belief in the elusive goal of treatment and cure.

Tuberculosis had reached such endemic proportions in the damp, overcrowded institutions that the Inspector of Mental Hospitals began to collate separate statistics for TB-related deaths and repeatedly highlighted the need to provide appropriate spaces for the segregation and treatment of infected patients. Whether built as extensions, as at Killarney, or detached structures, as at Limerick, these light-filled TB wards with their south-facing glazed verandas remain, even in dereliction, some of the most pleasant spaces ever built for mental health. But that they were even necessary

18. Henry Thomas Wright in *Dictionary of Scottish Architects*, www.scottisharchitects.org.uk/architect_full.php?id=205393, accessed on 27 Oct. 2019.
19. Wright's organisational layout bears several similarities to the English 'economic asylum' design used by London's Metropolitan Asylums Board at Caterham and Leavesden 50 years earlier. See illustration in Jeremy Taylor, *Hospital and Asylum Architecture in England 1840–1914: Building for Health Care* (London, 1991), p. 142.

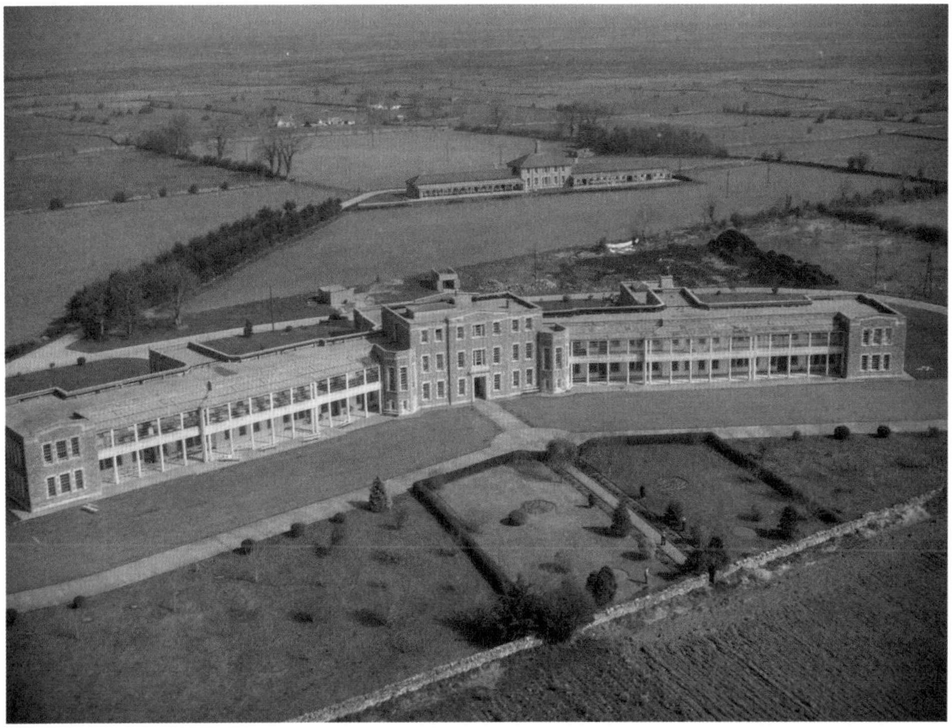

6.09 Ballinasloe: The few new buildings of the mid-twentieth century echoed contemporary sanatoria in promoting health by maximising sunlight and ventilation. *Image courtesy of the National Library of Ireland (NPA MOR1086).*

speaks of the two-fold failure of the institutions: their inability to cure underlying mental illnesses led to patients' long term committal, dwelling in conditions detrimental to their physical health and leading in all too many cases to death from preventable, communicable diseases. And while new vaccines and antibiotics from the late 1940s would succeed in preventing and eventually eradicating TB, progress in the treatment of patients' underlying mental illnesses remained fitful.

The advent of the 'Admissions Hospital' was an altogether more hopeful development. Central government may have failed to bring mental health policy into the twentieth century, but several individual hospital committees – spurred on by reform-minded superintendents – took matters into their own hands. Instead of commissioning another barn-like extension to warehouse yet more patients, new units were created to categorise and treat mental illness in its early, acute stage. Their ambition was to achieve improved cure and discharge rates and ultimately reduce the numbers whose stay would be measured in decades rather than days. The emergence in the 1930s of new medical treatments including insulin coma therapy, malarial therapy, electroconvulsive therapy (only some of which proved effective) was enough to rekindle the hope that mental illness could be treated medically, much like any other physiological disorder, and ultimately cured.

It seems to have been an unspoken rule that the new admissions units would stand apart from the original asylum buildings, albeit usually within the same secure perimeter. Modern architectural language further distinguished them from their parent institution, resulting in buildings akin to contemporary sanatoria – albeit several

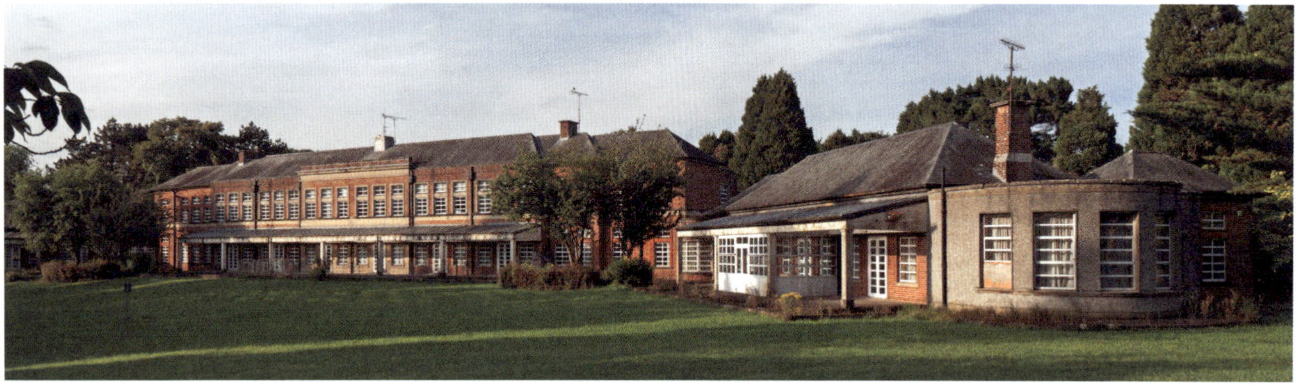

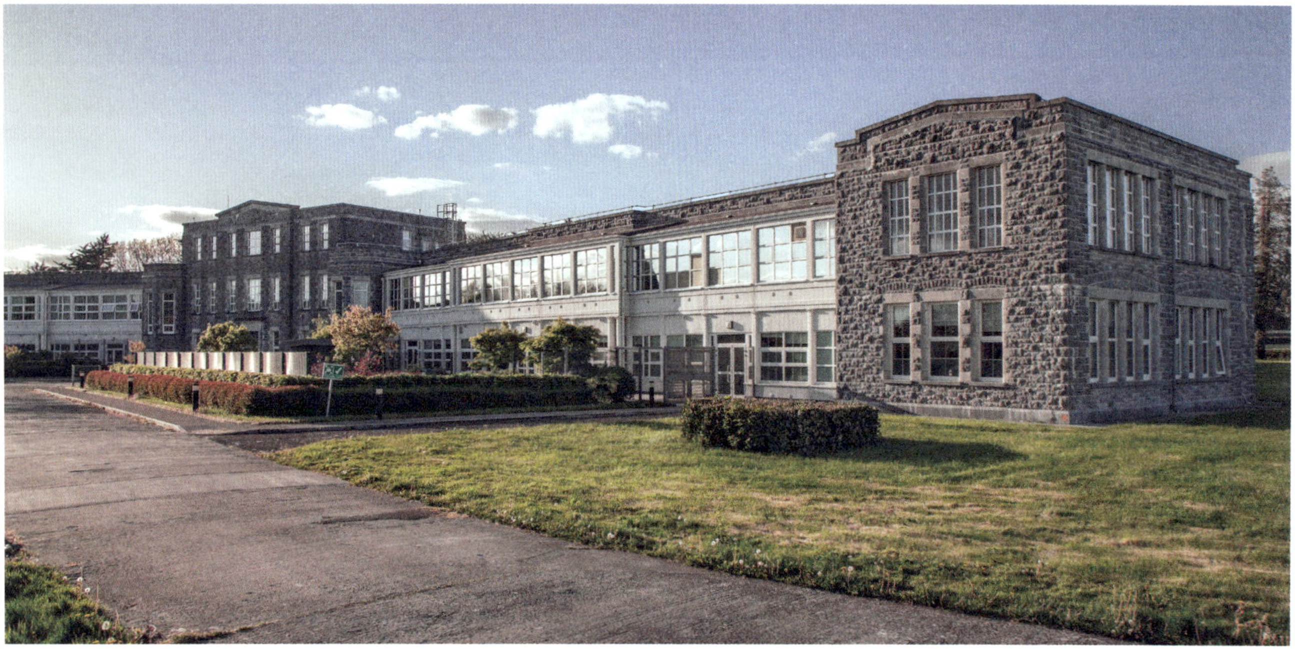

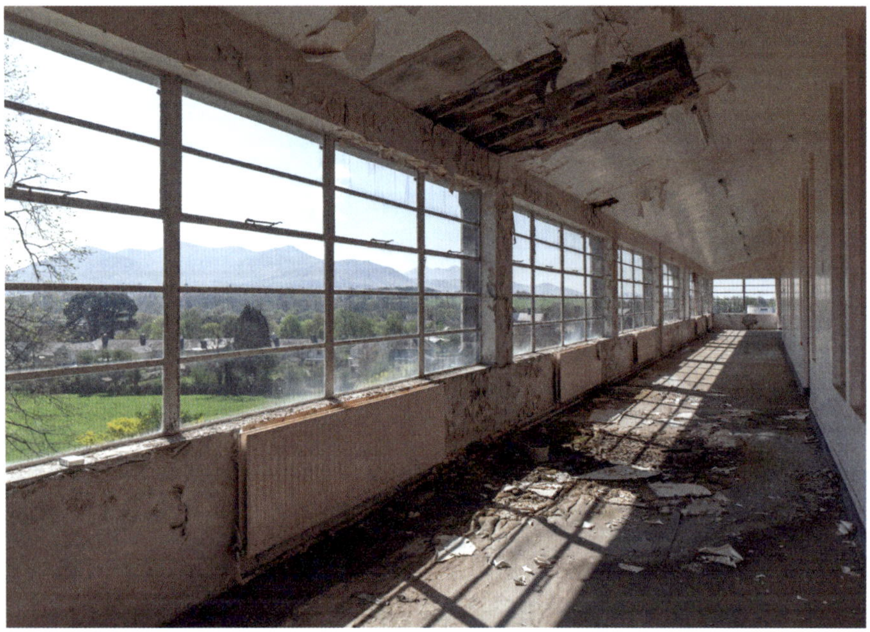

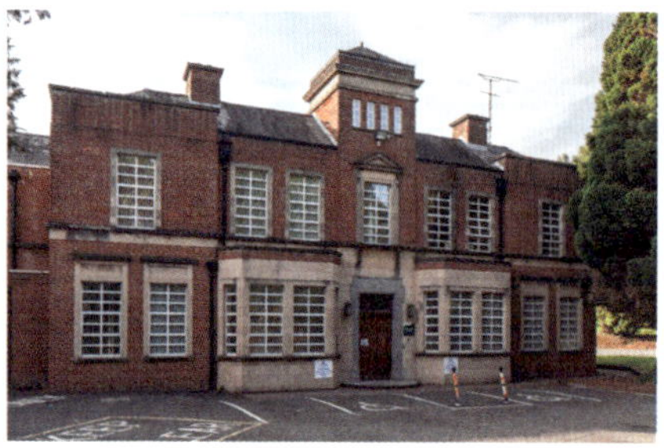

6.10 Monaghan: McLynn's Admissons Hospital is arguably the finest mental health building of the period - the now-familiar details of contemporary sanatorium design married with attractive stone and brick detailing, *Photograph by David Killeen, 2019.*

6.11 Ballinasloe: Boyd Barrett's Admissions Hospital is indistinguishable from contemporary TB sanatoria and general hospitals, *Photograph by David Killeen, 2019.*

6.12 Killarney: Bathed in sunshine and with spectacular views of the Macgillycuddy Reeks, even in dereliction these TB verandahs are amongst the most pleasant spaces to be found in any asylum, *Photograph by David Killeen, 2019.*

6.13 Monaghan: A much-reduced tower still commands the entrance, *Photograph by David Killeen, 2019.*

6.14 Grangegorman: Vincent Kelly's spare and solid nurses home, opened 1938, demolished 2014. A similar block was erected at the nearby Mater Hospital in 1952, demolished 2008, *Image courtesy of TU Dublin, 2012.*

6.15 Ballinasloe: Utilitarian nurses' home, now empty like the hospital it was built to serve, *Photograph by David Killeen, 2019.*

6.16 Monaghan: Nurses home designed in conjunction with new Admissions Hospital, 1940, *Photograph by David Killeen, 2019.*

6.17 Gransha: The quality of accommodation for nurses at the new Gransha Mental Hospital was lauded in the hospital's promotional video, *Image copyright of Terence McDonald Collection, reproduced by kind permission of the McDonald family and the IFI.*

6.18 Gransha: Improved accommodation for staff reflected improvements in their own status, arising from a greater emphasis on training and qualifications, *Image copyright of Terence McDonald Collection, reproduced by kind permission of the McDonald family and the IFI.*

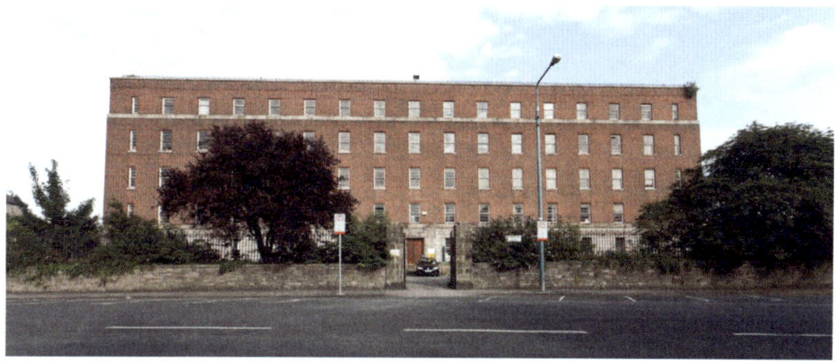

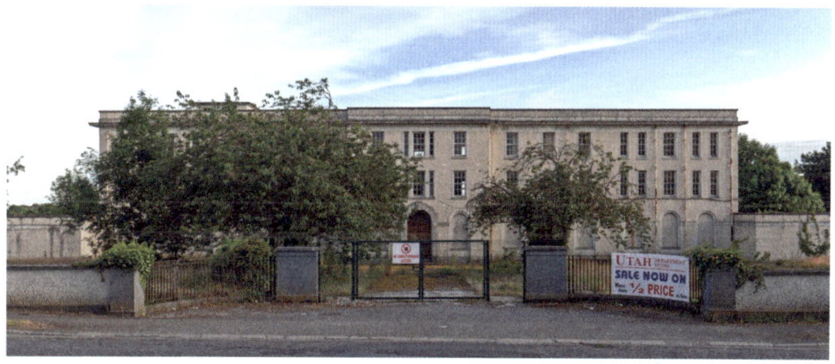

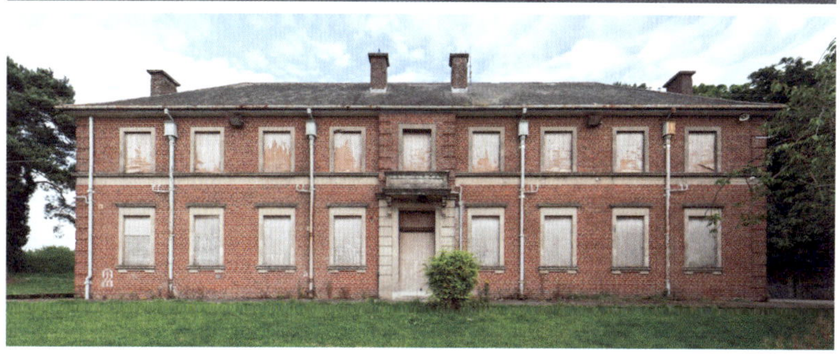

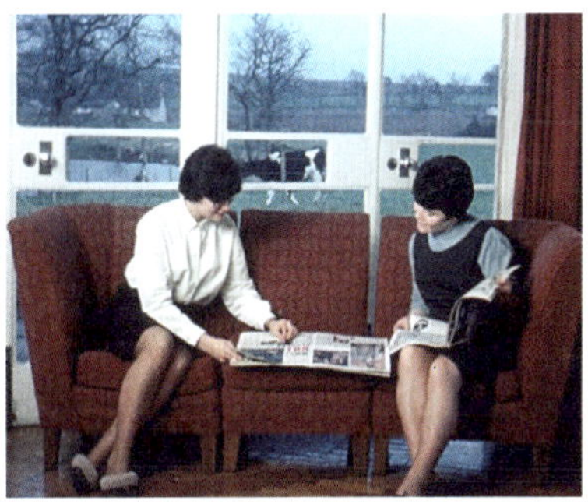

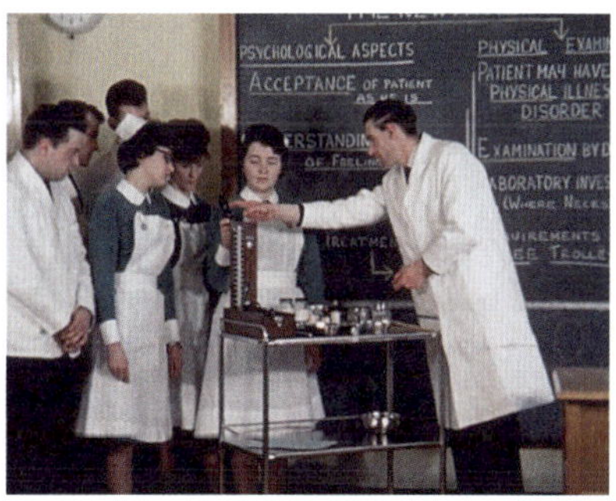

still felt obliged to sport the customary clocktower. Typical features included southerly orientation and cranked plans to maximise solar exposure, glazed verandas, a shallow open-plan layout with high-level clerestory windows to maximise natural cross-ventilation. Significant examples of this typology are found at Sligo, Ballinasloe and most especially Monaghan – buildings of exceptional quality whose internal finishes include decorative terrazzo, inlaid woodblock floors and bespoke ironmongery. These bright, airy, hygienic and distinctively modern hospital buildings must have seemed a world apart from the historically laden structures of the old asylums. They provide built evidence that local initiatives were still possible even in the face of government apathy and decades in advance of official policy.[20]

Nurses' homes and attendants' cottages

In Georgian and Victorian asylums, lower ranking 'keepers' (later known as attendants and nurses) were housed in rooms on the patient wards, a situation that pertained for decades even after their superior officers decanted into their own detached lodgings. The dramatic five-storey towers added at either end of Kilkenny in the 1890s were an early example of purpose built staff quarters, while the miniature town that was Portrane (1899–1903) included separate blocks for male and female staff in the heart of the complex; detached houses for married employees would follow in the 1920s and 30s. At Limerick, a terrace of ten houses for married staff was erected in the 1910s, each provided with their own door through the secure boundary wall; clearly anyone whose family home was dependant on their employment could be trusted not to facilitate an escapee. The years prior to Independence were marked by serious industrial unrest amongst asylum workers seeking better pay and conditions, including several prolonged strikes and, in the celebrated case of Monaghan, the declaration of a workers' soviet.[21] The pay rises achieved would soon be reversed by post-independence austerity, but workers had found their voice, and their influence would eventually lead to the widespread construction of purpose-built staff accommodation from the 1930s through to the 1960s.

It is a central thesis of this book that the quality of buildings is reflective of the priorities of those in power. By this measure, accommodation for subordinate staff appears to have been grudgingly accepted as a necessity rather than celebrated as an expression of pride or progress – even when the Sweepstakes was helping to foot the bill. Most staff blocks are Spartan internally and of limited appeal externally; those at Letterkenny and Monaghan reflected the detailing of the adjacent hospitals while the smattering of classical details are insufficient to relieve the monotony of larger blocks at Ballinasloe and Mullingar. The daddy of them all was Vincent J. Kelly's home for 173 nurses at Grangegorman (1938–40), a monumental five-storey, seventeen-bay brick edifice, which was demolished in 2014 despite being in good condition and potentially adaptable to new uses. Modestly modern nurses' homes at Monaghan (1958) and Portrane (1965) would be amongst the last major buildings erected to serve the old institutional regime, constructed just as the system began its long decline. Interestingly, staff north of the border were forced to suffer inferior lodgings for far longer, with large, purpose-built nurses' homes only beginning to appear there from the 1960s.

20. The published accounts of the period broadly agree that 'nothing much else happened during the first half of the twentieth century' and make no mention of these specific initiatives. Dermot Walsh and Antoinette Daly, *Mental Illness in Ireland 1750–2002: Reflections on the Rise and Fall of Institutional Care* (Dublin, 2004), p. 32; Brendan Kelly, *Hearing Voices: The History of Psychiatry in Ireland* (Dublin, 2014), pp 189–242.

21. Anton McCabe and Ciaran Mulholland, 'The red flag over the asylum: The Monaghan Asylum Soviet of 1919', in Prior, *Asylums, Mental Health Care and the Irish*, pp 23–43. Strikes also took place at Clonmel (1919), Castlebar (1923), and Letterkenny (1924).

Farms, farmyards and farmers

By 1900, the annual reports of the Inspectors of Lunacy could have been mistaken for the accounts of an agri-business conglomerate, including as they did detailed returns for every asylum farm. Receipts were booked for potatoes, root crops, other vegetables, grain, hay and straw, pigs, other livestock, milk, bacon, butcher meat, hides, skins and wools. The nationwide estate had by now expanded to 3,164 acres, giving an average holding of 137 acres per asylum compared to the 10 to 20 acres with which the first asylums had been endowed.[22]

In contrast to the architectural effort invested in some other parts of the asylum, the farmyards built to serve these activities were fairly utilitarian affairs, possessing neither the charm of the vernacular nor the formal trappings encountered on the demesnes and home farms of the gentry. Piggeries – identifiable on historic mapping by the individual enclosed yards for each sow and her litter – were ubiquitous, along with a byre, dairy and stabling for working horses. Portrane and Mullingar both featured unusually extensive and well-designed farm buildings as befitted their larger acreage, but architectural quality has not spared them the slow onset of dereliction experienced by their more modest counterparts. Only the farm buildings at Monaghan and, surprisingly, Dundrum remain in reasonable condition and active agricultural use – the sight of a tractor and freshly cut hay makes the latter feel like an especially exotic survivor deep within the mature suburbs of south Dublin.

If local hospital committees were generally reluctant to spend on patient accommodation during the inter-war period, they made up for it in the purchase of agricultural land; and if the land happened to include an old mansion that could be adapted at minimal cost to accommodate patients, so much the better.[23] The combined landholdings of all asylums on the island stood at 4,182 acres on the eve of Independence; holdings in the Republic alone would expand to peak in excess of 6,846 acres in the 1950s. Farming activities were described as 'a most valuable opportunity for providing a suitable form of occupational therapy for the patients, particularly in this country where so many are engaged in agricultural pursuits in ordinary life'.[24] Experts from Tuke's day onward agreed on the therapeutic value of exercise and fresh air to patient well-being, but it may have been more honest to acknowledge that their labour was also an economically valuable commodity, not just within the asylum, but also when 'farmed out' for a fee to neighbouring farmers.[25] But such discussions of landscape values – whether therapeutic or economic – related almost exclusively to male patients. The most common landscape feature unique to the female side of the house remained the laundry drying ground, and insofar as female patients feature in photographs of asylum landscapes, as often as not they are attending to flapping bedsheets.[26]

For hospital committees of the 1920s, 30s and 40s – on which farmers were usually well represented – the therapeutic value of landscape was secondary to the potential of productive farmland to reduce future operating costs and the burden on the rates.[27] The increasing emphasis on self-sufficiency at local level reflected national policy during the Economic War, but it was during the chronic shortages and rising commodity costs of the Emergency that these commercially motivated acquisitions

22. These accounts would represent a fascinating statistical resource for anybody researching agricultural production and economics through the late nineteenth and early twentieth centuries. *Forty-Ninth Annual Asylum Report 1899*, HC 1900 [312] xxxvii, pp 54–6.
23. A useful means of securing additional accommodation in an era when large mansions were valued at little more than their demolition value; examples of such adaptive reuse include Clonmel's Heywood House, Sligo's Hazelwood House, Dublin's Portrane House, amongst others. See also Emer Crooke, *White Elephants: The Country House and the State in Independent Ireland, 1922–1973* (Dublin, 2018).
24. *Report of the Inspector of Mental Hospitals, 1950*, p. 32.
25. The author's father recalls patients from the local mental hospital assisting with harvest on the family farm in the 1950s, and buttons bearing the name of 'Clonmel Lunatic Asylum' turn up in tillage fields to this day. An anecdote related from another farm described a normally quiet patient working at threshing when, without warning, he threw a pitchfork, javelin-style, at the doctor who visited to supervise proceedings. The doctor escaped unscathed; the implications for the patient's hospital career are not recorded.
26. It is interesting to note that in the absence of male inmates, women at some Mother and Baby Homes undertook agricultural work. *Final Report of the Commission of Investigation into Mother and Baby Homes* (Dublin, 2021), Chapter 5, p. 10, p. 16 Chapter 19, pp 4–5. See also Oonagh Walsh, 'Landscape and the Irish asylum', in Úna Ní Bhroiméil and Glenn Hooper (eds), *Land and Landscape in Nineteenth Century Ireland* (Dublin, 2008), p. 165
27. This sentiment is consistently echoed throughout Inspectors' annual reports and hospital minutes as cited in individual institutional histories. With less evidence but no less certainty, I might also credit the irresistible compulsion, innate within every Irish farmer, to purchase land adjacent to their own whenever the opportunity arises.

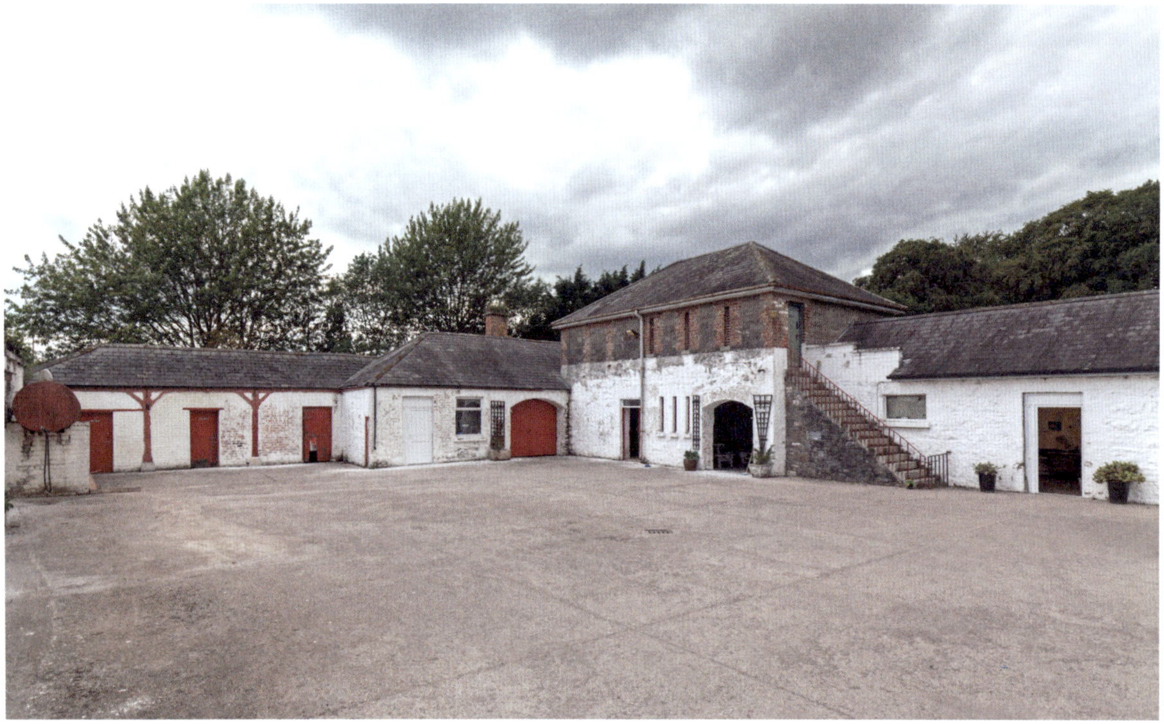

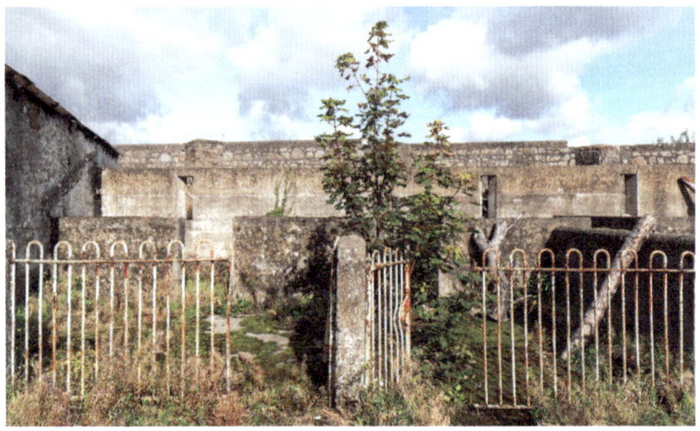

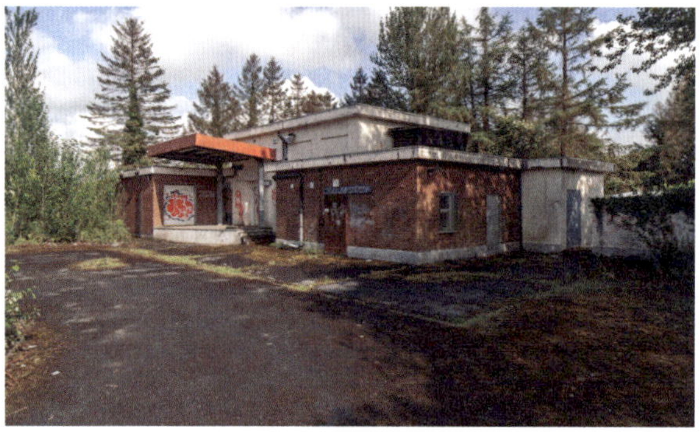

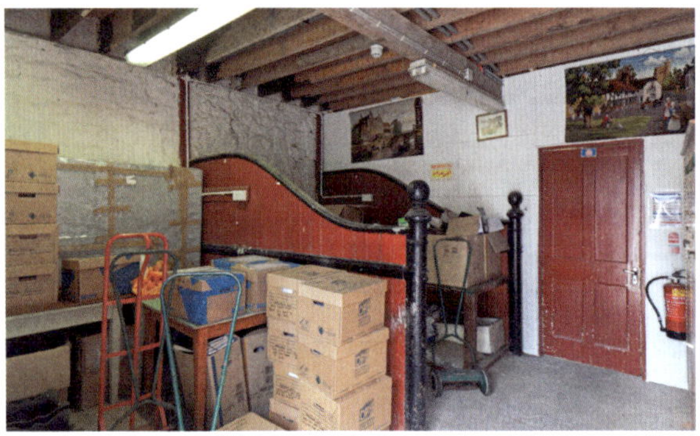

6.19 Monaghan: Farmyard was planned and built in parallel with the main asylum and remains in good condition, *Photograph by David Killeen, 2019.*

6.20 Dundrum: A range of nineteenth and twentieth century farm buildings survive on site. The later piggeries have lost their roofs but retain their arrangement of separate yards for each sow, *Photograph by David Killeen, 2019.*

6.21 Portlaoise: Many hospitals added their own abbatoirs to butcher meat raised on their own farms, *Photograph by David Killeen, 2019.*

6.22 Monaghan: Interior fittings are a rare survival, *Photograph by David Killeen, 2019.*

6.23 Cork: Cultivating vegetables on such steeply sloping ground must have been back-breaking work, 1955, *Image courtesy of the National Library of Ireland (NPA MOR979).*

6.24 Grangegorman: In the midst of the capital city lay a productive landsape of hay meadows, tilled fields and orchards, 1955, *Image courtesy of the National Library of Ireland (NPA MOR1490).*

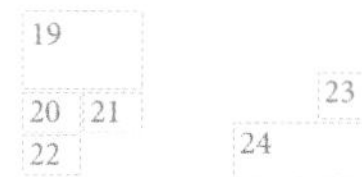

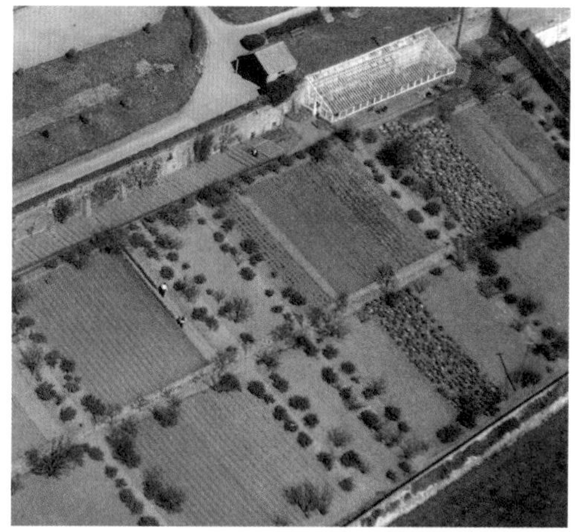

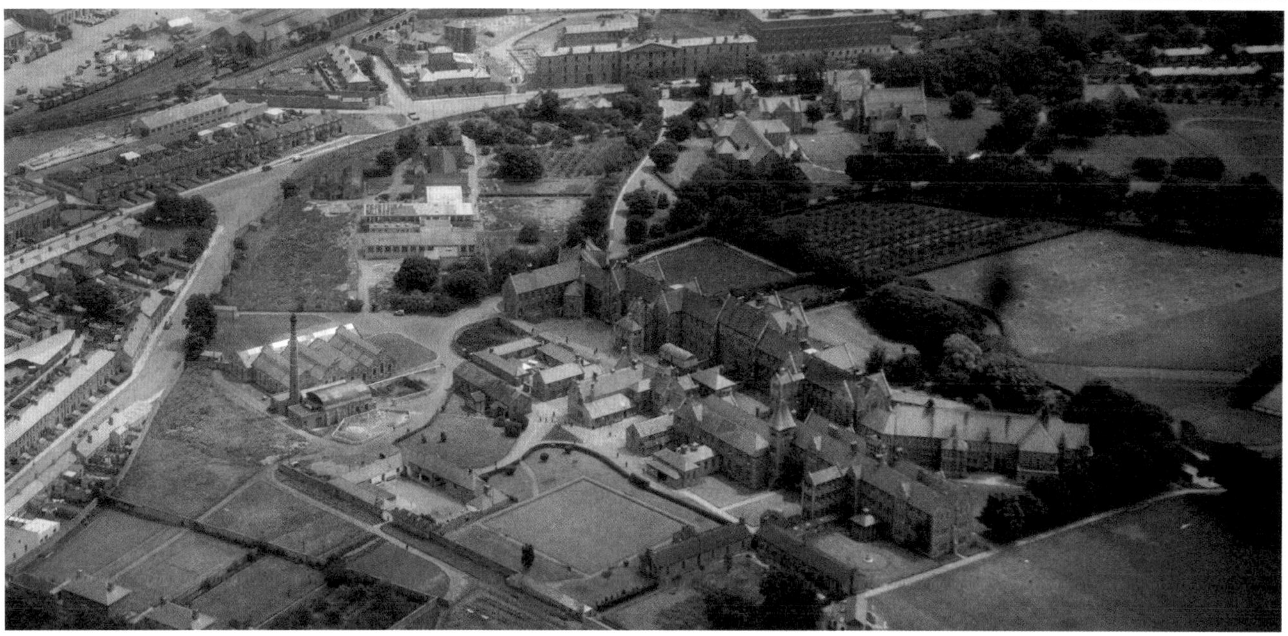

truly did benefit the patients. Not being a high political priority at the best of times, the mental hospitals risked being near the bottom of a long list of competing interest groups had they been entirely reliant on the discretion or goodwill of the Minister for Supplies.[28] But endowed with large, productive farms and plentiful labour, the hospitals were able to maintain good standards of nutrition, while many boilers were converted to burn turf cut from their own bogs.[29] Even as improvement projects on the core hospital buildings slowed to a halt, the hospital farms during the 1940s bustled with construction activity, with new silos and stores, cattle-fattening sheds and piggeries, dairies and abattoirs further boosting their already impressive food production capabilities.[30] Where the institutional landscapes had once been carefully cultivated to create an image of gentility, the priority now was to cultivate its way towards self-sufficiency, and beyond.

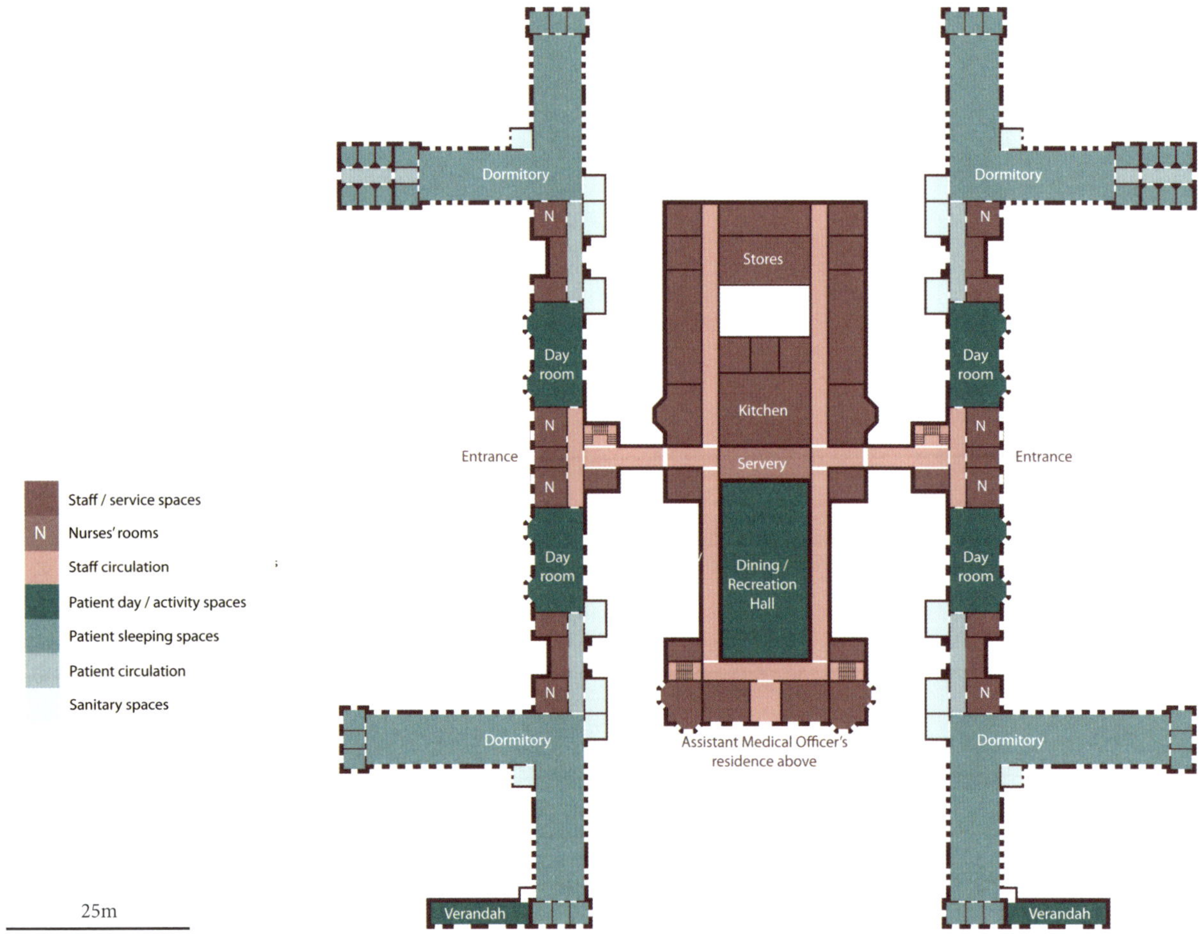

6.25 Plan diagram of Ardee Mental Hospital with key uses annotated. A compact and economic plan of 8 wards arranged around a central spine. *Drawn by the author.*

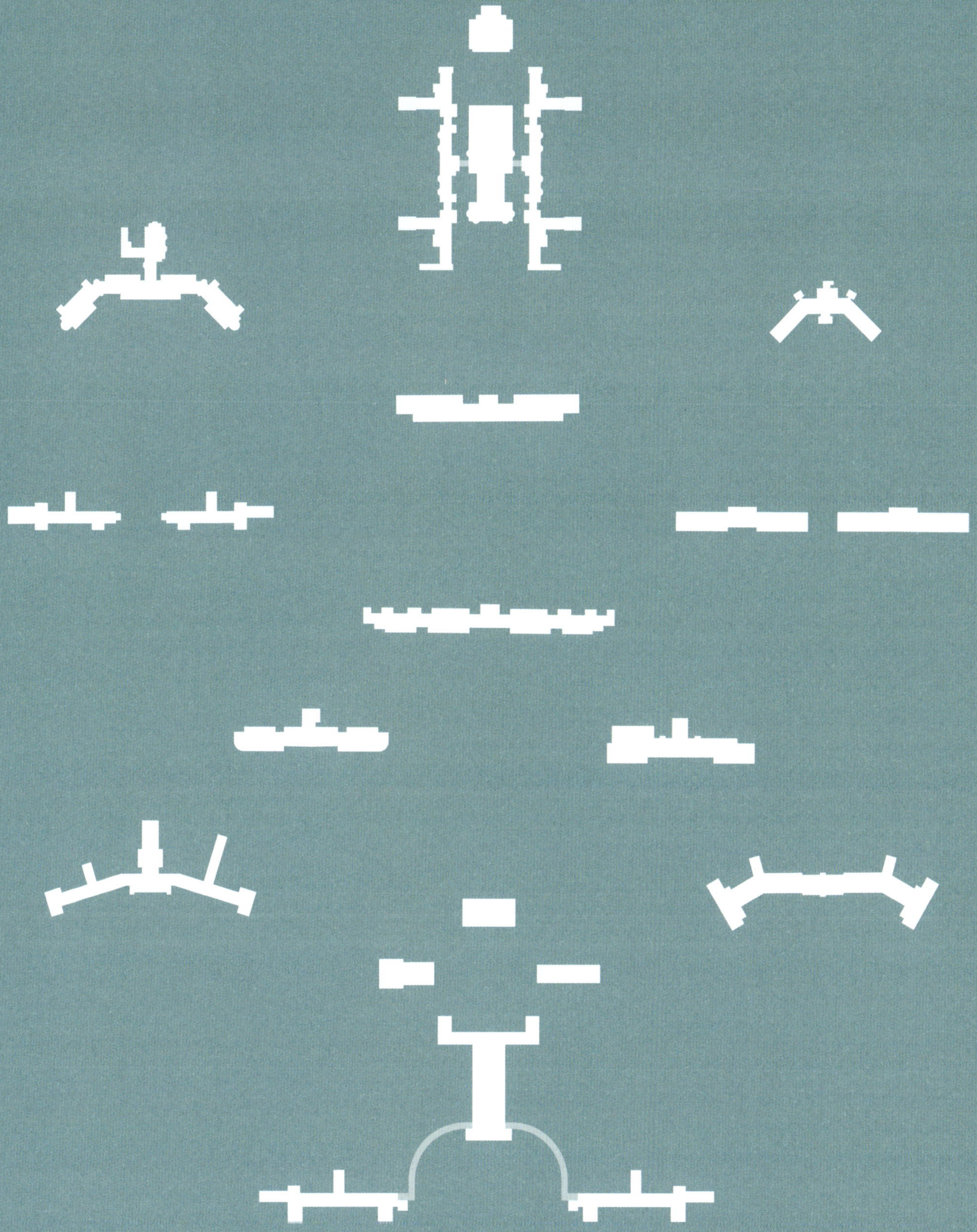

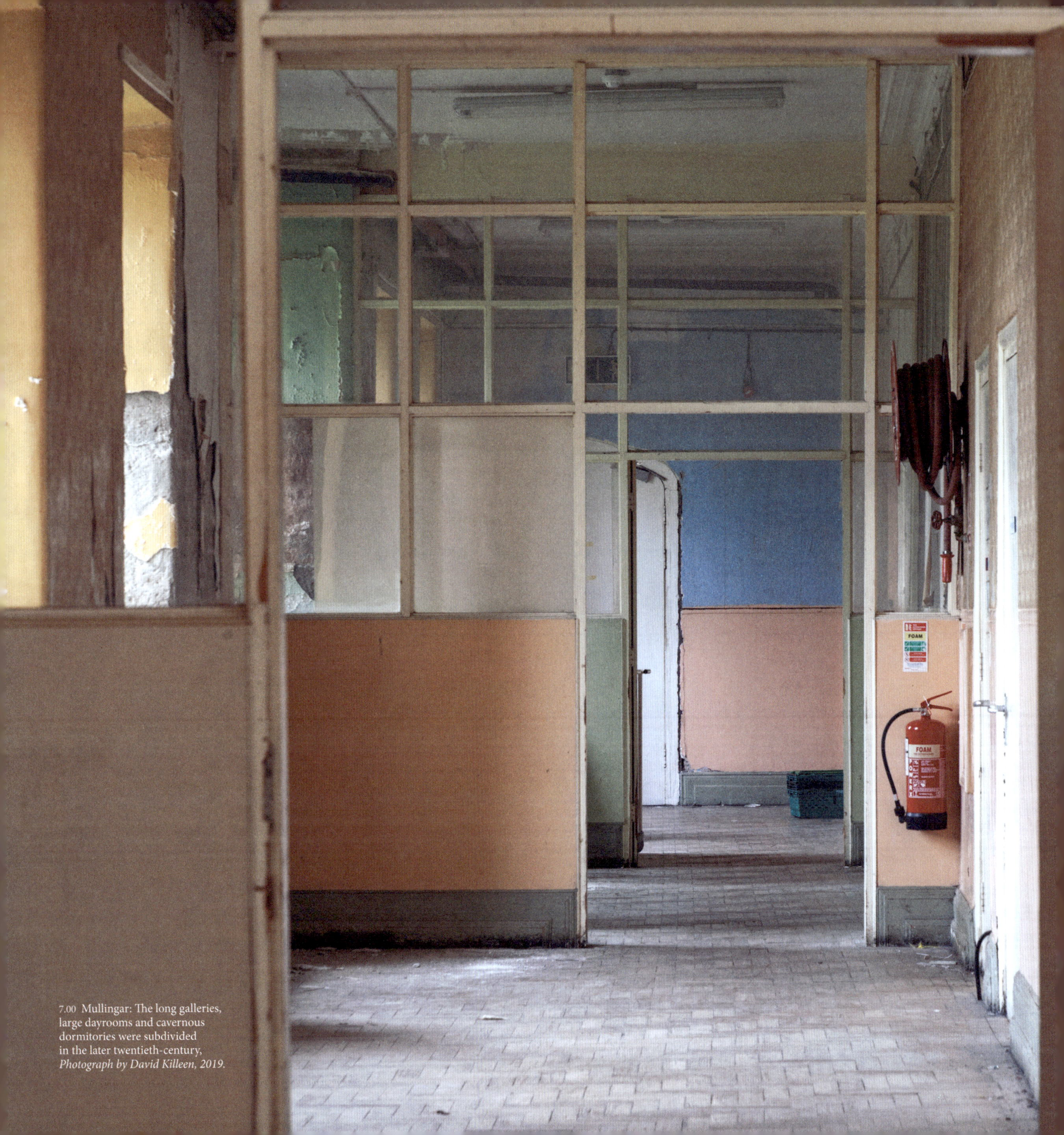

7.00 Mullingar: The long galleries, large dayrooms and cavernous dormitories were subdivided in the later twentieth-century, *Photograph by David Killeen, 2019.*

Continuous Progress, Intermittently

unsuitable in design and lacking facilities for the proper treatment of patients [1]

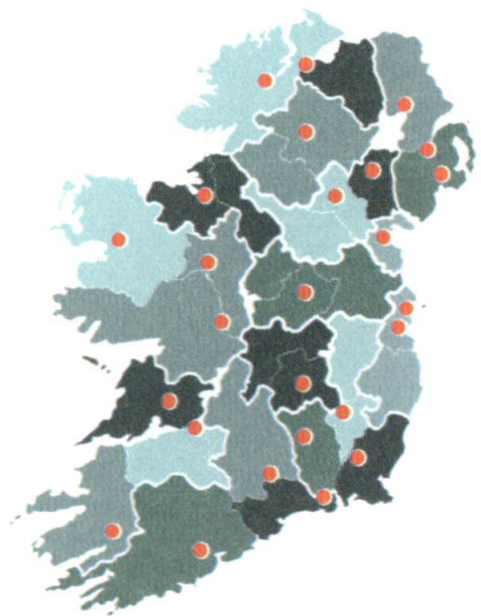

Mental hospital distribution in Ireland, 1945, *Drawn by the author.*

Whatever one's views on the motives underlying nineteenth-century insanity law or the desirability of its outcomes, the very quantity of legislation indicates that it was at least accorded a higher priority than in the twentieth century.[2] Almost half a century would pass before the long overdue reform of Ireland's archaic lunacy law, in the form of the 1945 Mental Treatment Act, would come to pass.[3] The legislation finally broke the link between the judicial system and insanity. Henceforth admissions – whether temporary, voluntary or compulsory – were dependant on medical certification in accordance with internationally standardised criteria.[4] The continued detention of compulsory patients would also become subject to periodic review, placing at least a theoretical check on the all-too-common incidence of life residency in a mental institution. The nineteenth-century language of lunacy too was reformed – medical terms replaced references to lunatics, idiots and imbeciles, attendants became nurses, and inmates became patients.[5] The reform was necessary and welcome, but tweaking a running tap while leaving the stopper in place can only slow the rate at which a vessel fills, not reduce its contents. And so the population of the Republic of Ireland's public mental hospitals continued to grow, peaking in 1958 at 21,075, at which point the country had the dubious boast of the highest per capita provision of psychiatric beds in the world, ahead of the USSR and the USA. Northern Ireland and Scotland occupied fourth and fifth places – perhaps the only league table before or since where three Celtic nations ranked shoulder-to-shoulder with global superpowers.[6] As will be seen in the coming chapters, the institutional system had acquired a life and a logic of its own, which would take more than legislation, commissions and reports to change.

Apogee...

It is sometimes difficult to reconcile conflicting views of life in an Irish mental hospital as the system reached its apogee in the 1950s. The benign view lauds a system of self-

1. *Report of the Commission of Inquiry on Mental Illness* (hereafter *1966 Commission Report*) (Dublin, 1966), p. 22.
2. Prior cites 20 statutes affecting mental disorder in the Republic of Ireland between 1800 and 1899; the 1945 Mental Treatment Act was only the third of five in the twentieth century. Pauline M. Prior 'Mental health law on the island of Ireland, 1800–2010', in Pauline M. Prior (ed.), *Asylums, Mental Health Care and the Irish 1800–2010* (Dublin, 2012), pp 317–18.
3. Mental Treatment Act 1945, No. 19 of 1945. Similar legislation passed 13 and 15 years earlier in Northern Ireland and England, respectively.
4. *Report of the Inspector of Mental Hospitals, 1977–1979*, pp 38–40; Damien Brennan, *Irish Insanity, 1800–2000* (Oxon, 2014), pp 96–8.
5. Prior, 'Mental Health Law on the Island of Ireland', p. 326.
6. Brennan, *Irish Insanity*, p. 9, p. 33, p. 120.

7. *Report of the Inspector of Mental Hospitals, 1950*, p.32, p. 60. A further 905 acres occupied by buildings, airing courts and woods brought the total landholding of the national asylum estate in the Republic to 6,846 acres.
8. Annie Ryan, *Walls of Silence* (Callan, 1999), p. 17.
9. Gillian McClelland, 'Speedwell Magazine: An insider view of Holywell Psychiatric Hospital, Antrim, 1959–1973', in Prior, *Asylums, Mental Health Care and the Irish*, pp 44–73.
10. Dermot Dwyer, (ed.), *St. Finan's Hospital Killarney: A Medical, Social & Sporting History 1852–2002* (Killarney, 2002), pp 55–9, 95–6.

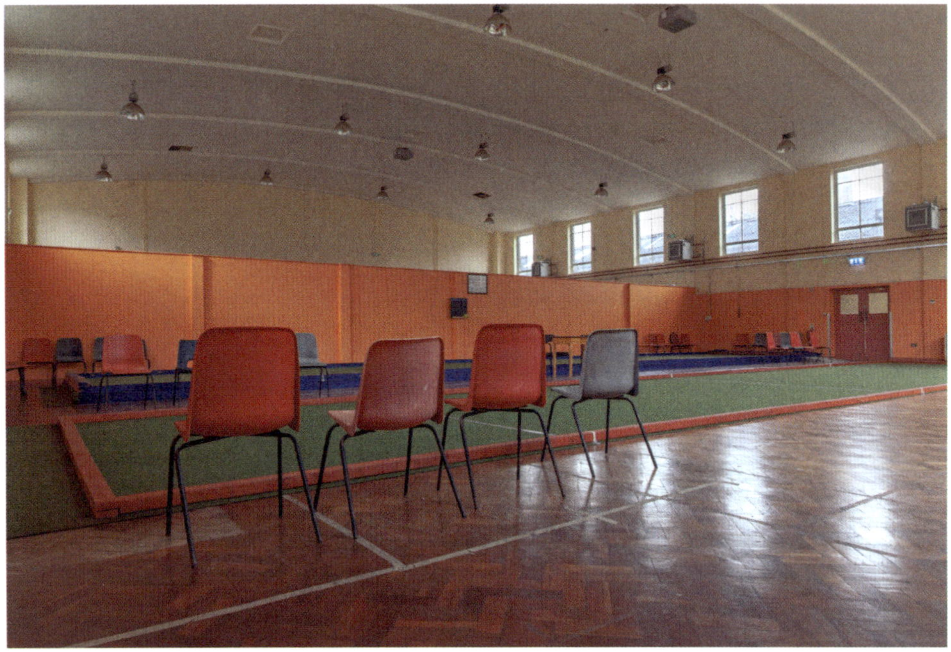

7.01 Kilkenny: Of the vast 1950s recreation halls built at Carlow, Portlaoise and Kilkenny, only the latter still serves something approaching its original function, *Photograph by David Killeen, 2019.*

sufficiency that was operating to its maximum potential with almost 6,000 acres under grass or cultivation, producing cereals, milk, meat, fruit and vegetables.[7] Patients who were willing and able to do so worked on the farm, in the laundry, or in workshops producing most of the requisites for use within the institution, including clothes, shoes and furniture. While the primary focus was on basic necessities, there were occasional tidings of comfort and joy: 'At Christmas in Portrane they had so many chrysanthemums in their glasshouses that the nurses were able to decorate all the wards with richly coloured blooms.'[8]

Extracts from hospital magazines of the time offer the 'official' account, portraying social clubs, concerts and weekly dances played by local or touring show-bands, cinema screenings, and seaside outings with packed picnics for patients.[9] Victorian dining halls on several sites were replaced by vast hangar-like recreation halls, complete with stages for drama productions and cinema screenings, and sprung sports floors designed for dancing, basketball and badminton. The wider landscape also offered outlets for those of more active disposition. Tennis courts and bowling greens appeared on many sites from the late nineteenth century, while the growth of the Gaelic Athletic Association (GAA) would see handball alleys added to the mix early in the twentieth. Full-size playing pitches attest to hospital populations sufficiently large, youthful, and (physically) healthy to sustain Gaelic football teams – gradually displacing soccer or cricket, which remained popular in Northern Ireland – with both staff and patient teams competing in inter-hospital competitions.[10] Pitch and putt courses were established on many hospital grounds in the 1960s, several of which remain in public use to this day. Indeed, life in a

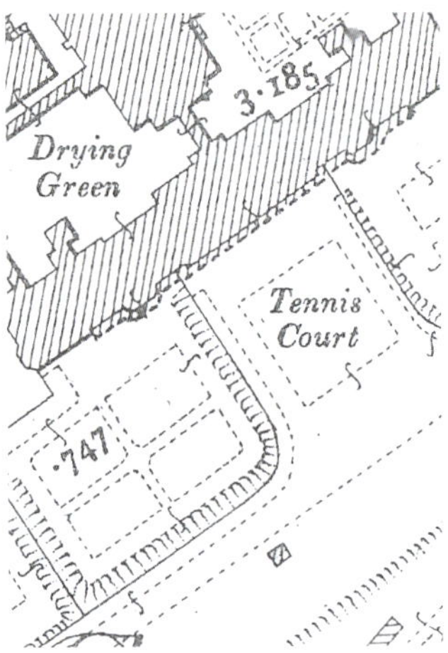

7.02 Monaghan: Tennis court to the south of the asylum building, separated from the adjacent airing yards by ha-has., *Reproduced courtesy Trinity College Dublin (OS-Monaghan-2500-Sheet 9:11-1908).*

district mental hospital – or rather, life for patients in better hospitals whose co-operation with the system earned them such privileges – was arguably a more sociable existence than that open to many in 1950s Ireland, and bore comparison to the pattern of life in a respectable boarding school or enclosed religious order. And given that both latter types of institution were home to many more people than the mental hospitals at their peak, we are reminded that voluntary submission to the discipline of an enclosed community was a relatively common lifestyle in mid-century Ireland – before even considering those less willingly confined in laundries, industrial schools and the like.[11]

Later developments within the walls reflected society without. As the cultural dominance of the Catholic church reached its zenith, all of the hospitals in the Republic underwent yet another rebranding, in keeping with the 'general sanctification… of every phase of personal, social and national life'.[12] And just as the Catholic bishops exhorted parishes to erect shrines to commemorate the Marian year of 1954,[13] hospital committees, staff and patients would proudly erect their own grottoes within the walls, with attractive examples surviving at Carlow, Mullingar, Kilkenny and Castlebar. Needless to say, institutions in Northern Ireland proved less fertile terrain for such conspicuous displays of Catholic piety, but some did look to the heavens for other forms of diversion, with enclosed aviaries found at Downpatrick and Armagh. The irony of the caged patients deriving therapeutic benefit from gazing at caged birds cannot have been lost on anybody.

And nadir

At the same time, conditions in some hospitals, or parts thereof, had fallen closer to what might be expected of a nineteenth-century workhouse. The modern reader may observe that the mental hospital was not the only major institution capable of perpetuating and concealing a range of abuses whilst at the height of its powers.[14] What is remarkable, however, is that the sector was already the subject of a long tradition of independent oversight in the form of the Inspector of Mental Hospitals. This office succeeded the Inspectors of Lunacy who had in turn assumed these duties from the Inspector of Prisons under the 1845 act. Collectively these bodies had generated well over a century of annual reports in almost unbroken run. The Inspectors did generally succeed in protecting patients from overt abuses while championing the continuous improvement of their amenities and physical comfort, even if they may justifiably be accused of complicity in the perpetuation of a deeply flawed institutional system that was itself a source of harm for many.[15] Yet the truth of conditions of some hospitals in the 1950s would prove so inconvenient to the body politic that this valuable safeguard would itself be side-lined.

The rot may be seen to begin in the 1959 Inspector's Report, where the traditional practice of providing a detailed, if understated, narrative on the conditions in every hospital was eschewed in favour of a generic, high-level commentary.[16] This shift also coincided with suppression of a special report on the Clonmel District Mental Hospital, which identified conditions that would have been unacceptable a century earlier:

11. Membership of religious communities reached 29,984 in 1967; most lived in congregated, and often enclosed, settings prior to the reforms of the Second Vatican Council. The numbers in boarding schools easily exceeded this number. Daithí Ó Corráin, 'Catholicism in Ireland, 1880–2016: Rise, Ascendancy and Retreat' (Unpublished draft paper, 2018), p. 732, www.researchgate.net/publication/325486860_Catholicism_in_Ireland_1880-2015_Rise_Ascendancy_and_Retreat, accessed 02 Nov. 2020.
12. Several hospitals in Northern Ireland were also renamed, but only Armagh was named for a saint. Louise Fuller, *Irish Catholicism Since 1950: The Undoing of a Culture* (Dublin, 2004), p. 24.
13. Ibid, p. 29.
14. After troubling reports have laid bare the harsh institutional regimes in Ireland's industrial schools, Magdalen Laundries and Mother and Baby Homes, it remains to be seen whether similar inquiries will one day be directed at the shortcomings of the mental hospital system.
15. Prior offers a useful overview of the role and concerns of the inspectorate and Brennan points to their role in advocating and perpetuating the system, but their anomalous role as independent watchdog, ex-officio board members of every local asylum board, and advocates of policy to power, could usefully be subjected to further study. Pauline M Prior, 'Overseeing the Irish Asylums: The Inspectorate in Lunacy, 1845–1921', in Prior, *Asylums, Mental Health Care and the Irish*, pp 221–45; Brennan, *Irish Insanity*, pp 63–4.
16. *Report of the Inspector of Mental Hospitals, 1959.*

> *In the kitchen, cabbage is taken out of the boiler by means of an ordinary farm-yard fork… it is then chopped up with a garden edging tool. The potatoes for patients are mashed and distributed in ordinary zinc buckets.' [The patients were put to bed at 6.30 in the evening]: '…patients undress in the day room downstairs. They then make their way up a stone staircase to the dormitories… they have no clothing on them except their day shirts and in several cases they are naked.*[17]

While Department officials in 1958 failed to remedy the situation, they did succeed in keeping the contents of the report secret – even from members of the local committee responsible for funding and running the hospital. This decision was ostensibly taken to prevent the contents causing 'great distress to the relatives of patients who were in the hospital' – the distress to the patients themselves seemingly of secondary importance.[18]

If even the Inspector was silenced, there was little chance of the voice of individual patients being heard. With few exceptions the succession of individual hospital histories published over the last three decades perpetuated the official, staff-centric view of their respective institutions, making the rare first-hand accounts of two women, Hannah Greally and Kate Millett, especially valuable. Greally's recollections of her almost 20 years as a patient in St Loman's, Mullingar dwell less on physical privations than on the unremitting monotony, despair and hopelessness of being powerless in a situation not of one's making:

> *I thought of people in prison, they at least knew their sentences. I had gone into hospital for a 'rest' and look at the 'rest' – fourteen years gone already, and very little rest at that… for I cannot leave, legally, without their help. I would soon become another dependant in the Legion of the Lost… a life prisoner… It was a deadly monotonous routine of work, sleep, eat… I had sewn thousands of garments, and ironed thousands of shirts, among other things, yet I seemed no nearer liberty than when I did my first days work, gratis.*[19]

Millett – already a veteran of involuntary sojourns in several American psychiatric institutions – offers an even more striking description of the material and intellectual poverty of the institutional regime that pertained in Our Lady's Hospital, Ennis. Her status as a university professor and celebrated writer was no defence against the dehumanising and debilitating effects of an institutional regime where, as late as the 1980s, the patient was expected to meekly comply with the dictates of unaccountable authority whose methods of control now also included a range of pharmaceuticals.[20] Millett and Greally both evinced a genuine terror of never again seeing freedom, and while both were discharged – after weeks and years respectively – the sad fate of many with whom they shared a ward validated their fears. During a 2014 visit to one hospital, the author's attention was drawn to an elderly gentleman who was admitted in 1947 and whose life spent behind the walls spanned 40% of that institution's long history.[21]

17. Report cited in Ryan, *Walls of Silence*, p. 26.
18. Ibid.
19. Hanna Greally, *Bird's Nest Soup* (Cork, 1987), p. 95, p. 117, pp 122–3.
20. Millett, Kate. *The Loony-Bin Trip* (New York, 1990).
21. The gentleman in question would have been admitted under the provisions of the new Mental Treatment Act that came into effect on 1 January 1947. If he had been referred just a few months earlier, it is statistically likely that his admission would have been made under the provisions of the 1867 Lunacy Act and hence warranted a claim to being Ireland's last living 'dangerous lunatic'. The safe distance from which we usually ponder such uncomfortable aspects of our history compresses dramatically when we consider that in the second decade of the twenty-first century, it still remained possible to meet living witnesses to the effects of involuntary detention under such a flawed legislative relic of Victorian social paranoia.

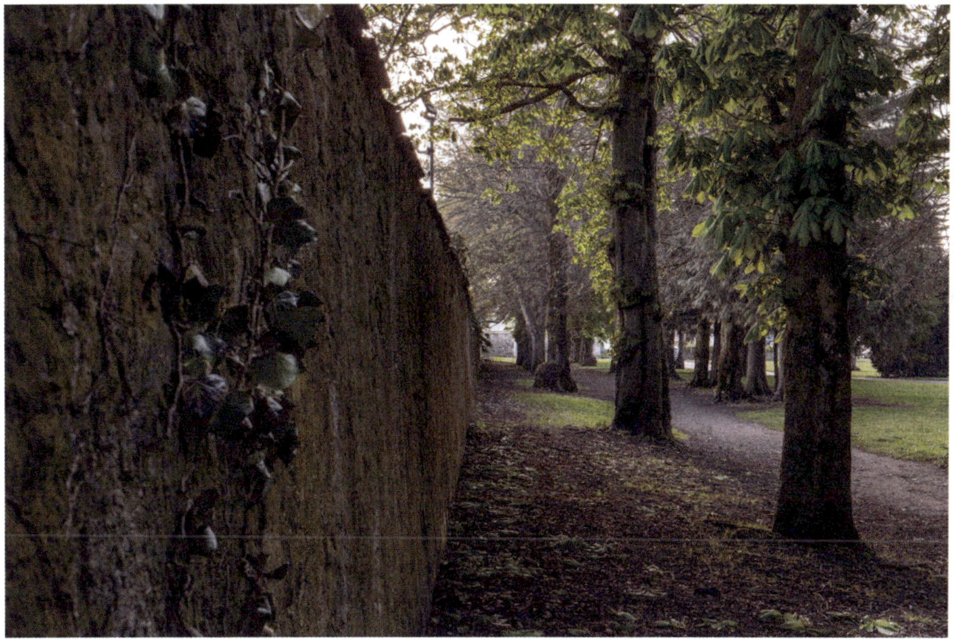

7.03 Carlow: A stretch of wall standing to original height with mature boundary woodland, *Photograph by David Killeen, 2019*

Falling walls

For most of their existence, the asylum wall was the most visible manifestation of the institution, enclosing and defining a place apart, both physically and psychologically. The wall served an explicit function of safely protecting the insane from the taunts and cruelties of an intolerant world outside, and an implicit function of protecting the world from the insane securely contained within.[22] Whichever motivation held the upper hand, the net effect was the same. Generations grew up regarding those who dwelt behind the asylum walls as potentially dangerous 'others'. Of course, asylum planners were not alone in presuming walls to be indispensable to the maintenance of institutional order within and moral order without; McKeith describes the erection of the boundary wall as an essential prerequisite to the opening of new Catholic seminaries in the nineteenth century,[23] while into the 1950s, the Catholic hierarchy still argued that the ideal situation for a Mother and Baby Home was somewhere 'quiet, remote and surrounded by high boundary walls'.[24]

As asylum lands expanded, minor feats of civil engineering were required to maintain the secure perimeter of the institution. Tunnels to connect newly acquired lands were excavated below the public road at Grangegorman and Londonderry and beneath the railway at Limerick; at Clonmel two tunnels, a 500-foot sunken walkway and an iron footbridge would be needed to maintain security as the complex sprawled across the town's western environs.[25] But from the 1950s, a generation of reforming RMSs, empowered by the success of new treatments, finally challenged the carceral imperative. In 1950 all but four district mental hospitals were already conducting regular outpatient clinics beyond the walls, at county and local hospitals.[26] Between 1955 and 1965 gates were unlocked and sections of boundary wall were lowered or demolished on almost every site around the country.[27] At Portlaoise the

22. Even the humanitarian Samuel Tuke did not question the necessity for a secure boundary around the asylum estate, but did argue for greater subtlety in its construction: '…the boundary should be so contrived as to intercept, as little as possible, the view of the surrounding country.' Samuel Tuke, *Practical Hints on the Construction and Economy of Pauper Lunatic Asylums* (London, 1815), p. 52.
23. Martin McKeith, 'The architectural development of the Irish diocesan major seminary – from 1782 to 1900' (unpublished MUBC Thesis, 2012).
24. *Final Report of the Commission of Investigation into Mother and Baby Homes*, (Dublin, 2021) p. 10.
25. For Limerick, see: *Fifty-Second Annual Asylum Report 1902*, HC 1903 [1762] xxvii, p. 32. The purchase and conversion in 1877 of the former House of Industry as an auxiliary asylum provided a cheap and ultimately unsatisfactory solution to Clonmel's accommodation needs, but necessitated over £3,000 of civil works to link the two. Eamon Lonergan, *St Luke's Hospital Clonmel 1834–1984* (Thurles, 1984), pp 32–3.
26. *Report of the Inspector of Mental Hospitals, 1950.*
27. Joe McDermott, *St Mary's Hospital Castlebar: Serving Mayo Mental Health from 1866* (Castlebar, 1999), p. 154; Lonergan, *St Luke's Hospital Clonmel*, p. 77.

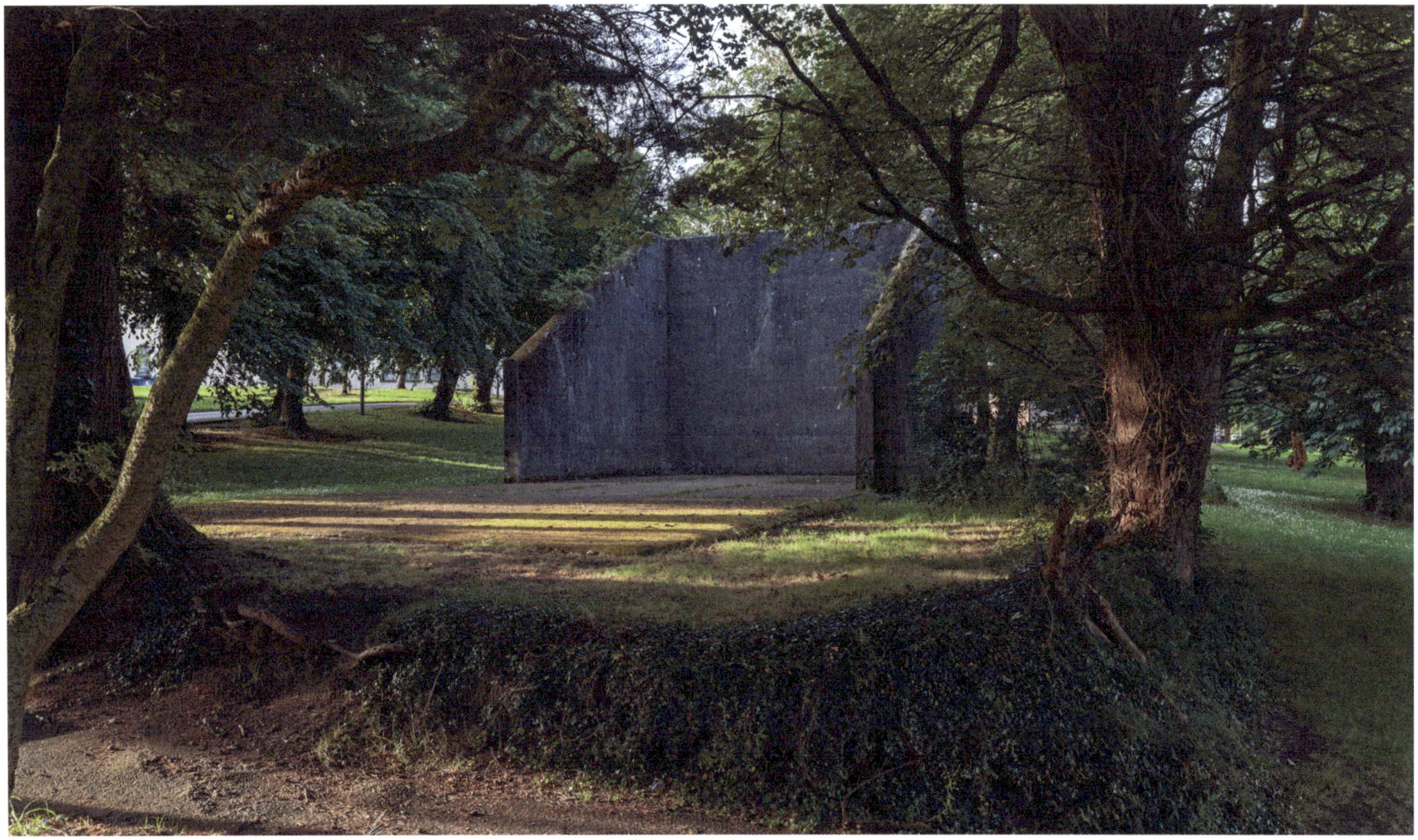

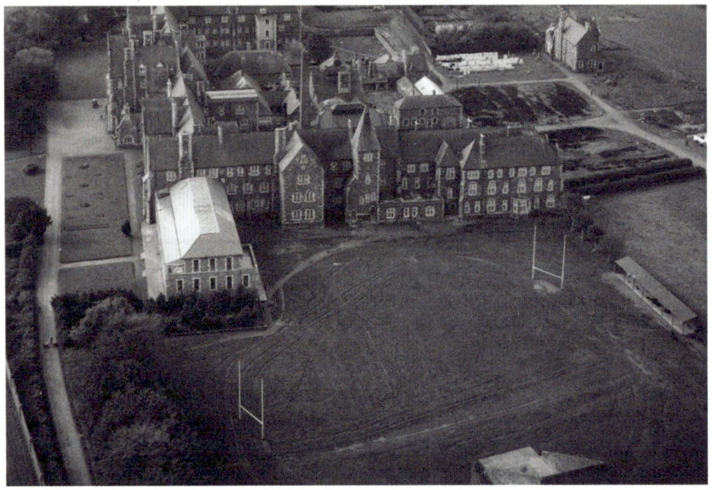

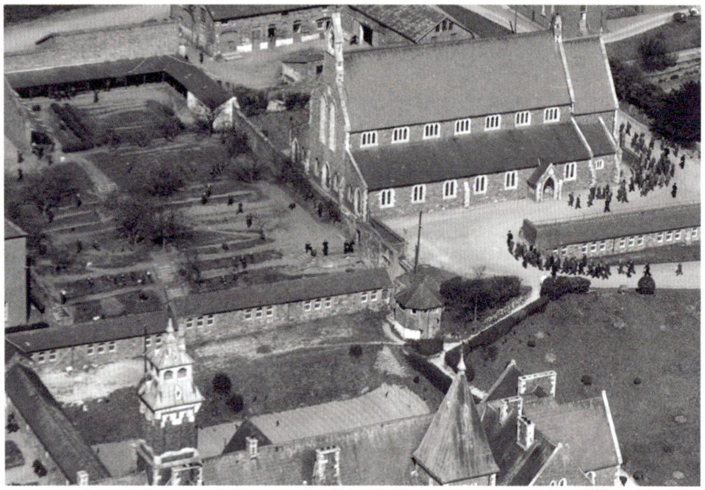

7.04 Monaghan: Handball alleys were a feature on most sites in the Republic, *Photograph by David Killeen, 2019.*

7.05 Killarney: Sporting landscape on the male side of the asylum includes a handball alley and football pitch, overlooking Fitzgearld GAA Stadium, which was constructed with patient labour. The only structured outdoor activity on the female side was hanging out the laundry, *Image courtesy of the National Library of Ireland (NPA MOR618).*

7.06 Cork: Aerial photograph, 1955, showing some patients confined to airing yards, others permitted a closely supervised walk around the grounds, *Image courtesy of the National Library of Ireland (NPA MOR980).*

7.07 Gransha: The only new hospital of the era was built as the long-awaited replacement for the city centre asylum, *Image copyright of Terence McDonald Collection, reproduced by kind permission of the McDonald family and the IFI.*

7.08 Gransha: As hospital farms fell out of use, pitch-and-putt courses opened on many hospital sites, *Image copyright of Terence McDonald Collection, reproduced by kind permission of the McDonald family and the IFI.*

7.09 Gransha: Occupational therapy which prioritised the recovery of the patient...

7.10 ...gradually replaced patient labour which prioritised the economic operation of the institution, *Images copyright of Terence McDonald Collection, reproduced by kind permission of the McDonald family and the IFI.*

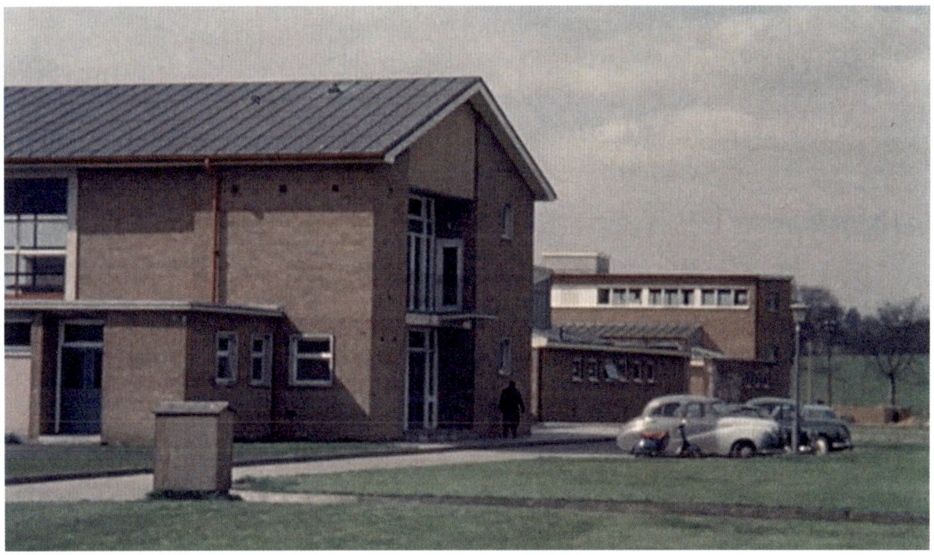

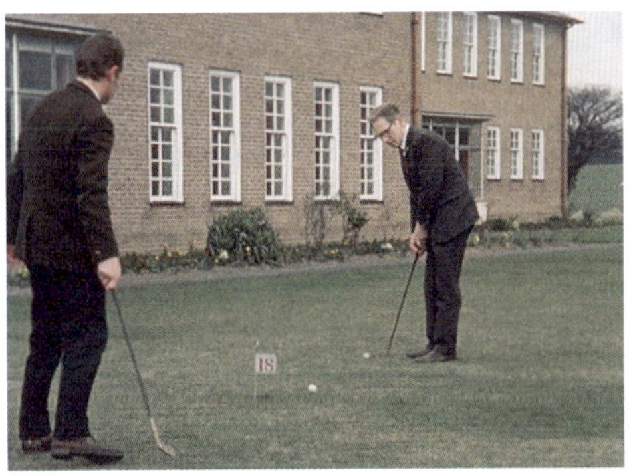

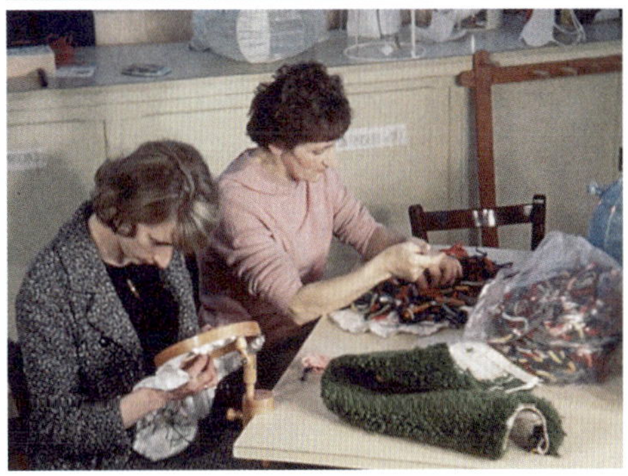

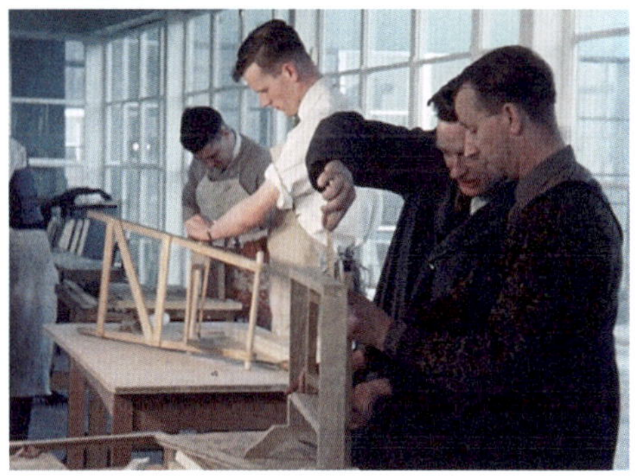

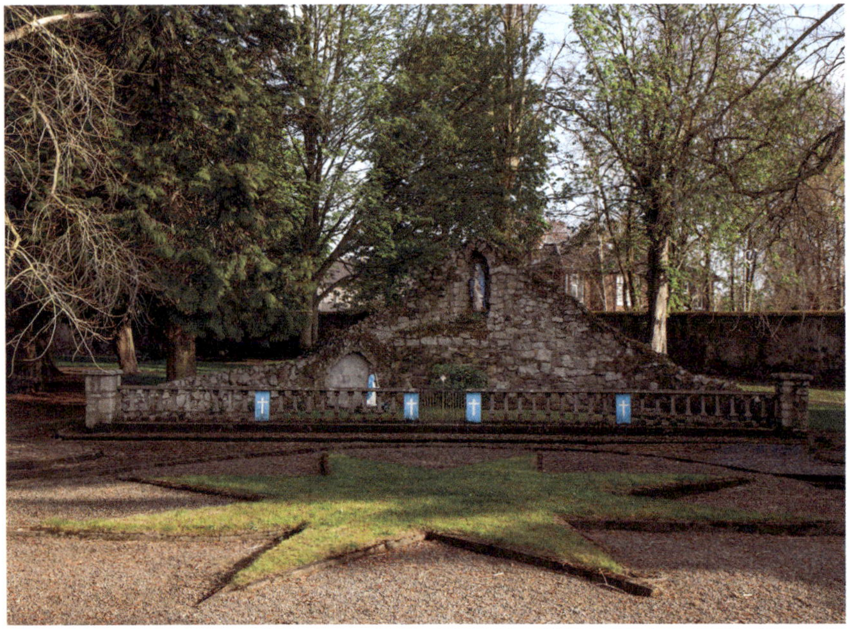

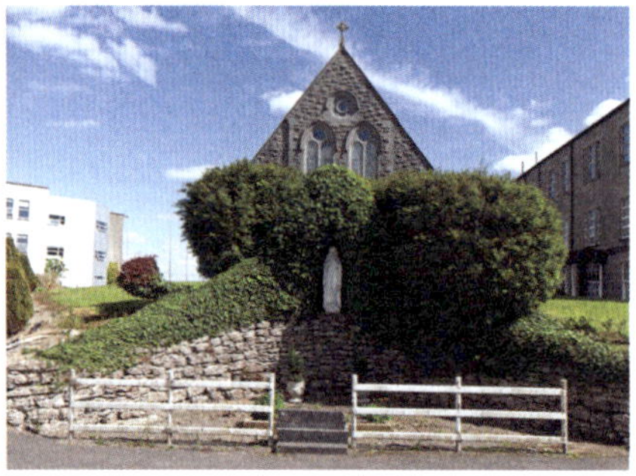

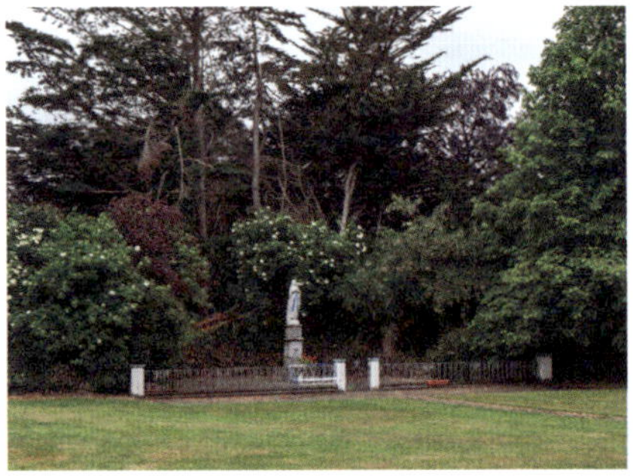

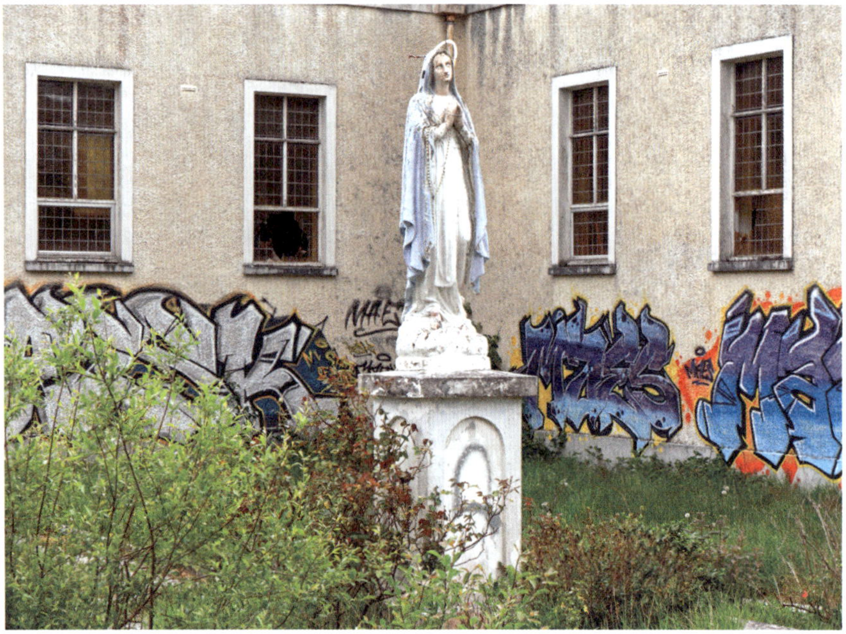

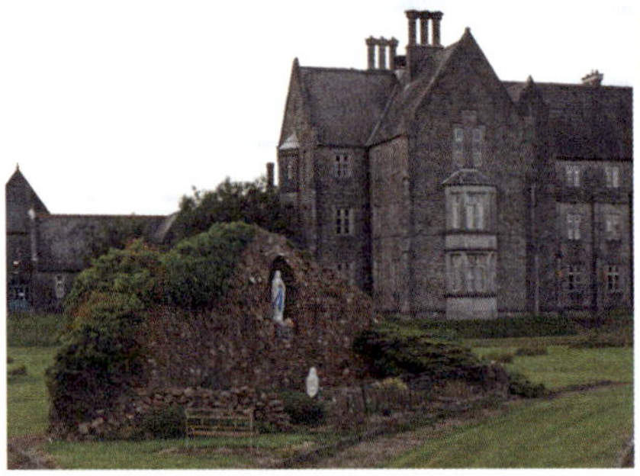

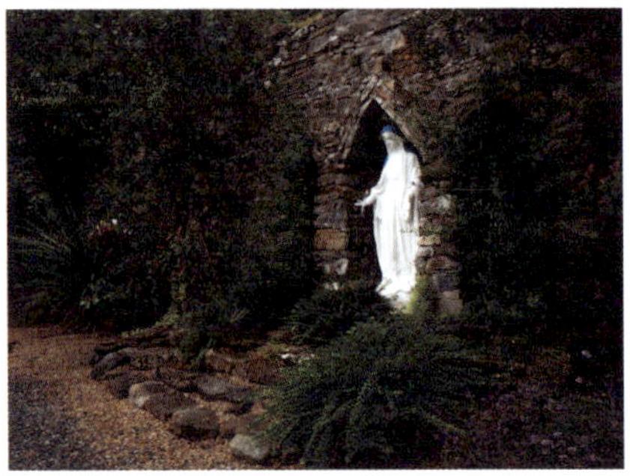

7.11 a-f Marian shrines at Carlow, Castlebar, Kilkenny, Mullingar, Ennis, Castlerea, *Photographs by David Killeen, 2019.*

7.12 Mullingar: Kitchens, laundries and central heating systems all saw improvement in the period, *Photograph by David Killeen, 2019.*

7.13 Ballinasloe: Sanitation may have improved in the twentieth century, but privacy remained in short supply. The imperative was to reduce the risk of suicide, even at the price of dignity, *Photograph by David Killeen, 2019.*

7.14 Portrane: The practicalities of distributing supplies across a complex like Portrane demanded vehicular assistance, *Photograph by David Killeen, 2019.*

7.15 Mullingar: Later cubicles and lashings of sunshine yellow paint cannot disguise the depressing character of the ward that Hannah Greally knew as 'No Hope Hold.', *Photograph by David Killeen, 2019.*

7.16 Killarney: New buildings after the 1970s were rare, which given the quality of the few that exist, may be just as well, *Photograph by David Killeen, 2019.*

11

12 13 14
15 16

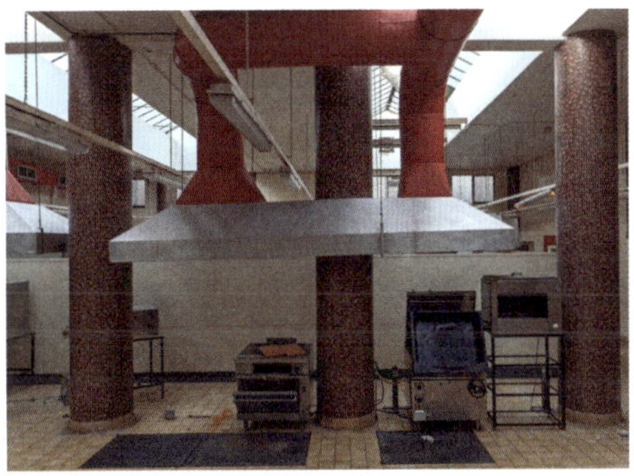
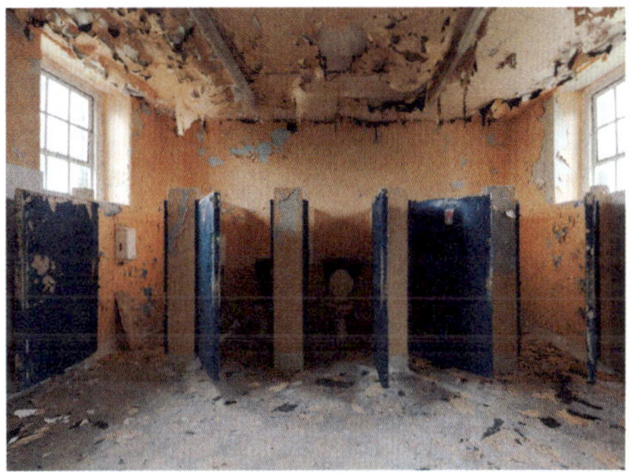
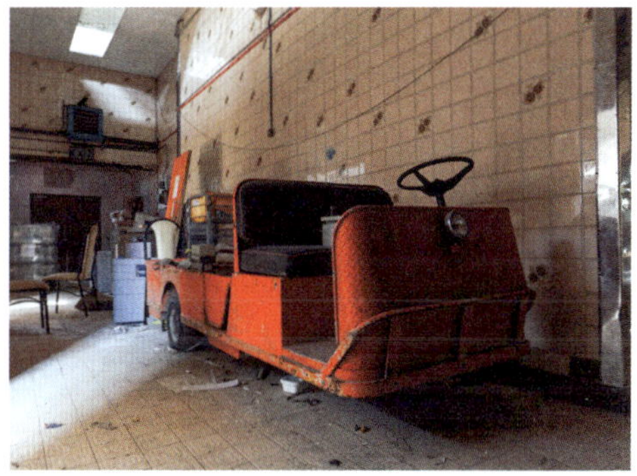
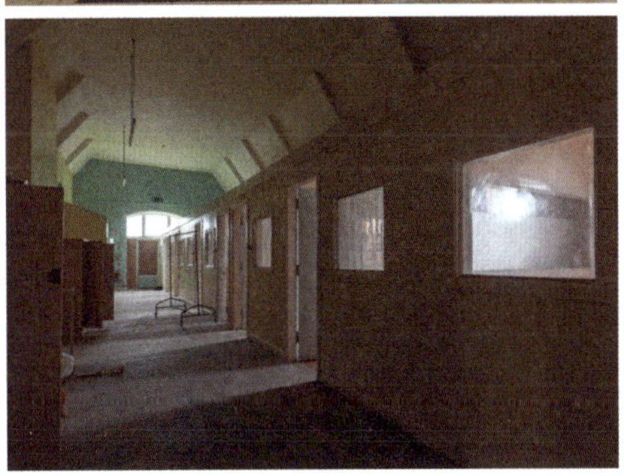
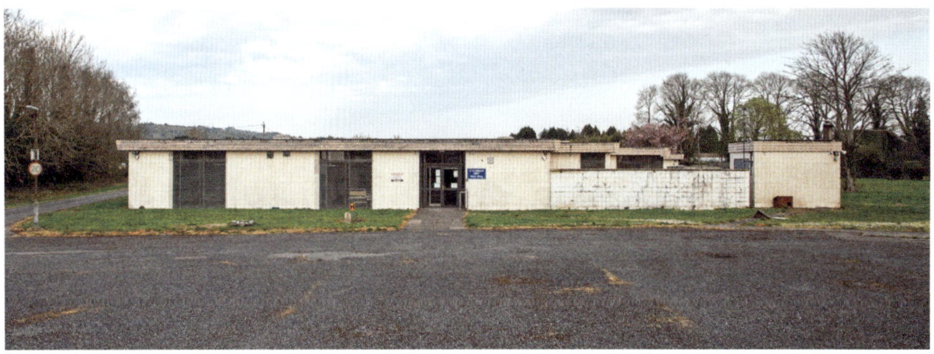

28. Donal Murphy, *Tumbling Walls: The Evolution of a Community Institution, St Fintan's Hospital Portlaoise, 1833–1983* (Portlaoise, 1983), p. 55.
29. The murder rate in both the Republic and Northern Ireland through the 1950s and 60s remained consistent with preceding decades, rising only in the 1970s with the outbreak of the Troubles. Brewer, John, Bill Lockhart and Paula Rodgers, 'Crime in Ireland since the Second World War', in *Journal of the Statistical and Social Inquiry Society of Ireland* 27:3 (1995–6), p. 147.
30. Sean Kelly, *A Grand Old Lady: A History of the Downshire Hospital, 1869–2014* (Dundonald, 2012), Chapter Six (no pagination).
31. *Report of the Inspector of Mental Hospitals, 1977–1979*, pp 6–8.
32. Michel Foucault, *Madness and Civilisation* (tr. Richard Howard; New York, 1965) p. 278. The same year saw influential publications by Szasz and Laing, which also became core texts for the anti-psychiatry movement.

RMS insisted that the grounds were fully landscaped and looking their best before the walls were lowered to ensure a positive first impression of the institution amongst a public who had never seen what lay within.[28]

The enormous significance of the boundary wall in popular perceptions of these institutions is difficult to appreciate more than fifty years after the momentous decision was first taken to breach them. A long-serving staff member at one site recounted to the author how townspeople feared that they would be murdered in their beds once the walls came down. Needless to say, the murder rate remained reassuringly stable.[29] Even in Northern Ireland, where something approaching an 'open hospital' regime had existed at Purdysburn for almost fifty years, the walls elsewhere would remain in place until the 1950s, and similar fears accompanied their eventual demise.[30] Opening hospital grounds to public use was part of an effort to erode the stigma that the high walls had helped to create, and habitual public use over many decades has doubtless helped to change the perception of these places. An unintended consequence is that the health service today carries the cost of maintaining grounds that have in some cases become de-facto public parks; the author certainly encountered many more dog-walkers than patients on hospital grounds. Only at Letterkenny has this organic change been formalised, with the town council taking a lease on the former asylum grounds to create a new urban park – an example worthy of wider emulation.

Revolutions: pharmacological and otherwise

Just as the modern mental hospital buildings of the 1930s and 40s had proven eminently adaptable for use as TB sanatoria, the unexpectedly sudden defeat of that epidemic saw the borrowed buildings returned, and with interest. Former TB sanatoria at Ballyowen (Lucan) and Crooksling (Saggart) were adapted to relieve overcrowding at Grangegorman in Dublin, as were sanatoria at Sarsfield Court (Glanmire) and Heatherside (Doneraile) in Cork. In 1966, the former Royal National Hospital for Consumption at Newcastle would be repurposed as a District Mental Hospital for County Wicklow, the last 'district mental hospital' as legally defined.[31]

In 1961 the Irish Government established a Commission of Inquiry on Mental Illness to investigate, inter alia, the startlingly high hospitalisation rate in Ireland compared to international norms. But 1961 internationally would prove to be a highly significant year for psychiatry, for other reasons. French philosopher Michel Foucault published the fruits of his doctoral thesis as *Madness and Civilization: A History of Insanity in the Age of Reason*. Foucault deconstructed the founding myth that modern asylum care was guided by humanitarian and scientific principles, instead denouncing the 'gigantic moral imprisonment' of individuals whose madness, far from being an objective fact, could be seen as a result of the prevailing social constructs of any given era, and whose penalty for deviating from society's moral code was incarceration.[32] In March of the same year UK Health Secretary Enoch Powell, in what may rank as his second-best known speech, dramatically called time on England's asylums. His address to psychiatric clinicians gathered at their annual conference dripped with powerful imagery and rhetoric, capturing the now classic image of the asylum as 'isolated, majestic, imperious, brooded over by the gigantic water-tower and chimney combined, rising unmistakable and daunting out of the countryside' before invoking his stunned audience to rise to the challenge of eliminating 'by far the greater part of this country's mental hospitals as they exist today'.[33]

The following year, Erving Goffman published *Asylums: Essays on the Social Situation of Mental Patients and Other Inmates*, a blistering attack on the contradiction between the 'officially avowed and officially approved ends' for which mental institutions were created and what they had become: a 'storage dump for inmates' operated in a manner that hypocritically served the interests of officialdom, rather than the needs of the patient.[34] Based on a year spent 'undercover' in a major American mental hospital, Goffman's observations of the *modus operandi* of a 'total institution' and the institutional neurosis[35] of its inmates could equally have applied here. The fuse had been lit on the modern international anti-psychiatry movement, which would shake the foundations of the profession and assist in hastening the demise of the institutional regime to which psychiatry owed its existence.

But if the official record is to be believed the debates that reverberated internationally from the 1960s and 70s somehow sank beneath the waves of the Irish Sea before reaching our shores. Members of the 1961–66 Commission, who proved to be enthusiastic advocates for evolutionary reform, neither acknowledged nor rebuffed the devastating critiques made by the revolutionary forces of anti-psychiatry. Individual institutional histories too remain silent on the matter, just as most ignore or downplay the less edifying aspects of their own stories in favour of a conventional narrative of continuous progress. Perhaps more surprising is that recent, authoritative histories of Irish psychiatry and healthcare should reinforce these omissions.[36] Certainly, contemporary research paints the rise and fall of the Ireland's national asylum system as a product of messy, complex, reciprocal and contingent interplay of numerous factors rather than the product of any single doctrine.[37] But if Ireland's mental health sector and the professionals who controlled it genuinely did remain aloof from the pressing international discourses of the day, that in itself seems worthy of further comment.

The Commission's report, published in 1966, was the first official document in 150 years to deviate from the national policy of institutionalisation, although as noted by Brennan, the Commission was belatedly endorsing an evolving reality, not leading it.[38] For by 1966 the monolithic mental hospital was already losing its status as the sole venue for the delivery of mental health services. A growing network of outpatient clinics and community-based care sought to prevent the need for inpatient admission and to help rehabilitate former patients back into the community. The report recommended that long-stay patients incapable of rehabilitation should be moved from the large hospitals into smaller residential units, with the ultimate aim of reducing inpatient hospital beds to 5,000 by 1981. Inpatient services for new admissions would be delivered in acute psychiatric units – successors to the 'Admissions Hospitals' – which would where possible be attached to public general hospitals in order to integrate the delivery of both medical and psychiatric care.[39] The goal of these units – as with almost every previous adventure and misadventure in this field – was to admit, treat and discharge patients in weeks rather than years.

33. Enoch Powell MP, Address to the National Association of Mental Health Annual Conference, 9 Mar. 1961.
34. Erving Goffman, *Asylums: Essays on the Social Situation of Mental Patients and Other Inmates* (Chicago, 1962), p. 74.
35. The term 'Institutional Neurosis' was coined by Russell Barton in his book of the same name two years earlier.
36. Most notably Brendan Kelly, *Hearing Voices: The History of Psychiatry in Ireland* (Dublin, 2014), pp 300–2. Dermot Walsh, a former Inspector of Mental Hospitals who has written prolifically on this period, also remains largely silent on the matter.
37. The most convincing, for this author, being the 'contingent model' put forward by Damien Brennan, *Irish Insanity, 1800–2000* (Oxon, 2014).
38. Ibid, pp 99–101. The 1927 Commission's recommendation for 'boarding-out' still presumed that patients would be admitted in the first instance.
39. The *1966 Commission Report* endorsed this approach and identified the optimal locations for 'short term' units for each county; over half were to be new facilities constructed alongside general hospitals. *1966 Commission Report*, pp 29–40.

40. *Report of the Commission of Inquiry on Mental Handicap* (Dublin, 1965), pp 50–1.
41. Joseph Reynolds, *Grangegorman: Psychiatric Care in Dublin since 1815* (Dublin, 1992), p. 197.
42. Ibid, p. 292
43. *Fifty-Third Annual Asylum Report 1903*, HC 1905 [2262] xxxv, p. 133.
44. 'Hospital building in Northern Ireland', in *The British Medical Journal* 1:5176 (19 Mar. 1960), p. 874.
45. Seán McEntee TD, Dáil Éireann, 6 Nov 1957, 164:4. The pair of units were built for £810 per bed, by far the cheapest of any new-build hospital beds cited. Second cheapest, at £1,200 per bed, was a new children's unit, also at Portrane, which compared to an average of ca. £2,000 per bed for additions to general hospitals. The absence of complex medical fittings is one explanation, though it is also possible that free patient labour played a role.
46. A standalone facility, 'Grahamholm', was also built at Purdysburn to cater to the psychiatric needs of ex-servicemen after World War II. Stephen Hamilton and David Martin, *The Burn, The Fever and Beyond* (Belfast, 2016), p. 74, p. 131.

Meanwhile, a parallel commission, which reported in 1965, addressed the distinct needs of the mentally handicapped and emphasised the therapeutic superiority of community care for the vast majority.[40]

That the new acute mental health services actually began to achieve their objective owed less to the character or location of the latest buildings than to a revolution of a different sort. From the 1950s new pharmacological treatments such as chlorpromazine (schizophrenia), imipramine (depression) and their successors would prove decisive in finally reversing the century-long trend of increasing institutionalisation, and allow people with even severe psychotic illnesses to live relatively normal lives beyond the walls.[41] The pharmacological revolution profoundly changed the nature of the patient population; by 1966 the RMS at Portrane was rueing the administrative challenges of losing 'the type of good, long-stay [and deeply institutionalised] patient which was a well-established [and economically imperative] feature of all mental hospitals.'[42]

A shell… to contain certain processes

The only green-field initiative of the era is found in Northern Ireland – the construction of an entirely new hospital to replace the old Londonderry District Lunatic Asylum. The central location of the old asylum saw it quickly hemmed in by the growing city, inhibiting expansion. A large estate was purchased across the river at Gransha where a satellite unit was opened in 1905,[43] but it was not until 1960 that the main elements of a major replacement hospital would open. Designed for up to 800 patients and described as the United Kingdom's first new mental hospital since the war, it would also be the last.[44] It was a late iteration of the villa-colony system, but the utilitarian design, uninspired layout and flat, minimally landscaped site made it a poor successor to Ireland's first villa-colony at Purdysburn.

As the population graph passed its peak and chronically overcrowded spaces slowly emptied out, there would be little need for large, new buildings. Vincent Kelly's pair of starkly minimal and exceptionally cheap 124-bed, flat-roofed pavilions at Portrane (1955–6, demolished 2015) would represent both the first truly modernist structures, and amongst the last traditional inpatient wards, to be built on an asylum site in the Republic.[45] A phenomenon unique to hospital sites in Northern Ireland – where the patient population peaked several years later than in the Republic – was the 'dual purpose unit', utilitarian single-storey blocks built in the mid-1950s for regular use by geriatric patients, but which would be made available to US military forces if needed in the event of outbreak of conflict in cold-war Europe. Happily, they were never called upon to serve their second purpose, and most continue to fulfil their first to this day.[46]

New acute psychiatric units presented the only real opportunity for architectural innovation, with moderately interesting buildings commissioned at Cork (1965) and Clonmel (1968), again with the assistance of the Sweepstakes. The former was an exercise by Boyd Barrett in economic, mildly modernist, healthcare design – flat-roofed, brick-built, sparsely detailed. The new unit at Clonmel was a freestanding building whose southerly orientation and articulation as a series of connected

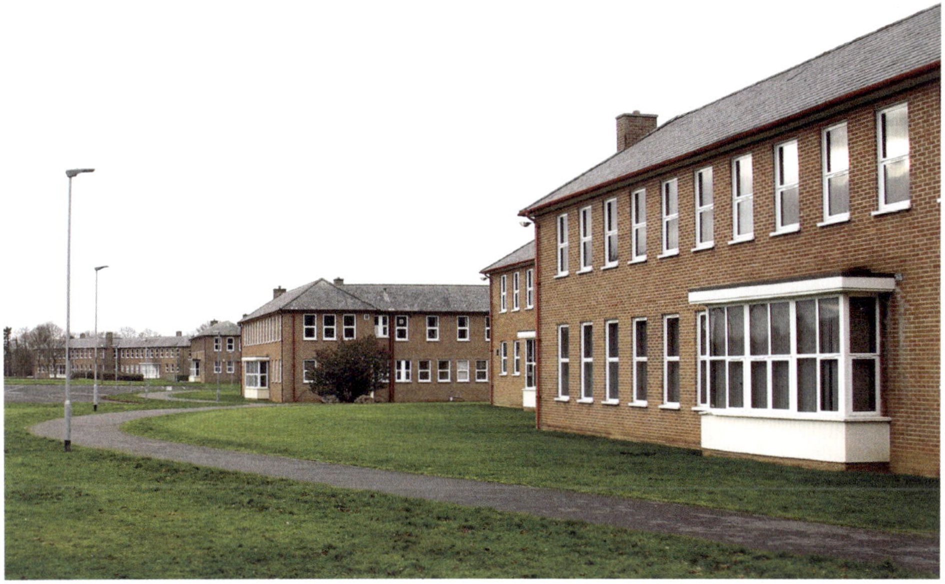

7.17 Gransha: The new hospital was built on a promise of openness, but struggles with a reality of bleakness, *Photograph by the author,*

pavilions derives from earlier sanatoria, but with more expressive mid-century external detailing and finishes, not least a dramatically angular, asymmetrically placed entrance foyer.[47] Notably, neither featured a tower of any description. But far from being the brave pioneers of a new family of psychiatric spaces optimistically reflective of an era of reform, these would instead prove to be amongst the last, modest monuments to a 160-year tradition of specially commissioned psychiatric buildings.[48] Under the Health Act of 1970, eight regional Health Boards assumed authority and budgetary responsibility for the operation of most public hospitals in the Republic, including the mental hospitals.[49] Institutions that had operated as independent entities for well over a century and whose continued existence seemed like an end unto itself would suddenly find themselves reclassified as just one element of a wider healthcare 'system'.

This shift in governance was reflected in the next generation of psychiatric spaces, which would henceforth be subject to the same utilitarian logic that governed general hospitals.[50] New wards were housed either in rudimentary extensions barely distinguishable from the general hospitals to which they were attached, or in the low-grade, repurposed space within them – in both cases visually discreet so as to suppress any sense of the service having a separate identity. Moreover, decisions by some hospitals to locate their new psychiatric wards at the rear or in basements at best conveys a sense of mental health ranking last among equals;[51] at worst it offers unsettling echoes of Francis Johnston's hidden basement cells for 'dirty and ungovernable' patients. Psychiatry had swapped the infamous 'back wards' of its own asylums for the back wards of the general hospital. Changing the location of mental health service delivery alone could not change attitudes that had been generations in the making.

47. Eamon de Barra (ed.), *Irish Hospitals 1956–1971* (Dublin, 1971), p. 60.
48. The mental hospital sector received a slightly larger share of the capital grants allocated between 1956 and 1969 than in the previous period (£2.7 million or ca. 6 per cent). Most of the money was spent on pragmatic improvements rather than new buildings. Only two mental health buildings would feature in the photographic parade of flagship projects: Clonmel's acute psychiatric unit and Portrane's new nurses' home. ibid. pp 66–76.
49. 1970 Health Act, S.I.1 of 1970. Eamon Lonergan, *The History of the South-Eastern Health Board, 1971–2004* (Kilkenny, 2004), pp 10–12. Mental hospital committees in the main cities had already been superseded by 'Health Authorities' under the 1960 Health Authorities Act, S.I.9 of 1960.
50. This being an era that few in the field of general hospital design would regard as a golden age.
51. Including at University Hospital, Cork, the Mercy Hospital, Cork, the Mater Hospital, Dublin and Cavan General Hospital. Also observations by Aisling Campbell, Consultant Psychiatrist, in a panel discussion following the Thomas Davis lecture: *Houses in Motion: Architecture and Patterns of Dwelling*, RTÉ Radio 1, first broadcast 16 Feb. 2020, and in subsequent conversation with the author.

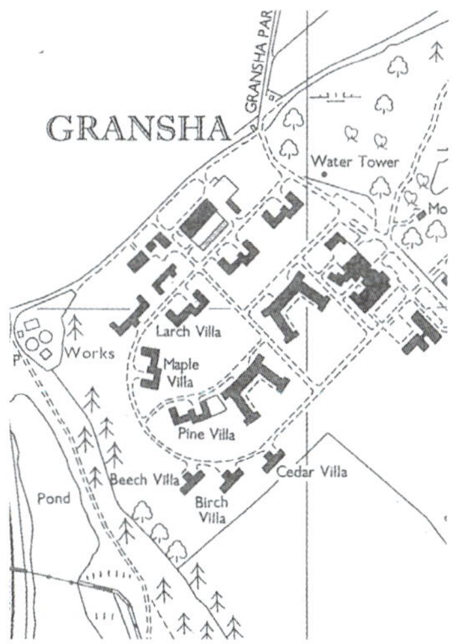

7.18 Gransha: A landscape of dispersed villas, a world away from the cramped confines of the city asylum, *Reproduced courtesy of Trinity College Dublin (OSNI-100000-Sheet027-1979).*

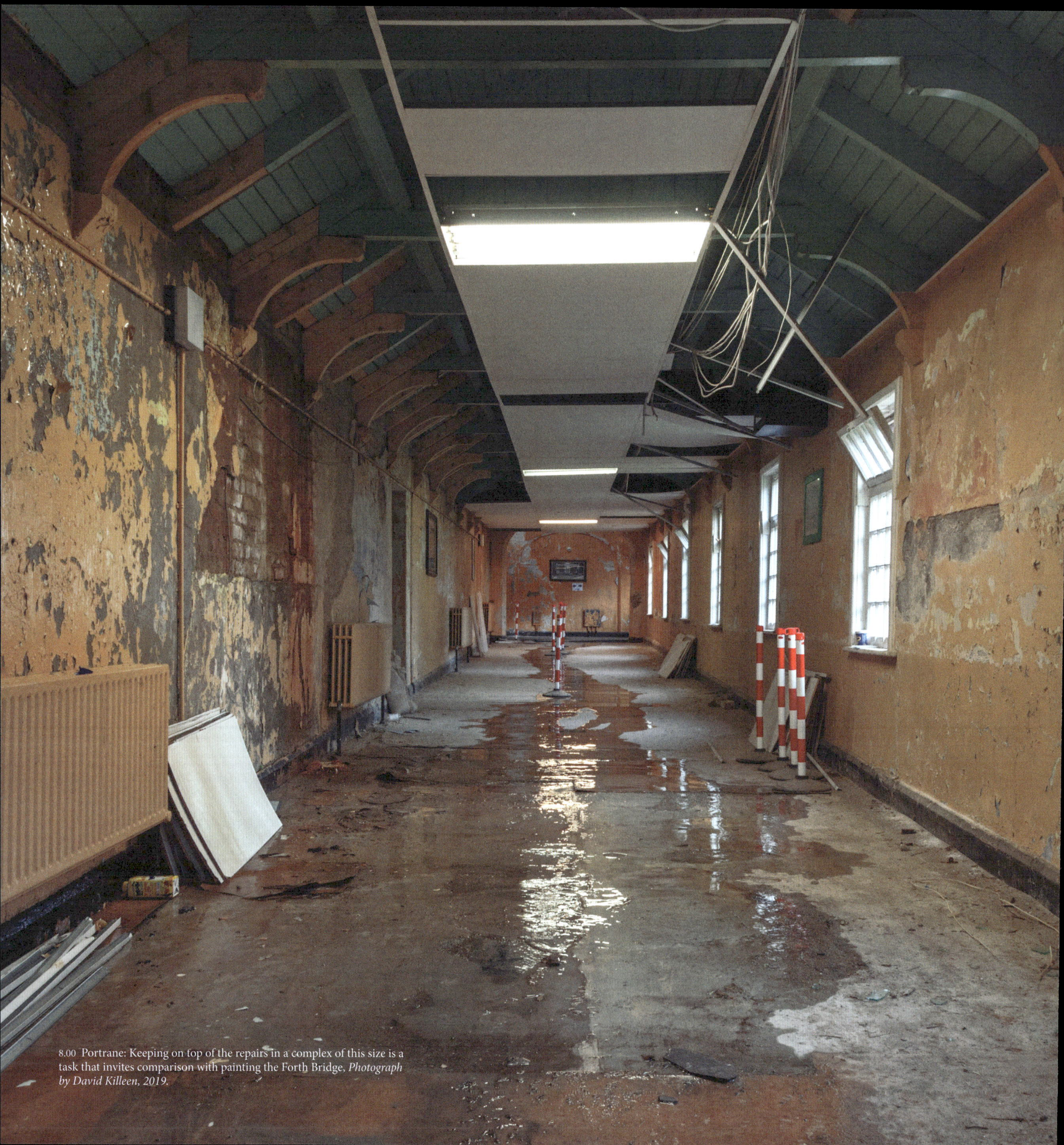

8.00 Portrane: Keeping on top of the repairs in a complex of this size is a task that invites comparison with painting the Forth Bridge. *Photograph by David Killeen, 2019.*

1980 - 2006

Inertia of Mind and Matter

the psychiatric hospitals must not become forgotten places [1]

The goal of complete integration of acute psychiatric services within densely developed general hospital sites left little space – physically, organisationally or conceptually – for architecture or landscape to contribute to the new model of care. Perhaps that is understandable: clinicians armed with new therapies were at last able to treat and discharge patients at rates that had long eluded their predecessors who were endowed with fine buildings and pleasing landscapes, but little else. With the old institutions in decline, the narrative of Ireland's asylums and mental hospitals as places of architectural innovation and progress, where landscapes and buildings were designed as vehicles for contemporary therapeutic theories, as expressions of civic pride, or as showcases of technical innovation, arguably concludes at this point. But the story of the institutions and their buildings continues.

By the 1980s progress had undoubtedly been made in shifting the delivery of mental healthcare to community and acute hospital settings, positive developments that delivered drastically improved life outcomes for very many service users. The numbers resident in the old mental hospitals had dropped to levels last seen in the 1890s, but still remained double that targeted by the 1966 Commission.[2] The population was radically different from the 1950s, now overwhelmingly comprising 'geriatric, psycho-geriatric and mentally handicapped patients,'[3] which created major problems for a system whose economic operation had relied on copious amounts of patient labour. The atmosphere of the places had also changed profoundly – the sense of dynamism and activity created by a population of mentally-ill but physically healthy patients who had once laboured in the farms and laundries, danced at dances and fielded football teams, was long gone, replaced by a cohort of chair- and bed-bound patients in many cases lacking stimulation or activation beyond the dayroom television set.

It reflects poorly on the Irish body-politic that it took 13 years for any elected representative in either chamber to notice, and then ask, why no report from the Inspector of Mental Hospitals had been laid before the Oireachtas in all of that time.[4]

1. *The Psychiatric Services – Planning for the Future: Report of a Study Group on the Development of Psychiatric Services* (hereafter *1984 Planning for the Future Report*) (Dublin, 1984), p. xiv.
2. The *1966 Commission Report* had targeted a long-stay inpatient population of 5,000 by 1981, compared to an outturn of 13,342. Aileen O'Hare and Dermot Walsh, *Irish Psychiatric Hospitals and Units 1981* (Dublin, 1983), p. 10. But even these figures can be misleading: it was not uncommon for the same people to continue to occupy the same beds in the same wards but, by virtue of the process of 'de-designation' of certain categories of patient, some were removed from the remit of the Inspectorate and hence the statistics.
3. *Report of the Inspector of Mental Hospitals, 1977–1979*, p. 9.
4. Barry Desmond TD, Dáil Éireann, 23 Oct. 1979, 316:3.

5. Helen Connolly, 'The scandal of the mental hospitals', in *Magill*, 30 Oct. 1980.

When a combined report for the years 1977–79 was finally presented, it probably should have made for grimmer reading than it did. Dolphin opened the report with a very large fig leaf for his political masters by stating that, save for the specific adverse comments: 'I am satisfied otherwise with the standard of care, welfare and treatment of persons of unsound mind…' He carefully confined his choice of adjectives to a narrow range between 'satisfactory' and 'unsatisfactory', enlivened only with the occasional 'unsightly' or 'outdated'.

In her explosive article for the investigative magazine *Magill* in 1980, Helen Connolly walked the same corridors as Dr Dolphin, but reached a rather different conclusion:

> *We have found that most of the larger hospitals are in a state of physical disintegration, oppressive congestion, demoralisation, often squalor and inadequate staffing, and that conditions were entirely inadequate to begin to cope with the problems of the patients… A pervading stench of urine, excrement and sweat confronts the visitor to the sleeping areas of many of the psychiatric hospitals in the country, most notably Our Lady's Hospital, Cork, and sections of St. Brendan's Hospital, Dublin.*[5]

Even allowing for stylistic differences between statutory inspectorate and investigative journalist, a quarter century in post appears to have inured the Inspector to the worst conditions encountered on his rounds. When the Minister for Health was called upon to defend the service from the outcry generated by the *Magill* report,

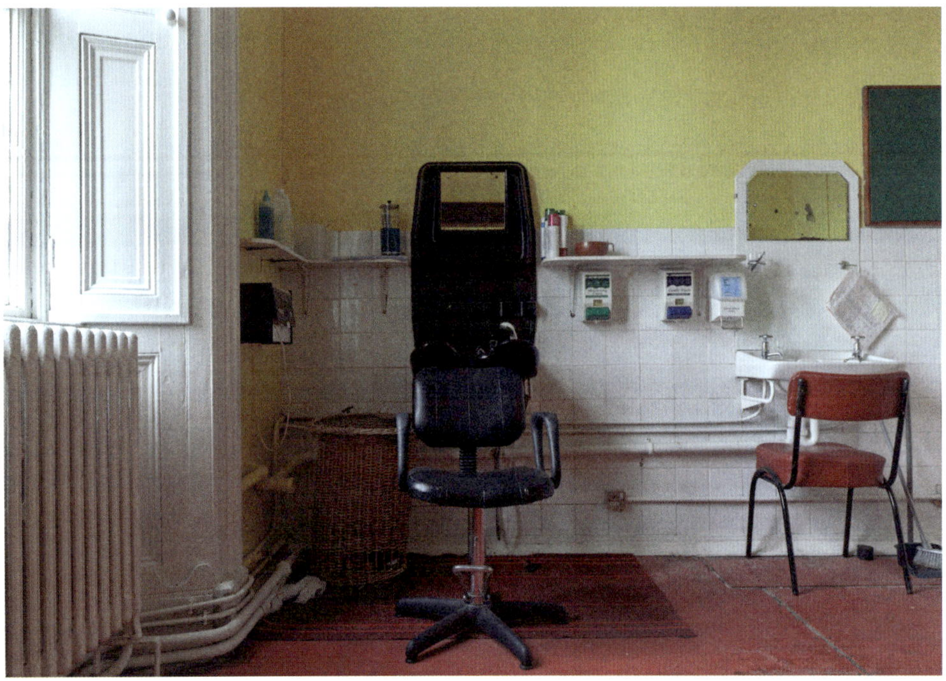

8.01 Mullingar: Efforts to restore patient individuality included the introduction of hair salons to many hospitals, *Photograph by David Killeen, 2019.*

he observed that the reporters had neither visited nor commented upon the well-run facilities, which at this time would have included the upgraded wards at St Dympna's, Carlow – 'as good as modern private psychiatric hospital accommodation' – and the star pupil, St Davnet's, Monaghan, with its swimming pool used by both patients and local school groups and a growing tally of 20 supported hostels in the community.[6]

It was clearly galling for the psychiatric profession to hear the Minister, as representative of a political system that had consistently neglected the sector,[7] invoke a handful of examples of good practice in individual hospitals, examples that had been achieved through the commitment of reforming clinicians in the face of political apathy and chronic underfunding.[8] Yet authors of the modern history of mental health services frequently fall into the same trap – eulogising the individual reforming pioneers without pausing to ask the valid question implicit in the Minister's lame response: if service improvements were possible in some localities even in spite of the unfavourable backdrop, what prevented others from pursing the same path?[9] If for no other reason than to investigate the gulf between the best hospitals and the worst, or to explain how some sites have evolved into thriving multi-purpose health campuses while others have been left to rot, I cannot avoid the sense that the history of our mental health services during this period is ripe for a critical re-appraisal, albeit by scholars better qualified for the task than I.

An Inspector Calls

The publication of the Inspector's report for 1977–79 would prove to have been an isolated event, with another gap in reporting occurring between 1979 and 1988.[10] In a bitter parable of political life, the opposition deputy whose question to the then Minister for Health forced the latter to publish the reports for 1977–79, now found himself as minister defending the very same failings, using the same words, quite probably prepared by the same civil servant:

Minister for Health, Charles Haughey TD, October 1979:

> *There is not the same need for such reports now as there was when the mental hospitals were closed institutions. The inspector of mental hospitals carries out the statutory inspections required by section 236 of the Act… Reports on these inspections are furnished to me by the Inspector and appropriate action is taken by my Department as required in relation to matters raised in the reports.*[11]

Minister for Health, Barry Desmond TD, April 1984:

> *There is not the same need for such reports as there was when the mental hospitals were closed institutions. However, the inspector of mental hospitals continues to inspect each district and private mental hospital as required by law. Reports on these inspections are furnished to me and appropriate action is taken by my Department.*[12]

6. *Report of the Inspector of Mental Hospitals, 1977–1979*, pp 9–12.
7. Magill canvassed the views of psychiatrists to the Minister's response, who described it variously as 'an insult' and 'offensive, unworthy of any Minister'. 'The Woods cover-up', in *Magill*, 30 Dec. 1980.
8. This, the inference from reading the accounts of later twentieth-century developments in Irish psychiatry, especially Brendan Kelly, *Hearing Voices: The History of Psychiatry in Ireland* (Dublin, 2014), and Dermot Walsh and Antoinette Daly, *Mental Illness in Ireland 1750–2002: Reflections on the Rise and Fall of Institutional Care* (Dublin, 2004), is that most progress in the psychiatric services resulted from the initiatives of reform-minded psychiatrists in individual hospitals, and not as a result of central planning or co-ordinated action.
9. The unspoken corollary of attributing progress to the actions of notable individuals is that equivalent failures of local leadership must at least be considered as a factor in shortcomings elsewhere. As with most aspects of asylum history, the most convincing discussions of this period will ultimately acknowledge the influence of multiple factors rather than a single simplistic cause, but insufficient time has elapsed to allow for the thoroughly critical review that this period deserves.
10. Annie Ryan, *Walls of Silence* (Callan, 1999), pp 2–6.
11. Charles Haughey TD, Dáil Éireann, 23 Oct. 1979, 316:3.
12. Barry Desmond TD, Dáil Éireann, 10 Apr. 1984, 349:9.

13. *Report of the Inspector of Mental Hospitals, 1988–1989*, p. 155.
14. Ibid., pp 143–9.
15. *Report of the Inspector of Mental Hospitals, 1990*, p. 100.
16. Ibid., p. 21.
17. Walsh and Daly, *Mental Illness in Ireland*, p. 79.
18. Ryan, *Walls of Silence*, p. 88.

The defence fielded by both Ministers was more damning than perhaps either realised. Both had effectively admitted that health officials at the highest levels, themselves included, were fully aware of the conditions that pertained in some hospitals, and indeed sought to prevent the details of same entering the public domain. The belated resumption of annual reporting by a newly installed Inspector of Mental Hospitals for the years after 1988 finally laid bare the implications of such callous disregard for transparency, revealing both shambolic conditions and specific abuses – not least the egregious use of mechanical restraint: 'a young man of 21 years… restrained on his bed for 9 years, and another [whose] arms were pinioned behind his back for an equally long period of time.' That both examples corresponded with the duration for which no reports were published proved – as if proof were still needed – that external oversight remained as critical to the prevention of abuses in the late twentieth century as it was in the early nineteenth.[13]

Falling ceilings

Of all the hospitals inspected, it was Our Lady's Hospital, Cork that moved the new inspector to break the protocol of decorous language that had characterised his office for generations. Physical conditions were 'filthy… litter in profusion… windows grimed with opaque matter and walls peeling'. And unlike many of his predecessors, Walsh looked beyond the broken toilet seats and faeces-encrusted floors to diagnose the organisational root causes of such malaise. The report identifies a bureaucracy whose 'inability or unwillingness to direct the service in the interest of patients', married with an 'inexplicable attitude to the transfer of resources' on the part of a trenchantly unionised – if themselves long-suffering – staff, perpetuated 'the worst form of custodial care'. The net result was that patients were 'forced to continue to live in poor, or more correctly, squalid, conditions'.[14]

The Southern Health Board, under whose remit the hospital now fell, could not ignore such a bluntly devastating report, and the 23 wards visited by Walsh in the 'Grey Building' (Atkin's 1852 building) in February 1988 had been cut to 7 within 18 months. By the time the reports for 1988–89 were actually published in 1992, the building had closed completely. No repairs or decorative touches could have remediated the 'indescribable filth, dirt and sub-human conditions that prevailed' at Our Lady's,[15] but at other less discredited sites, the Inspector's recommendations did result in gradual improvements, with the 1990 report expressing satisfaction that many previously poor ward environments now ranged from 'moderate' to 'high domestic standard', alongside an increasing provision of supported hostels, outpatient clinics, day centres and rehabilitation units.[16] The growth of purpose-built accommodation options for intellectually disabled and senile elderly persons in the private and voluntary sectors in this period also helped to reduce reliance on the large mental hospital as a 'convenient catch-all' for various vulnerable groups in Irish society,[17] although it remained the final destination for the most challenging of cases, which these new settings declined to accept.[18]

Throughout the 1970s the new acute units at the general hospitals had absorbed the majority of government capital spending in the sector. The meagre capital funding

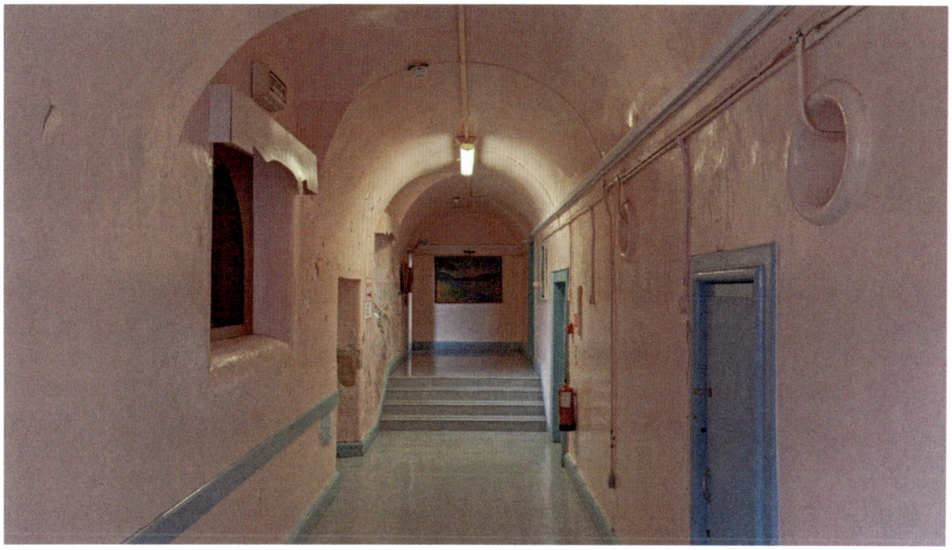

8.02 Waterford: The colour choices of the later twentieth century may jar, but represented a genuine effort to brighten previously drab interiors, *Photograph by David Killeen, 2019.*

left for the old asylum buildings – £11 million spread across 22 hospitals over 10 years, or £50,000 per hospital, per year – was insufficient to arrest their continued physical deterioration, let alone contemplate major improvements.[19] Priority was accorded to projects that maintained the basic necessities of life for a resident population declining in numbers but advancing in years, most commonly the refitting of kitchens and laundries, the renewal of hot water and heating systems, the installation of lifts and the upgrading of sanitary annexes. Long-standing water supply issues on many sites were finally rectified with the construction of reinforced concrete water towers – perhaps the only architecturally notable projects of the period. But in early 1980 cuts to the Public Capital Programme saw all mental health capital projects that were not already approved for commencement halted.[20]

That news seems to have been the last straw for one plaster ceiling in St Brendan's Hospital, Grangegorman, which shortly afterwards surrendered its tenuous grip on the rotten joists above; the sleeping patient on whom it landed fortunately lived to tell the tale. By the time the omnibus report for 1977–79 was actually published much later in 1980, the section on St Brendan's revealed Dolphin's unexpected expertise as a building surveyor: 'In the older buildings (on the west side), there is some evidence of dry rot in wooden ceilings and floors which in one location has caused sagging.'[21] The uncanny prescience of this observation – and the pointed inclusion of other specific failings identified by *Magill* – make it hard to avoid the suspicion that the document was concocted *ex post facto*. That ceiling was not the only element of the architectural fabric succumbing to the combined forces of gravity and neglect. The Chief Psychiatrist of the Central Mental Hospital, on taking up his post at the dawn of the new millennium, was genuinely terrified that loose masonry on the tall chimney stacks was in imminent danger of falling through the roof into the wards below.[22] His counterparts at St Loman's in Mullingar must have shared the same fear, where to this day an assortment of metal braces prevent similarly slender stacks from falling to earth.

19. Michael Woods TD, Dáil Éireann, 12 Nov. 1980. 234:2.
20. 'The scandal of the mental hospitals', *Magill*, 30 Oct. 1980.
21. *Report of the Inspector of Mental Hospitals, 1977–1979*, p. 6.
22. Prof. Harry Kennedy, in conversation with the author, June 2019.

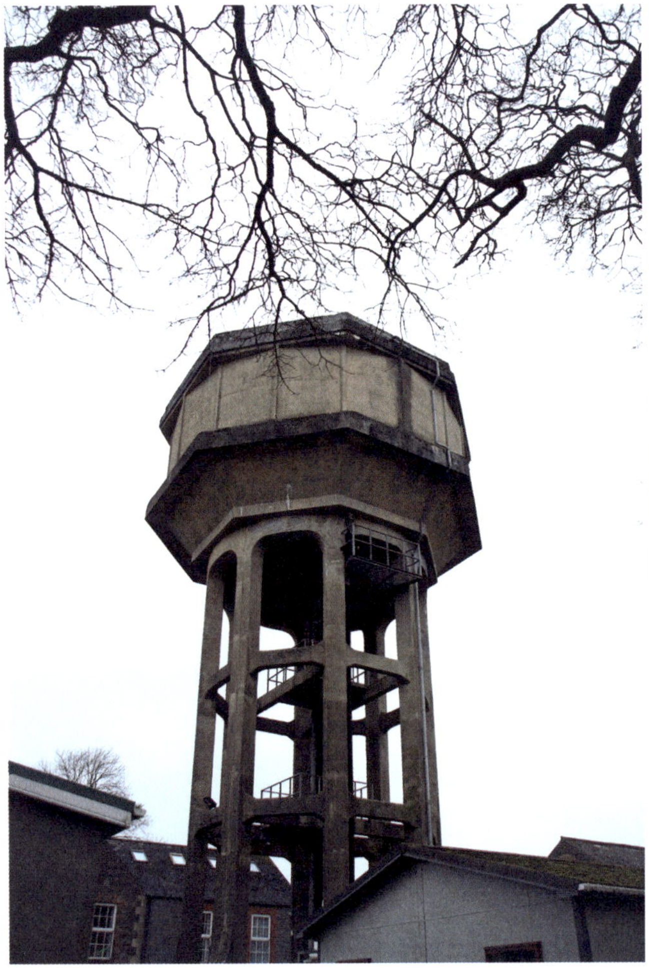

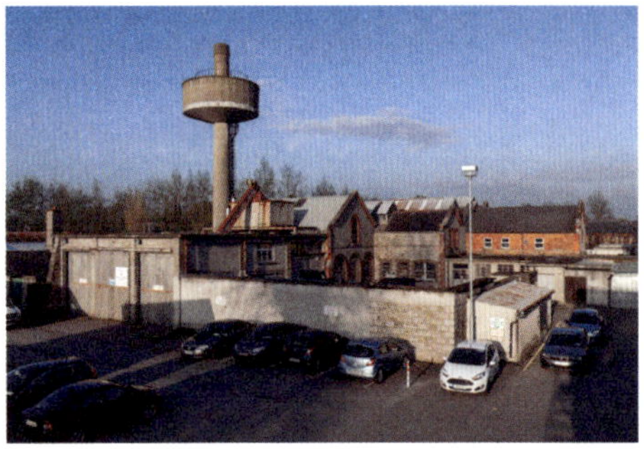

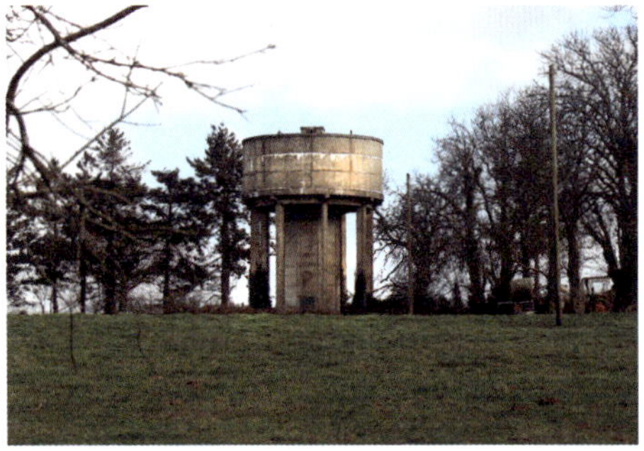

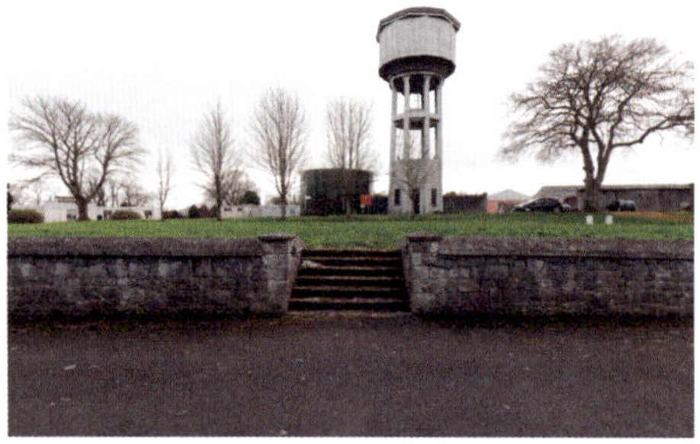

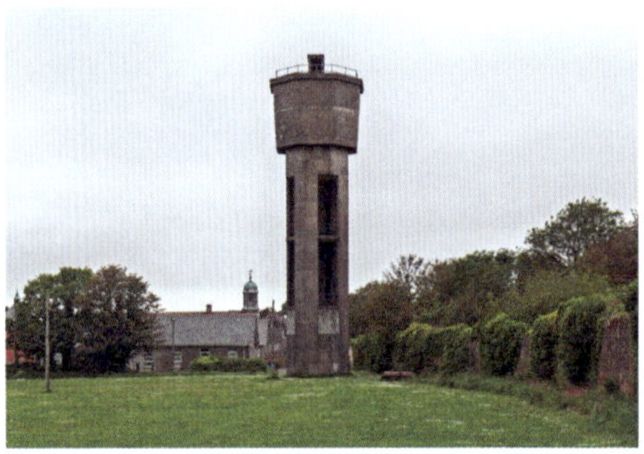

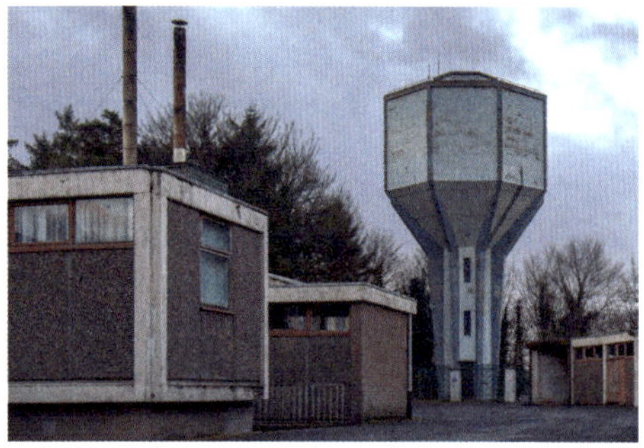

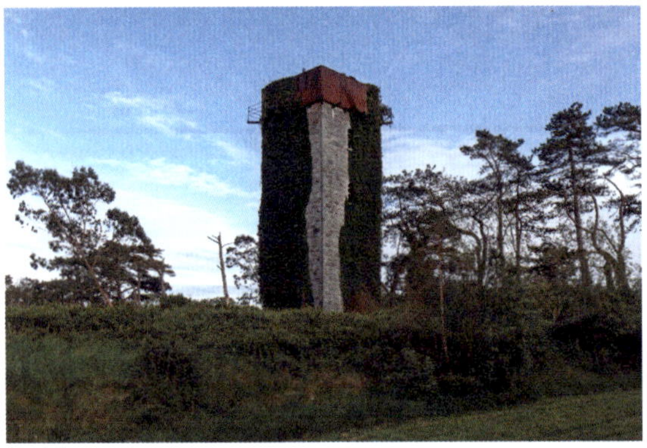

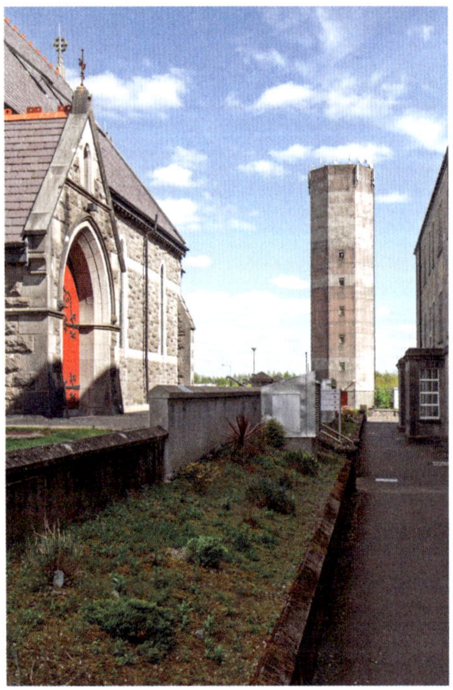

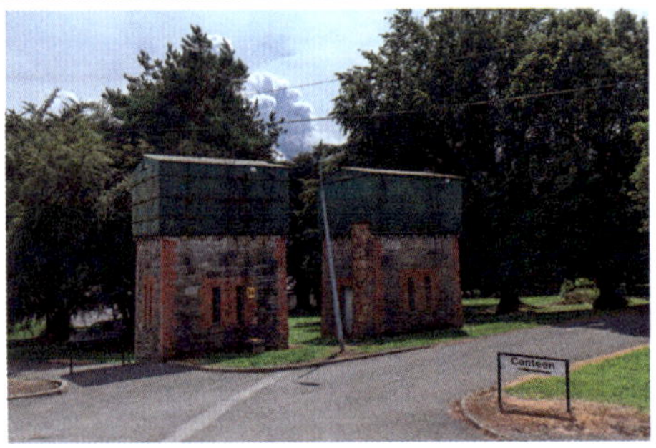
Canteen

8.03 a-i Reinforced concrete water towers are rare visible markers of progress in the period, becoming landmarks in their own right, *Photographs by David Killeen, 2019, and the author, 2013, 2020.*

8.04 Limerick: Terrazzo finishes were tiled over in a vain attempt to create a sense of domesticity, *Photograph by David Killeen, 2019.*

8.05 Mullingar: Ward interior, *Photograph by David Killeen, 2019.*

8.06 Mullingar: Curtains and vinyl tiles are indicative of wider efforts to improve patient comfort, *Photograph by David Killeen, 2019.*

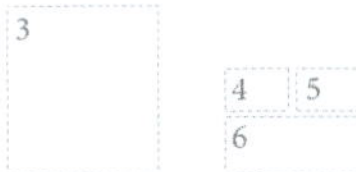

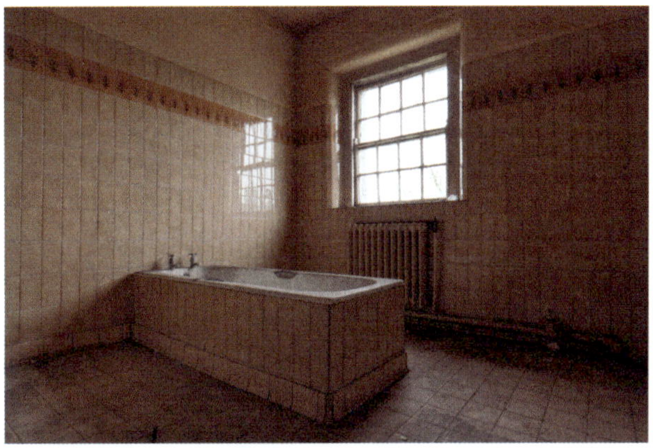

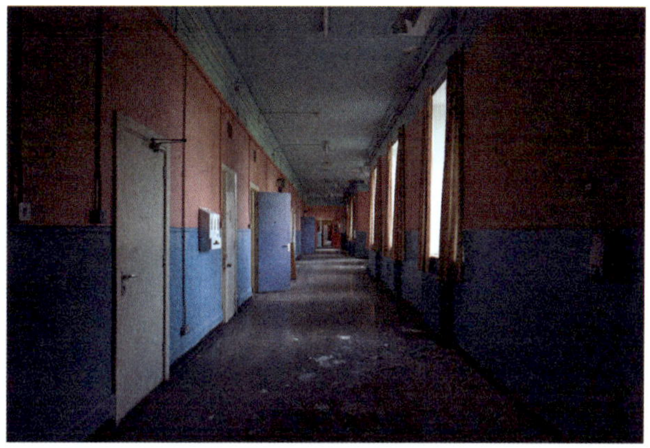

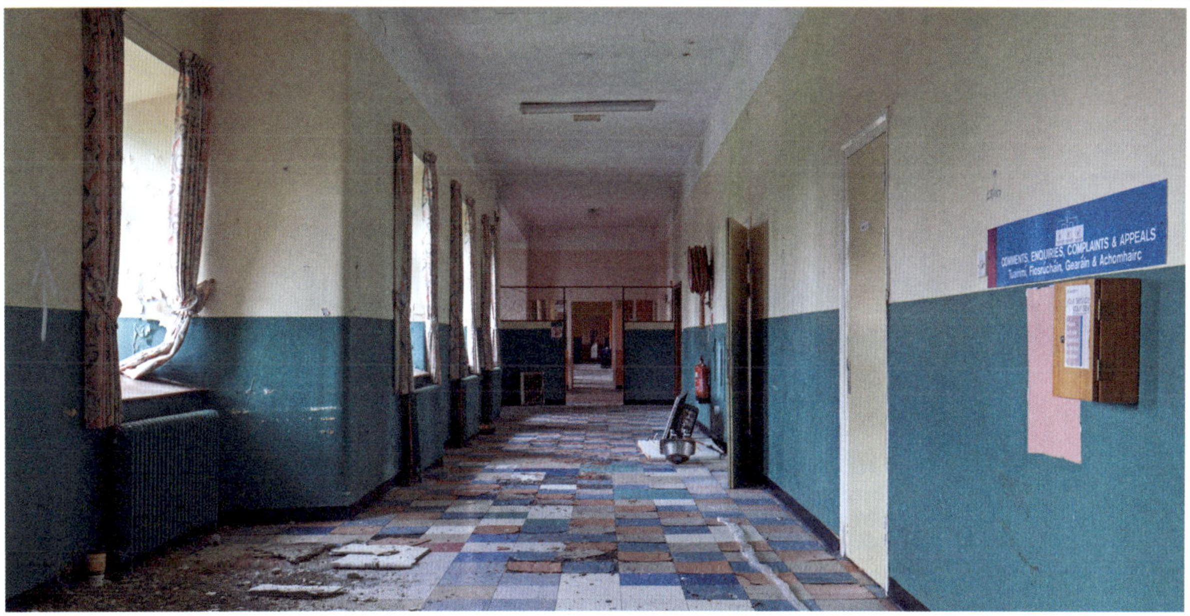

Do not underestimate their powers of resistance to our assault

Whether a response to the outcry surrounding the *Magill* expose or otherwise, (another) new Minister for Health in November 1981 appointed (another) expert group to examine existing psychiatric services and to 'clarify their objectives and draw up planning guidelines for [their] future development'.[23] Their report, published in 1984 as *Planning for the Future*, set out a vision for a community-orientated, sectorised service, with admissions to what were now referred to as psychiatric hospitals minimised. Existing patients were to be transferred, where possible, to alternative units in the community including high-support hostels, digs, staffed blocks of flats and group homes. All were important developments for service-users whose impact should not be overlooked, but insofar as they contribute anything to our narrative, it is in how starkly their non-architectural disposition contrasted with the monumental asylums of old.

The report still did not explicitly recommend the final closure of the old hospitals – even as late as 1984 such a proposal would have been politically toxic.[24] The cliché that 'there are no votes in mental health' offers a convenient explanation for the neglect of the sector, but it is only partly true. The staff and suppliers of an average mental hospital, together with their families, could easily number over a thousand voters – an enormous pool of potential first preferences and vote transfers, which any prospective politician in Ireland's multi-seat, proportional representation electoral system would be unwise to ignore. Campaigning on a ticket of investing additional resources for mental health services may not win many votes, but confronting vested interests by supporting unpopular reform or outright closure was a certain way to lose them. In any case, straitened government finances of the 1980s militated against a 'big-bang' implementation of the recommendations of *Planning for the Future*; instead, change continued to occur incrementally and at wildly differing paces in different regions. In many places the sheer weight of institutional inertia made it inconceivable for local communities, staff, and perhaps even some patients themselves, that the large mental hospital as they knew it would cease to exist.

Instead the authors sought to achieve the same ends by more subtle means, allowing natural mortality rates to erode the population of older long-stay patients while restricting the admission of new long-stay patients.[25] While acknowledging that the hospitals would need to remain open for some time to come, it was noted that the risk of improving them too much would generate increased admissions to a care setting that was no longer deemed appropriate.[26] This paradox was reflected at local level, where health boards diverted capital and maintenance budgets away from buildings that were ultimately destined for redundancy, while remaining conceptually and operationally committed to the outdated model of care practiced therein. The exhortation that 'the psychiatric hospitals must not become forgotten places', thus represented as much a critique of the status quo as a warning for the future.[27]

The six mental hospitals in Northern Ireland had been integrated into the new National Health Service in 1948, coming under the day-to-day management of the Northern Ireland Hospital Service and with political leadership from Health Ministers of the Northern Ireland Parliament until the reintroduction of direct rule

23. *1984 Planning for the Future Report, p. 3.* For completeness, it should be noted that a new Act, whose principal effect was to reform the area around involuntary detention, the Health (Mental Services) Act of 1981, passed all stages and was signed into law in May 1981, but never implemented. After three changes of government in 18 months, the new Minister for Health declared its provisions 'inoperable'. For more, see Kelly, *Hearing Voices*, pp 215–20.
24. As evidenced by the success with which local communities resisted Minster for Health, Barry Desmond's shock announcement in 1987 that hospitals at Carlow and Castlerea would close. Dermot Walsh, 'Mental health services in Ireland, 1959–2010', in Pauline M. Prior (ed.), *Asylums, Mental Health Care and the Irish 1800–2010* (Dublin, 2012), p. 82.
25. *1984 Planning for the Future Report*, pp 46–7.
26. Ibid., p. 8.
27. Ibid., p. xiv.

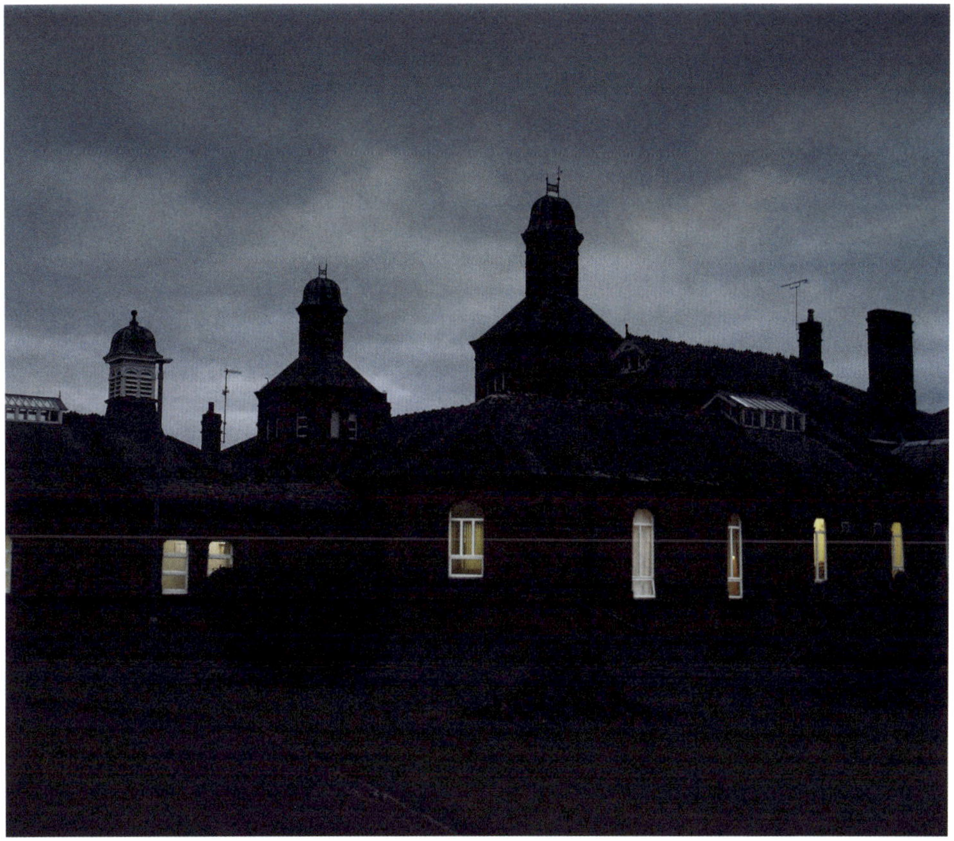

8.07 Holywell, Antrim: Lights shining as dusk settles – now a rare sight in Ireland's asylums, *Photograph by author, 2020.*

from Westminster in 1972. While the province had taken most of its policy leads from the British mainland,[28] the continuing primacy of the large hospitals well into the later twentieth century implies that local forces remained at least as protective of their social and economic value as their southern counterparts, and, if anything, were more inclined to maintain capital investment levels.[29] Northern Ireland's uniquely integrated health-and-social-care administrative structures were at least theoretically better placed to deliver a smooth transition from hospital to community care, though also burdened with the mental health fallout of the Troubles.[30]

Ritual demolition

The 'inertia of mind and matter' that Powell predicted would resist his attempts to close Britain's 'old but somehow cherished institutions' would prove to be an even more formidable force on this island, and the ruthless political will needed to 'light the funeral pyre' of the old asylums was almost – though not entirely – absent.[31] As the largest, oldest and arguably most notorious of Ireland's former asylums, St Brendan's Hospital, Grangegorman became the stage where the mettle of reform-minded psychiatrists would be pitted against the full weight of institutional inertia. Professor Ivor Browne and others made it their mission to end the continued dominance of that institution in the capital's mental health landscape. A new assessment unit helped to

28. Pauline M. Prior, 'Mental health law on the island of Ireland, 1800–2010', in Prior, *Asylums, Mental Health Care and the Irish*, p. 324.
29. One example of which was the significant investment in new nurses' homes and facilities for nursing education through the 1960 and 70s.
30. Prior gives a comprehensive account of the interaction of politics and health policy up to 1993 in *Mental Health and Politics in Northern Ireland: A History of Service Development*. (Aldershot, 1993). As of 2020, all six of Northern Ireland's historic asylum sites continue as important locations for the delivery of mental health services, as will be seen in Chapter Nine. See also Jim Campbell, 'Mental health policy, care in the community and political conflict: The case of the integrated service in Northern Ireland', in Peter Bartlett and David Wright (eds), *Outside the Walls of the Asylum: The History of Care and Community 1750–2000*, (London, 1999), pp 227–43.
31. Enoch Powell MP, Address to the National Association of Mental Health Annual Conference, 9 Mar. 1961.

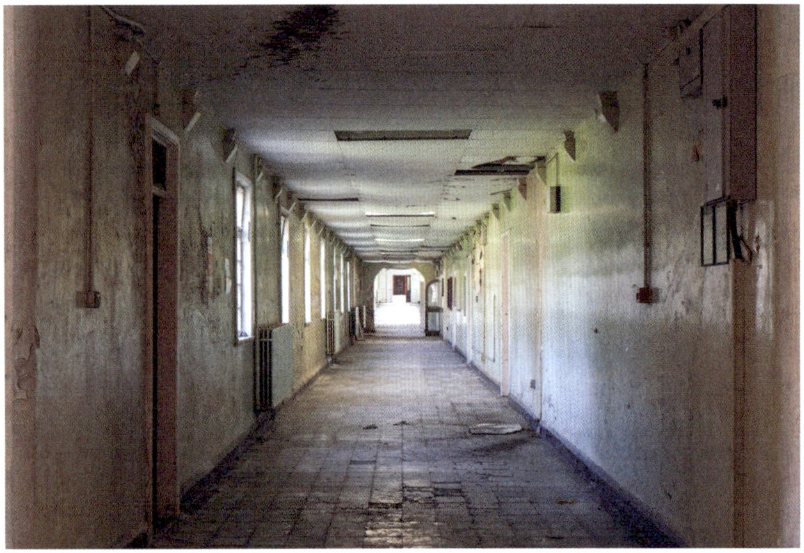

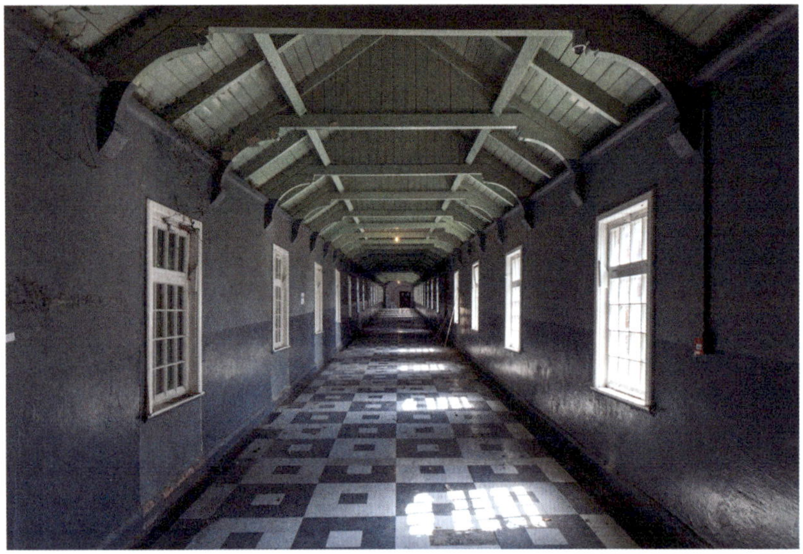

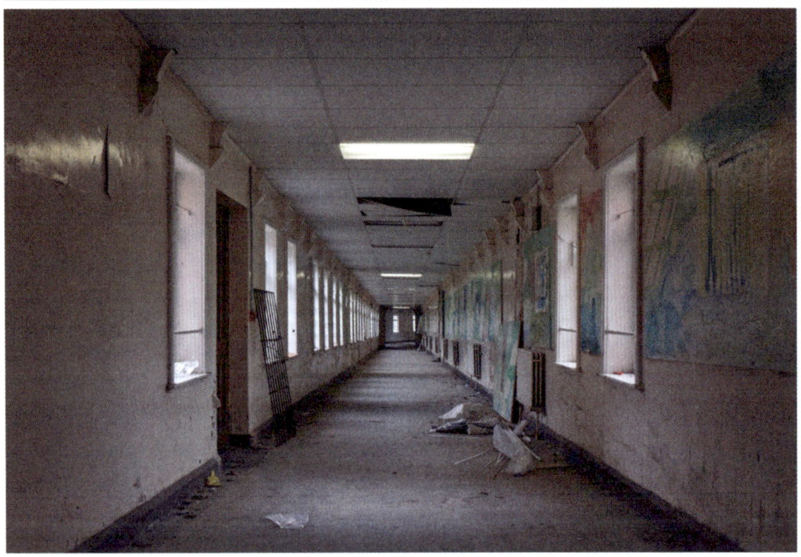

8.08 Portrane: Communication corridor, *Photograph by David Killeen, 2019.*

8.09 Portrane: Communication corridor, *Photograph by David Killeen, 2019.*

8.10 Portrane: Communication corridor, *Photograph by David Killeen, 2019.*

8.11 Grangegorman: Demolition of portion of the original Richmond Asylum ('Lower House'), 1986, *Photograph courtesy of Brian O'Connell.*

8
9
10
11

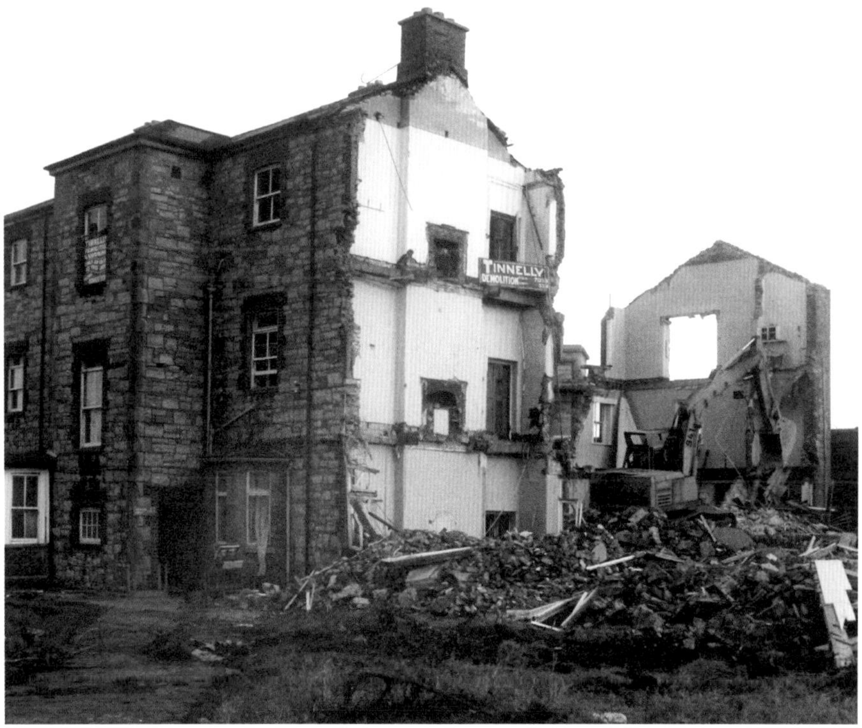

substantially reduce the number of admissions, while a 'resettlement programme' saw long-stay patients decanted en mass into accommodation 'in the community', which in this case meant dozens of rather dingy hostels and bedsits just outside the wall on the North Circular Road.[32]

Changing models of care are not always obvious to wider society, but at Grangegorman the change was visibly manifested with the demolition of many of the old asylum buildings. Plans for demolition were prepared in 1984 and two years later, the bulldozers moved in on parts of the 'Lower House' (Johnston's Richmond Asylum of 1814), of which only the entrance block would be left standing. All but a few annexes of the 'Upper House' (Murray's New Richmond of 1854 and site of the infamous sagging ceiling) was demolished, pointedly creating a void at the former heart of the site and erasing the landmark that had dominated the asylum landscape and lent the institution its visual identity. The demolitions were justifiable on the pragmatic grounds of dangerously decayed fabric, but the event was also highly symbolic, presided over by a local politician in her chains of office who took the controls of the excavator in the ceremonial inverse of laying a foundation stone.[33]

That such changes could be achieved at Grangegorman should have sent a powerful message to underperforming mental health services in other regions, but wholesale demolition of hospitals was as yet far from the agenda.[34] The process of de-institutionalisation proceeded fitfully. Even where nineteenth-century buildings were closed, as at Sligo (1991) and Cork (1992), services continued to be provided in other buildings on the same site. Castlerea – the last purpose-built mental hospital in the Republic – would in 1994 also become the first to completely close: something politically palatable only by virtue of a commitment to locate a new prison on the site. Patients would continue to reside in the old asylum buildings at all other hospitals into the new millennium, and at all but three of those into the decade after that.

The old hospitals were refusing to dwindle away quietly as policymakers had hoped. Some retained only a 'residual' population of geriatric or mentally handicapped patients, but others were continuing to receive admissions, a proportion of whom would inevitably become new long-stay patients.[35] Sceptical communities were loath to allow even the most unsatisfactory inpatient services to close before their replacements had actually materialised, knowing that political promises of future funding are like post-dated cheques that cannot always be cashed. And even as mental health services and frontline staff dispersed beyond the walls, administrators and senior clinicians often retained their offices at the heart of the old hospitals, subtly reinforcing the 'inertia of mind and matter' identified by Powell, which saw the old institutions stumble on, almost zombie-like, not fully alive but seemingly impossible to kill.

32. Kelly, *Hearing Voices*, pp 210–11. The resettlement programme has itself been subject of more recent criticism: Damien Brennan, *Irish Insanity, 1800–2000* (Oxon, 2014), p. 103
33. I am grateful to Una Sugrue for noting the existence of demolition drawings dated 1984, and especially for drawing my attention to rare archive footage of the 1986 demolition. *St Brendan's Demolition*, RTÉ 1 Television, first broadcast 26 Nov. 1986, www.rte.ie/archives/collections/news/21232208-st-brendans-demolition, accessed on 28 Oct. 2020. Record photographs in the Irish Architectural Archive suggest that the Upper House survived until at least 1993. The surviving front block of Johnston's Lower House was finally emptied of its last patients in 1989 on fire-safety grounds. Rory O'Hanlon TD, Dáil Éireann, 30 Jan. 1990, 394:8. It survived in a state of increasing dereliction, not helped by its use as a film set representing another of Johnston's landmarks – The General Post Office – in the 1996 film 'Michael Collins'.
34. The location of St Brendan's within the more economically diversified capital city, with employees spread across several parliamentary constituencies, may have made it a less politically charged location than rural towns where the hospital remained the dominant employer.
35. *1984 Planning for the Future Report*, p. 1, pp 50–1.

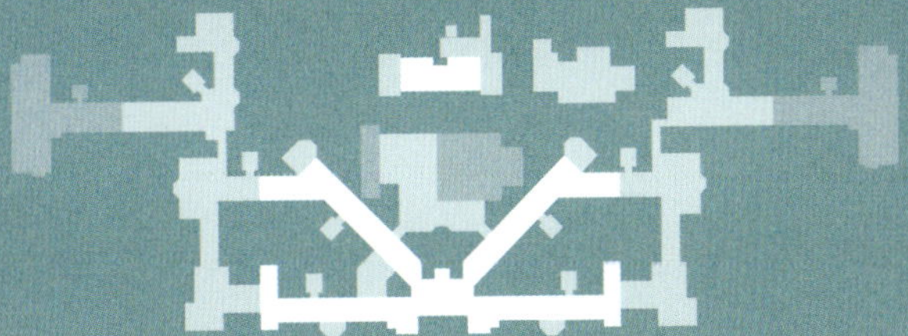

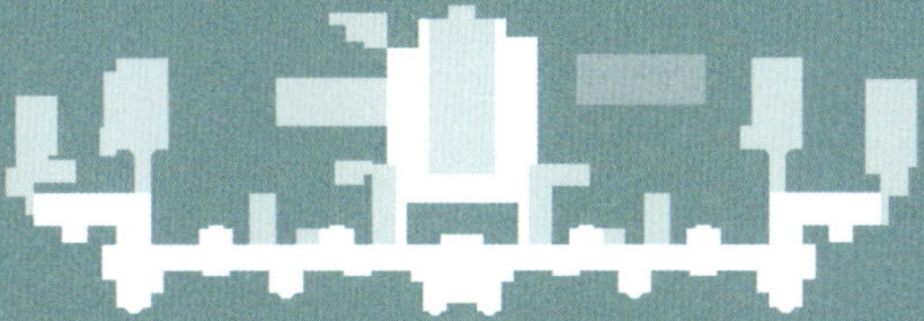

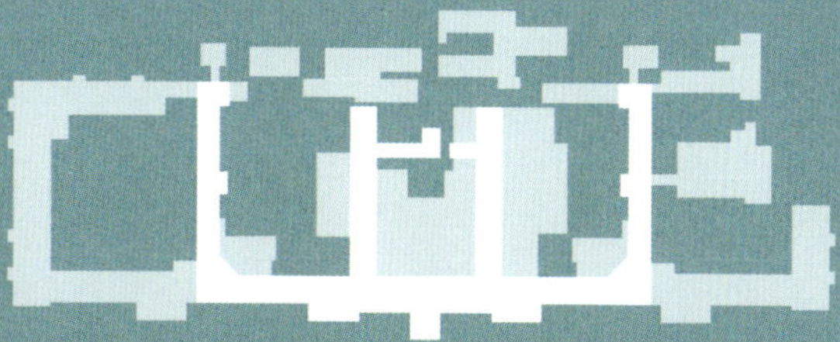

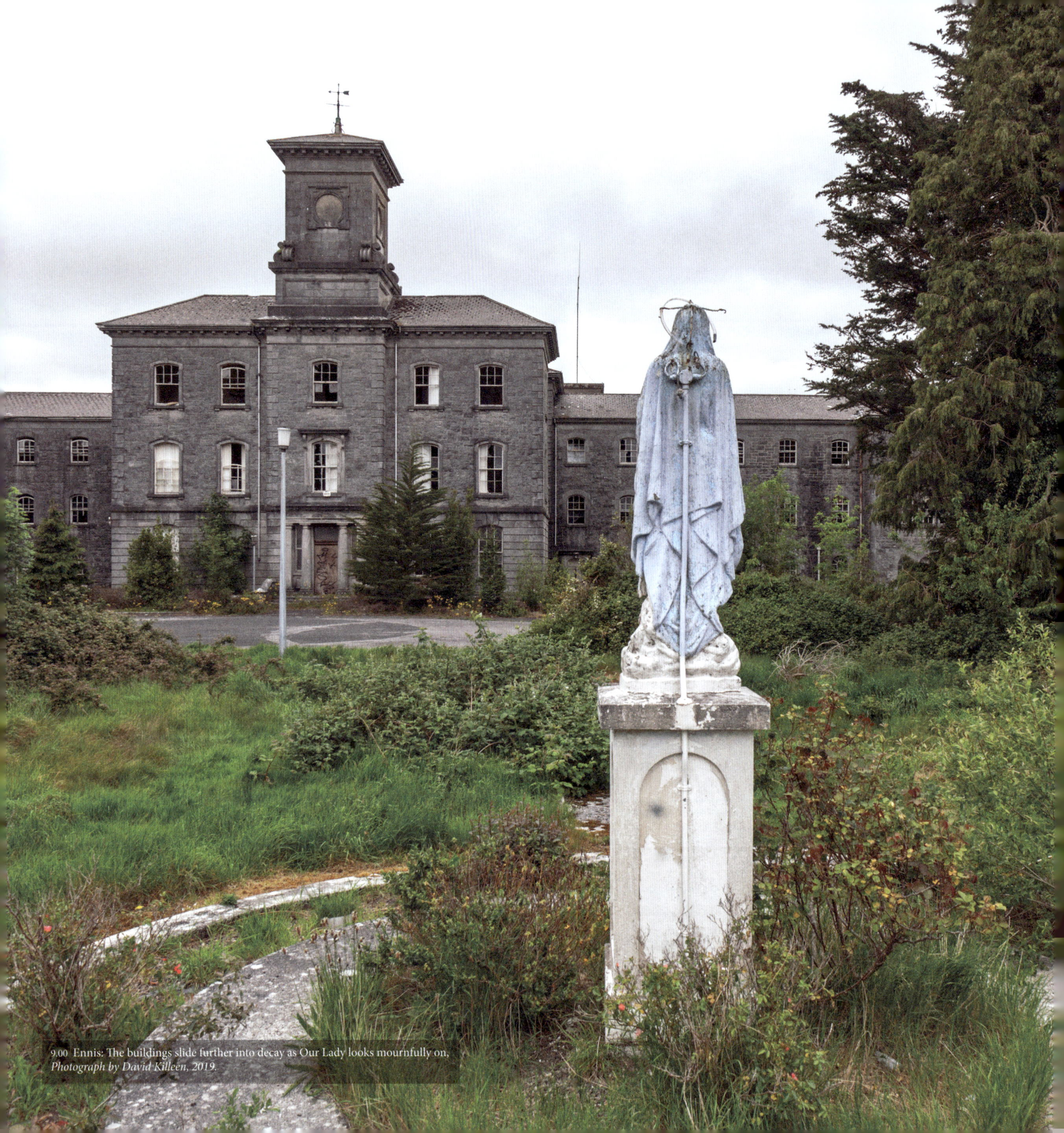

9.00 Ennis: The buildings slide further into decay as Our Lady looks mournfully on.
Photograph by David Killeen, 2019.

A Vision for Change?

more than blame levelled at dilapidated piles of bricks and mortar[1]

Fresh impetus was clearly needed if the objectives of *Planning for the Future* were ever to be realised, and it came in the form of another expert group on mental health, and another report. *A Vision for Change*, published in 2006, was hailed as the 'blueprint for a modern, comprehensive, world class service', but at its core it was built upon many of the themes that had underpinned mental health policy since 1966. At the risk of gross over-simplification: if *Planning for the Future* was the *1966 Commission Report* with the addition of a roadmap for delivery,[2] *A Vision for Change* could be seen as *Planning for the Future* with robust measures to monitor that delivery, and the expectation that the fruits of a booming economy would at last prove equal to the costs.[3]

The existing hospitals were universally condemned as 'institutionalised and stigmatised structures' completely unsuited to the delivery of modern mental healthcare. The inappropriateness of the old buildings was first flagged in the *1966 Commission Report* and continuously repeated over the following 40 years, such that their irredeemable unsuitability became both received wisdom and self-fulfilling prophecy. In terms of architecture and construction, very few of the old buildings are truly impossible to reconfigure to accommodate new models and standards of care, evidence for which may be seen in the continued ability of highly regarded private and voluntary providers in the Republic of Ireland and public Health and Social Care Trusts in Northern Ireland to deliver satisfactory care within similar historic structures.[4]

Rather, the prospect of finally achieving the closure of all former lunatic asylums in the Republic seems to have been as conceptually attractive to the twenty-first-century Mental Health Commission as the completion of a full county-based asylum system was to their predecessors, the Inspectors of Lunacy, in the 1860s. Doubtless, the deplorable conditions that pertained in the likes of St Brendan's, Grangegorman and Our Lady's, Cork into such recent times cast a shadow over the entire sector, and underpinned the Commission's determination to eradicate the last vestiges of the *ancien regime*. In 2011 the Commission issued a special progress report focused on the sole objective of closing the last remaining wards in each of the historic buildings. The report concluded with the recommendation that 'closure of the above hospitals

1. Markus Reuber, 'The architecture of psychological management: the Irish asylums, 1801–1922', in *Psychological Medicine*, 26 (1996), p. 1188.
2. Dermot Walsh, cited in Brendan Kelly, *Hearing Voices: The History of Psychiatry in Ireland* (Dublin, 2014), p. 227. Elsewhere, Walsh describes the 1966 recommendations as 'so visionary that that they are hardly bettered, in principle or in sprit, by their successors. Dermot Walsh, 'Mental health services in Ireland, 1959–2010', in Pauline M. Prior (ed.), *Asylums, Mental Health Care and the Irish 1800–2010* (Dublin, 2012), p. 78.
3. For a detailed account of the structural reforms proposed by the report, see Kelly, *Hearing Voices*, pp 249–53.
4. Private patients at St Patrick's Hospital and St John of God's Hospital, both in Dublin, continue to occupy nineteenth-century buildings, and have received satisfactory reports from almost every inspection in their respective histories. Patients remain resident in three of Northern Ireland's four surviving nineteenth-century asylums. Former workhouses form the

should also include changing the name of the new services that will be established in their place', a measure as superficial as it was unoriginal.[5] The dominant view from the centre discounted the possibility that some longstanding and quality mental health services might by now be highly regarded within their local communities, regardless of the trappings of their physical setting.

Even with acute psychiatric care fully integrated with the general hospital system, and well-developed options for care in the community, it was acknowledged there would always be a cohort of 'service users' in need of longer term residential care in a supported setting.[6] *A Vision for Change* thus unleashed a late flurry of projects across the land, mostly low-rise, low-key buildings that made a virtue out of their domestic scale and welcoming, non-institutional appearance. While many are of higher quality than much of what was built in the sector over the previous 60 years, it is too soon to offer a balanced critique of these most recent additions to the portfolio of Irish psychiatric architecture. But if the story told in these pages offers any lessons, it is that new buildings are often invested with more power – whether to cure illness or change culture – than is within the gift of architecture alone to deliver. If the services delivered within these new units disappoint, these newest buildings may in turn find themselves as the latest devalued, stigmatised and redundant relics of Ireland's mental healthcare system.[7]

5. Most services having already changed name three or four times in their existence. Mental Health Commission, *Under the Clock Towers – An Overview of Remaining Nineteenth-Century Public Psychiatric Hospitals due for Closure* (Dublin, 2011), p. 23.
6. *A Vision for Change: Report of the Expert Group on Mental Health Policy* (hereafter *2006 A Vision for Change Report*) (Dublin, 2006), p. 182
7. The most dramatic example of treating buildings as disposable 'containers' is at Gransha (see Case Study 29).

Adapting the asylum

As the inpatient population dropped, many local health leaders took the initiative to repurpose empty wards to serve other needs, providing appropriate and sustainable new uses for the old buildings while also allowing the health service to relinquish privately rented properties locally. The least taxing transition is to administrative uses, as seen at Kilkenny and Clonmel. Portlaoise, Carlow and Ardee feature a wider mix of public services, including primary care centres and clinics for ophthalmology, physiotherapy, speech and language and occupational therapies. Letterkenny and Monaghan are perhaps the best examples, where an even wider range of public health uses co-exist alongside an array of community, voluntary and sporting organisations, from GAA clubs and theatre groups to sheltered workshops and 'Mens' Sheds', bringing new life to under-utilised grounds and buildings. These local initiatives have allowed these sites to evolve and even to fulfil a modified version of their original purpose – improving the health and wellbeing of the communities they were built to serve – and doing so today within an open rather than secure setting. The formal adaption of the grounds at Letterkenny as a town park is merely the most visible example of a trend that has seen formerly closed landscapes reintegrated into local community life.

The six asylum sites in Northern Ireland have evolved along slightly different lines. All continue as important bases for the provision of mental health services, with patients still resident in original Victorian buildings on three sites. Indeed, far from divesting legacy mental health assets and decanting services to general hospitals and the wider community, the hospitals have instead come to the asylum. New community and general hospitals have been erected in recent years on asylum sites

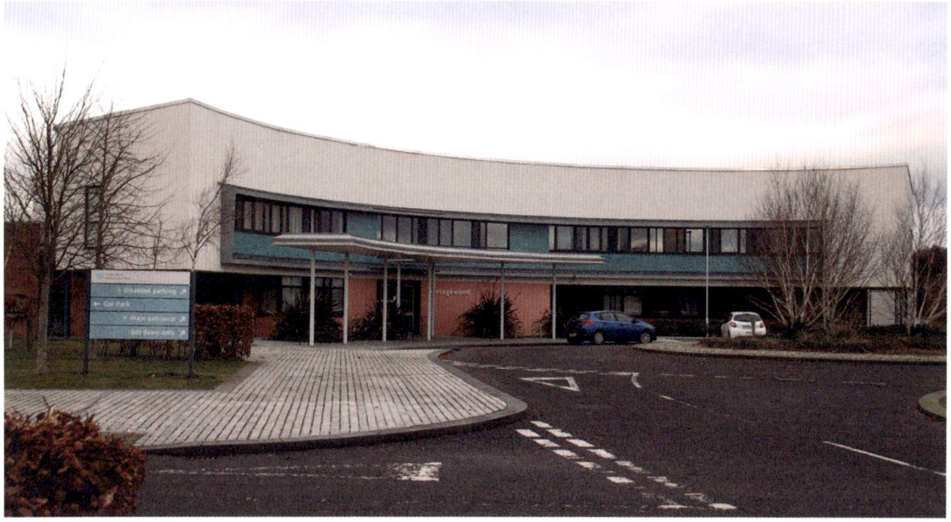

9.01 Gransha: Grangewood Acute Unit, *Photograph by the author, 2020.*

at Armagh, Downpatrick and Omagh, while a new acute inpatient unit opened on Derry's Gransha site as recently as 2012 – running precisely contrary to policy south of the border. The 50 buildings of the former villa colony at Purdysburn, now rebranded as Knockbracken Healthcare Park, are home to a bewildering array of health services which – if the car parks are any guide – employ and serve more people now than the asylum ever did.[8]

Those sites that have successfully adapted to serve new public goods may be said – to borrow a concept much in vogue – to have achieved a 'just transition' for communities who might otherwise have regarded the closure of the hospital as a catastrophe. Yet such transitions are not universally welcomed. For some psychiatrists in the Republic, the re-use of former asylum sites for other ends is a form of asset-stripping that unjustly short-changes the mental health service.[9] Given that many of the voluntary groups thus accommodated contribute positively to the mental health of the community, such attitudes may seem unduly trenchant, but the psychiatrists' frustration must be understood in the context of a decades-long process that saw mental health assets repeatedly raided to plug budget deficits across the health service. Political representatives on hospital committees also saw their holdings as cheap land-banks to be diverted as necessary for other public goods – as seen in the development of local authority housing and IDA industrial units on former hospital lands. And while few would consider it equitable that stretched mental health budgets should be burdened with the costs of maintaining vast legacy complexes for the use and benefit of other organisations, the surplus space can still serve public goods in the most unexpected ways, as seen in 2020 when the grounds at Mullingar and Ardee were adapted to serve as drive-through Covid-19 test centres.

New institutions for old

Through the latter half of the twentieth century the population of two very different types of institution swelled almost as dramatically as the number of mental hospital

8. The historical geography of mental health care in Northern Ireland thus appears to be have evolved quite distinctively from the other countries of the UK, and from the Republic of Ireland. The causes and effects of this divergence seem worthy of further enquiry and comparative analysis.
9. Siobhán Barry, Justin Brophy and Dermot Walsh, *The Lie of the Land: Psychiatric Service Land Disposal & Failures and Delays in Capital Development of Community Based Mental Health Services* (Blackrock, 2008).

patients declined. In a period when the numbers resident in psychiatric institutions fell 94%, the Irish prison population rose by 400%. This correlation – known as Penrose's Hypothesis – has been observed across many other jurisdictions that experienced a similar pattern of psychiatric deinstitutionalisation, although what, if any, causal relationship links both trends remains the subject of debate beyond the scope of this book.[10] The closure of beds may not have directly caused former patients to fall into homelessness or prison, but by eliminating the 'residual social accommodation role performed by long-term psychiatric institutions', the policy certainly reduced the options available to future marginalised individuals.[11] The construction of a 340-bed prison may have compensated the electorate of Castlerea for the economic fallout arising from the closure of their 400-bed mental hospital, but at least 10% of inmates currently incarcerated in the former have needs that would probably be better met in the latter.[12]

No hypothesis links the deinstitutionalisation process with the second graph – the 700% increase in the number of students enrolled in third-level education in the same 40-year period – but this trend serendipitously generated demand for new accommodation just as the old hospitals were emptying out.[13] Third level institutions were thus ideal occupiers of former hospital buildings, but early initiatives met with little success: the historic buildings at Cork and Sligo were sold on the open market after discussions between their respective health board owners and prospective educational institutions failed.[14] The concept proved more successful at Letterkenny and Castlebar, with Regional Technical Colleges occupying parts of both hospitals.[15] The former was a temporary arrangement but the latter has proven permanent, transforming more than half of the old hospital into a lively home for what is now the Galway Mayo Institute of Technology (GMIT). The GMIT campus at Castlebar shows how former asylum spaces can be positively transformed when clients have the will and vision to do so, even with relatively modest budgets.[16]

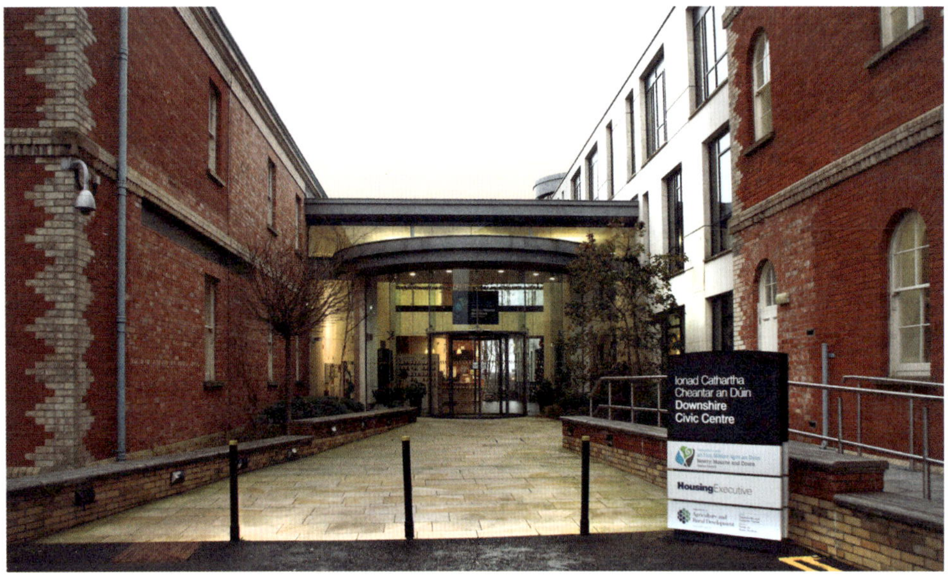

9.02 Downpatrick: Asylum repurposed as new civic centre, *Photograph by the author, 2020.*

10. The theory linking the two trends is known as the Penrose Hypothesis. In Ireland's case, at least part of the rise in prison population in the 1970s and 1980s can be attributed to the outbreak of the Troubles. Irish Penal Reform Trust, www.iprt.ie/prison-facts-2/, accessed on 27 Dec. 2019. The hospital population fell from 15,392 to 893 in the same period. For a more rigorous statistical analysis, see: C. J. Smith, Brendan Kelly and Harry Kennedy, 'A 25-year dynamic ecological analysis of psychiatric hospital admissions and prison committals: Penrose's Hypothesis updated', in *Irish Journal of Psychological Medicine*, pp 1–4. doi: 10.1017/ipm.2018.40.
11. Simon Communities of Ireland, 'Health Strategy 2001: Submission by the Simon Community of Ireland to the Department of Health on its review of the Health Service', (2001).
12. I am grateful to Castlerea Prison Governor Martin O'Reilly for this insight.
13. Over the same 1970–2011 period, students enrolled in higher and further education grew from 24,496 to 196,187. Department of Education, *Statistical Report 1968–72* and Higher Education Authority, https://hea.ie/statistics-archive/, accessed on 27 Dec. 2019.
14. University College Cork seriously considered taking over the 'Grey Building' at Our Lady's in Cork. *Southern Health Board Annual Report 1995*, p. 38. The North-Western Health Board offered St Columba's, Sligo to the Sligo Vocational Educational Committee, but no deal was reached. Mary O'Rourke TD, Dáil Éireann, 17 Apr. 1991, 407:1.
15. *Reflecting on the North Western Health Board 1970–2004* (Manorhamilton, 2004), p. 98.
16. The term 'trans-institutionalisation' has been used to describe this phenomenon in other jurisdictions. Graham Moon, Robin Kearns and Alan Joseph, *The Afterlives of the Psychiatric Asylum: Recycling Concepts, Sites and Memories* (Farnham, 2015), pp 87–106.

This success pointed the way for a much more ambitious institutional transformation – the reinvention of Grangegorman as a twenty-first-century university campus. In 1998 an Eastern Health Board report to consider the future of the Grangegorman site identified an opportunity to co-locate the disparate departments of the Dublin Institute of Technology on the site.[17] The project won political backing with the creation of a statutory agency to oversee the development in 2006. The first major act of the new Grangegorman Development Agency was to announce an international competition to create a masterplan for the site, which was won by a suitably international consortium comprising architects Moore Rubel Yudel (USA), landscape designers Lutzow (Germany), and a supporting cast of British and Irish consultants.

The completed masterplan went on to scoop six major international awards – generating an extraordinary amount of coverage for a place which, for most of the twentieth century, struggled even to register on the local political agenda. Such high-profile exposure probably helped to maintain momentum in the face of the subsequent recession. Money was provided for an impressive new mental health facility known as the Phoenix Centre, which was officially opened on 28 February 2013 – 199 years to the day since the first admission to the original Richmond Asylum – allowing the last patients to finally depart the historic hospital complex. In the same year the Government committed some €188 million to the project as part of a wider stimulus package for the battered economy, and after a few false starts, construction work on several major new academic buildings got underway in 2017. At time of writing, the site of Ireland's largest asylum is now home to thousands of students of what may one day become Ireland's largest third-level institution, the Technological University, Dublin.[18]

Amidst these new structures, many of Grangegorman's historic buildings are being repurposed for university use. The surviving wing of Francis Johnston's original Richmond Asylum of 1814 – long a roofless shell – has been stabilised and is on course to become a new 'student hub'. These efforts extended beyond the obvious landmark buildings to include a range of secondary structures from the later nineteenth century – infirmaries, ward extensions, the hospital laundry and mortuary – whose retention helps to preserve more subtle aspects of the institution's history for future generations. In a curious twist, the buried remains of Murray's 1854 'New Richmond' building became the subject of a detailed archaeological excavation, its fragmentary foundations acquiring a greater heritage value than that ascribed to the whole building when the decision was taken to demolish it less than 30 years earlier.[19]

The open parkland with its views over Dublin has been largely preserved, but within a radically changed context. Several public routes now weave through a site once characterised by the closed face it turned to the city. The iconic boundary wall is retained, but deliberately punctured to improve permeability. Within the walls, the original hierarchy of a dominant central building approached via a sweeping avenue through a demesne-like landscape has been completely erased. In its place a new pattern of paved streets, enclosed quadrangles and green links mix historic collegiate precedents with more modern campus typologies in pursuit of the masterplan's ambition of creating 'an urban quarter with an open future'.

17. Eastern Health Board, *Draft proposal for the future of St Brendan's Hospital, Grangegorman* (unpublished report, 1998).
18. Enda Kenny TD, Dáil Éireann, 23 Apr. 2013, 799:4. *Grangegorman Development Agency Newsletter*, Dec. 2019. As of Sept. 2020 Technological University, Dublin claimed 29,700 student enrolments compared to UCD's 32,000.
19. Teresa Bolger and James Hession, *Grangegorman Dublin 7, Report on investigation and recording of structural remains at proposed site for Central Quad* (unpublished report, 2013). I am grateful to Una Sugrue, Grangegorman Development Agency, for sharing this report.

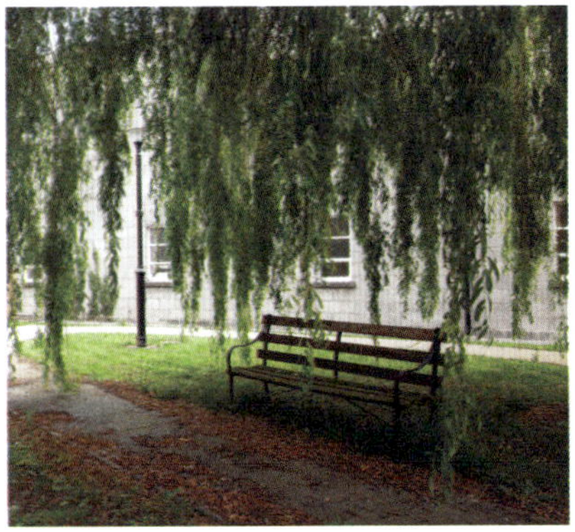

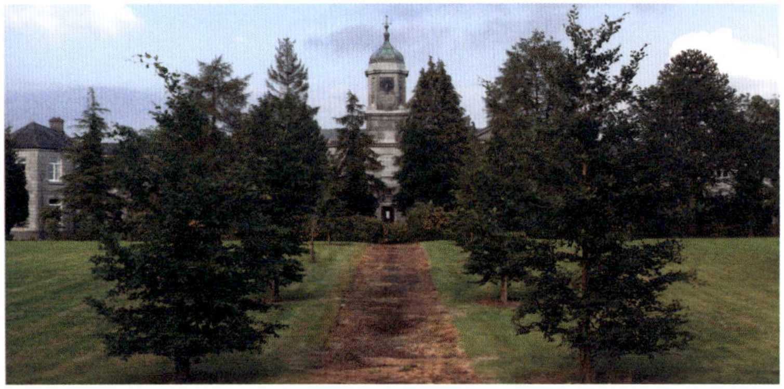

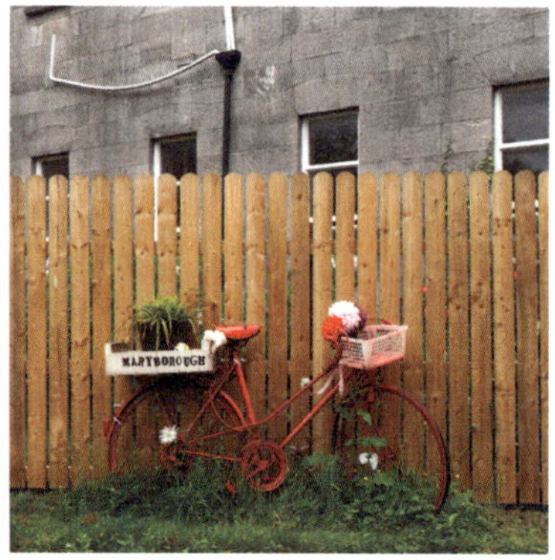
MARYBOROUGH

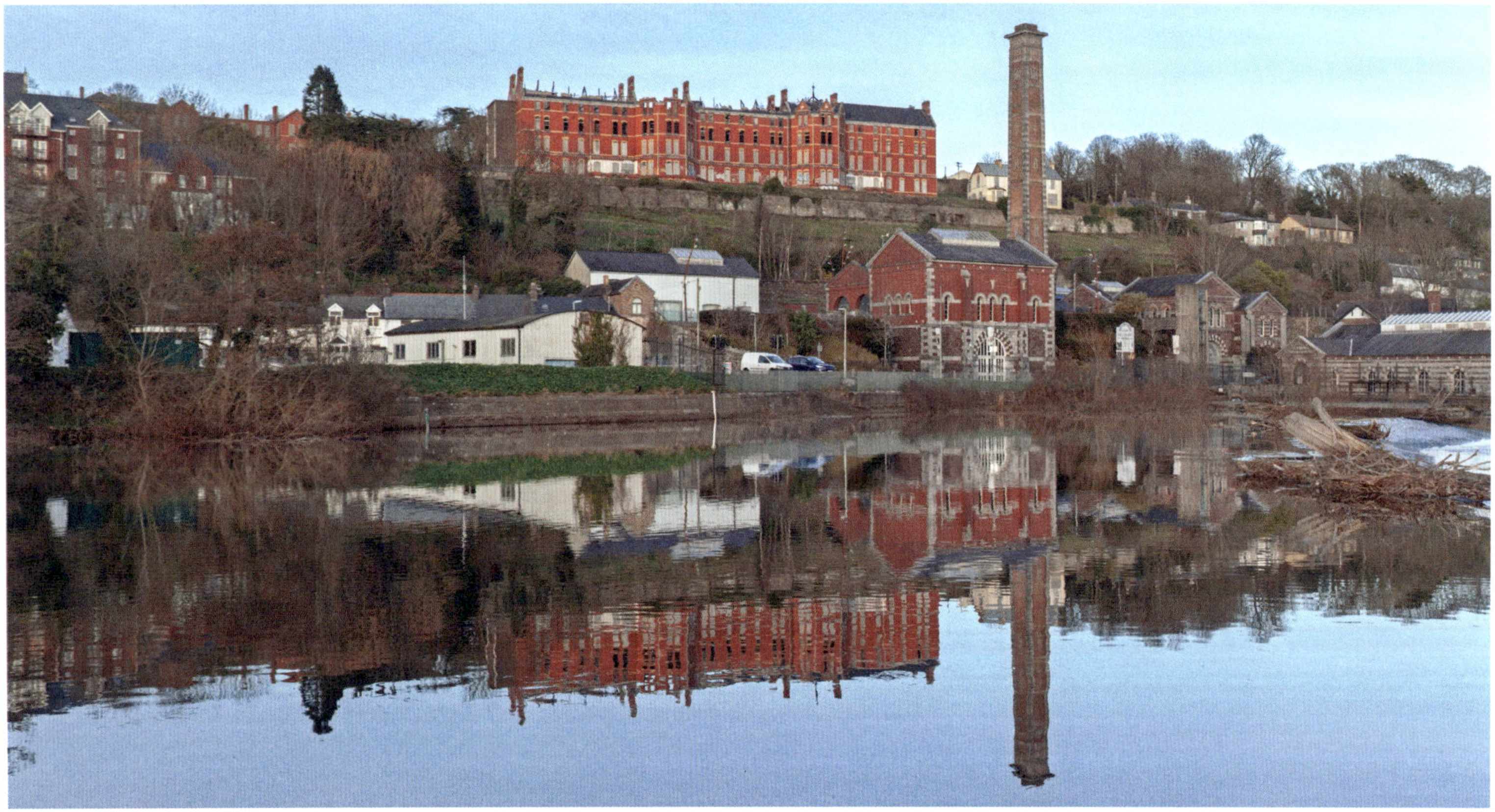

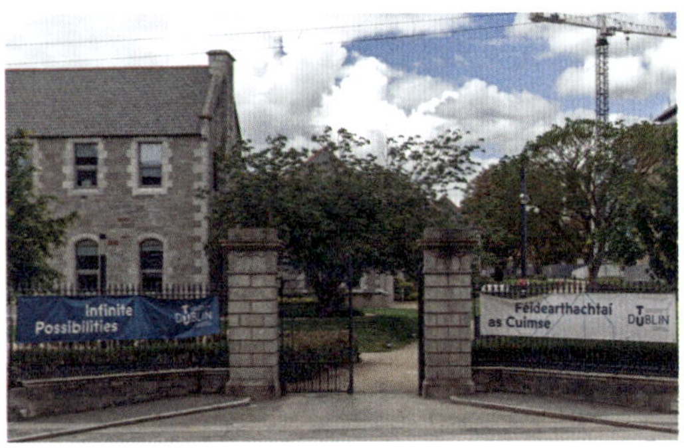
Infinite Possibilities
T DUBLIN
Féidearthachtaí as Cuimse
T DUBLIN

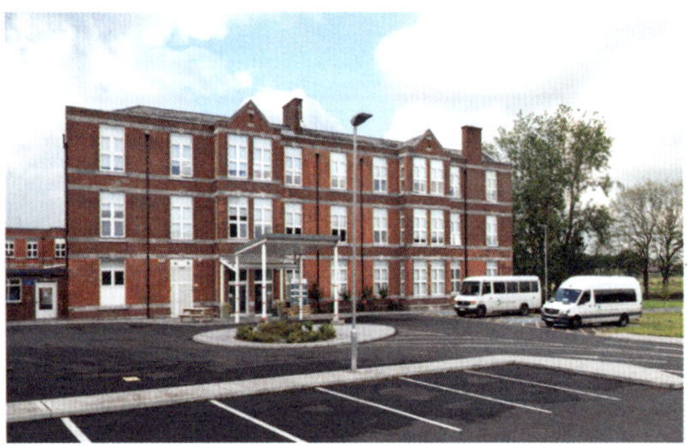

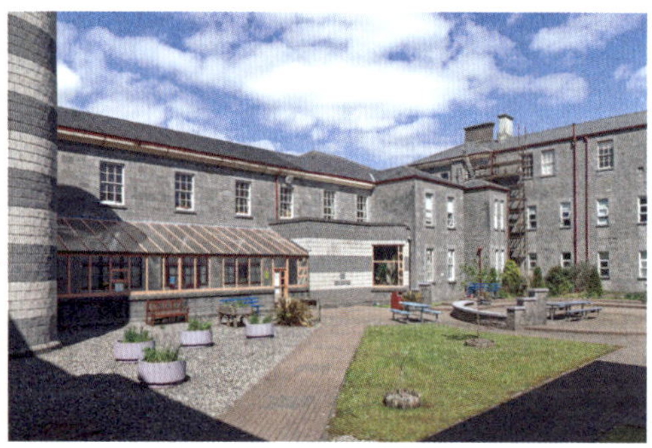

9.03 Portlaoise: The grounds of the last remaining inpatient ward have been attractively landscaped, *Photograph by David Killeen, 2019.*

9.04 Portlaoise: The historic parkland landscape continues to be maintained and enhanced, *Photograph by David Killeen, 2019*

9.05 Portlaoise: Memories of 'Maryborough' live on, *Photograph by David Killeen, 2019.*

9.06 Cork: Detached pavilion for 400 patients, completed 1894. Better known locally as St Kevin's, the building stood empty since 2002 and finally succumbed to arson in 2018, *Photograph by David Killeen, 2019.*

9.07 Grangegorman: 'Infinite Possibilities', *Photograph by David Killeen, 2019.*

9.08 Portlaoise: Even the long-vacant extremities have been brought back into modern healthcare use, *Photograph by David Killeen, 2019.*

9.09 Castlebar: Successful reuse of former asylum spaces as a third level college, *Photograph by David Killeen, 2019.*

9.10 Portlaoise: A space which once reverberated with the sounds of sport and dancing now plays silent host to the archives of its past life, *Photograph by David Killeen, 2019.*

9.11 Waterford: Peripheral parts decay even as the core of the building remains in use, *Photograph by David Killeen, 2019.*

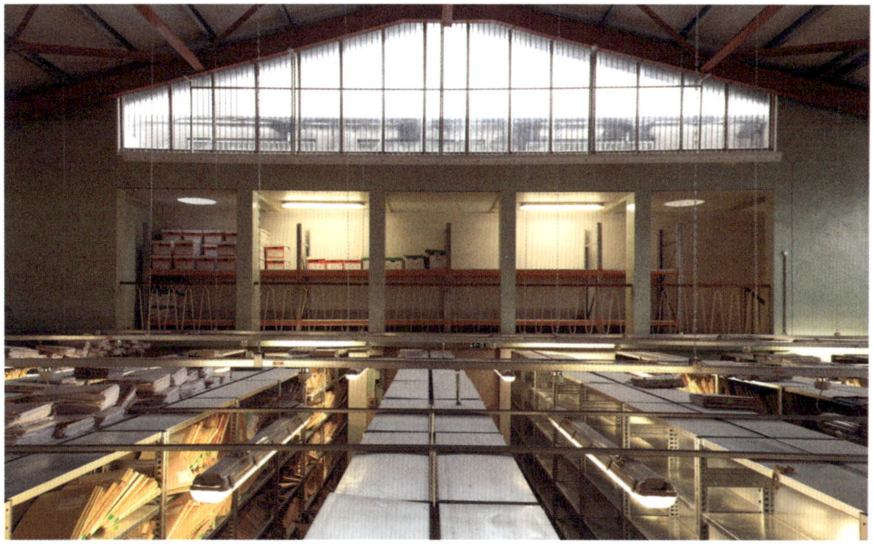

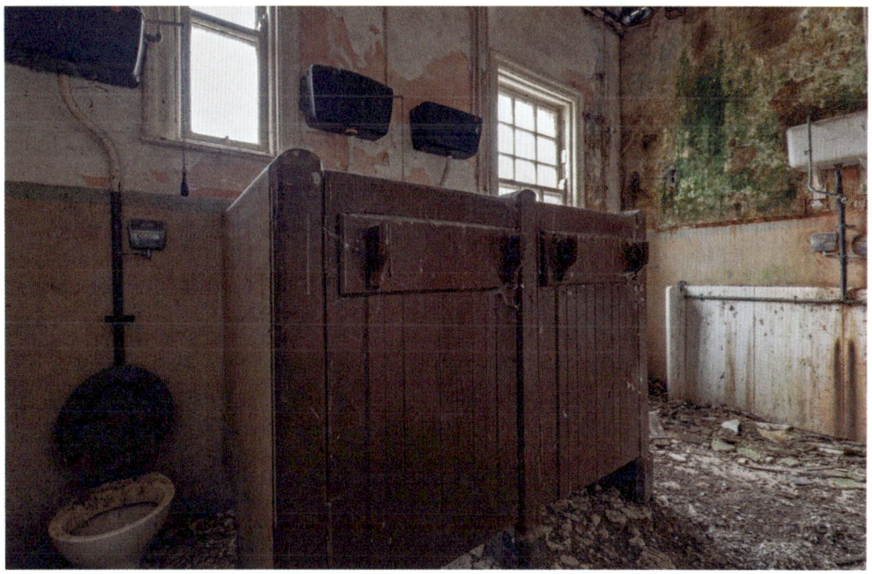

Decay and dereliction

As an example of central government intervention to secure the future of a former asylum, Grangegorman stands alone. None of the three major policy documents between 1966 and 2006 offered any vision for the future of the enormous swathe of publicly owned real estate that would be rendered redundant by the closure of the old asylums. Like so much of the twentieth-century history of the psychiatric service itself, the successful transitions already encountered were the product of local circumstance and initiative rather than central policy. Sites that failed to encourage new uses eventually passed a tipping point beyond which it made little sense to allow prospective occupiers a foothold in a building or complex likely destined for outright divestment. On such sites, five decades of contraction saw peripheral wards and secondary structures decline into decay and dereliction, but the continued presence of a small cohort of patients and staff kept the lights of the main building shining, the central heating boilers firing and the roof more watertight than not. The author was privileged to visit many of these places in their final days, when one could still meet the men and women who had worked a lifetime on the grounds or in the workshops, in the kitchens or laundries, who knew its every nook and cranny, and who could repopulate its empty spaces by recalling with striking clarity the adventures and mishaps of long-deceased patients and colleagues, albeit through sometimes rose-tinted glasses. It was the last moment when a walk through endless empty wards could still conclude with a steaming cup of tea in a comfortable canteen at the heart of the complex, humming with the chatter of staff conscious that they were the last of their kind, and counting the days until they too would follow their patients out the door.

The departure of the last patients and administrative staff in the years between 2011 and 2015 saw these old buildings, sites of such intensive human habitation and

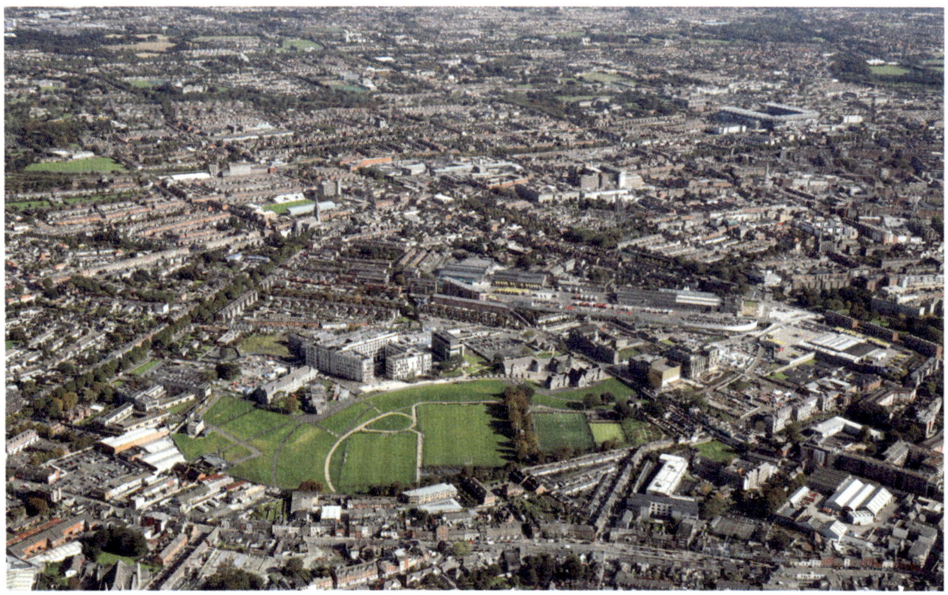

9.12 Grangegorman: Aerial photograph of a place transformed, 2020, *Photograph by Barry Coakley, 2020, reproduced courtesy of the Grangegorman Development Agency.*

activity spanning three centuries, fall finally and completely silent. Windows soon adopt the blank stare that is particular to the abandoned building. There is a distinct sense of melancholy: the layering of dust and cobweb on glass, the forgotten articles fading on window sills, the sad absence of lights on dark winter evenings. And that is before the more obvious evidence of decay and vandalism – the peeling paint, the broken glass, the tags of the spray-can artist, the gutters groaning under the weight of vegetation.

The natural processes of decay accelerate once the radiators fall cold. The Irish climate is hard on buildings, and harder yet the further west one goes. Killarney's former asylum is one of the most climatically exposed anywhere in the British Isles, a point made abundantly clear when one observes the pace of deterioration in a well-secured building that has escaped the vandalism seen at other sites. If the combination of poor workmanship and horizontal Atlantic rain could lead to rampant dry rot in a brand-new building in 1852 (see Chapter Four), its recurrence should be no surprise in an unoccupied, unheated veteran of almost 170 winters.[20] But it is the spectre of vandalism that poses the most immediate threat to Ireland's empty asylums. Low-grade damage such as graffiti and broken windows, left unchecked, advertise the building's vulnerability and act like a public invitation for worse. Copper pipework, electric wiring and stainless-steel kitchen fittings are all appealing to thieves, but most of all it is base lead that seems to gleam like gold. The theft of lead sheeting, valleys and flashings causes damage a hundred times more costly than the scrap value of the metal taken, rendering habitable spaces derelict and unsafe within a couple of winters. Only arson achieves the task of destruction more quickly. Thus far, incidents of the latter have been thankfully rare, limited to the brigade of Cork pyromaniacs who have successively gutted each of the landmark nineteenth-century institutions that commanded the northern slopes of the Lee valley.

20. Individual asylum sites in the UK experience higher rainfall or wind exposure, but not Killarney's combination of both.

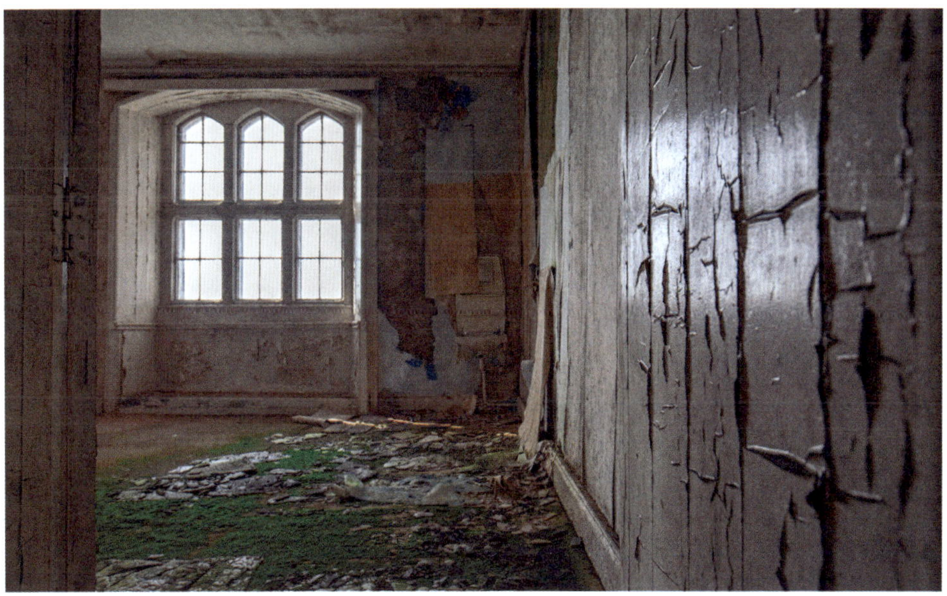

9.13 Killarney: A building which leaked buckets when newly opened is even more vulnerable in its unoccupied and unheated state, *Photograph by David Killeen, 2019.*

21. *A Vision for Change Report*, p. 8, pp 179–85.

At the time of writing, nine significant former asylums stand almost or entirely empty and deteriorating. Those at Waterford and Limerick, by virtue of prime locations within major cities, are well placed to find commercially viable new uses, most likely enabled by private residential development. The same will eventually hold true at Cork, where a developer has been slowly converting William Atkin's 285-metre behemoth into a private apartment scheme, arson and recession impeding but not preventing progress. The state's Land Development Agency has prepared a masterplan for the residential redevelopment of the remaining lands at Cork, including the gutted shell of the late-nineteenth-century ward block better known locally as St Kevin's. The same agency is preparing a similar plan for the pristine historic buildings and landscape at Dundrum, which hopefully will not stand empty long enough to suffer the indignity of dereliction.

It was a core assumption of *A Vision for Change* that the 'considerable equity in buildings and lands within the current mental health system' could be realised through open market sale to meet the almost €800-million cost of replacement facilities.[21] Even without the property crash of 2008–2012, anticipating multi-million valuations for such complex entities was both naive and optimistic. With the notable exception of Dundrum already mentioned, the presence of numerous protected structures in various states of disrepair depresses the potential value of the wider holding; their restoration and reuse is a challenge to which few developers active in the Irish market will be equal. The hidden long-term costs of decades of underinvestment in maintenance and repair have finally crystallised.

So it has proven at Ennis, which was put on the market again in 2020, having passed through several hands since being sold into private ownership in 2002. None have even secured the building against trespass, let alone attempted to halt its continued deterioration. Only the watchful presence of a lonely statue of Our Lady, halo askew, seems to stand between the building and its total destruction at any moment of the vandal's choosing. A happier story appears to be playing out at

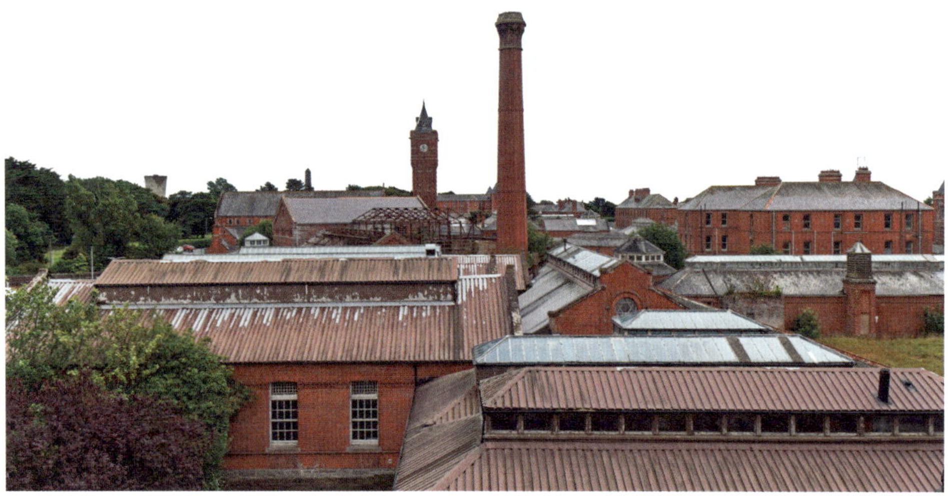

9.14 Portrane: How do you solve a problem like...?, *Photograph by David Killeen, 2019.*

Enniscorthy, where a local consortium in 2017 purchased the 12,000-square-metre building on 46 acres of potentially developable land, for little more than might be paid for a five-bedroom house on a similarly sized farm.[22] Commendably, the new owners invested significant funds in securing and conserving the fabric from the outset while appointing a design team via competition and obtaining planning consent for a development of 71 retirement apartments. If this venture succeeds it may embolden others to consider pitches for similarly challenging opportunities at Mullingar or Killarney. Even so, local conservation officers may need to accept that protecting a structure in law does not mean that it is possible, or even desirable, to preserve it in its entirety. Long derelict extensions, like frostbitten extremities, may need to be amputated to save the patient.

The great metropolitan asylum of Portrane is a challenge on an altogether different scale, not helped by its location on an isolated peninsula site 13 miles distant from the city it was built to serve. Precedents from Britain, where dozens of similar 'pavilion echelon' asylums were divested by the National Health Service during the 1980s and 1990s, point to private residential redevelopment as the only approach likely to save even a fraction of the original buildings, but at the cost of destroying most of the features that lend the building its historic, architectural, social and technical interest. But the most challenging site of all is undoubtedly Ballinasloe. Built to serve a whole province, at its peak the hospital comprised over 2,000 patients and staff in a town with a population of only 5,711.[23] Today, the majority of the campus, including the main building of 1833, stands empty and in a state of advanced dereliction, having been subject to repeat visits by the nocturnal salvage teams. Analogous with the rustbelt factory, Ballinasloe has lost not just a hospital, but its largest industry, albeit stranded by political, rather than economic, forces. Here, more than anywhere, political will at regional and national level is needed to resolve an intractable problem far beyond the capacities of any coalition of local public and private sector actors. All the while, the scavengers continue to ply their destructive trade.

22 *Irish Examiner*, 12 Jan. 2017, www.irishexaminer.com/property/victorian-building-guiding-just-euro6-a-square-foot-at-enniscorthy-438812.html, accessed on 27 Dec. 2019.

23 Total patient numbers resident in Ballinasloe through the 1950s generally exceeded 1,550 (discounting Ballinasloe patients lodged at other hospitals, which are sometimes erroneously included when this example is cited in other sources). Staff headcount in 1954 (the last year for which staff statistics were recorded by the Inspector of Mental Hospitals) was 434. Town population from Census of Ireland, 1961.

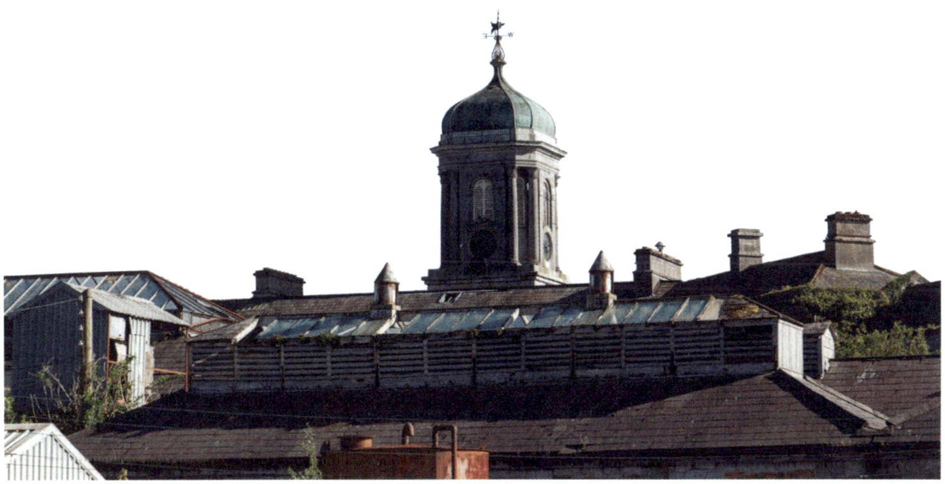

9.15 Ballinasloe: Redundant relics of a once-mighty 'industry', *Photograph by David Killeen, 2019.*

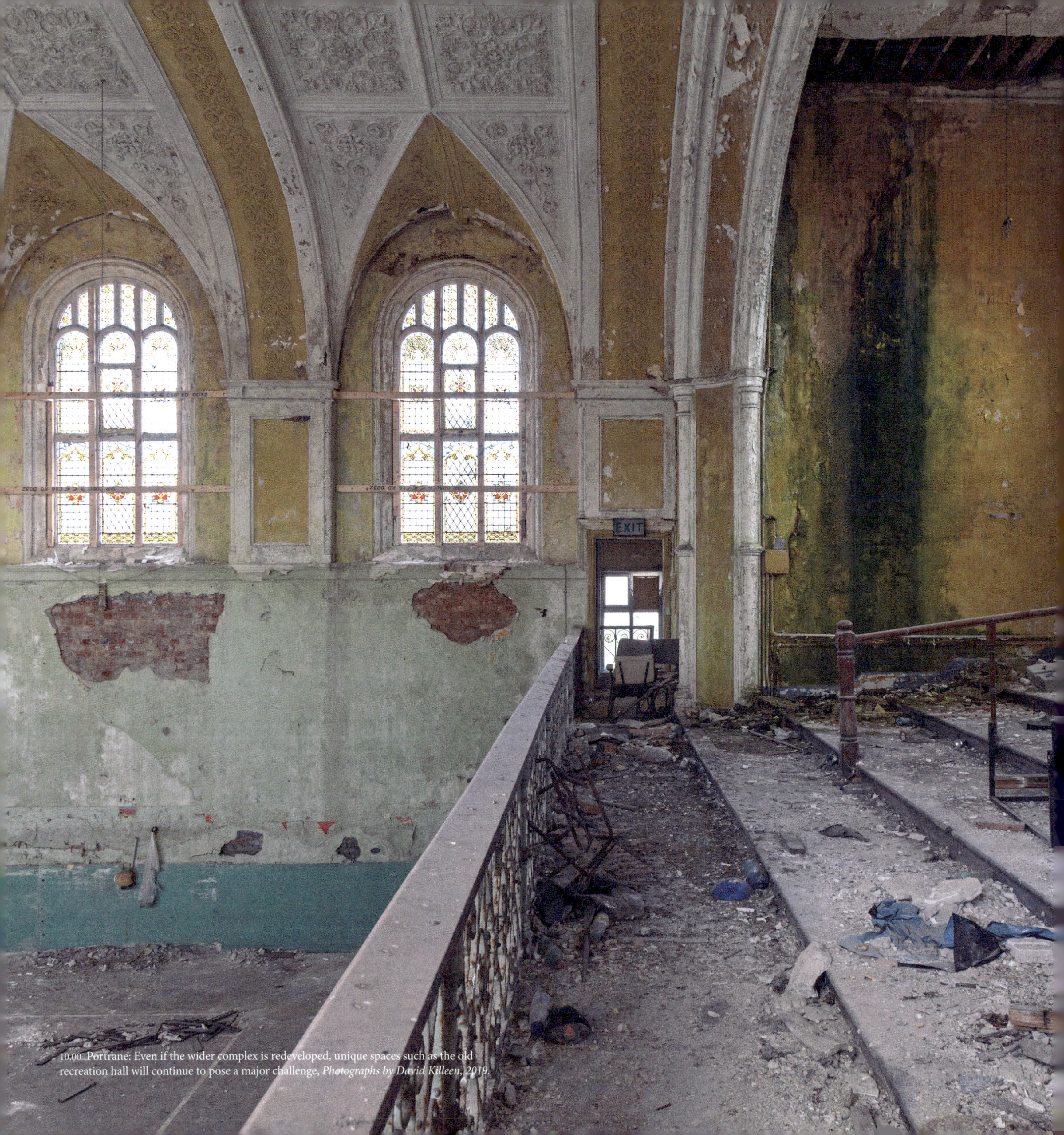

10.00 Portrane: Even if the wider complex is redeveloped, unique spaces such as the old recreation hall will continue to pose a major challenge, *Photographs by David Killeen, 2019.*

Conclusion

> *The centre is an ideal model for the type of modern facility required to provide services over the 21st Century. It reflects both the ideology and implementation of mental health policy agreed under 'A Vision for Change' and clearly reinforces the commitment of the Government to progress a more flexible and patient-centred focus by our changing mental health services.*[1]

On the 28 February 1814, the first patients took up residence in an experimental new institution on the north-eastern outskirts of Dublin City. The Richmond Lunatic Asylum was built in a spirit of optimism as a national solution to the shameful conditions in which insane persons had theretofore been held – in prisons, bridewells and houses of industry all over Ireland. Precisely one year shy of the two-hundredth anniversary of that day, the great and the good again gathered in a spirit of optimism to unveil the latest solution to the shameful conditions in which Grangegorman's mental health service users had historically been accommodated – a repurposed prison, cholera- and tuberculosis-stricken wards, chronically crowded tin-and-timber sheds, packed into 70-bed dormitories in structures on the verge of physical collapse.

For those familiar with these less auspicious aspects of Grangegorman's twentieth-century history, the day was one to celebrate, and the new facility was a fitting expression of a shared hope that for those afflicted with mental illness, the future would be a better, kinder place. Most of those gathered probably regarded the event as a transformative break with a long and sometimes unhappy past. Probably fewer reflected on how closely their aspirations echoed those of their predecessors, who had initiated their own new ventures with similar optimism and zeal. And perhaps none realised that, in explicitly portraying the building as a living embodiment and advertisement for a new ideology in mental health care, a wheel that was set in motion two centuries earlier had in fact come full circle.

At the outset of this book, I invited readers to think of the asylum as a trinity of *idea, institution* and *place*. The *idea* of asylum rested on a premise that a combination of architecture, kindness and moral guidance could cure insanity. The *institution* emerged as an organisational structure to deliver those cures. And the *place* provided the physical setting that was supposed to make it all possible. I observed that while all three have been the subject of research on the international stage, Irish scholars have, with limited exceptions, neglected the third component. This book was intended to remedy that shortcoming and, by allowing them to be

1. Minster of State for Mental Health, Kathleen Lynch TD. Speech at the official opening of the Phoenix Care Centre at Grangegorman, 28 Feb. 2013, www.dit.ie/newsandevents/news/archive2013/officialopeningofthephoenixcarecentreatgrangegorman/, accessed 11 May 2020.

more widely understood and appreciated, to restore the buildings and landscapes to a level of prominence in today's historical debates that reflects their importance to the societies that created them.

Built to cure

The original idea of the asylum was intimately bound up with the concept of 'environmental determinism' – that buildings have the potential to materially influence the lives of those who use them. This application of Enlightenment thinking was expressive of a new-found optimism in the potential of architecture to help to cure insanity – the potential of reason to cure un-reason. Johnston's innovative design for the earliest asylums embodied such modern theories of moral treatment within their very fabric, but as panoptic architecture became irrevocably associated with prison design, these innovative buildings would soon come to be seen as too prison-like to offer a real therapeutic environment; their genesis as a genuine attempt to 'scale-up' the curative potential of moral management was soon forgotten. Individual cells lit by tiny, high and inaccessible windows may long have been a staple of asylum design, but by the 1840s they too seemed irredeemably carceral. Changing therapeutic priorities discarded the curative potential of the 'all-seeing eye' and in its place invited patients to rest their own eyes on the view outside their windows. While undoubtedly more pleasant for the inmates, the latter would alas prove no more curative than the former.

Despite early rhetoric that repeatedly promoted the idea of the asylum as an idealised version of a family home, the very act of congregating so many strangers into a single location under the control of an unrelated paternal figure created something that was ultimately neither familial nor domestic, but a professionally structured residential institution. By the third wave of asylum building, most architects simply regurgitated more economic versions of the corridor plan of the second phase. The idea that buildings could contribute to the cure of the insanity had all but died, not least because the latest architecture had repeatedly failed to live up to the claims made on its behalf. Ever more complex ancillary spaces and systems were necessary to accommodate historically unprecedented numbers of people in a single building, within which continuously improving levels of physical comfort masked the creeping dilution of any sense of individual dignity. However, this research actually reveals that the old dream continued to resurface in various guises, sometimes in the most unexpected of places. It is one thing to see the newly created asylum committee of a thriving and confident metropolis (Belfast) look past the received wisdom of conventional English designs to mainland Europe for inspiration. More surprising altogether is the discovery that, 40 years earlier, the governors of a far less affluent rural district (Monaghan) undertook their own benchmarking exercise, prescribing an excellent competition brief and committing to a pioneering design in the face of resistance from a conservative central bureaucracy – and all this at a time when some of their peers in other counties were happy to settle for the tired reheats of a superannuated workhouse architect. Not content to rest on past glories, their successors repeated the trick two generations later.

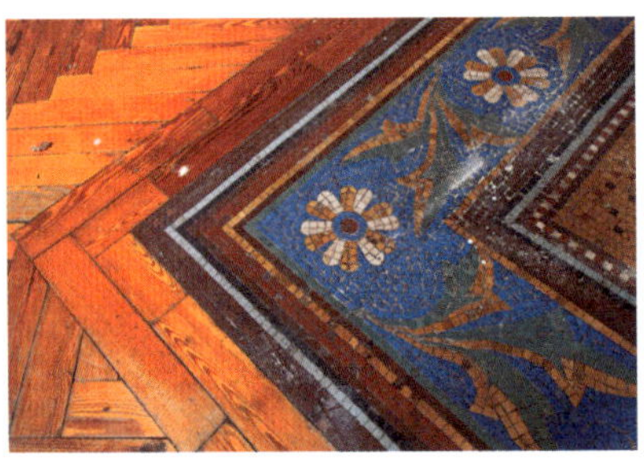

10.01 Portrane: Late nineteenth-century decorative mosaic, *Photograph by David Killeen, 2019.*

Even enthusiastic cheerleaders for the power of good architecture should hesitate before attributing Monaghan's generally high institutional reputation over time to the qualities or properties of its buildings – even if we accept that the fine doctor's residence may have succeeded in attracting a better calibre of RMS as the governors had hoped. It is safer to suggest that excellent buildings may be the physical expression of a positive culture that permeates other aspects of how an institution conducts its affairs. And if buildings offer irrefutable evidence that *something* happened, then Armagh's exceptional Hill Building of 1898 suggests that hope and aspiration could still blossom even in a desert of disillusionment. The point is proven more strongly in the scattering of rare but wonderful new buildings built in the 1930s and 40s. Paradoxically, it was depressingly high mortality from tuberculosis that inspired structures where the curative powers of sunlight and fresh air were once again paramount. More optimistically we encounter similarly sun-soaked admissions hospitals for the reception and treatment of acute cases of insanity appearing in some localities decades earlier than the generally accepted narrative, implying that those lean decades when we are told that 'nothing much else happened' warrant a fresh look.

After the 1970s the imperative to swap the discredited setting of the asylum for the brave new world of the general hospital aligned with the pharmacological revolution to send 'environmental determinism' into a medically induced coma from which it would only emerge in the twenty-first century. Most recently, a new generation of buildings commissioned to finally euthanise the old asylums and to replace that first dismal generation of acute psychiatric units have re-awakened the notion that good spaces can have positive effects on their occupants. Only time will allow us to determine the effects and longevity of this latest swing of the pendulum.

Built to communicate

Ireland's asylum buildings – especially those built during the first two phases – clearly reflect the line of thinking pursued by Stevenson and Topp: that the asylum was never merely a container for the processes of the *institution*, but also an advertisement for the very *idea* that underpinned it and the powers that sponsored it. In adding a cupola at Armagh and every one of his asylums thereafter, Johnston was proclaiming the civic credentials of the building to an audience beyond the walls. But for those within the walls – patients and subordinate staff alike - the cupola conveyed more than just civic values: it acted as a symbolic marker of the authority of the moral governor at the centre of the institution. It mattered not that the cupola was functionally blind and housed nothing more sinister than the asylum clock – its dominant position astride the governor's house made it a physical proxy for the 'all-seeing eye' on which this early brand of moral management depended.

Symbolic central towers were less compatible with the picturesque aesthetic sought by architects of the second phase of asylums, but the appearance of these buildings was no less loaded with meaning. With layouts constrained by a prescriptive brief, the private sector architects instead indulged their creative egos in the design of elaborate façades. In doing so they were responding to the brief set by the Board of Public Works, but also showcasing their skills at a time when architecture

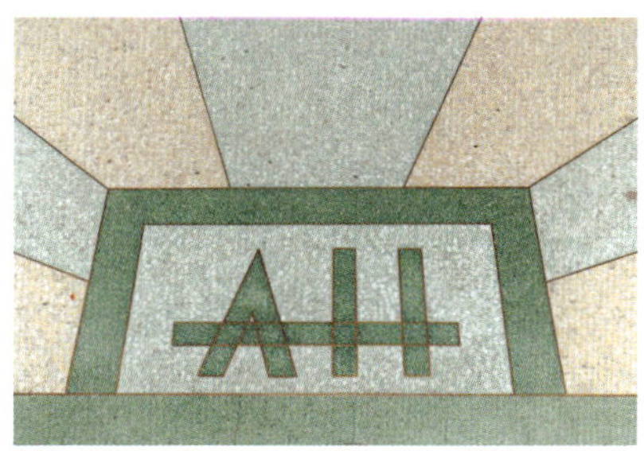

10.02 Ballinasloe: Mid twentieth-century decorative terrazzo, *Photograph by David Killeen, 2019.*

was beginning to organise itself as a profession. Their efforts also succeeded in positioning the asylums alongside other respectable institutions of the age, not least the new colleges and seminaries erected by both church and state. However, theirs was a triumph of form over function: the criticisms that soon attended their extravagant detailing, defective workmanship and depressing airing courts imply that the lessons of London's Bethlem, old and new, had been too easily forgotten.

After a brief absence from the second generation of buildings, the clocktower returned as a central focus of asylums of the third phase and beyond. At Monaghan the tower followed the RMS to his newly detached quarters, a none-too-subtle reminder that the boss might still be watching even when not in the building. The clocktower or cupola was a motif that designers of the 1930s mental hospitals at Ardee and Castlerea felt obliged to include, and it continued to feature on several of the modern admissions units built right into the 1940s. The latter buildings would have been indistinguishable from general hospitals and sanatoria of the period were it not for these towers: architectural markers of central authority had no place in a modern general hospital, but were seemingly indispensable in a mental hospital.

In the early days of the system, officials and designers invoked domestic associations of the asylum as a model family home. But in truth, and even without the rhetorical flourish of the tower, the formality, rigid symmetry and sheer physical presence of the asylum were sufficient to endow it with an intimidating sense of power and purpose far removed from any sense of home. Perhaps it is in this respect that Wilkinson's economic designs for Castlebar and Letterkenny deserve some credit – his conscious effort to downplay the domineering centrality and symmetry of conventional asylum design made for aesthetically mediocre, but also less intimidating, buildings. Wilkinson aside, it was not until the brief flowering of modernist admissions units in the 1960s that the tyranny of architectural symmetry and its overtones of hierarchy and control would finally be overthrown in favour of less formal, more approachable design.

Built to care

The utilitarian layout and appearance of the buildings after the 1860s are evidence of a system that had surrendered its original curative aspirations in favour of a policy of care and containment. Building sponsors and designers became more focused on meeting the functional needs of the 'asylum-as-institution', and ever less concerned with the original curative aspirations of 'asylum-as-idea'. The latter could be said to have died amidst the anonymous pauper graves that most powerfully symbolise its failure, but the loss of its founding ideal was no impediment to the continued expansion of the institution, and so too, its buildings. As belief in the power of architecture to 'mend muddled minds' faded, so too did any willingness to spend money on architectural façade treatment as an end in itself. Instead, professional designers turned their attention towards the enormous practical and technical challenges of accommodating unprecedented numbers of people at close quarters, creating buildings where stylistic treatment was of secondary importance to the rigorous resolution of complex programmatic requirements. Kitchens, laundries, workshops and boiler houses all grew in size and complexity. In an era before mains

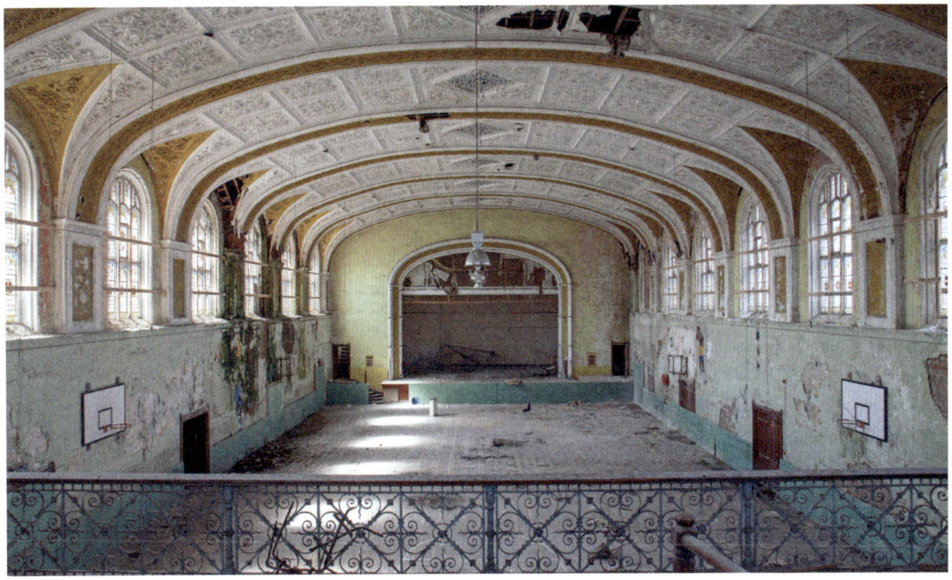

10.03 Portrane: Over a century on, the recreation hall still ranks as one of the largest indoor spaces in any public building in Ireland, *Photograph by David Killeen, 2019.*

services, water supply and sewage disposal represented continuing challenges that demanded capital investment at least once in every generation. Sanitary annexes containing rows of half-height cubicles were more convenient and hygienic than the single privies of old, but at the expense of dignity and privacy. The latter attributes were in short supply as individual sleeping cells gave way to dormitories of 10, then 20, 50 and as many as 80 people in a single space. By day these patient hordes were shepherded into cavernous day rooms, thence to large, central dining halls where cacophonous mealtimes reverberated with the noise of hundreds of chairs scraping across floors and hundreds of spoons clattering on enamelled plates.

Throughout the history of the asylum, there had been an inevitable tension around the standard of accommodation deemed appropriate for the 'pauper class'. For many of those admitted to an asylum, especially before the famine, these solid masonry buildings with private sleeping accommodation, glazed windows, planked floors, enclosed fireplaces and rudimentary sanitation would have represented a dramatic improvement compared to their domestic living arrangements, an argument that parsimonious local governors were not shy to invoke. However, it must be recorded to the credit of the Inspectors of Lunacy that, whatever their other failings, they did drive continuous improvements in the standards of material comfort within the asylums throughout every era. By the dawn of the twentieth century, asylums with their gas or electric lighting, indoor sanitation, forced ventilation and (frequently though not universally) central heating systems employed technologies that would not appear in the average Irish home for several more generations.

Technical improvements could not make up for the general absence of other trappings of domesticity that contribute to psychological comfort, not least homely furnishings, wallpaper, curtains, pictures and plants. It is dangerous to draw firm conclusions in the absence of internal photography (and the few photographs as do exist are explicitly staged and therefore hardly representative), but on balance the

2. Kate Millett, *The Loony-Bin Trip* (New York, 1990), p. 202.

Inspectors' reports infer that initiatives to introduce such home comforts tended to be both rare and short-lived. Kate Millett, during her brief sojourn in Ennis in the 1980s, observed that the 'large, ugly, shabby, bilious yellow' walls were enlivened only by that ubiquitous Sacred Heart picture, 'the one in every home and refectory in Ireland'.[2]

Looking past the barnlike dormitories and dayrooms which offend our modern sensibilities of privacy and dignity, other developments on asylum sites allow for some intriguing observations. Governing boards dominated by the Protestant gentry proved to be willing builders of fine Roman Catholic chapels, even locating them in prominent positions at the expense of the landscape set-pieces devised by their grandfathers. Nurses' homes were tolerated as an unavoidable necessity, but the reticence of so many of the same governors to sanction detached houses for their most important employees – the Resident Medical Superintendents (RMS) – implies that Scull's theories around psychiatry's nineteenth-century project of self-aggrandisement did not entirely succeed on this island.

Built to contain

Notwithstanding the radical ambition to cure, which underpinned the design of Johnston's early asylums, closer examination reveals a more conservative commitment to containment. The most obvious example is in the design of his cell windows, whose conventional external appearance belied a more prison-like character internally. Lessons were learned, and each subsequent phase of buildings employed more and bigger windows than the last, allowing more daylight in and better views out. The second-phase asylums featured iron casements with small panes – the window discreetly integrating its own bars – but by the third phase paranoia around the risks of escape (or self-harm) had eased to the extent that conventional timber sash windows became the norm. Measured against the standard of a 'prison-like appearance', the generously fenestrated buildings of the later nineteenth century

10.04 Mullingar: The formal set-piece to the front...

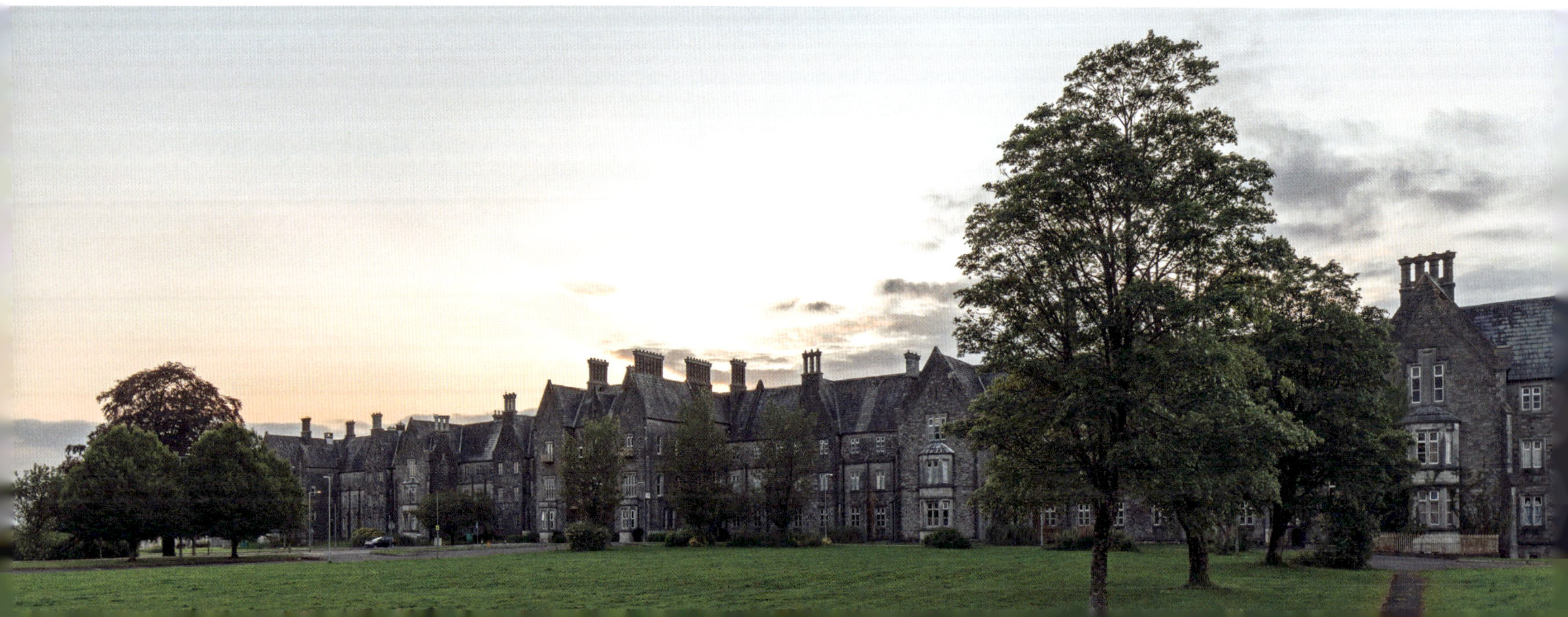

were as far removed from contemporary penal architecture as could be imagined, and not stylistically dissimilar from the new architectural vernacular of religious institutions that had sprouted across Ireland in the period. But in another paradox, it was these buildings whose appearance was the least objectively 'prison-like' that abandoned all pretence of cure and succumbed to 'containment' mode.

It was a founding thesis of moral management that patients had to be categorised and physically segregated according to their condition or behaviour. The logic of placing the 'noisy and refractory' in their own separate ward to minimise inconvenience to more 'tranquil' patients is understandable, but it is no coincidence that Johnston relegated these refractory wards to the rear of the institution. Worse still were the basement cells for the 'dirty and ungovernable'. In both cases, those patients most in need of the therapeutic effects of moral management were denied its supposed benefits by virtue of their disadvantaged location within the building.[3] While refractory patients enjoyed a brief promotion to the main ground floor wards in asylums of the second generation, a general trend of marginalising difficult cases recurs throughout the entire period under examination, from the grim and gloomy 'back wards' of Hannah Greally's Mullingar to *Magill* magazine's revelations of decrepit buildings full of hard-pressed staff struggling to care for 'residualised' patients deemed too challenging to decant to 'community' settings. Yet, the practice of locating so many of the new acute psychiatric wards in the basements and back-wings of general hospitals in the 1970s and 80s at least begs the question as to whether the general health authorities retained similar prejudices – conscious or subliminal – against the entire mental health enterprise.

For much of their existence, lunatic asylums were sealed societies, enclosed behind high walls, whose stated function was to protect the insane from the cruelties of an intolerant world, but whose lasting impact would be to convince the world that it needed to be protected from dangerous 'others' within. More so

10.05 ...conceals the complexity of what lies behind. *Photographs by David Killeen, 2019.*

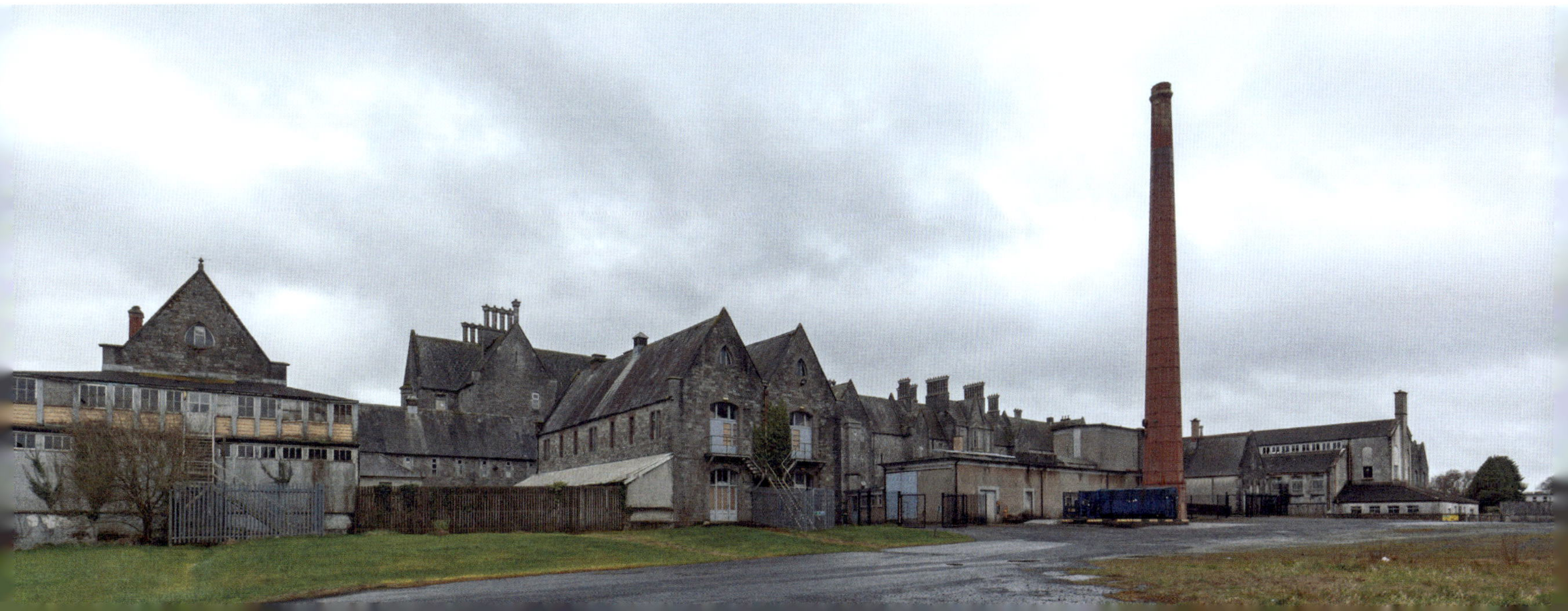

3. On the one hand, such odious features can seem to support narratives of the asylum as a repository for society's unwanted. However, I would consider the very starkness of the contrast between these marginalised spaces and the majority of the building could be seen to support the argument that the agenda of the earliest asylums was predominantly curative.

even than the clocktower, it was the stark face of its boundary wall that defined the asylum in most communities. Minor feats of civil engineering reinforced perimeters that for a century had to be secured at all costs, until one day, they did not. The walls were lowered, nobody died, and Irish society began the slow and fitful journey towards reintegrating those whom it had long been believed were better off inside an asylum.

Planted for pride and pleasure

Every asylum site includes a mix of buildings good, bad and indifferent, and even those designed along the most ostensibly curative lines can still be tainted by the bleaker aspects of the regime they facilitated and the meanings they came to embody. But of the many and various efforts to create therapeutic environments, I conclude that the most convincing and enduring are not buildings at all, but the landscapes that surround them. There is something quite revolutionary in the thought that pauper lunatics of the 1820s, 30s and 40s, most of whom were drawn from the ranks of the subsistence farmer or landless labourer, were at leisure to enjoy summerhouses and bowers, herbaceous borders and woodland walks – simply by virtue of their diminished or disturbed mental state. These were trappings of elite landscape culture, created at the public expense to benefit those at the opposite end of the social spectrum, generations before the concept of the public park gained currency. In my view, Ireland's asylum landscapes offer the strongest evidence that the powerful agents who initiated the asylum project were indeed motivated by the curative, benign and therapeutic aspects of their endeavour. While the set-piece of the monumental asylum building in its genteel parkland setting was undoubtedly manipulated to compose a particular image of the institution, this self-serving motive alone cannot begin to explain the extraordinarily rich landscape legacy with which the asylums were endowed.

Landscape tends to be overlooked on two accounts: landscape and garden history remains a relatively niche and underdeveloped discipline, while planted features and garden buildings are by their nature ephemeral and least likely to survive once insufficient labour remains to maintain them. Landscapes are especially vulnerable to change – while the historic asylum buildings now mostly enjoy statutory protection, landscape features survive only by the whim of their owners. The therapeutic value of landscape also suffered a similar decline in the eyes of those responsible for shaping our mental health services in the later twentieth century. Access to landscape was not a consideration during the long transition to general hospital settings: the new acute wards mostly had neither outdoor space nor a view worth drawing a curtain for. The lesson is most vividly portrayed at the Central Mental Hospital, behind whose foreboding boundary wall lies a veritable secret garden – a time machine that offers a glimpse of what most asylum landscapes looked like in a heyday of large, able-bodied patient populations. This garden will fade away like all of its peers when the hospital moves to its new quarters in Portrane, but we can hope that – just as the value of well-designed architectural spaces have latterly returned to vogue – so too might those who commission future mental health facilities re-discover the therapeutic potential of landscape.

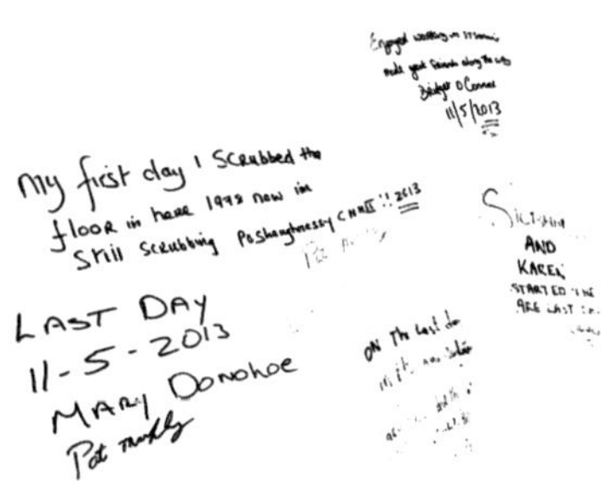

10.06 Enniscorthy: Past memories...

After the asylum

The mental hospital system is the last element of Ireland's institutional infrastructure that has not been subject to public enquiry, despite historically embodying many of the features that have been criticised in other state- and religious-run institutions – involuntary detention, humiliating and degrading conditions, unaccountable management regimes, and unmarked mass graves – even as it delivered an important public service to some of our most vulnerable citizens in permanently straitened circumstances. But the past is not the only place where the vulnerable are the 'cannon-fodder of social change'.[4] Rather than stoking the fires of moral outrage by raking over a past deemed shameful by modern standards, Irish society may be better served by taking an honest look at our conduct in the present.

In concluding his analysis of Ireland's historic asylums more than 25 years ago, Reuber cautioned that 'care in the community needs to be founded on more than blame levelled at dilapidated piles of bricks and mortar'.[5] Yet as the 50-year project to de-institutionalise Ireland's mental health services has finally achieved its goal, it is becoming apparent that the pendulum may have swung too far. From a position in the 1950s when Ireland had the highest number of psychiatric beds per capita in the world, our provision today is less than half the European average and barely 5 per cent of that former peak.[6] Clinicians and local communities report real difficulties in accessing crisis services,[7] the true capacity of twenty-first-century families and communities to deliver effective care in the home is probably declining,[8] and vulnerable people with mental health issues are now at much higher risk of finding themselves homeless or in prison.[9] Even the word 'asylum' has re-entered daily usage, though now by reference to asylum seekers living in another discredited residential setting, 'direct provision'. The Government's latest policy document, *Sharing the Vision*, has belatedly acknowledged capacity constraints in the mental health sector and committed, amongst many other important initiatives, to review inpatient bed numbers.[10] With the announcement in Budget 2020 of the first net increase in mental health inpatient beds in many years,[11] the wheel has indeed turned.

The places of asylumdom represent a national infrastructure of historic buildings comparable in quantum only to the workhouse system, and of considerably greater architectural interest, quality and variety. By my count, the 27 sites surveyed include at least 400 individual structures or features, contain over 20 kilometres of corridors and more than 45 hectares of accommodation – equivalent to almost 5,000 three-bedroom semi-detached houses. For these places, which traced a common trajectory through the nineteenth and twentieth centuries, the only certainty in the twenty-first is that their individual stories will diverge dramatically. The best examples have already transitioned gracefully to accommodate diverse public uses. Some will undergo a jarring metamorphosis to serve commercial ends, with mixed outcomes for their historic and landscape legacies. For others the picture is more challenging. Buildings that once exuded power and permanence became suddenly vulnerable when their doors close for the last time. Vacancy invites vandalism, which leads to decay, dereliction and ultimately destruction. Even routine maintenance places a heavy burden on strained health budgets; the eight kilometres of gutters and roof valleys at Portrane, if laid end-

4. John Farrelly, CEO of the Mental Health Commission, In conversation with the author, 24 Jan. 2020.
5. Markus Reuber, 'The architecture of psychological management: The Irish asylums, 1801–1922', in *Psychological Medicine* 26 (1996), p. 1188.
6. Ireland 1955: 710 beds / 100,000. EU Average 2018: 72 beds / 100,000. Ireland 2018: 35 beds / 100,000. Source: Eurostat, https://ec.europa.eu/eurostat/statistics-explained/index.php?title=File:Hospital_beds_per centE2 per cent80 per cent94_psychiatric_care_beds,_2013_and_2018_(per_100_000_inhabitants)_Health20.png, accessed 29 Oct. 2020.

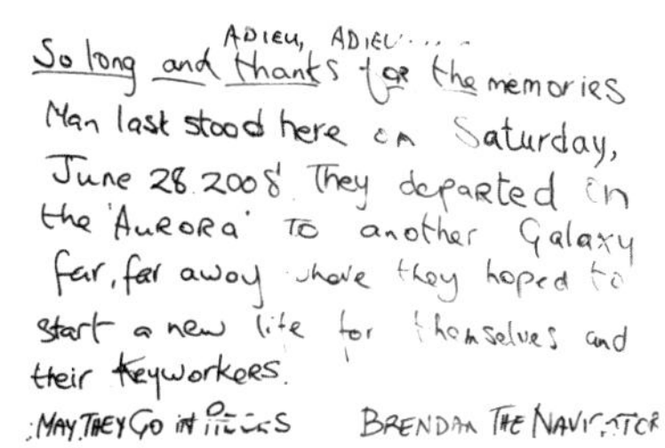

10.07 Limerick: ...and future hopes, *Photographs by David Killeen, 2019.*

to-end, would stretch down the coast to Portmarnock. In the absence of viable new uses, a very rich architectural legacy faces a deeply uncertain future.

Final Reflections

The architectural history of Ireland's lunatic asylums is a complex tale, littered with paradoxes. We have seen that the buildings that most closely resembled prisons actually best embodied the curative ideals on which the system was founded, while the most innocuous were conceived in a time of failure and despair. The most aesthetically accomplished façades were designed to impress but short-changed the patients who lived behind them and the communities who had to pay for them. The pharmacological revolution did more to allow patients to resume their normal lives than a century of architectural endeavour, but just as psychiatry was fleeing the back wards of its old asylums for the supposedly un-stigmatised setting of the medical hospital, general medicine would in turn consign psychiatry to its own back wards. The health-enhancing value of light, air and view waxed and waned and waxed again. The therapeutic potential of landscape is surely next to be 'rediscovered', but sadly not before the 'for sale' signs will be raised over many of the landscapes that did the most good, and the least harm, over the longest time, for those who were committed to the asylum system.

These paradoxes are reflected in how these places are perceived today. Each asylum site holds a unique, if contested, place in the consciousness of the local community it was built to serve, generating responses ranging from pride, affection, nostalgia, or gratitude through indifference and ambivalence to antipathy, fear or loathing. What for one person may be an irredeemably stigmatised structure fit only for the wrecking ball is, for another, a historically, socially and architecturally significant aspect of local heritage deserving of recognition and respect. The validity of both viewpoints must be recognised, though the co-existence of such seemingly incompatible visions of stigma and significance is a conundrum that will form the next chapter of my continuing research adventure.

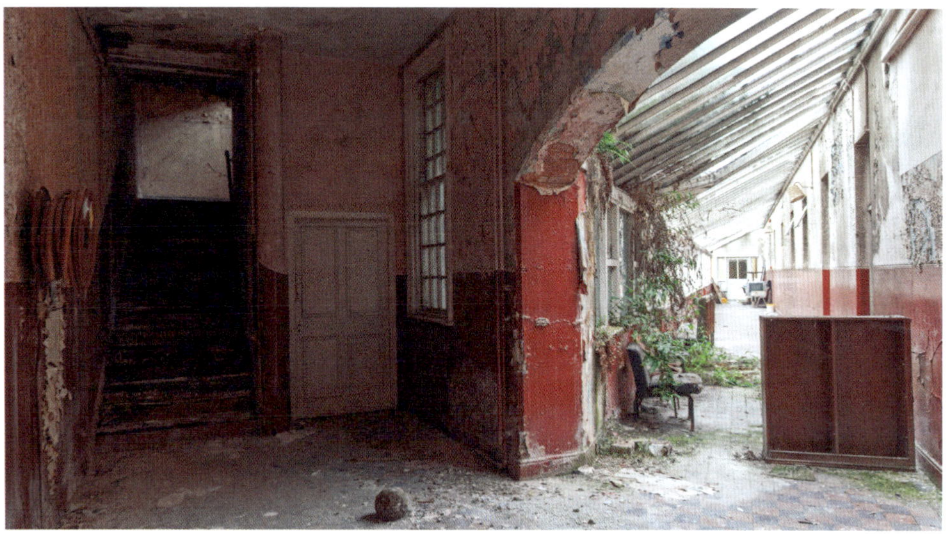

10.08 Waterford: Local flora breaking, entering...

7. Brendan Kelly, *Hearing Voices: The History of Psychiatry in Ireland* (Dublin, 2014), pp 275–6.
8. Damien Brennan, 'Family care provision for psychiatric patients in post-institutional Ireland' (unpublished conference paper). *Prisons, Asylums, Workhouses: Institutions in Ireland.* 15 Jun. 2019.
9. Kelly, *Hearing Voices*, p. 305.
10. *Sharing the Vision: A Mental Health Policy for Everyone.* (Dublin, 2018), pp. 48–9.
11. Mary Butler TD, Dáil Éireann, 15 Oct. 2020, 999:4.

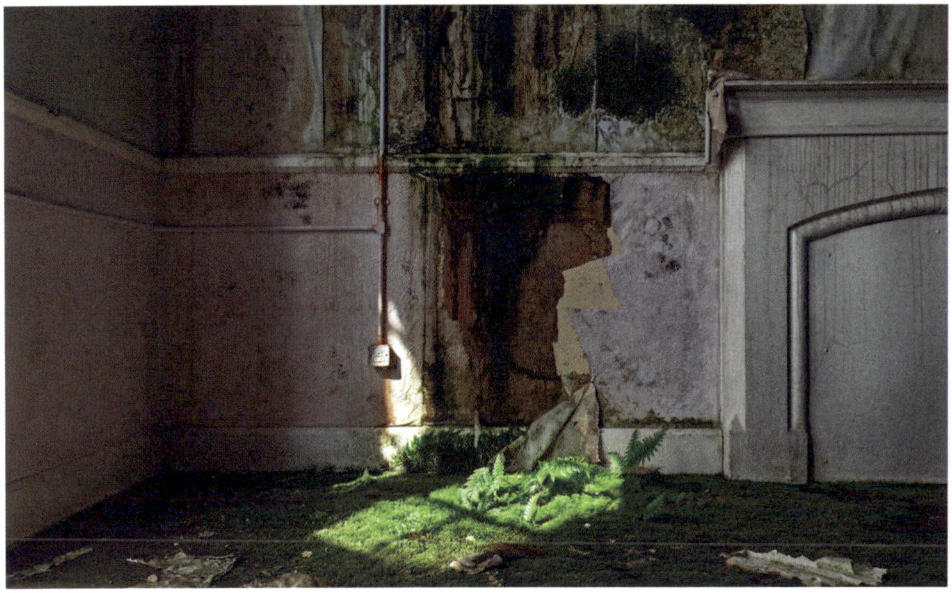

10.09 Killarney: ... and putting down roots, *Photographs by David Killeen, 2019.*

The curiosity that was kindled in that north Dublin field nine years ago has led me on a fascinating journey around a significant but largely overlooked aspect of our island's built heritage. In the time it has taken to write this book, that field in Portrane has been transformed into Ireland's newest mental hospital – a once-in-a-century project that will in time become no less worthy a subject for research than the greatest buildings in this book. However, flagship projects can only ever be part of the picture. Buildings endure, and as the state of the art evolves, a growing stock of older buildings must adapt to changing circumstances. So it was that I felt compelled to tell not just how Portrane Asylum and its ilk initially came to be, but no less importantly, the intervening chapters of how it was used or abused, and how it ultimately came to be as I found it on that May morning: sullen, empty, desolate.

The very act of not building, of not maintaining, and even of demolishing a building, is no less a part of its story than an analysis of its architectural details or the philosophical debates that presaged its construction. Churchill's old cliché about first shaping and ever after being shaped by our buildings may ring true in the ossified grandeur of the Palace of Westminster, but for asylum and hospital buildings, the relationship between shaper and shaped is a reciprocal and ever-evolving affair. The long life story of Ireland's lunatic asylum buildings, from ambitious birth and arrogant adolescence, through bloated and complacent middle age to frail decline and involuntary euthanasia, suggests that architectural historians – no less than architects – may benefit from engaging more deeply with the long and messy reality lived out by their subjects. And whether the future stories of Ireland's asylums tell of fiery destruction, prolonged limbo or glorious resurrection, I hope that this book will encourage communities to look again at these buildings 'which our forefathers built with such solidity to express the notions of their day', and appreciate them anew in all of their complex, contradictory grandeur.

10.10 Enniscorthy: If the sympathetic redevelopment of this most challenging of buildings proves successful, then there is hope for many others (next page), *Photographs by David Killeen, 2019.*

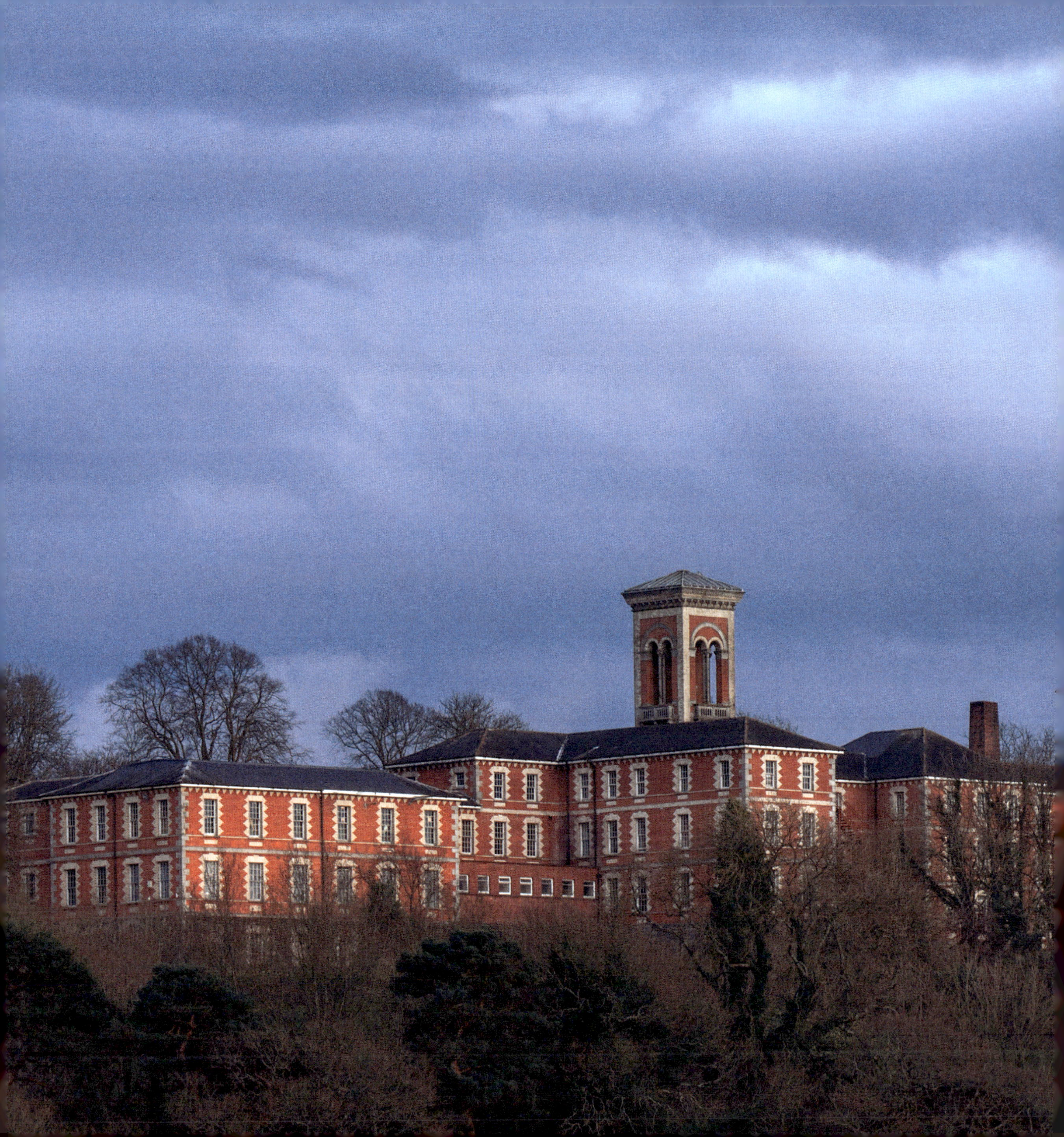

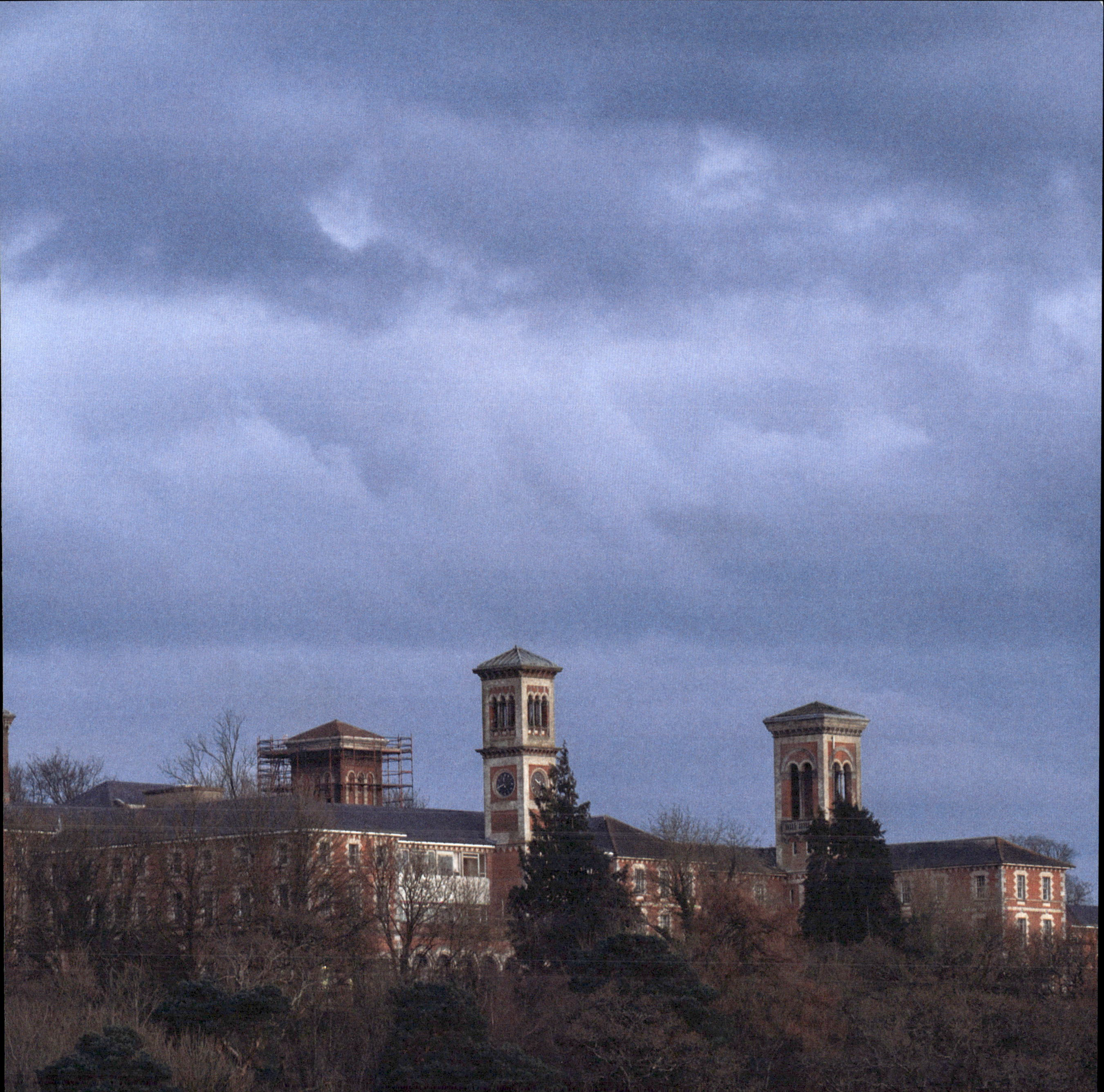

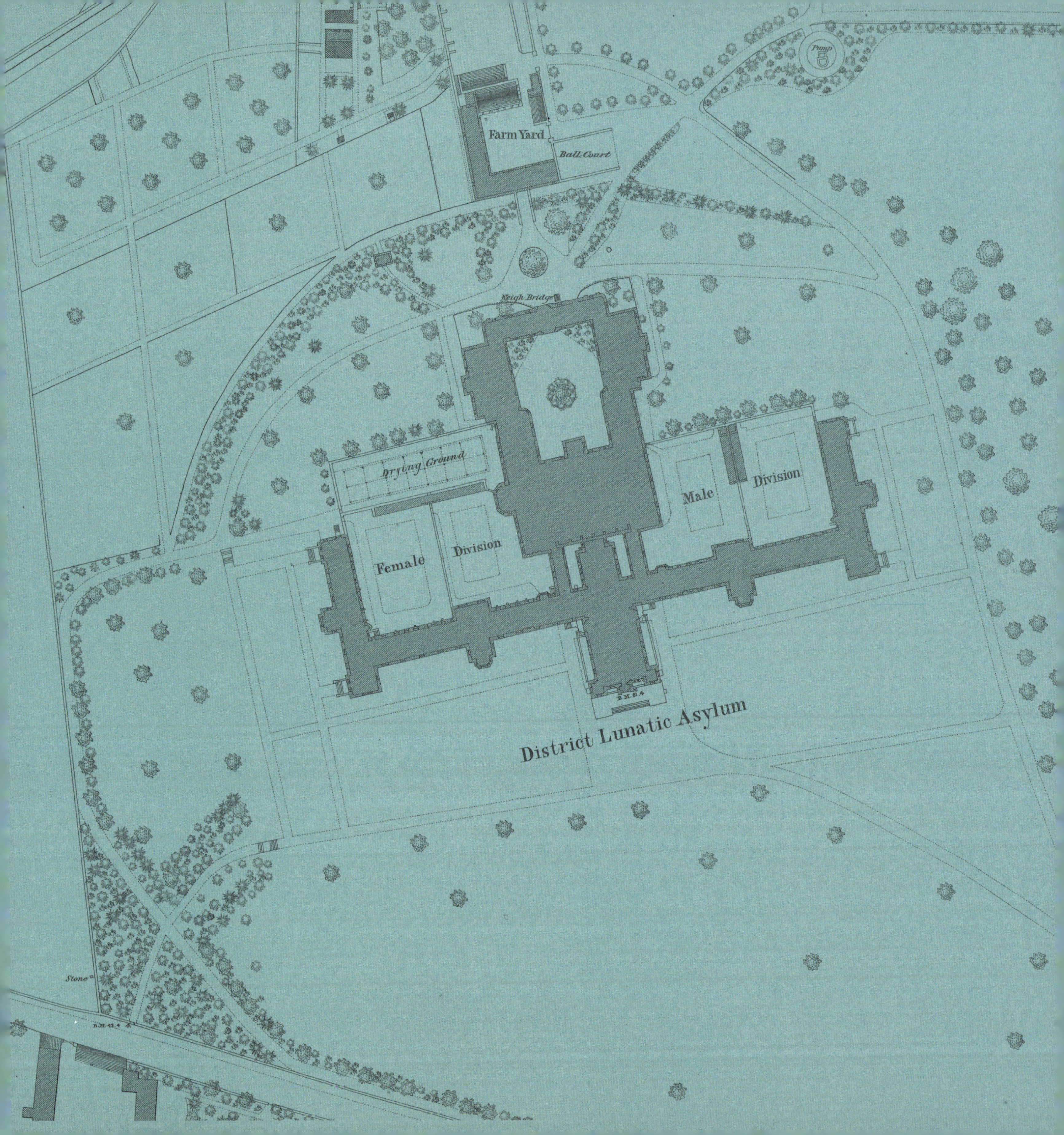

Pump
Farm Yard
Ball Court
Weigh Bridge
Drying Ground
Male
Division
Female
Division
B.M. 61.4
District Lunatic Asylum
Stone
B.M. 42.4

Case Studies

This section comprises individual profiles of each of the 29 publicly-funded, purpose-built asylum sites in Ireland. In defining this list, it has been necessary to draw certain limits to the type of site considered. So despite the existence of earlier asylum facilities erected at the initiative of various local authorities – ranging from ad-hoc cells to the large, late-eighteenth-century structure of the Cork City and County Asylum – our story starts with The Richmond, as the first institution established on a statutory footing.

Arranged in chronological order by date of opening, we first encounter the nine asylums built to the designs of Francis Johnston and completed in collaboration with his cousin, William Murray, including two sites which are no longer extant. The seven asylums of the second phase of construction, and the six asylums of the third, follow. The architect of the primary building is cited, with a necessarily subjective selection of other key designers from amongst the many who contributed later work on each site.

Holywell was the last new 'District Lunatic Asylum,' in the sense of being a new building created for a newly formed, self-governing institution, but developments thereafter require more careful definition. So despite Portrane being a mere auxiliary to Dublin's Richmond Asylum, it is included by virtue of being 'purpose-built' and hence of architectural interest. Auxiliary institutions which re-appropriated existing buildings, from workhouses and infirmaries to country mansions and TB sanatoria, are omitted. It is for this reason that readers will not encounter St Raphael's in Youghal, St Loman's in Ballyowen, or Newcastle Hospital in Wicklow between these pages. Finally, the three new twentieth-century green-field mental hospitals never actually bore the title 'asylum,' but they remained committed to the concept in all but name, and so merit inclusion.

Prepared by reference to historic and contemporary maps, drawings, photographs and documentary records, the diagrams that follow attempt to clarify the evolution of highly complex sites which have been subject of continuous change over many decades. And while the principal buildings and features are self-evident, these diagrams also identify smaller buildings and landscape features which are more easily overlooked. Buildings are coloured by relative age, with the darkest colour denoting the earliest phase of construction and the lightest reserved for late-twentieth-century additions. Demolished features denoted by dotted lines and italic labels. An undertaking of this nature is limited by the best available information and prone to error and omission and the author warmly welcomes corrections.

Legend:

ab:	Abbatoir
ac:	Airing court or airing yard: walled area for patient exercise
ah /au:	Admissions hospital / unit: separate units for reception and treatment of acute cases
bg:	Burial ground
bw:	Bowling green
bh:	Boiler house
ch:	Chimney
coi:	Church of Ireland chapel
dg:	Drying green or bleaching green for laundry
dh:	Doctor's house (generally for Assistant Medical Officer or other senior officer)
fg / kg:	Formal garden / kitchen garden (enclosed, intensively cultivated area)
fy:	Farm yard
g:	Gasworks
gh:	Greenhouse or glasshouse
gl:	Gate lodge
ha:	Handball alley
i / ih:	Infirmary / isolation hospital (detached ward for the infectious or medically unwell)
l:	Laundry
m:	Mortuary
ms:	Marian shrine or grotto
nh:	Nurses' home (for unmarried staff, both male and female)
ot:	Occupational or industrial therapy unit
pp:	Playing pitch
r:	Reservoir
rc:	Roman Catholic chapel
rms:	Private dwelling for the Resident Medical Superintendent
sc:	Staff cottages (for married attendants and their families)
sh:	Summer house or gazebo
t:	Tunnel
tb:	Tuberculosis sanatorium (specialist ward for isolating cases of TB or other infectious diseases)
tc:	Tennis Court
vm:	Viewing mound (to allow views over airing yard walls)
w:	Ward (generally detached pavilion wards)
wb:	Weigh bridge
ws:	Workshops
wt:	Water tower

CASE STUDY 01

St Brendan's Hospital

(previously Richmond Lunatic Asylum, latterly Technological University, Dublin)

Years in operation
1814–2013 (main buildings vacated c.1989)

Original cost
£49,859 (Richmond Asylum) + £25,617 (New Richmond Asylum)

Capacity (min /max)
200 (Richmond Asylym), 160 (New Richmond) 2,170 (entire)

Architect(s)
Francis Johnston, William Murray, Murray & Denny, George Wilkinson, William Kaye-Parry, W. H. Byrne, P. J. Munden, Vincent Kelly

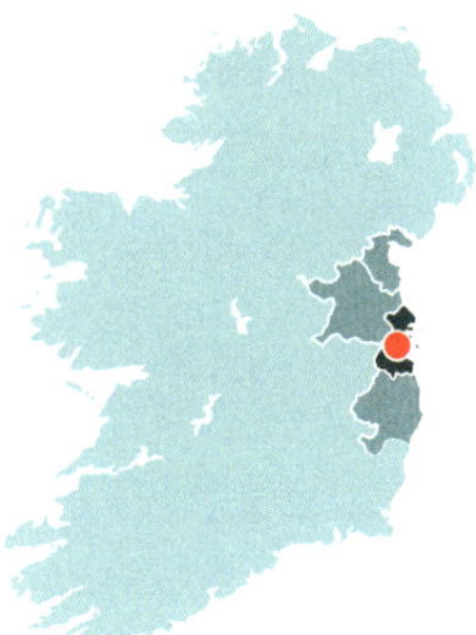

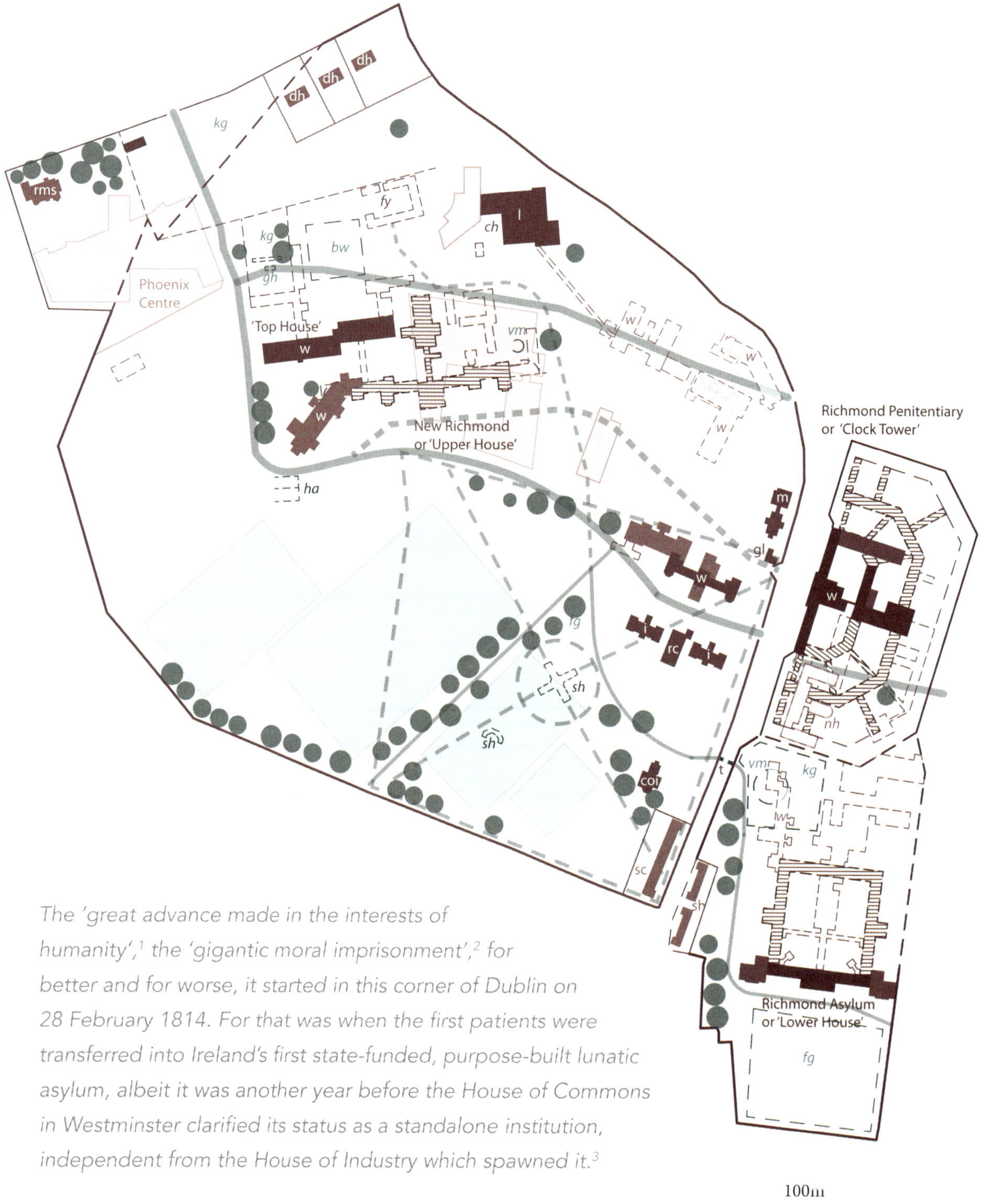

The 'great advance made in the interests of humanity',[1] the 'gigantic moral imprisonment',[2] for better and for worse, it started in this corner of Dublin on 28 February 1814. For that was when the first patients were transferred into Ireland's first state-funded, purpose-built lunatic asylum, albeit it was another year before the House of Commons in Westminster clarified its status as a standalone institution, independent from the House of Industry which spawned it.[3]

The Richmond Lunatic Asylum could be said to have been born in a stable. For that would be a fair description of the lunatic cells attached to the rear of the House of Industry, which represented the earliest dedicated accommodation for the insane on this site. The evolution of a separate, specialist institution for the insane represented just one of a fascinating array of structures for health, welfare and reform that came to colonise this quarter of Dublin. From the nucleus of the House of Industry, which was established in 1772 (known after 1839 as the North Union Workhouse), would emerge the Hardwicke Fever Hospital (1803),[4] the Bedford Asylum for Industrious Children (1808),[5] the Richmond Surgical Hospital (1810), the Whitworth Medical Hospital (1816) and the Richmond Penitentiary (1820). But it was the Richmond Lunatic Asylum that would ultimately prove to be the longest lived and most significant institutional entity of all – seeing 199 years of continuous service before being replaced by a new facility with a new name that nonetheless continues the tradition of caring for Dublin's mentally ill on part of the site to this day.

Francis Johnston's Richmond Lunatic(k) Asylum of 1814 might have been the first building of an entirely new typology, but as seen in Chapter One, its design owed more to archaic precedents of the eighteenth century than to the growing international discourse in asylum design at the dawn of the nineteenth. Before it was even complete, changes were afoot to incorporate the recommendations of Alexander Jackson, the first physician appointed to the new institution, including the erection of corridors to link the individual blocks and create separate airing yards.[6] But within two years of opening, the house was already full. Johnston was engaged to provide extensions for convalescent patients at either end of the main block, while the governors petitioned the Lord Lieutenant to relieve them of the burden of accommodating lunatics from all corners of the island by instituting a nationwide network of district asylums.

The pioneering buildings that Johnston and his partner William Murray went on to create for this national network of asylums would serve to highlight the many shortcomings of the original facility at the Richmond, not least its constrained urban site. The Richmond governors thereby purchased 16 acres of open countryside from Lord Monck on the opposite side of Grangegorman Lane in 1836, which they laid out as a landscaped garden and linked to the main institution via a tunnel under the public road.[7] Further acquisitions expanded this gently rolling landscape, whose views south over the city to the Wicklow Mountains beyond rendered it an ideal site from the point of view of the next generation of asylum builders in the late 1840s. And so, as the second major phase of asylum construction got underway nationwide, the Richmond would be endowed with an entirely new building, unimaginatively dubbed the 'New Richmond'.

Architect William Murray was well embedded with the institution and had already produced designs for some detached infirmary blocks and a chapel on the new lands. His architectural practice of Murray and Denny was therefore well placed to retain the commission for the 'New Richmond' project even after his own untimely death from cholera in 1849. The brief effectively prescribed a standalone facility, designed in accordance with the 'Instructions to Architects' issued by the Commissioners of Public Works. While identical in layout to the other asylums of the era, the design for the New Richmond appears to have been more successful than most in achieving a genuinely picturesque effect and downplaying the underlying symmetry and formality of the building.

Murray & Denny's highly articulated neo-Gothic edifice in its salubrious and scenic parkland setting stood in stark contrast with Johnston's cramped, sombre and unhealthy Georgian pile, and must have looked like a panacea for many of the ills that afflicted the earlier structure. High-minded optimism is an essential precondition for commissioning the best new buildings, but as has been seen time and again throughout this book, the sweeping vistas of the possible soon telescope into the blinkered tunnels of reality. The New Richmond would be no less prone to overcrowding than the old, its drains no less liable to contaminate the once-healthy soil on which it was built, its inmates hardly less susceptible to the resulting infectious diseases. But most importantly of all, its resident physicians were no better able to effect elusive cures, nor to resist the tidal wave of admissions forced upon the institution by society outside the walls.

And so the numbers continued to grow. By the close of the nineteenth century, the Richmond - Upper, Lower, and all parts in between - was home to over 2,000 patients in the most unbelievably overcrowded conditions, dwarfing the workhouse from which it had grown. Beds overflowed from the grotesquely large dormitories of the 200-bed ward block added in the 1870s, piling up in the corridors and day rooms, workshops and dining spaces, leaving the institutional

The three iconic faces of Grangegorman

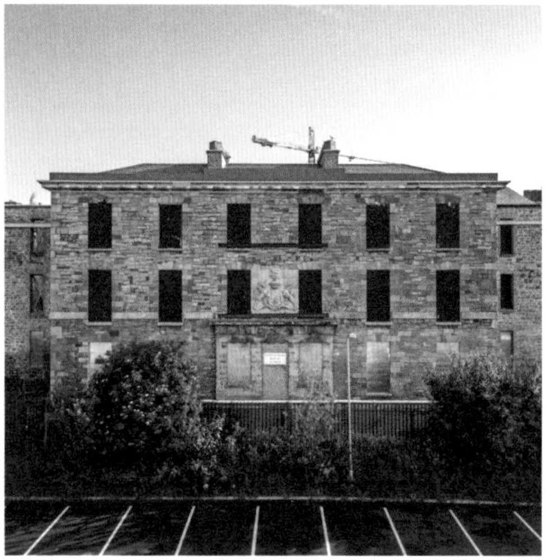

Francis Johnston's Richmond Asylum (1814)
Photograph by David Killeen, 2019

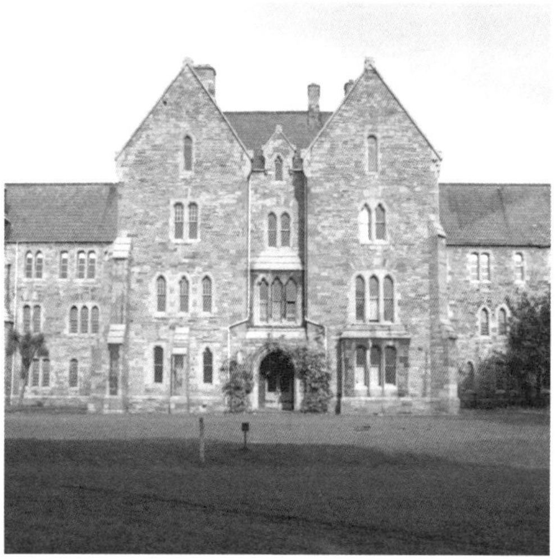

Murray & Denny's New Richmond (1854, demolished)
Image courtesy of the Irish Architectural Archive (Photographic Collection, 052_034_X_01_08)

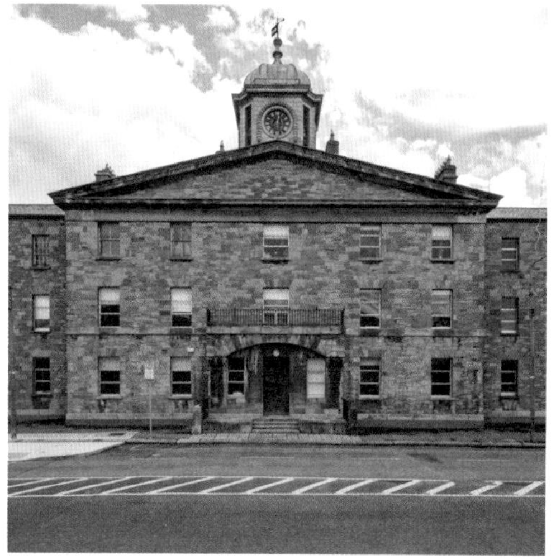

Johnston's Richmond Penitentiary (1816)
Photograph by David Killeen, 2019

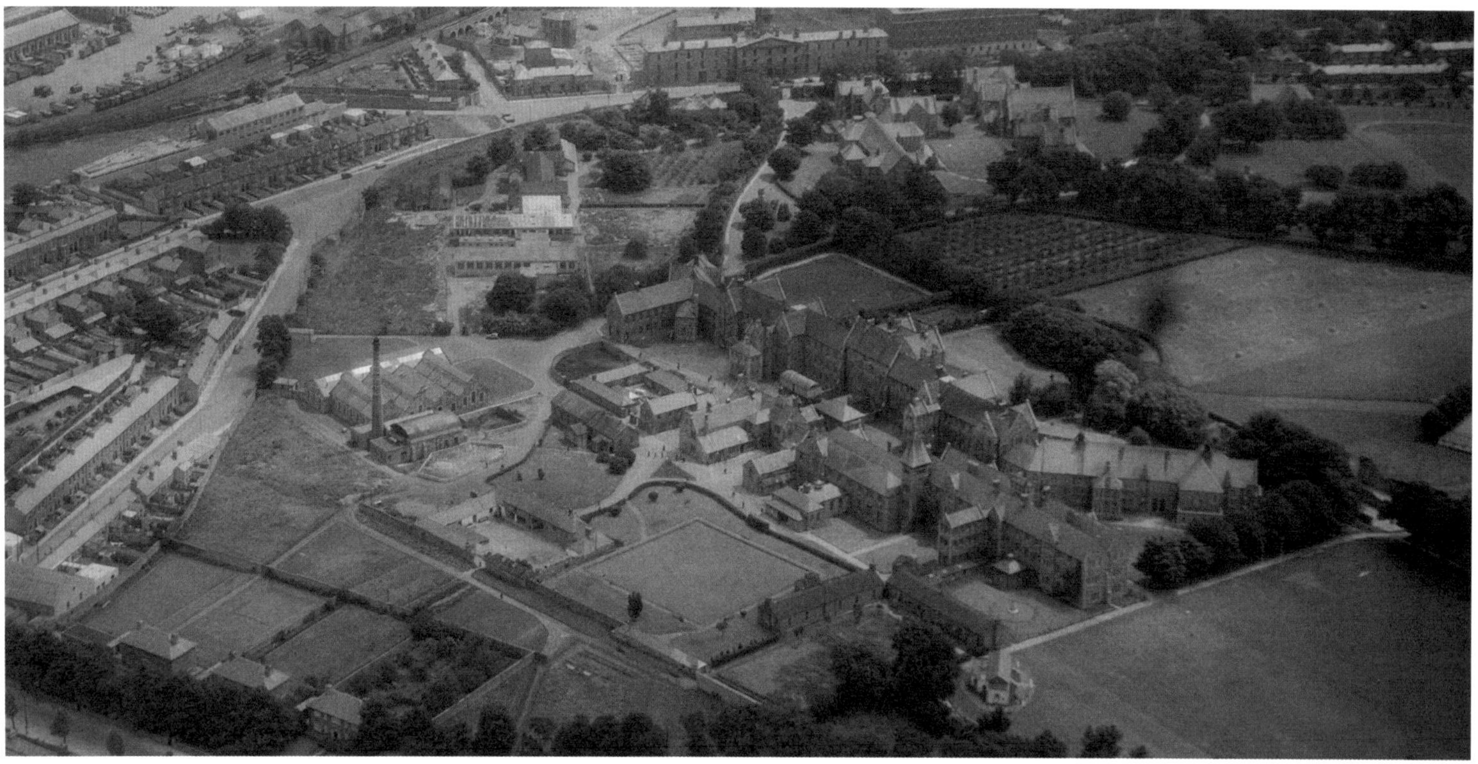

In the midst of the capital city lay a productive landsape of hay meadows, tilled fields and orchards, 1955.
Image courtesy of the National Library of Ireland (NPA MOR1490)

regime barely able to meet patients' most basic needs, let alone aspire to therapeutic respite.

Partial relief was at hand in the form of the new auxiliary asylum (see Case Study 25), but before the sod was even turned in Portrane, it was becoming clear that the despatch of 1,200 patients to the remote north Dublin peninsula would not solve all of the institution's problems. Concerns about conditions in The Richmond were aired at length in the House of Lords on several occasions in 1895, albeit central government was actually powerless to dictate solutions in what was strictly a local responsibility.[8] Calls to sell the Grangegorman site and reinvest the proceeds in a second modern asylum on the lands at Portrane came to naught,[9] so architect W. H. Byrne was commissioned to prepare plans to overhaul the existing buildings. His most ambitious scheme would have turned the New Richmond back-to-front and wrapped it in a mesh of corridors and ancillary spaces to produce a hybrid pavilion-echelon layout similar in principle to the new facility at Portrane.

This unusual vision failed to progress, perhaps falling foul of the scepticism with which cost estimates for Irish construction projects were greeted, then as now: 'In Ireland it was the universal practice of architects to spend twice the amount of their original estimate.'[10] Instead, make-do-and-mend was taken to its limits, with timber and corrugated-iron appendages added haphazardly to various extremities of the institution during 1895. In a measure of how far the asylum project had fallen from its optimistic heights earlier in the century, the asylum governors urgently petitioned the Lord Lieutenant to take over the old Richmond Penitentiary and, in 1897, refashioned what the Inspectors acknowledged was a 'very unsuitable building' to form a 'useful annexe' to the main asylum.[11] Whether patients fared better lodged between the cold masonry walls of a 90-year-old prison or the timber sheeted walls of a new tin shed is moot.

In the same period and in an attempt to improve hygiene and reduce the incidence of infectious diseases (which had repeatedly ravaged the overcrowded institution with fatal consequences), a modern disinfecting laundry was erected alongside a new mortuary – just in case clean linen proved insufficient inoculation against recurrence. It would doubtless seem curious to those who originally commissioned it that a humble laundry today appears as the best surviving building of this period; rather appropriately, it continues to promote public health in its new use as a primary care centre.

The RMS was finally given some respite from the 'carking cares' of his role with the construction of a substantial new dwelling with its own entrance from the upper-middle-class boulevard of the North Circular Road. Terraced houses for married attendants would follow in the lower-rent environs of Grangegorman Lane, where in 1938 a five-storey, seventeen-bay behemoth of a nurses' home to the designs of Vincent Kelly would be erected – a structure of enormous solidity built for the ages and largely paid for by the Sweepstakes. The latter was regrettably and rather unnecessarily razed in 2014, not long after the demolition of its twin at the nearby Mater Hospital.

As with so many other asylums, the landscaped grounds at Grangegorman did much to improve the quality of life for those patients allowed to use them. Nineteenth-century mapping reveals some intriguing garden buildings – clear evidence that leisure and pleasure were encouraged, at least in the early days. Unlike many buildings, a well planted landscape also has the welcome quality of improving with age, as seen in finely wooded parkland that enveloped the main buildings in mid-twentieth-century aerial photography. The same photographs also record a wider productive landscape of pastures and hay-ricks, orchards and vegetable fields, which would not have been out of place in this locality a century earlier, but which by now seem strangely alien in the midst of the densely packed artisan terraces of Stoneybatter. Gaelic football pitches, handball alleys and bowling greens point to a more active, if less genteel, interpretation of patient leisure in the twentieth century than the curious summerhouse of the nineteenth. Of all of the different roles that this landscape has played during its institutional history, it is this latter role as a sporting landscape that has taken on a central importance in the masterplan for the new Grangegorman.

The later twentieth-century history of what became known as St Brendan's Hospital is not edifying. Despite valiant efforts to improve the service and modest investment in new admissions units in the 1970s, investigative reporting in the 1980s revealed to what depths conditions in older parts of the institution had sunk.[12] If asylum buildings were vaunted in their heyday as being part of the cure, then it is probably inevitable that they would also be seen as contributing to the system's failure. Following this logic it is perfectly understandable that the generation of psychiatrists who undertook the Herculean task of reforming St Brendan's Hospital should have attributed symbolic

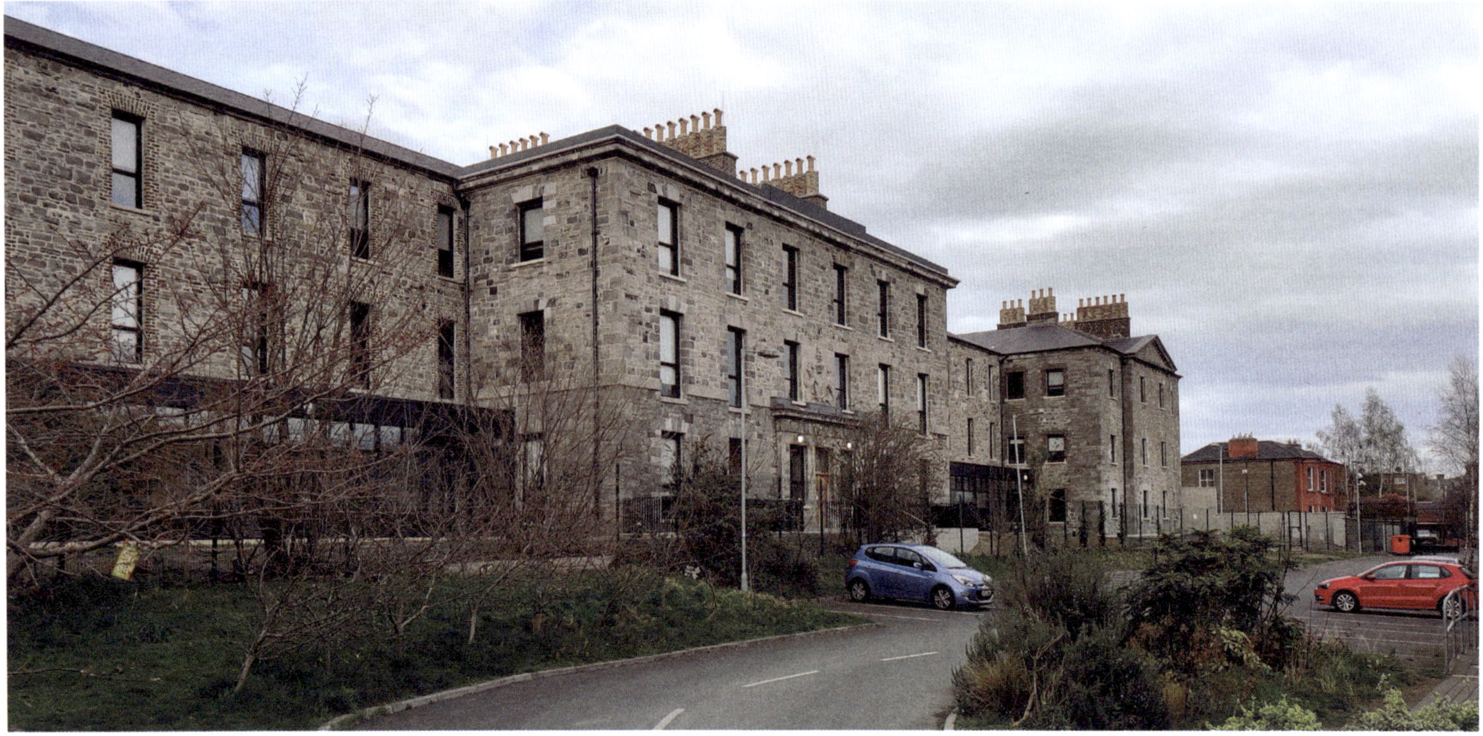

Since being vacated by patients in 1989, Johnston's Richmond Asylum fell into deriliction and large sections were demolished. Now, after a major conservation project, it stands ready to write the next chapter in its history. *Photograph by David Killeen, 2021.*

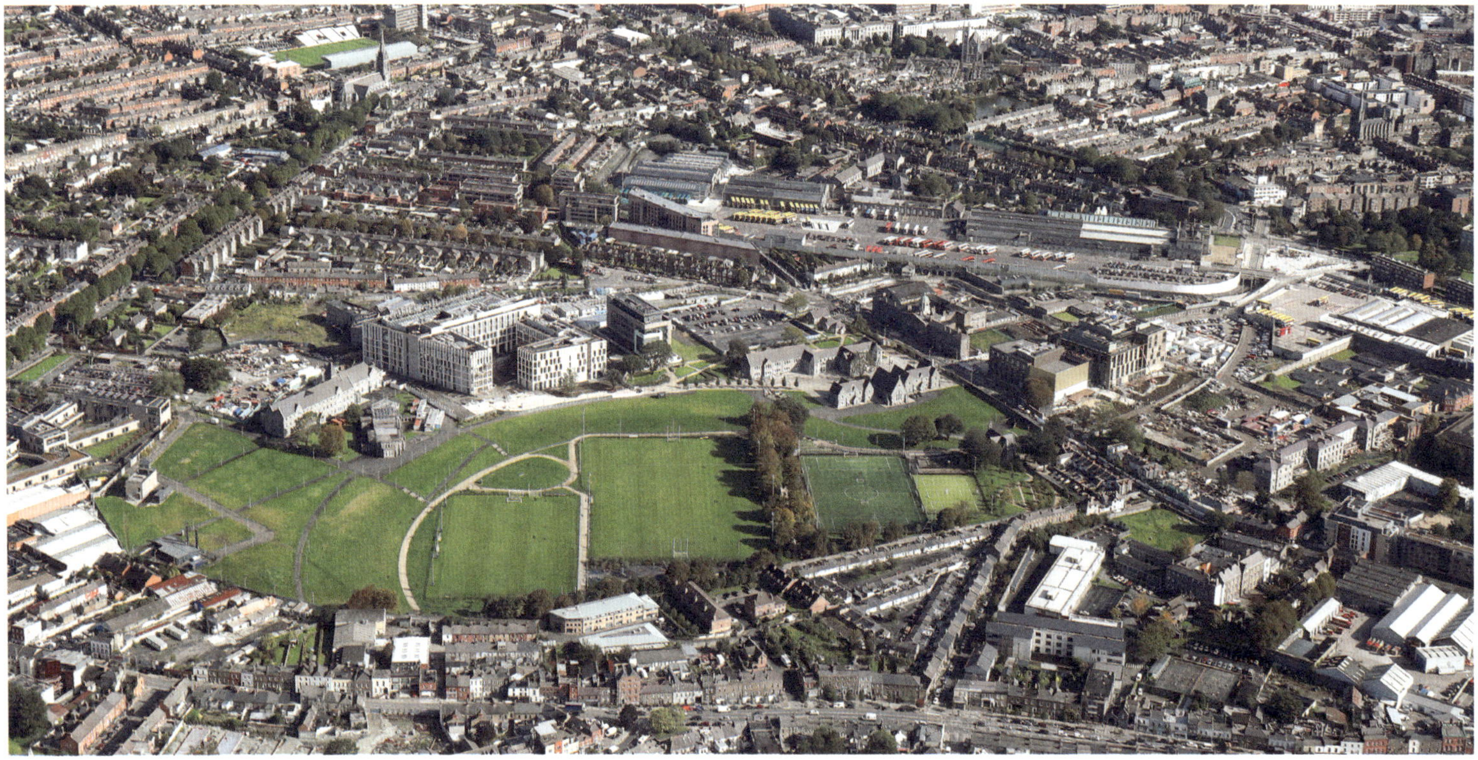

Few places in Ireland can have witnessed such a dramatic physical and reputational transformation in this century. *Photograph by Barry Coakley, 2020, reproduced courtesy of the Grangegorman Development Agency.*

value to erasing the built relics of the ancien regime. And so, as the de-institutionalisation express pulled out of the asylum station bound for the sunnier uplands of care in the community (or at any rate the hostels and bedsits of the North Circular Road), the wrecking ball came for the spaces they left behind. Three quarters of Johnston's 'old' Richmond and the entirety of Murray's New Richmond came crashing down, the latter leaving a tangible void at the centre of the landscape it had been built to command.

When the site became the subject of an international competition to devise a masterplan for a new university, this void at the heart gave a much freer hand to prospective designers than might otherwise have been the case. The winning masterplan integrated individual historic buildings and landscape features and adapted them to serve new educational uses, albeit as isolated features within a radically altered context. A public investment unmatched since the construction of Portrane has transformed Grangegorman from a concealed, enclosed backwater to 'an urban quarter with an open future' as the permanent home for the Technical University, Dublin (formerly the Dublin Institute of Technology). Few places in Ireland can have witnessed such a dramatic physical and reputational transformation in this century.

Further Reading

Joseph Reynolds, *Grangegorman: Psychiatric Care in Dublin since 1815* (Dublin: Institute of Public Administration in association with Eastern Health Board, 1992)

Christine Casey, *The Buildings of Ireland: Dublin* (London and New Haven: Yale University Press, 2005) pp 256-60.

Grangegorman: An urban quarter with an open future (Dublin: GGDA, 2008)

References

1. *Report of the commission for inquiring into the erection of district lunatic asylums in Ireland*, HC 1856 [9] LIII.367, p. 4.
2. Michel Foucault, *Madness and Civilisation* (tr. Richard Howard; New York,1965) p. 278.
3. Richmond Lunatic Asylum (Ireland) Act 1815, 55 Geo. 3, c. 107
4. Eoin O'Brien, Lorna Browne and Kevin O'Malley, *The House of Industry Hospitals: The Richmond, Whitworth and Hardwicke (St Laurence's Hospital); A Closing Memoir* (Dublin, 1988).
5. Actually operating from 1798 within the main institution, this date refers to the purpose built structure. See Katherine Fennelly, 'The Bedford Asylum: Building for the "industrious child" in early-nineteenth century Dublin', in Jane Eva Baxter and Meredith Ellis, eds, *Nineteenth Century Childhoods in Interdisciplinary and International Perspectives* (Barnsley, 2018)
6. Markus Reuber, 'Public Lunatic Asylums, 1800–1845', in Elizabeth Malcolm and Greta Jones (eds), *Medicine, Disease and the State in Ireland, 1650–1940*, (Cork, 1999), p. 213; Irish Architectural Archive, Murray Collection, 1814, Richmond Asylum, 92/46, Sheets 0411, 0412, 0413.
7. Sixteen additional acres purchased in 1836. *Fifteenth Report of the Inspectors-General of Prisons 1837*, HC 1837 [123] xxxi, p. 18.
8. 'The Richmond Lunatic Asylum,' *The Irish Builder*, 1 June 1895, pp 142–3.
9. House of Lords (HL) Debate, 16 May 1895, vol. 33, cc. 1299–1306.
10. Ibid.
11. *Forty-Seventh Annual Asylum Report*, HC 1898 [8969] xliii p. 23; *Forty-Eighth Annual Asylum Report*, HC 1899 [9479] xl, pp 33–4.
12. See Chapter 8.

CASE STUDY 02

Years in operation
1827–2014

Original cost
£20,899

Capacity (min /max)
104

Architect(s)
Francis Johnston
& William Murray,
J. J. Phillips & Son.

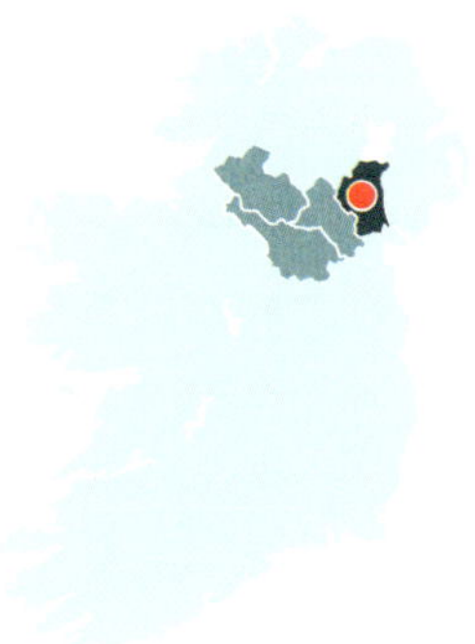

St Luke's Hospital

(previously Armagh District Lunatic Asylum)

St Luke's Hospital claims to be the first asylum in the western world that was established under mandatory national statute – an entirely legitmate if ever-so-slightly niche claim. That makes it no less a source of local pride than the fact that this institution – whose founding legislation was passed in the reign of George III – remains relevant to the community is serves in the twenty-first century.

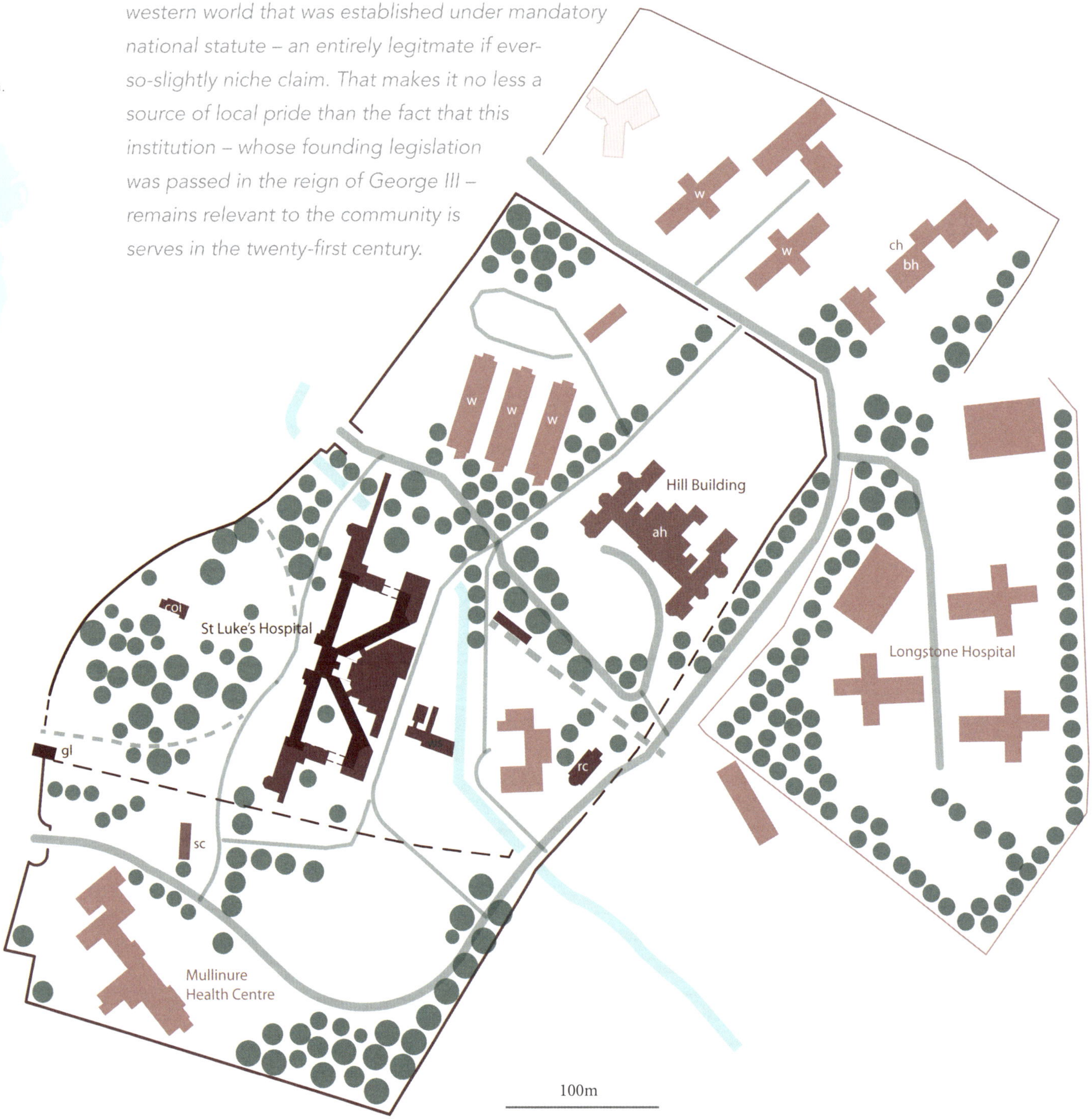

The Armagh District Lunatic Asylum was the first of Francis Johnston's standard-plan asylums to be constructed, completed in 1824 at a cost of £20,900. While superficially identical to six more built over the following decade, a comparison of the prototype and its facsimiles does reveal some design refinements along the way. Armagh was constructed of rubblestone rather than finely tooled ashlar, and featured camber-headed rather than square windows in the patient wings, subtleties that together lend the building a softer, less formal countenance than its later siblings. Indeed, the initial design intent for Armagh was less formal yet – the crowning cupola was an afterthought added when construction was already underway. The cupola would go on to become a defining feature of the type, emphasising the important civic nature of the building to a largely illiterate populace beyond the walls.

For the Board of Control in the 1820s, a more immediate lesson from Armagh is that the original four-acre site was far too small for an institution of this nature, and all subsequent asylums of this phase were endowed with three to five times as much. The 1824 building sat just metres from a fast-flowing stream that initially formed a moat-like northern boundary to the site, but was later integrated as an attractive feature within the extended grounds, albeit one that was never without risk to patients.

In 1837, William Murray was tasked with designing ward extensions across the rear of the building but these were not implemented at that time,[1] and the asylum would grow increasingly crowded until relieved by the removal of patients from counties Cavan and Monaghan to the new Monaghan Asylum in 1870. Major extensions in the 1880s executed at a total cost of £25,000 included a dining/recreation hall, laundries, stores and ward extensions at either end of the main block executed in a sympathetic, if by then slightly outdated, Georgian style. Probably around the same time, the centre block was reordered with the insertion of additional windows and a projecting bay window, spoiling the classical proportions of Johnston's façade, while a somewhat lumpy Italianate water tower behind the north wing undermined the overall symmetry of the composition.[2]

Chapter Five describes how overcrowding led to the construction of large freestanding pavilions on many asylum sites between 1890 and 1910. Armagh experienced faster growth than most: a doubling of patients from 250 to 500 over a 15-year period. In response the governors commissioned one of the finest buildings of the period, commended by the Inspectors of Lunacy in 1898 as the first in Ireland designed to cater specifically to the needs of acutely ill patients:

> *The Governors may be congratulated on the completion of the new asylum hospital, in the erection of which they took such a practical interest, and showed such a generous appreciation of the requirements of certain classes of the insane.*[3]

Known as the Hill Building for its siting on an eminence above the original asylum, the 1898 hospital is like the Victorian lovechild of an Elizabethan mansion and a French chateau, adorned with an array of bay windows and verandas, towers and turrets, chimneys and ventilators. It is all a bit much for Alistair Rowan, whose architectural guide describes architect J. J. Phillip's edifice as a 'disquieting Frenchified extravaganza in rock faced limestone' with a 'freakish silhouette' that punctures the skyline from its shroud of trees. Happily, the aforementioned panoply of high-maintenance features – so often vulnerable to decay and removal – have been successfully restored as part of a recent conservation project.[4]

Alas, the governors proved themselves more prescient in matters of architectural embellishment than staffing and management: the absence of an Assistant Medical Officer was identified by the Inspectors as one reason why the exemplary new facility was not being used for the class of patients for whom it was intended. Those readers who today express frustration at the hijacking of newly completed healthcare facilities for purposes other than that for which they were built may be forgiven a wry smile.[5]

Armagh was one of only two asylums in Ireland to have its own railway siding for delivering goods, albeit the need to manually rotate individual wagons through 90 degrees on a turntable before shunting the final 100 metres must have limited its utility, even in an era when rail was king. The later decimation of Northern Ireland's railways saw the numerous lines that converged on Armagh dismantled, though the route of the siding can still be discerned on site. Another vestigial trace in the landscape is the original front avenue, today only a grassed track curving through beautiful tree-studded parkland, but its location remains obvious from the surviving gate lodge.

The last residential patients departed the 1824 building 190 years after the first were admitted, but it continues to host teams delivering many mental health related services. The Hill Building provides offices for a

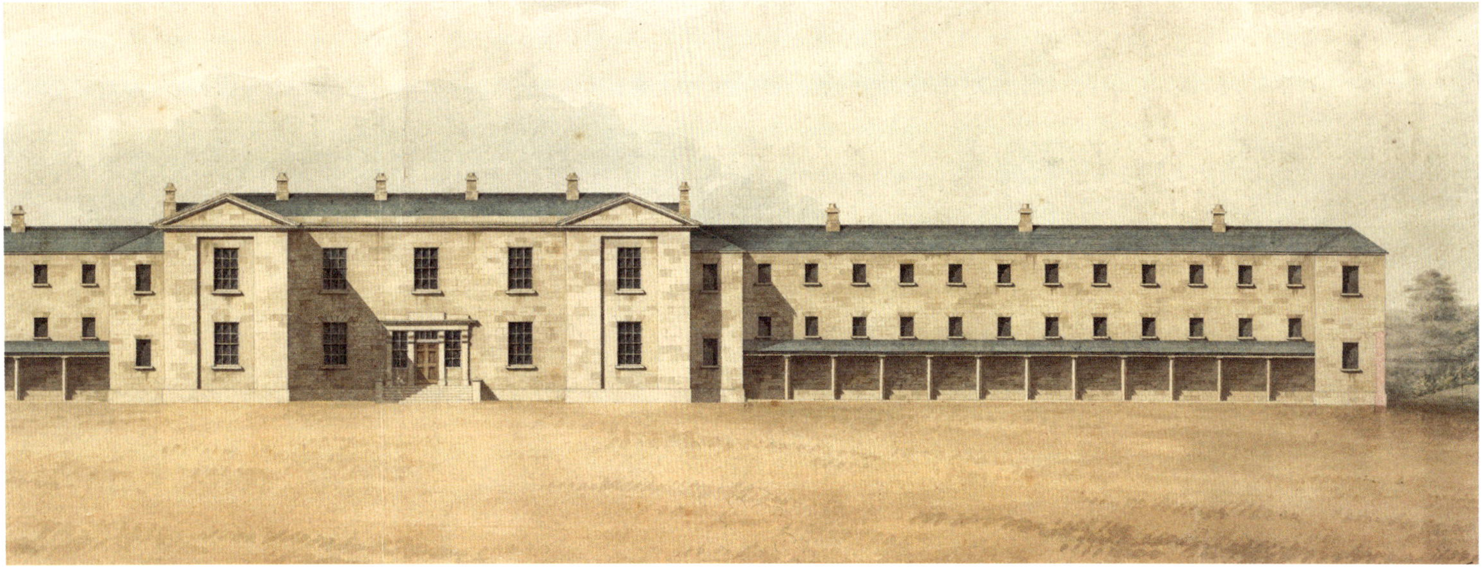

The centrepeice of Armagh's facade was clearly derived from domestic precedents. *Image courtesy of the Irish Architectural Archive (RIAI Murray Collection 92/46: 66)*

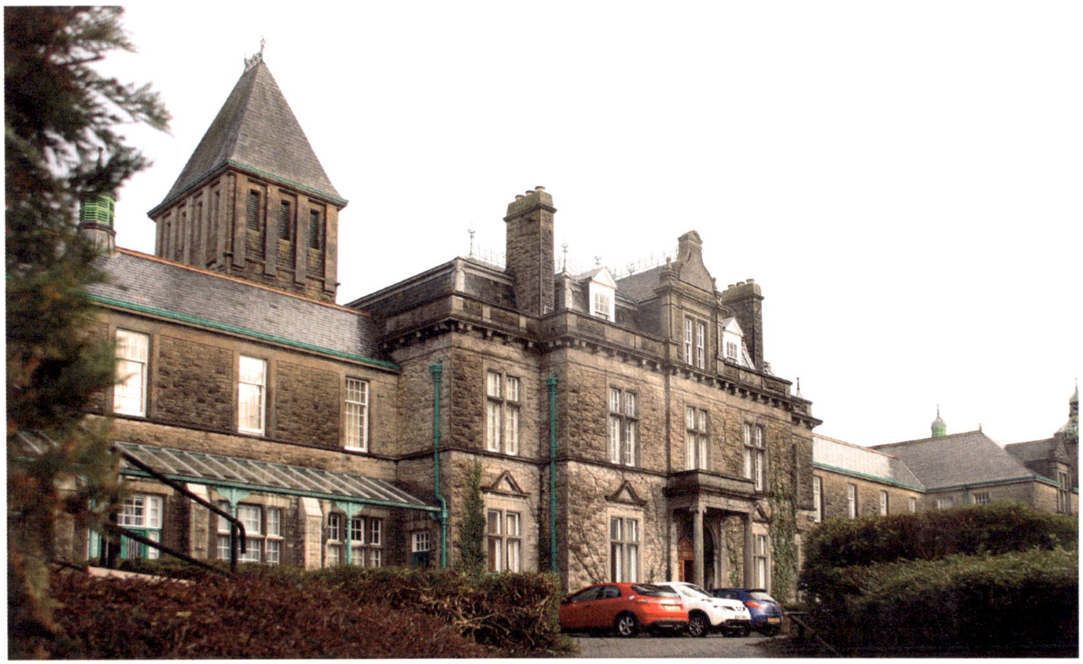

The 'Hill Building' of 1898 was an architectural extravaganza in an era of otherwise underwhelming buildings. *Photograph by the author, 2020.*

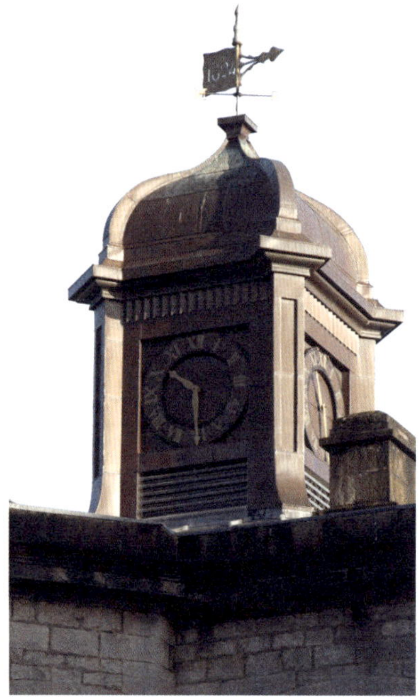

The cupola was a late addition, but became a distinguishing feature of the type. *Photograph by the author, 2020.*

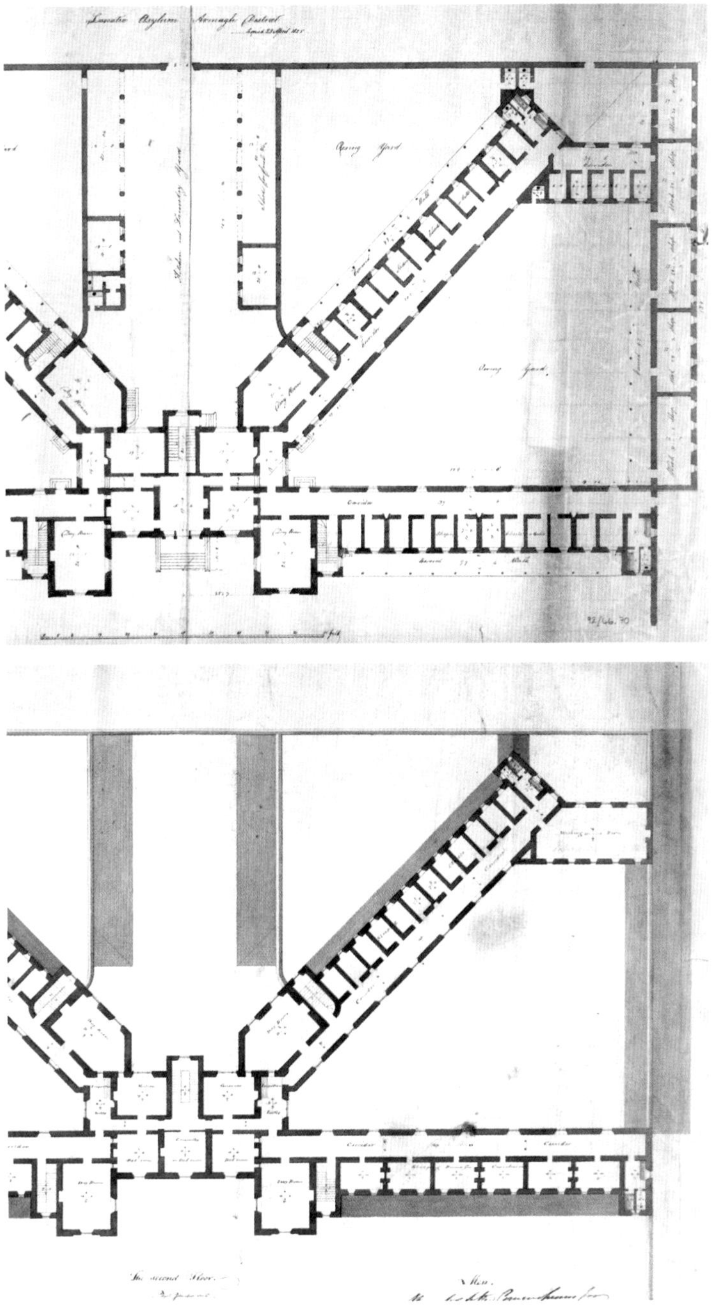

Ground and first floor plans, 1828. Kitchen, laundry and sanitary facilities were severely lacking in this early prototype. *Images courtesy of the Irish Architectural Archive (RIAI Murray Collection 92/46: 65, 70)*

range of health administration staff, while later buildings on the site include an autism centre and a community hospital offering outpatient services for general health and wellbeing. Strikingly, the site also hosts a horse-riding centre for disabled people, a living example of the continuing therapeutic value of former asylum landscapes. Today, the 'first asylum in the western world established under a mandatory national statute' presents as a thriving and intensively used community health facility, successfully reusing an impressive range of well-maintained historic buildings set in a stunningly landscaped setting.

References

1. Drawings hand annotated 'not approved'. Irish Architectural Archive, Murray Collection, 1837, Armagh District Lunatic Asylum, 92/46, Sheet 0071, 0072, 0073.
2. *Thirty-Seventh Annual Asylum Report 1887*, HC 1887 [5121] xxxix, p. 13.
3. *Forty-Eighth Annual Asylum Report 1898*, HC 1899 [9479] xl, p. 112.
4. Kevin V. Mulligan, *The Buildings of Ireland: South Ulster* (London, 2013) p. 138.
5. *Forty-Eighth Annual Asylum Report 1898*, HC 1899 [9479] xl, p. 112.

CASE STUDY 03

St Joseph's Hospital

(previously Limerick District Lunatic Asylum)

Years in operation
1827–2014

Original cost
£29,856

Capacity (min /max)
150 / 883

Architect(s)
Johnston & Murray, William Fogerty, George Wilkinson, Carroll & Batchelor, P. J. Sheahan.

As one of the most impressive witnesses called before the 1817 House of Commons Select Committee on the Lunatic Poor in Ireland, it would be no coincidence that one of the first new institutions built under the legislation that followed would be located in the local bailiwick of the prominent advocate for asylum reform, Thomas Spring Rice.

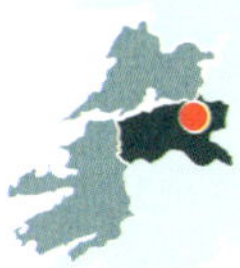

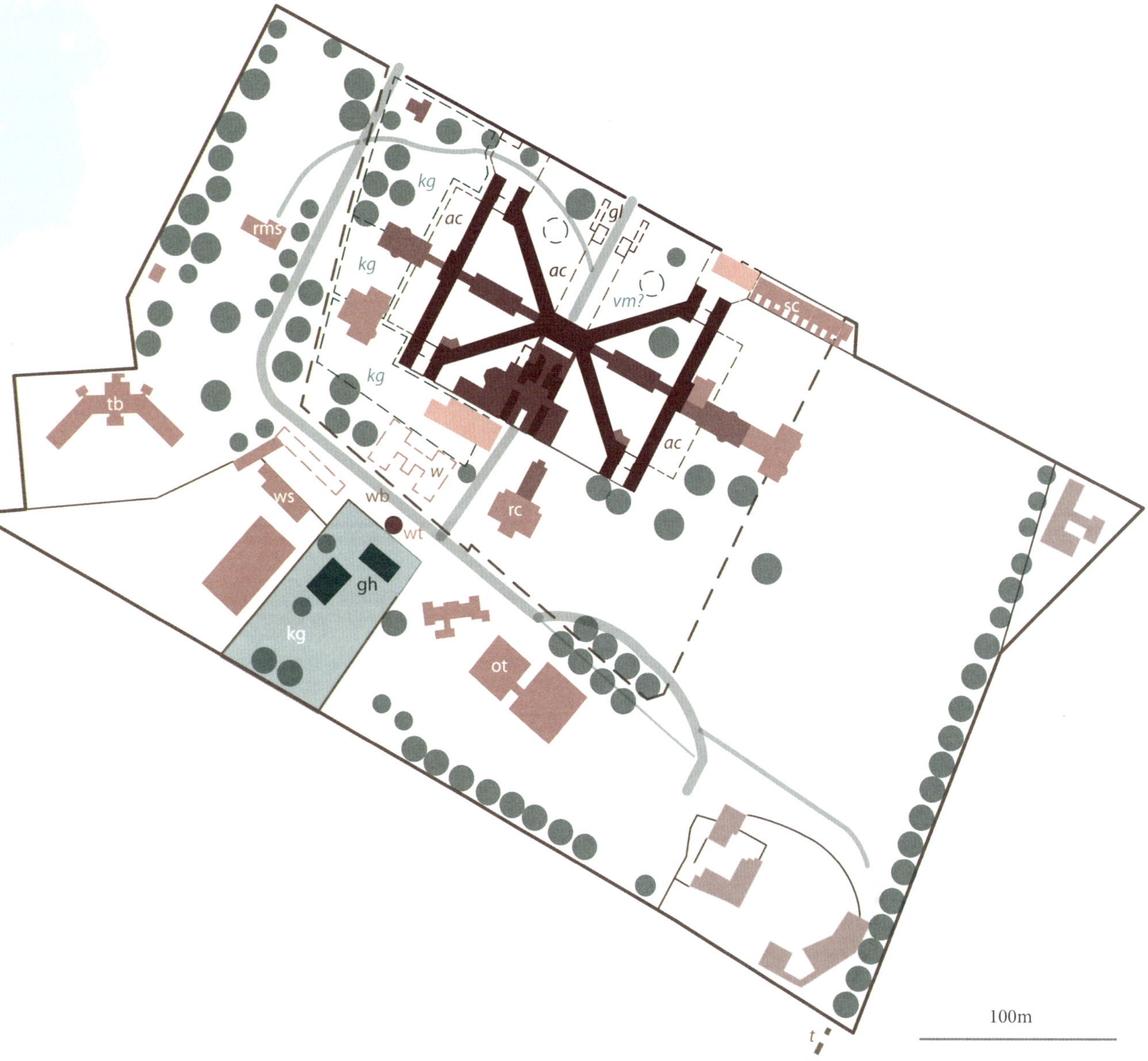

Even before launching his national political career, Spring Rice had taken it upon himself to conduct a detailed study of the existing arrangements for the care of the insane in Munster, which ranged from Dr Hallaran's highly respected asylum in Cork, via lunatic annexes at the Houses of Industry in Clonmel and Waterford whose operation occasionally fell short of their aspirations, to the shameful cells found at the Limerick House of Industry. Spring Rice was less prone to hyperbole than many reformers of his era, but his description of the lunatic department in Limerick was unequivocally damning:

> *accommodation [which would not be] appropriate for our dog-kennels; it consists of... an open arcade, behind which cells have been constructed with stone floors, without any mode of heating or of ventilating, and exposed during the whole of the winter to the extremities of the weather [frequently resulting in] mortification in the extremities [ie: amputation of limbs].*[1]

It must therefore have been a matter of some satisfaction for Spring Rice that within ten years of presenting his evidence, the city that he now represented as a Whig MP would become only the second to erect a district lunatic asylum under the new statutory legislation. It was also the first location where Johnston and Murray's larger 'first class' design for 150 patients was employed, but its opening was delayed by eight months as the new governor, Mr Jackson, sought to resolve shortcomings in the design and fitout of the establishment,[2] including concerns over the inadequacy of the water supply and the robustness (or otherwise) of the furnishings.[3] Worse was to come, as shortly after opening, several patients would deliver their own verdict on the institution by making good their escape over the boundary walls. Architect William Murray justified the 8-foot-6-inch height of the existing walls, which had been designed so that 'the surrounding country should not be shut out', but agreed to examine the feasibility of increasing their height at an estimated cost of £100.[4]

Before its younger twin at Ballinasloe had even commenced, the Limerick asylum was already facing the challenge of an accumulation of incurable inpatients which 'must eventually, if not remedied... put an end to the original object of such asylums, viz. treatment with a view to cure'.[5] Spring Rice, by now serving as chairman of the board of governors of the new asylum, pondered 'the propriety of opening some general house for reception of incurables', but the Inspector countered that '...an additional wing to each provincial asylum would answer all the purpose' at much less expense, and suggested in the case of Limerick 'that two of the present straw houses and yards could be economically fitted up for incurables'.[6] The single-storey ranges along the eastern and western flanks of the asylum were duly adapted and extended to accommodate an additional 140 patients, but at the cost of completely enclosing the original airing courts.

In 1863 the governors sought to enhance both the spiritual and temporal welfare of their patients with the construction of a detached Roman Catholic chapel and a Turkish bath. This single-cell chapel was nearly doubled in size in 1914 with the addition of a crossing and double transepts, supported internally on a fine limestone arcade that makes for one of the most spatially elaborate asylum chapels in the country. Patient accommodation would undergo several further expansions. In 1878 a matching pair of three-storey, double-pile blocks were added for chronic patients, with Georgian proportions and detailing that could have passed for a middle-sized country house were it not for the disconcerting absence of a central doorcase.[7] These were joined in the twentieth century by another pair of blocks of similar proportion but somewhat greater architectural pretension, the central bay of their principal façades sporting blind opes and a pedimented central niche. Internally, these buildings are characterised by enormous, open-plan dormitories and day rooms, improved only by some fine terrazzo finishes in the circulation areas. The 1890s saw the Resident Medical Superintendent retreat to a large new residence on the northern part of the site, its ungainly composition redeemed by some attractive arts-and-crafts detailing. His escape was timely-avoiding the chaos caused by the protracted reconstruction of the laundry, kitchen and stores in the opening years of the twentieth century.[8] In 1910 a new terrace of houses for married attendants was constructed fronting onto the public road.[9] Distinguished externally only by decorative cast iron railings, St Dympna's Terrace also concealed another surprising detail – each dwelling was provided with its own door directly into the asylum grounds. Attendants may have been unlikely to facilitate patient escapes, but at a time when live-in staff were only slightly more at liberty to leave the asylum grounds than their patients, these houses must surely have been a popular route for nocturnal sorties by unmarried colleagues.

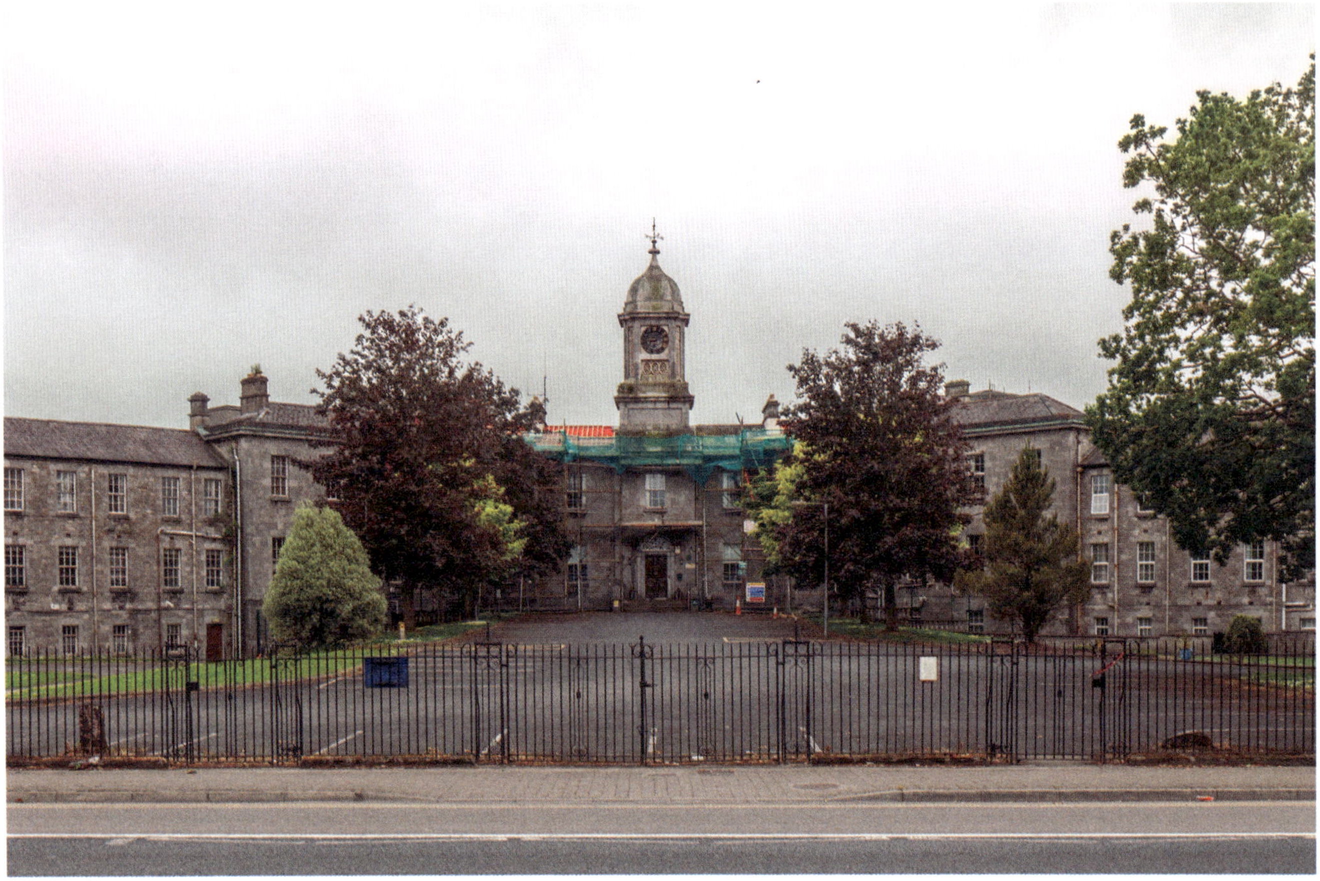

For a building whose future trajectory is uncertain, roof works can only be a positive omen. *Photograph by David Killeen, 2019.*

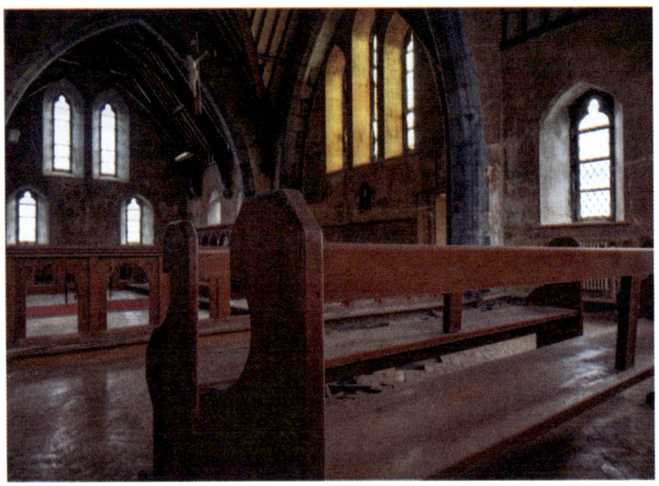

The asylum chapel was almost doubled in size in 1914 with the addition of new transepts and chancel. *Photograph by David Killeen, 2019.*

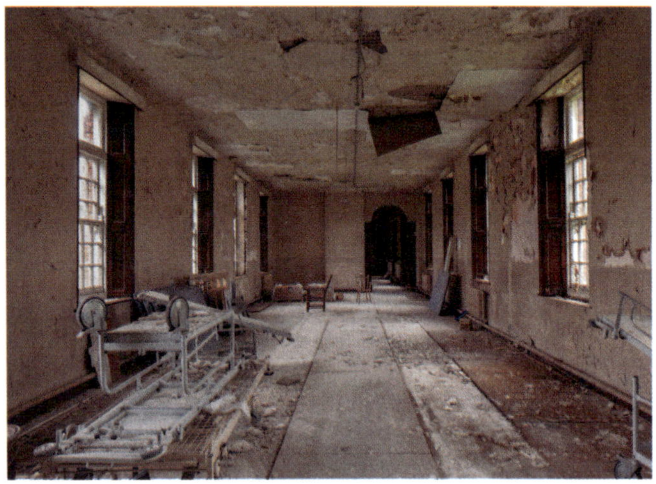

The earliest expansion (1830s) saw workshops and sheds adapted for use as patient accommodation. *Photograph by David Killeen, 2019.*

The grounds immediately surrounding the asylum at Limerick never expanded to the extent of many others around the country, being constrained from the outset by the county gaol to the west and the public road to the north. The governors agreed to sell a small part of the site to the Waterford and Limerick Railway for the sum of £2,870 – a healthy return given that the whole site had cost only £3,840 – but would thereafter be constrained to the south, while later again a new municipal cemetery blocked eastward expansion.[10] But the landscape was worked productively from the outset, with almost half of the site depicted under intensive cultivation on the first edition Ordnance Survey map. Horticultural activity would later shift to a walled garden to the south of the site which, unusually, remains in use at time of writing. In 1903, the asylum governors secured additional farmland to the south-east of the main asylum, access to which would necessitate a new tunnel under the tracks.[11]

Between the 1930s and 50s, the hospital benefited from improvements to the value of £105,999 funded by the Irish Hospitals Sweepstakes, the most architecturally notable of which was a single-storey TB sanatorium with a south facing verandah on a cranked plan.[12] As the inpatient population declined through the latter half of the twentieth century, the hospital contracted within its shell, but no new uses emerged to fill the empty spaces left behind. The large site less than a kilometre from the city centre will doubtless prove appealing for redevelopment; it remains to be seen if its new uses will be respectful of the two centuries of history embodied by this place, which, as well as being amongst the oldest asylums in Ireland, should be seen as a local monument to the wider achievements of one of Limerick's most influential sons.

References

1. *Report from the Select Committee on the Lunatic Poor in Ireland 1817*, HC 1817 [430], viii, p. 14.
2. *Fifth Report of the Inspector of Prisons 1827*, HC 1826–27 [471] xi, p. 54.
3. National Archives of Ireland (hereafter NAI), Chief Secretary's Office, 1826–27: *Letters between Limerick Board of Governors, Chief Secretary / Under Secretary, and William Murray, architect*, CSO/RP/1826/2352 and CSO/RP/1827/1089.
4. NAI, Chief Secretary's Office, 1827: *Letter from William Murray, architect, to William Gregory, Under Secretary, referring to letter from Rev Josiah Crampton, Chairman of the Limerick District Lunatic Asylum*. CSO/RP/1827/1373.
5. *Eighth Report of the Inspector of Prisons*, HC 1830 [48] xxiv, p. 49. Emphasis in original.
6. *Eighth Report of the Inspector of Prisons*, HC 1830 [48] xxiv, p. 59.
7. *Twenty-Eighth Annual Asylum Report 1879*, HC 1878–79 [2346] xxxii, p. 12.
8. *Fifty-Third Annual Asylum Report 1903*, HC 1905 [2262] xxxv, p. 128.
9. *Fifty-Ninth Annual Asylum Report 1909*, HC 1910 [5280] xli, p. 122.
10. *Sixteenth Report of the Commissioners of Public Works 1847*, HC 1848 [983] xxxvii, p. 146.
11. *Fifty-Third Annual Asylum Report 1903*, HC 1905 [2262] xxxv, p. 128; *Fifty-Fifth Annual Asylum Report 1905*, HC 1906 [3164] xxxix, p. 135.
12. Eamon de Barra and John O'Sheehan (eds), *Oispidéil na hÉireann: Ireland's Hospitals 1933–1950*. (Dublin, 1956), p. 58.

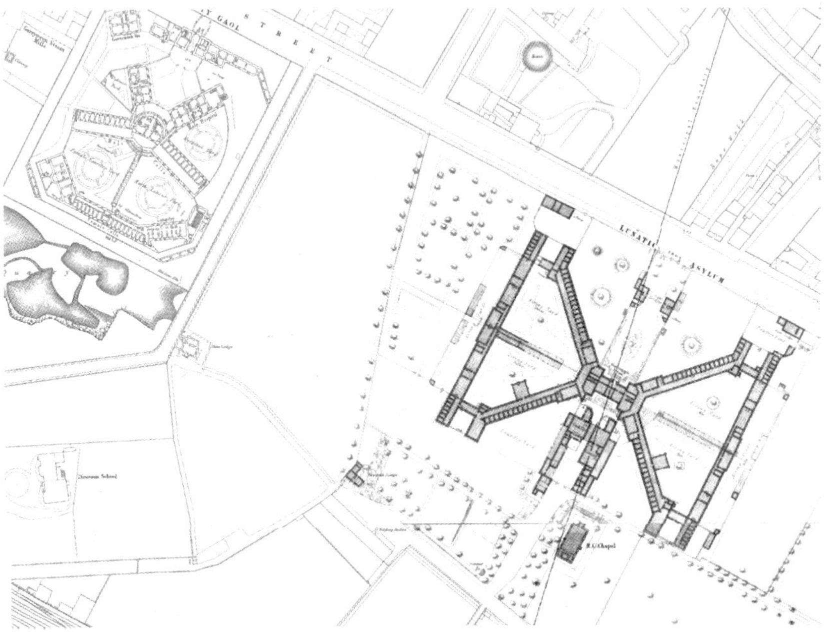

The asylum landscape was intensely productive from the outset. *Reproduced courtesy of Trinity College Dublin (OS-Limerick-1056-Sheet 5:76-1872)*

CASE STUDY 04

Belfast District Lunatic Asylum

(demolished, site now part of Royal Victoria Hospital)

Years in operation
1829–1919

Original cost
£25,319

Capacity (min /max)
104 / 800+

Architect(s)
Johnston & Murray,
Charles Lanyon

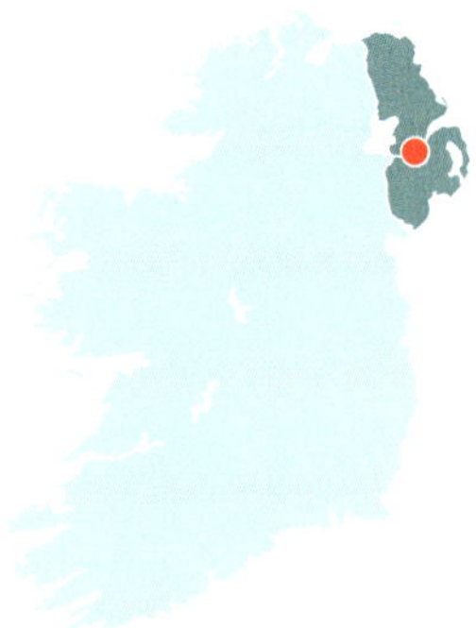

Whatever the future may hold for Ireland's asylums, it remains a fact that very few of the buildings in this volume have to date been demolished. Belfast holds the distinction as the first municipality to dispense with its original asylum after less than 90 years of service in favour of a pioneering new villa-colony asylum on the southern outskirts of the city.

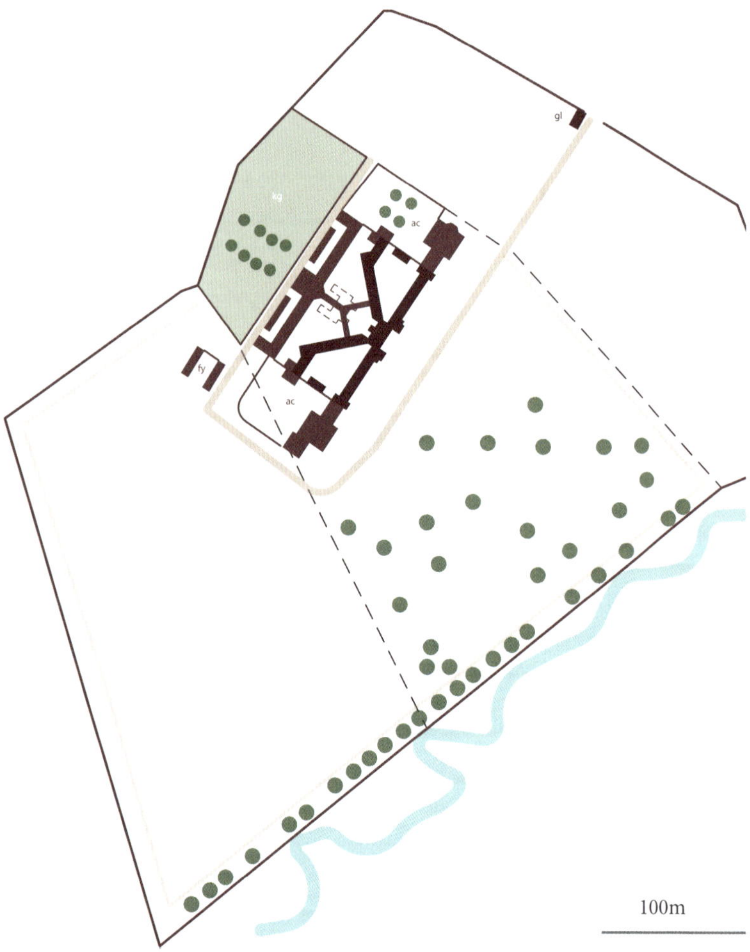

The original Belfast District Lunatic Asylum was completed in 1829 at a cost of £25,319, and was built to serve patients from counties Antrim and Down. The building was erected in parallel with the new asylum at Londonderry, such that some of the construction drawings used at Belfast are annotated for use on both sites.[1]

Erected on a rural site off the Falls Road, the asylum was soon engulfed by urban and industrial expansion. But even before the terraces and factories of the metropolis invaded its once-bucolic setting, the institution found itself overwhelmed by a different type of congestion. Within just four years of opening, the optimistic projections for moral management were already confronted with the stark reality of the accumulation of incurable cases, demanding a major expansion of the land and buildings.[2] And while the local board's 1833 proposals were initially rejected by the central Board of Control, plans were drawn up the following year for extensions to the rear to accommodate '100 incurable patients'.[3] When further extensions were added to the east and west of the main building in 1852–53, these earlier extensions were repurposed to provide improved ancillary uses, including a new laundry, kitchen and chapel.

By the 1850s all newly planned asylums were provided with chapels, and new chapels would in due course be added to most existing asylums. However, the provision of a dedicated chapel space in the Belfast asylum was of particular significance, occurring in the context of a long-running controversy that pitted the local asylum governors against the national inspectorate, the Lord Lieutenant and central government. The Belfast governors argued that the denominational diversity of their patient cohort created a risk that chaplains of multiple creeds might incite 'religious excitement' and sectarian tensions within the institution. For decades, the Belfast governors held firm in their resistance to the appointment of salaried chaplains, despite unanimous support for such chaplains amongst the Inspectors, all other asylum boards, and the hierarchy of the main denominations. Although ultimately vindicated at law, Belfast's victory proved short lived, as revised legislation in 1867 made the appointment of chaplains mandatory.[4]

The question of how to deal with the accumulation of 'incurable patients' challenged all involved in the asylum project for the best part of a century. The merits of provincial asylums for 'incurable cases' were discussed in the 1840s and occasionally thereafter, but this approach was rarely pursued in Ireland. Belfast provides a rare exception where in the 1880s, the distinct lunacy and poor law authorities co-ordinated to realise the economic benefits of making cheaper provision for 'congenital idiots and imbeciles':

> *the Guardians have just shown an example well worthy of imitation, and somewhat approaching the plan adopted in the London metropolitan districts. By erecting a separate receptacle altogether for 300 of the classes in question, suitably constructed in an open space, at an outlay of nearly £6,000, where paid attendants are employed, the cost of the establishment being derived from the usual poor rates.*[5]

In an era when the entire asylum project was trapped in the gloomy discourse of containing the ever-increasing burden of insanity, the Inspectors were keen to encourage any glimmers of progress. While hardly worse than any of the other Johnston and Murray asylums around the country, the Inspectors ratcheted up their criticism of Belfast's old asylum '...some parts of the buildings are dark, dreary and deficient in ventilation, and, above all, they are overcrowded to an extreme degree' while simultaneously flattering the egos of the asylum governors to do the right thing.[6] Ultimately, the solution to the challenges of the constrained Falls Road site lay in an entirely new asylum at Purdysburn (see Case Study 26), a project that would place the freshly minted city at the forefront of enlightened care for the insane in the new century.

As the last patients decanted to the new villa colony at Purdysburn (some via the less than salubrious setting of the Ballymena Workhouse), the old asylum buildings were requisitioned by the Ministry of War in 1915 to serve as the Belfast War Hospital.[7] The buildings would stand long enough to witness the formation of the new nation of Northern Ireland before succumbing to demolition soon afterwards. The new Royal Victoria Hospital had already opened on the adjacent site, and during the course of the twentieth century, its buildings would ebb and flow across the site, leaving no trace today of the old asylum or its landscape.

References

1. Irish Architectural Archive (hereafter IAA), Murray Collection, c. 1827, Belfast District Lunatic Asylum, 92/64, Sheets 0107, 0108.
2. National Archives of Ireland (hereafter NAI), Chief Secretary's Office, 1833, *Correspondence between Belfast Governors, Under Secretary and Lord Lieutenant*, CSO/RP/1833/1072; CSO/RP/1833/1941.
3. IAA, Murray Collection, c. 1830, *A Plan of the Belfast District Lunatic Asylum, shewing [sic] the proposed addition for the accommodation of 100 incurable patients*, 92/64, Sheet 0119.
4. Pauline M Prior & David V Griffiths, 'The "Chaplaincy Question" at Belfast District Asylum 1834–1870', in Pauline M. Prior (ed), *Asylums, Mental Health Care and the Irish 1800–2010* (Dublin, 2012) pp 167–84.
5. *Thirty-First Annual Asylum Report 1882*, HC 1882 [3356] xxxii, p. 11.
6. *Fifty-Fifth Annual Asylum Report 1905*, HC 1906 [3164] xxxix, p. 80.
7. *Sixty-Seventh Annual Asylum Report 1917*, HC 1919 [32] xxv, p. 19.

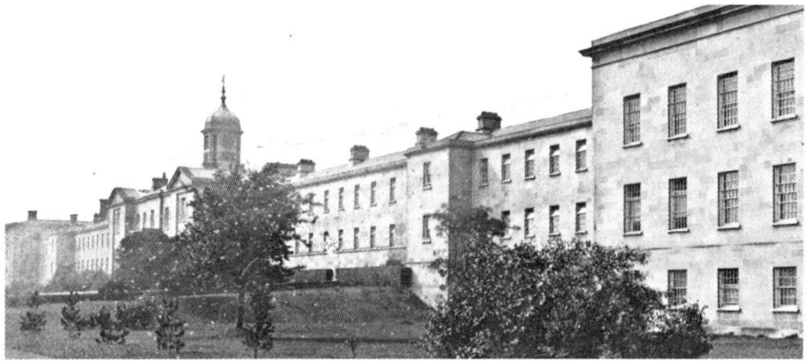

Image courtesy of the National Library of Ireland (L_CAB_00048)

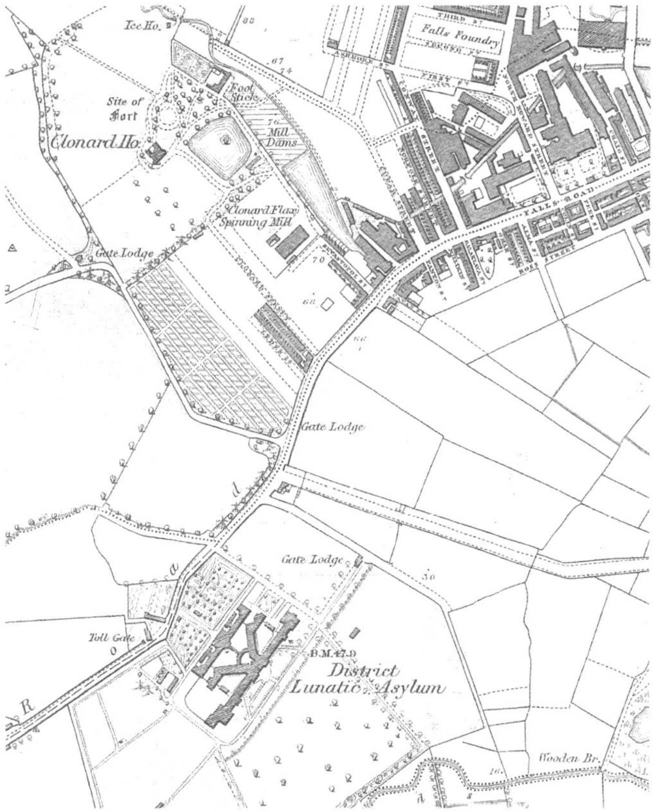

Reproduced courtesy of Trinity College Dublin (OS-Antrim-10560-Sheet 60-1859)

CASE STUDY 05

Years in operation
1829–1960

Original cost
£25,676

Capacity (min /max)
104 / 800+

Architect(s)
Johnston & Murray,
A. C. Adair

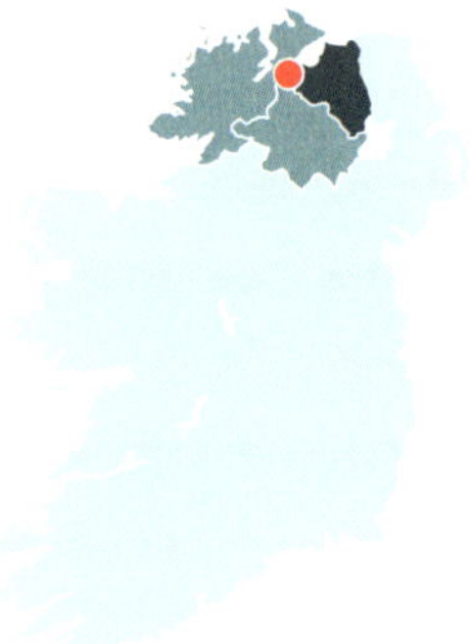

Londonderry District Lunatic Asylum

(demolished, site now in multiple ownership)

The board of governors of the Londonderry District Lunatic Asylum never quite seemed equal to their responsibilities. The enviable tax base of a thriving city should have afforded them ample resources to meet the needs of those in their care; instead, internal dissent and parochial interests time and again prevented progress and left the Inspectors indignant at their procrastination.

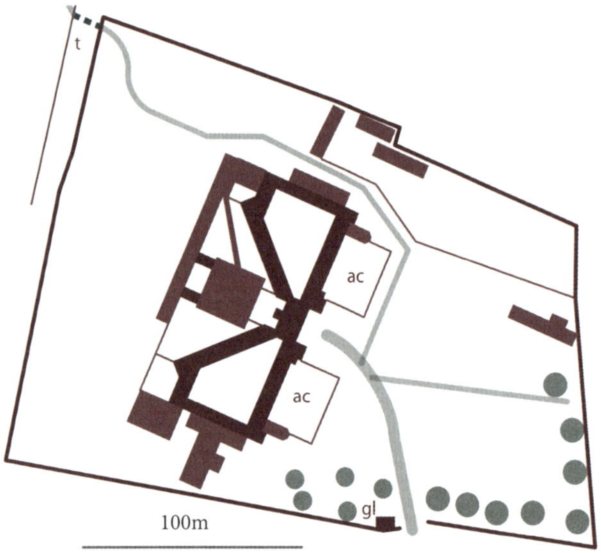

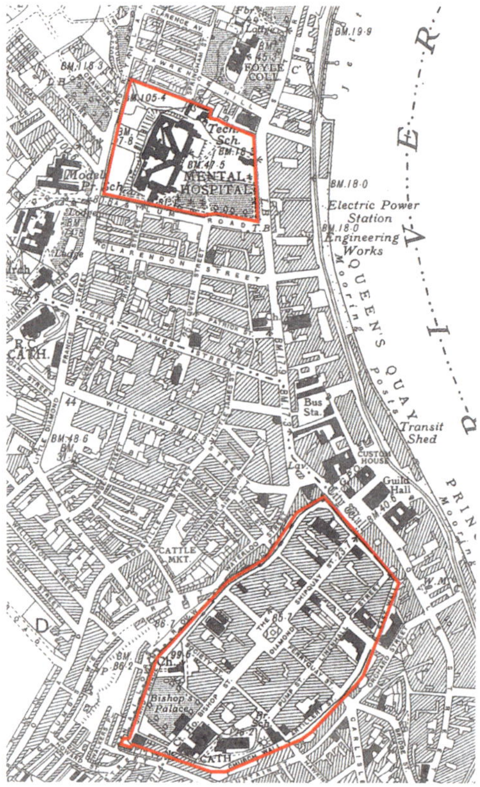

The asylum grounds were around two-fifths as large as the historic walled city, but for decades were criticised as woefully inadequate to the needs of the institution. *Reproduced courtesy of Trinity College Dublin (OSNI-LDerry-10560-Sheet 14-1954)*

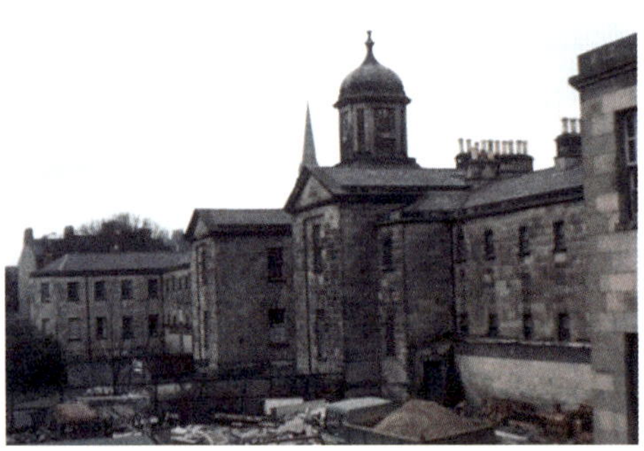

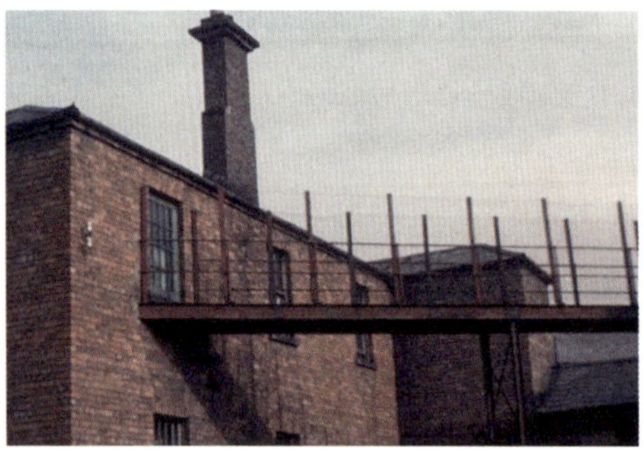

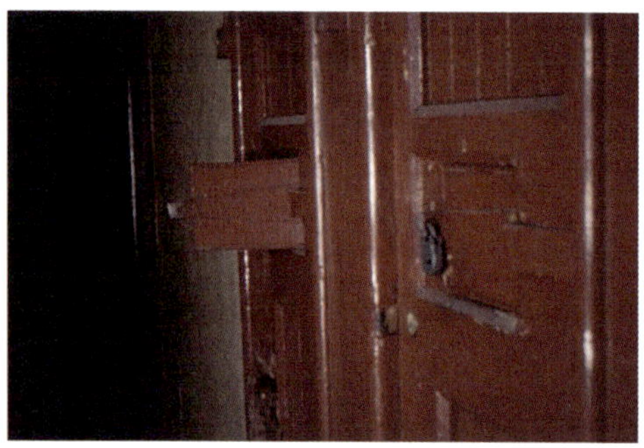

A promotional film for the new Gransha Hospital (see Case Study 29) recorded the old asylum in its final days before demolition. *Images copyright of Terence McDonald Collection, reproduced by kind permission of the McDonald family and the IFI*

The last of the three Ulster asylums to open during the first wave of asylum construction, the Londonderry District Lunatic Asylum entered service in 1829 with accommodation for 104 patients drawn from counties Tyrone, Donegal and Londonderry. Transferees from houses of industry and prisons threatened to fill the house from the outset, leading the Inspectors to warn that 'much discrimination' would be required in selecting only those with a reasonable chance of recovery, if the institution was to live up to its promise 'to become a serious blessing to the district'.[1]

Situated on an attractive site north of the city overlooking the River Foyle, the new asylum stood in similar proximity to the urban centre as most of its contemporaries. What few had anticipated was the rapid urban growth of an industrialising city, leading the Inspectors to early and sustained criticisms that 'the initial and irremediable fault' of the asylum was its location 'hemmed in by streets, wharves and private dwellings'.[2] As elsewhere, the site originally purchased for the asylum was too small, but increasing it was no easy task. In 1850 a small farm was purchased on the opposite side of Northlands Road to which the asylum was linked by a tunnel, but thereafter the governors struggled to compete in the local market for what was now valuable building land.[3] Aside from the difficulty of providing outdoor occupation for patients, the cramped site also constrained the expansion of the buildings. Overcrowding was a perennial problem, relieved only briefly by the opening of new district asylums at Omagh in 1853 (taking 67 Tyrone patients) and Letterkenny in 1866 (taking 113 Donegal patients). In 1870, the Board of Governors resolved:

> *that considering the dilapidated condition of the present lunatic asylum, the large sum necessary to put it into an adequate state of repair, and its general unfitness for the purpose of modern lunatic treatment, this board is of the opinion that it is desirable to construct an entirely new asylum.*[4]

Their proposal was confirmed by the Lord Lieutenant via an order in council in 1876, but by 1880 no progress had been made. The governors recoiled from the boldness of their plans, instead deciding in 1881 to borrow £20,000 to extend and improve the existing asylum, much to the horror of the Inspectors. The latter exhorted the governors to construct 'a new asylum altogether, on an open and cheerful site, so as to afford ample space for classified airing courts, and the erection of an adequate infirmary and dining hall; besides a recreation room and chapel, not included in the present plans.'[5] As the Inspectors foresaw, the £20,000 budget proved insufficient for the task in hand, with the final cost of the works coming to £29,000. This was not much short of the cost of a brand-new asylum, but for the money, Derry was stuck with a compromised building on a site that offered no possibility of expansion. The timidity of the governors ultimately did not serve their patients, or their ratepayers, well.[6]

In September 1893 the governors again resolved to act decisively where their forbears had not, but 'when the immediate locality came to be selected, differences of opinion arose between former advocates… ending in a do-nothing policy.'[7] In their report for 1899, the Inspectors came as close to exploding in frustration as the constraints of late Victorian professional prose would permit, setting out chapter and verse of the entire saga and exhorting the incoming asylum committee not to waste another decade by revisiting the decision of the old board of governors, but to proceed urgently to execute it.[8]

Their advice was heeded, but only in part. By 1905, 160 patients were accommodated in new buildings on land purchased on the east bank of the Foyle at Gransha, but there matters again stalled. The old asylum at Strand Road would continue to function through two domestic conflicts, partition and two world wars, enduring long enough to be subsumed into the National Health Service. When the new Gransha Mental Hospital finally opened in 1960 (see Case Study 29), the asylum buildings were vacated and demolished soon afterwards, though not before they were filmed as part of a promotional film for the new hospital. The asylum site was divided to accommodate a variety of public buildings, including a school, a social welfare office and an RUC station, the latter requiring that the secure boundary, originally designed to keep patients in, be raised even higher to keep a hostile citizenry out. Indeed, the timing of the move to the new, 'open-door' hospital at Gransha meant that that the boundary wall of the original asylum was never lowered or demolished, and survives today as the most complete historic boundary of any asylum site in the country, a trait it shares with the walled city it was built to serve.

References

1. *Eighth Report of the Inspectors-General of Prisons 1830*, HC 1830 [48] xxiv, p. 39
2. *Forty-Eighth Annual Asylum Report*, HC 1899 [9479] xl, p. 180.
3. Ibid., p. 180
4. *Forty-Eighth Annual Asylum Report 1899*, HC 1899 [9479] xl, p. 182.
5. *Thirty-First Annual Asylum Report 1882*, HC 1882 [3356] xxxii, p. 10.
6. By way of comparison, Wilkinson's new 260-bed asylum at Castlebar cost just under £35,000.
7. *Forty-Eighth Annual Asylum Report 1899*, HC 1899 [9479] xl, p. 182.
8. Ibid., p. 184.

CASE STUDY 06

Years in operation
1831–2011

Original cost
£22,552

Capacity (min /max)
104 / 542

Architect(s)
Johnston & Murray,
George Wilkinson,

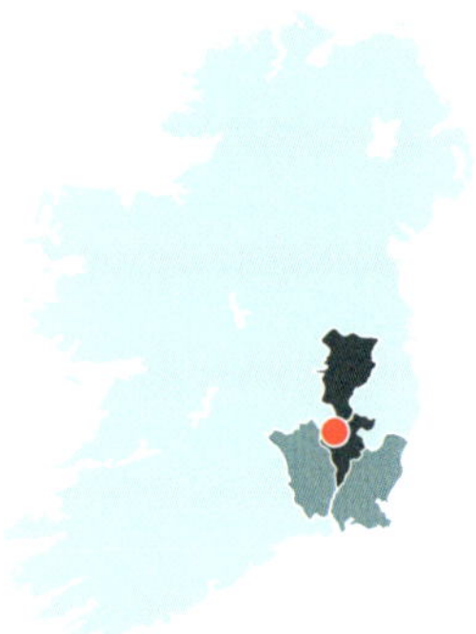

St Dympna's Hospital

(previously Carlow District Lunatic Asylum)

It is a measure of the physical wear to which these buildings have been subjected that eighteen decades of use leaves its mark on even the hardest granite stair treads. But herein also lies a truth: these early asylums are buildings of almost medieval solidity, built for hard service, stubbornly resistant to short-term alterations of convenience, but in the long term capable of outliving any of their more inherently flexible successors.

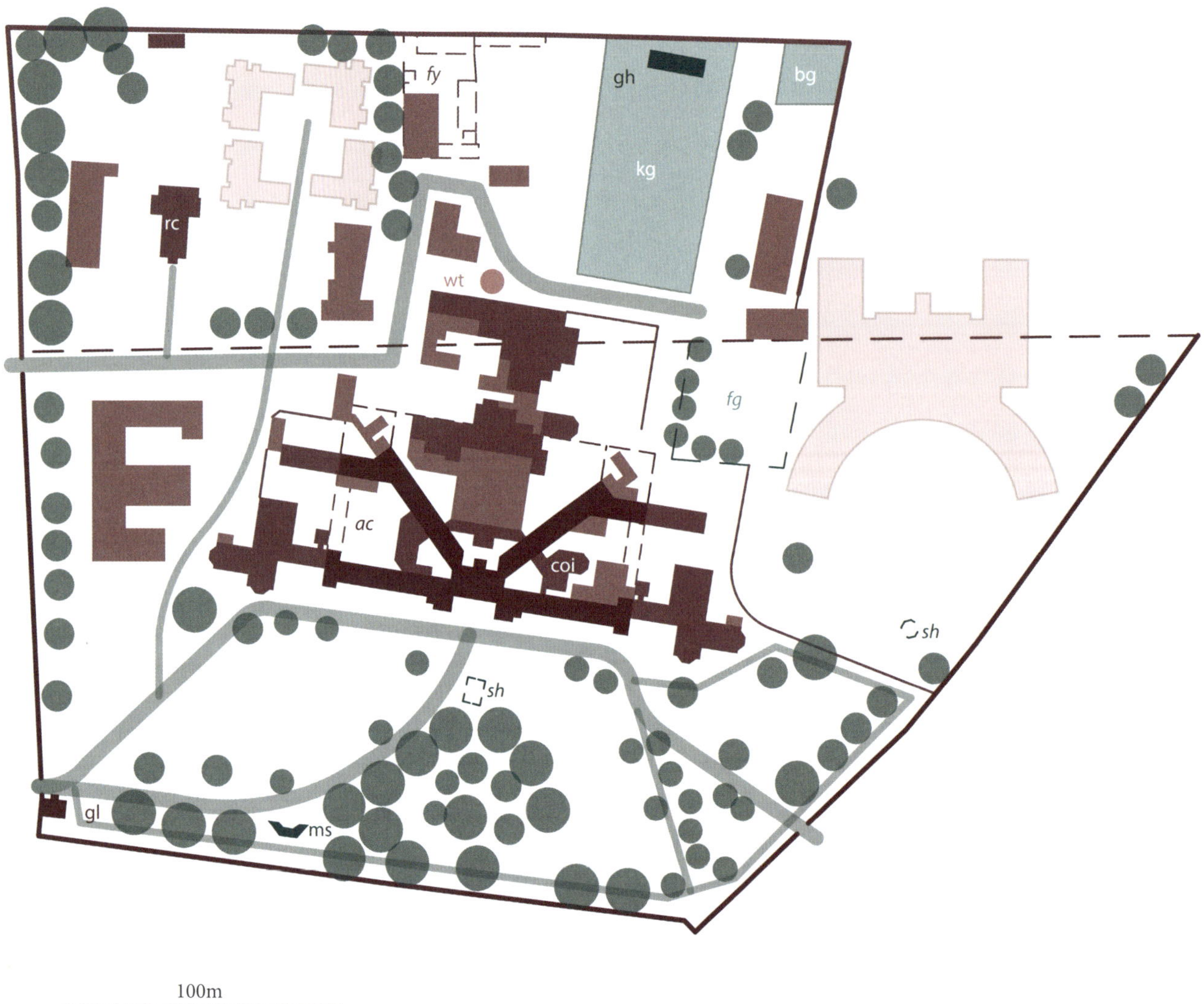

As the fourth 'second-class' asylum for 104 patients to roll off William Murray's drawing board, the model for the building was already well established and little change is evident from its predecessors. Contractors Williams and Cockburn completed the building in 1831 for the sum of £22,552, broadly in line with the Ulster triplets of the 1820s and nearby Maryborough a year later. Built to serve counties Carlow, Kildare, Kilkenny and Wexford, the latter two would be peeled away with the establishment of separate district asylums in 1852 and 1868 in Kilkenny and Enniscorthy, respectively. With a population that peaked only a little over 540 patients, the asylum remained one of the smallest on the island, which, architecturally speaking, was no bad thing. And in a country whose dominant geology predisposes towards buildings of grey limestone that stain dark navy after rain, the honey-coloured hues of Carlow's granite-built asylum are a rare treat. Its rich, mica-flecked texture seems to seek out and reflect light on even the dullest day; bathed in sunlight, it positively glows.

The need for extensions was first raised in 1836,[1] but the decanting of patients to the new district asylums meant that the Carlow Asylum, while not immune to overcrowding, managed to operate for 40 years without a major building programme. When the asylum governors finally acquiesced to the construction of major extensions in 1871, they turned to George Wilkinson, better known as the architect of Ireland's workhouses. Wilkinson's aesthetic judgement has been criticised elsewhere in this volume, but at Carlow, his pair of extensions flanking the main building are careful and respectful, executed in matching granite and continuing Johnston and Murray's finely detailed cornice and parapet. The Inspectors welcomed the completion of the extensions in 1873 (after delays due to worker strikes), but bemoaned the 'cold and cheerless' interiors throughout the asylum and exhorted the Board to commit 'a very trivial sum [compared to their already significant expenditure of £20,000] on homely comforts and ornamentation [to] render the institution perfect in its details'.[2]

Despite Wilkinson drafting plans for both Catholic and Protestant chapels, only the Catholic chapel was built at that time. Church of Ireland patients would have to wait almost 30 years for a diminutive chapel of their own, tucked into a courtyard on the eastern side of the institution. This latter chapel was but one element of a wide-ranging renovation scheme that again left the asylum 'in the hands of workmen' for several years in the late 1890s, and which included new male and female dining rooms, sanitary blocks, a new laundry and drying room, a boiler house and stores, staff accommodation, and the further expansion of Wilkinson's extensions.[3]

The Inspectors recommended the lowering of window sills to the front of the building at this time, work that was at least partially underway when prolific photographer Robert French visited the asylum.[4] His recording of a summer fête, attended by the great and the good of the county, is especially evocative as a piece of social history and shows that there were occasions when

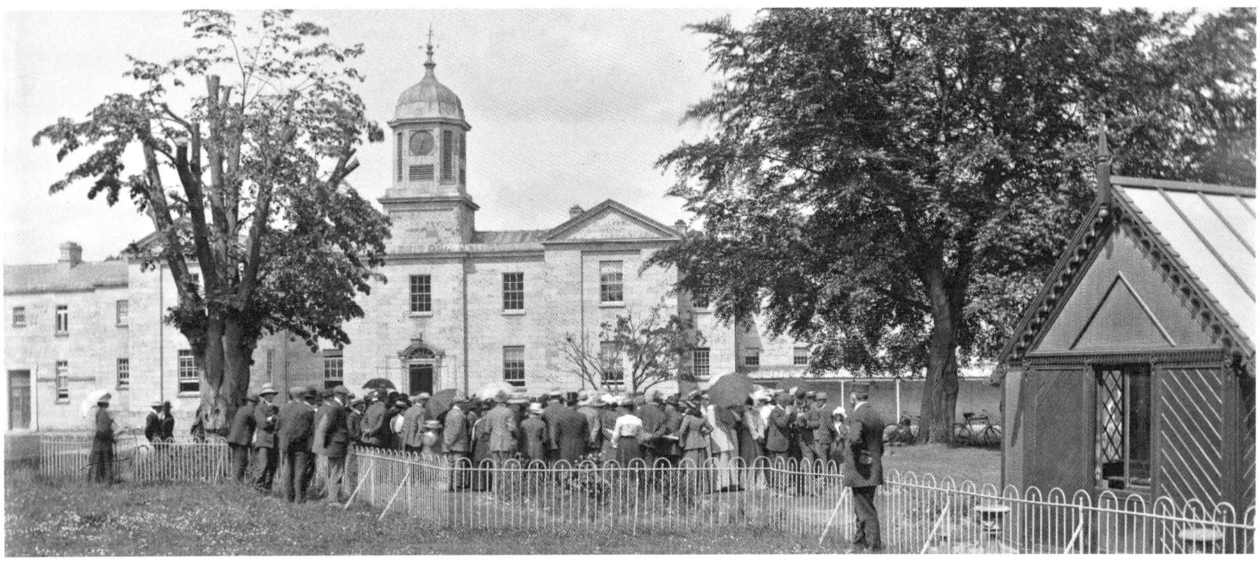

The great and the good of the county gathered in the grounds for festivities, *Image courtesy of the National Library of Ireland (L_ROY_07511)*

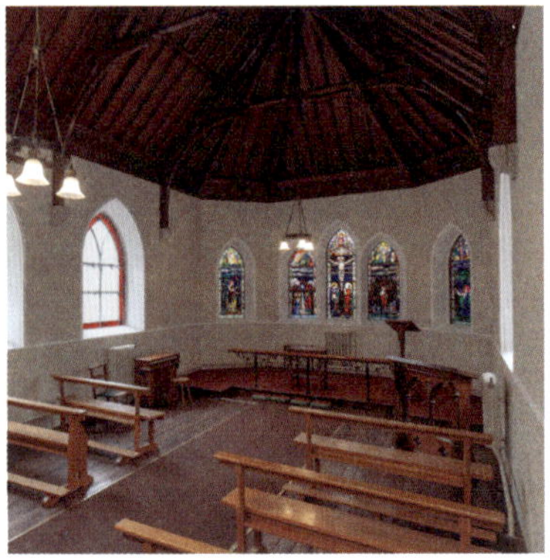

The dimunitive Church of Ireland chapel (above) was endowed with colourful twentieth-century glass. *Photograph by David Killeen, 2019.*

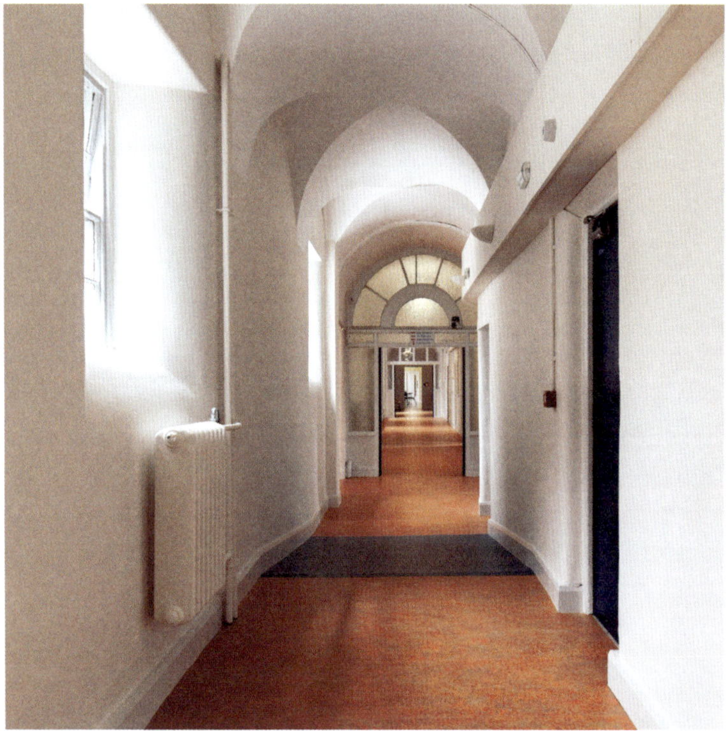

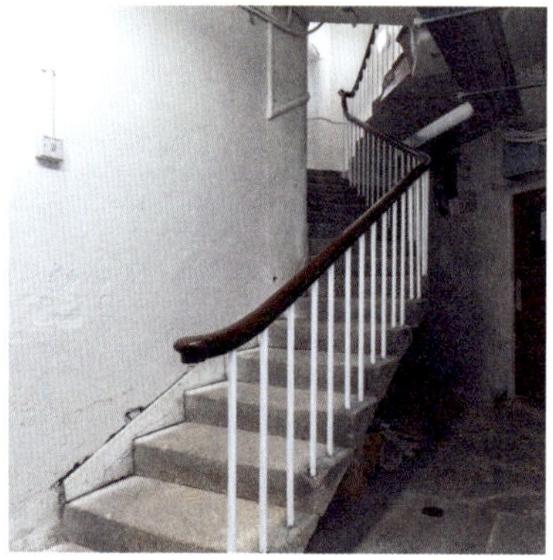

Masonry vaults and cantilevered stone staircases (above, opposite and left) make for buildings of quasi-medieval solidity, but stubbornly resistant to change. *Image courtesy of the Irish Architectural Archive (RIAI Murray Collection 92/46: 110), Photographs by David Killeen, 2019.*

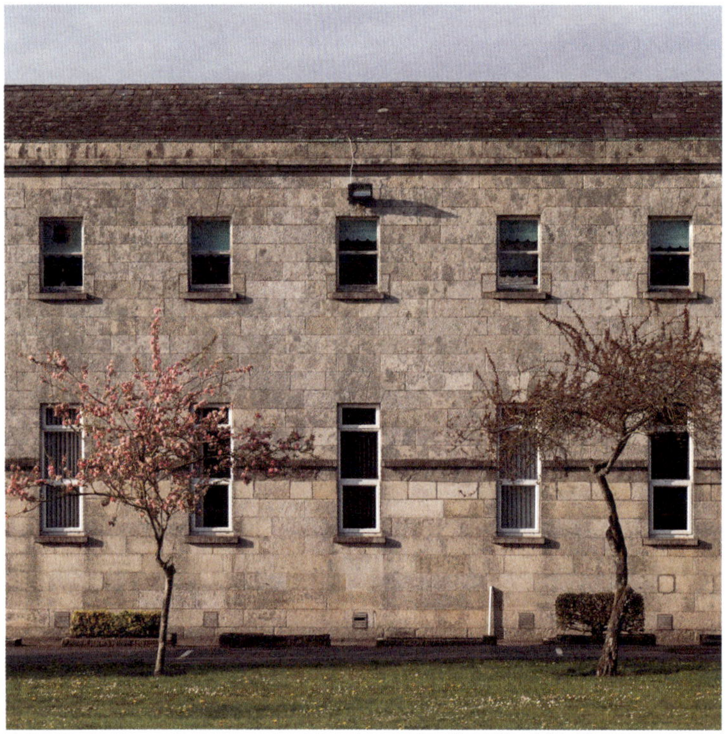

Honey-hued granite distinguishes Carlow from its contemporaries.
Note the differential weathering above and below the line of the former airing shed.
Photograph by David Killeen, 2019.

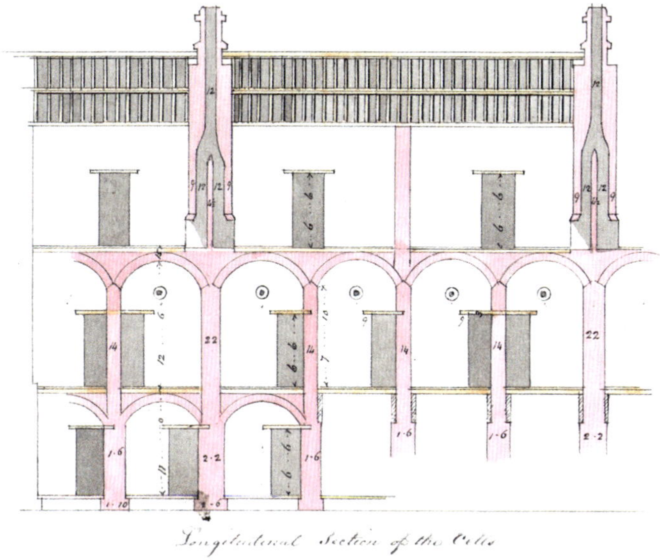

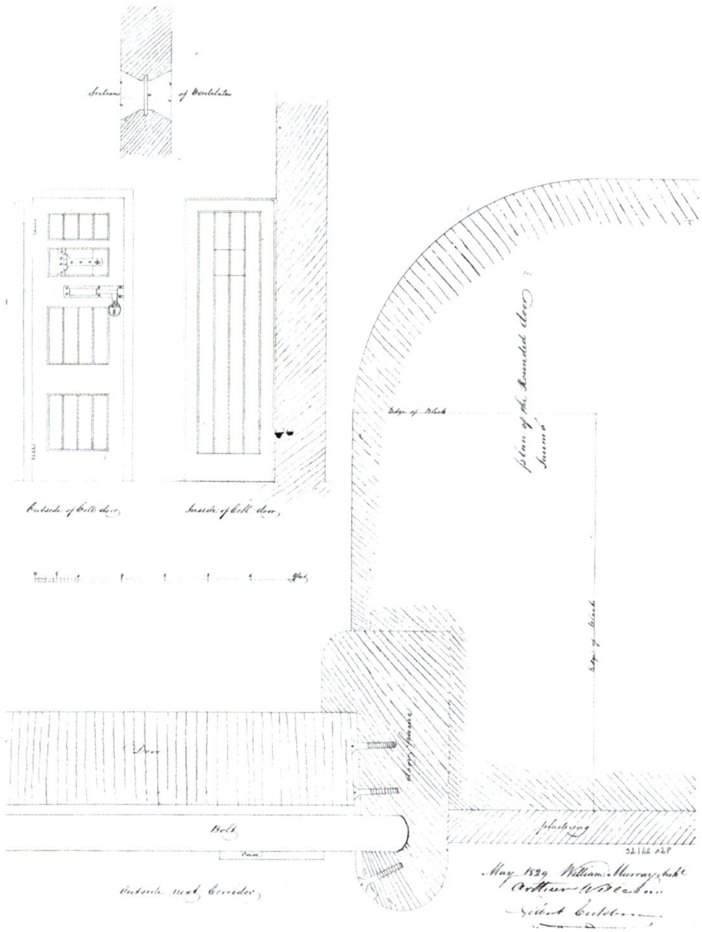

Detail of original cell door, 1829. *Image courtesy of the Irish Architectural Archive (RIAI Murray Collection 92/46: 128)*

the county at large was invited *intra muros* to sample the delights of the beautiful grounds. The patients, it would appear, remained safely indoors, avoiding the risk that the unscripted reality of insanity could undermine the positive impression that the festivities sought to foster.

Today, the building sits comfortably in a mature parkland setting studded with numerous specimen trees. The ornate summer house, decorative railings and 'living gazebo' in French's photographs are all now gone, but the 1950s saw the addition of a rather attractive Marian Grotto overlooking a distinctive star-shaped lawn. To the rear, a concrete water tower affirms that supply challenges pertained right into the second half of the twentieth century, a period that also saw the erection of a large, and distinctly modern, multi-purpose recreation hall in the heart of the complex.

More so than many of the other first-phase asylums, the historic interiors at Carlow remain, if not unaltered, at least substantially intact. Original masonry barrel- and cross-vaulting are exposed in cells and corridors, in many cases now accentuated with feature lighting rather than concealed above the depressing monotony of low-slung gridded ceilings. Early joinery, chimney pieces and plasterwork remain intact throughout the administration block, while in the rear wings, a handful of 1830s pivoting iron casement windows, once ubiquitous in all asylums of the era but now vanishingly rare, survived the Inspector's reconstructive recommendations. The evolution of the campus to serve a variety of public healthcare uses means that the stubbornly robust granite edifice of St Dympna's Hospital can look forward to a sustainable future serving the local community for whom it was built.

Further Reading

Catherine Cox, *Negotiating Insanity in the Southeast of Ireland, 1820–1900* (Manchester: Manchester University Press, 2012)

References

1. 'Some addition of Ground and Buildings are necessary to enable the Board to accommodate all of the Insane and Incurable of the District, and, as these Additions have been made by the Asylums in Belfast and Limerick, I beg to submit them to the consideration of the local board.' *Sixteenth Report of the Inspectors-General of Prisons 1838*, HC 1837–38 [186] xxix, p. 36.
2. *Twenty-Fourth Annual Asylum Report 1875*, HC 1875 [1293] xxxiii, pp 31–2.
3. *Forty-Seventh Annual Asylum Report 1898*, HC 1898 [8969] xliii, pp 116–17.
4. National Library of Ireland, Lawrence Collection, post 1871, Carlow District Lunatic Asylum, L_ROY_07510, L_ROY_07511. The photographer visited at least twice, as evidenced by changes in the buildings between each visit. The earlier picture dates from after 1871, as Wilkinson's extensions are visible but airing sheds to both sides of the asylum are intact. By the time the second picture was taken, the south-facing airing shed on the west side was already removed and some windows lowered, but those on the east remain in place.

CASE STUDY 07

St Brigid's Hospital

(previously Connaught District Lunatic Asylum)

Years in operation
1833–2011

Original cost
£27,128

Capacity (min /max)
150 / 1660

Architect(s)
Johnston & Murray,
Fuller & Kempster,
J. R. Boyd Barrett

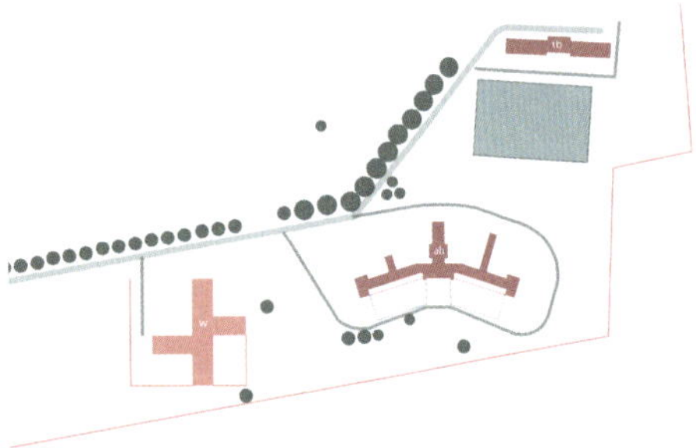

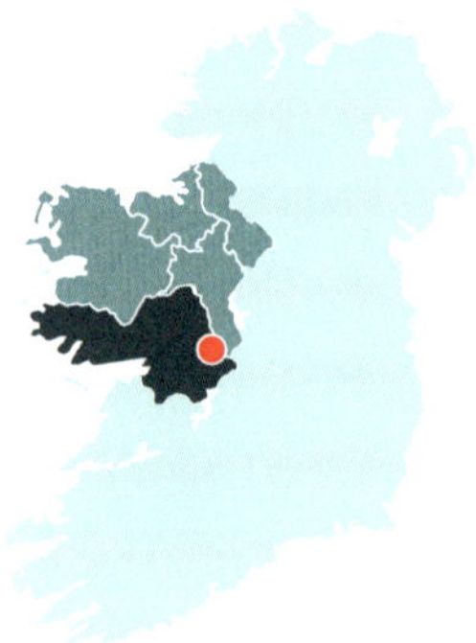

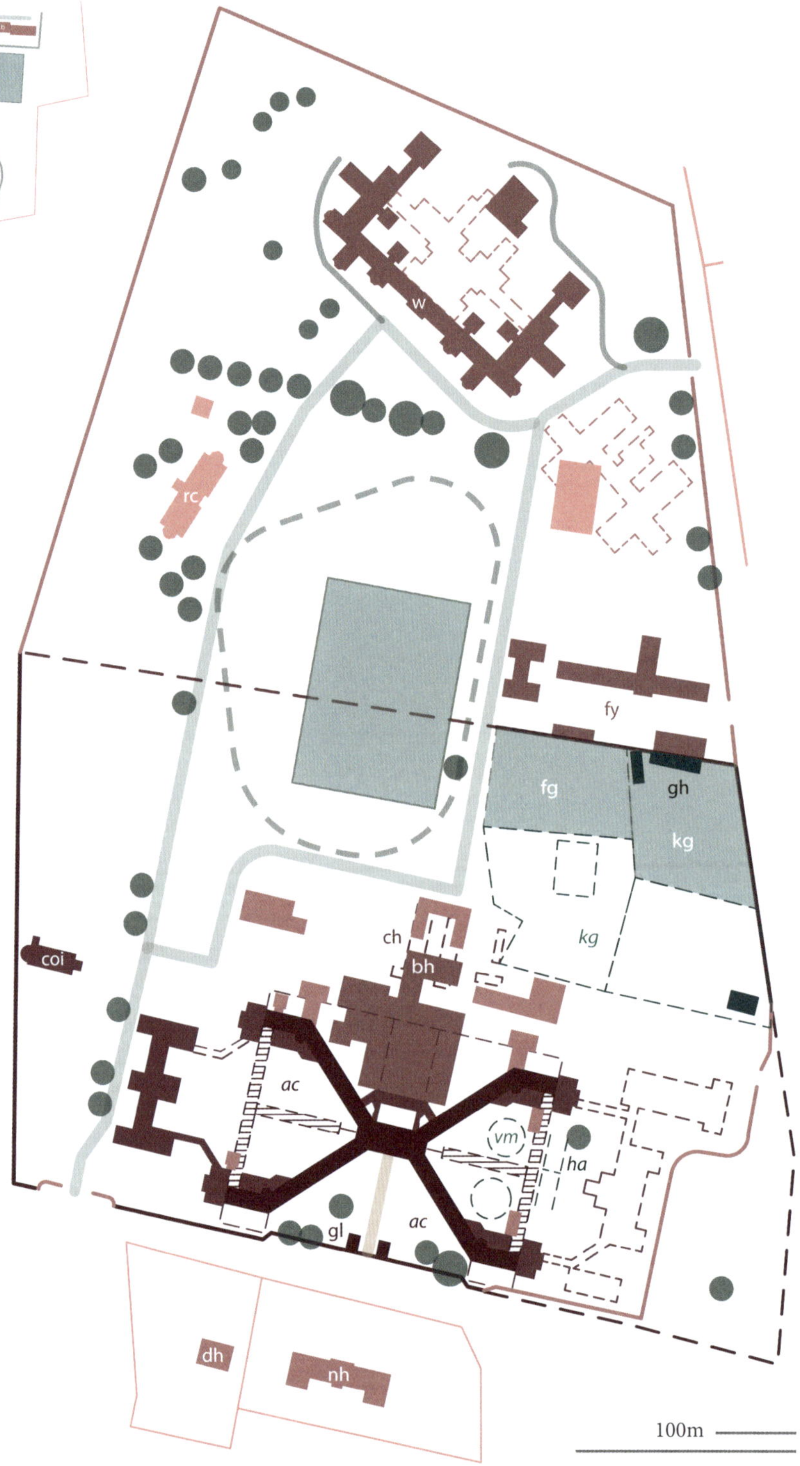

If the expansion of Ireland's lunatic asylums transformed them into major economic forces in their respective municipalities, it was inevitable that their closure risked causing an equivalent economic shock. The most dramatic example is seen at Ballinasloe, where one of the largest asylums in the country grew to dominate the economy of its relatively small host town, and whose closure leaves a challenging legacy of redundant institutional buildings on a post-industrial scale.

The primary legislation that created the lunatic asylum system gave the Lord Lieutenant the discretion to decide on the location of new asylums and the extent of their districts, opening the process to a level of canvassing and politicking. The result was a haphazard and inequitable distribution, with Connaught emerging as something of a second-class province. The single 150-bed asylum that opened at Ballinasloe in 1833 had to serve a peak population in excess of 1.4 million and a geographic terrain of over 6,800 square miles, by both measures the largest catchment of any asylum in the country.[1] The location of the asylum – in a small town on the eastern fringe of a poorly connected province – was too far from many prospective patients, a failing only rectified with the opening of new asylums at Sligo and Castlebar.

Ballinasloe was only the second asylum erected to the larger standard plan for 150 patients. William Murray – now in sole charge of design matters following Johnston's death in 1829 – made several modifications to the plan originally used at Limerick. The 'noisy' wards at the end of each wing were turned through 90 degrees, while the small 'straw sheds' at Limerick evolved into a range of outbuildings running the full depth of the building. Murray also indulged in a rare architectural flourish: enlarging and elaborating the cupola into an octagon with eight engaged Corinthian columns crowned by an entablature, cornice and shallow ogee dome. It is the only use of the higher architectural orders observed by this author in any Irish asylum, before or since.

The first major extension of the asylum was constructed in 1848 under the auspices of the Board of Works as part of their asylum expansion programme, creating an additional 80 beds for infirm patients.[2] The decanting of patients to new asylums in Sligo in 1855 and Castlebar in 1866 provided temporary relief of the perennial pressure of overcrowding, but by the 1880s, major investment could be deferred no longer. Alterations and extensions during the decade saw total capacity increased to 711 patients, supported by major improvements of the kitchen and dining areas and new heating boilers. The net result was that the original 'X' plan became fully enclosed at each end to create a labyrinthine figure-of-eight, rendering useless the 'viewing mounds' that had once allowed patients a view beyond the airing-yard walls. And whereas finely landscaped grounds helped to mitigate poor architectural decisions at many other asylums, the site at Ballinasloe was never well endowed in this regard – pretty flowers in the forecourt were an insufficient foil to the sobriety of the original structure and the scale of its later appendages.

The possibility of forming a separate Roscommon district with its own asylum was at this time discussed, but ultimately dismissed. Instead, a new detached block for 260 patients was constructed at the north of the site to the designs of Fuller and Kempster, bringing the total capacity to 1,004 by the turn of the twentieth century.[3] Large windows made for healthier levels of daylight than the main building, but the rock-faced ashlar finish lent it an austere institutional character that the smattering of Elizabethan-revival detailing at its centre was insufficient to relieve.

The new Free State brought a change of name to the Ballinalsoe Mental Hospital, but little material improvement for its patients who, by the 1930s, numbered in excess of 1,800. Change, when it eventually came, could not have happened without the largesse of the Irish Hospitals Sweepstakes. Grants of £203,354 helped to fund a new admissions hospital, TB hospital, chronic unit and nurses' home, making Ballinasloe the single largest recipient in the mental hospital sector even before counting the £163,509 allocated to the new hospital at Castlerea, which also came under Ballinasloe's management.[4] (See Case Study 28)

If the quality of a building reflects the aspirations of its sponsor, these new structures were conceived in a spirit of surprising optimism. Architect James Boyd Barrett's use of southerly orientation, wall-to-wall glazing, generous verandas, tall ceilings and high-quality internal finishes resulted in some of the best healthcare buildings of their generation. His admissions hospital in particular, opened in 1941, ventured further along the path of architectural modernism than any mental health building to date and contrasted starkly with the gloomy wards of the original asylum building.[5] And while pragmatic considerations doubtless played a role in the siting of the new buildings, the decision to erect them on virgin terrain, independently accessed and far removed from the core of the institution, also implies a desire for a fresh start, untainted by association.

At its peak, the hospital comprised over 2,000 patients and staff in a town with a population of only 5,711,[6] but thereafter would experience the same slow-but-steady decline as new services developed beyond the confines of the old institution. But when the Inspector of Mental Hospitals belatedly resumed inspections in 1988, he identified the 'continuing lack of a coherent approach to the problem of Ballinasloe', implying that decisions were driven by local instincts to create

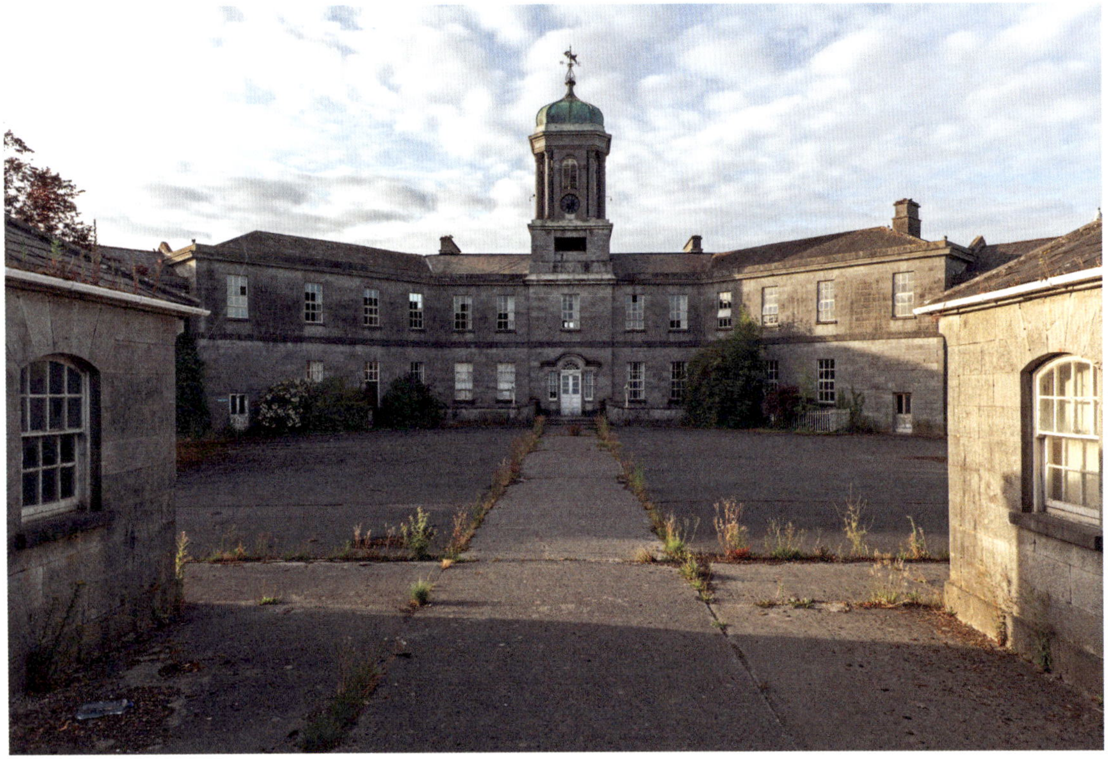

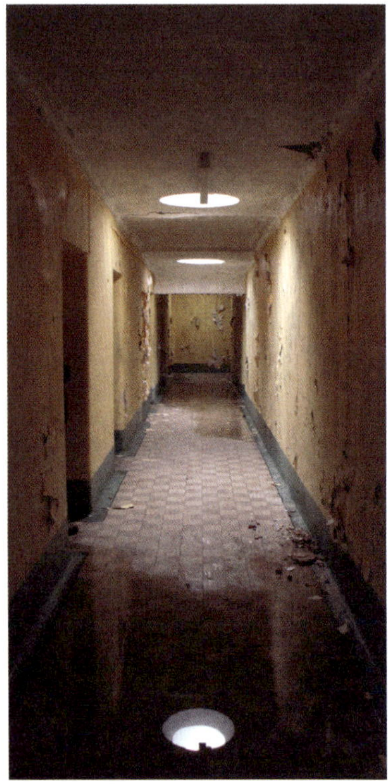

The solid and serene classicism of Ballinasloe's facade (above) belies the deterioration playing out within (above right). *Photographs by David Killeen, 2019, and the author, 2014.*

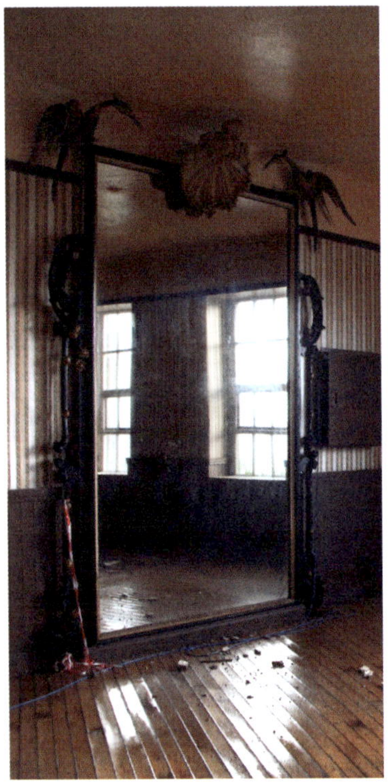

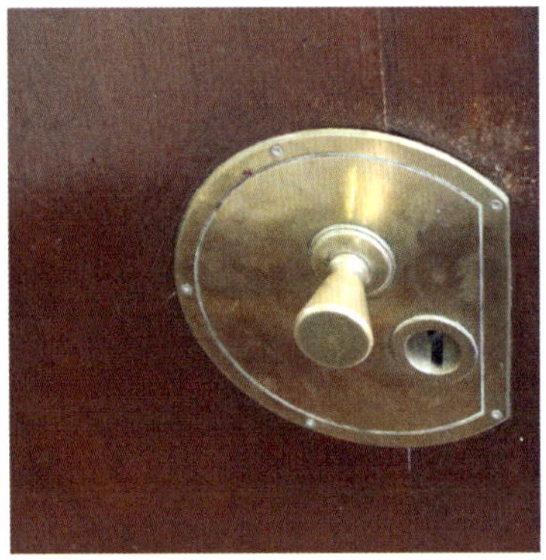

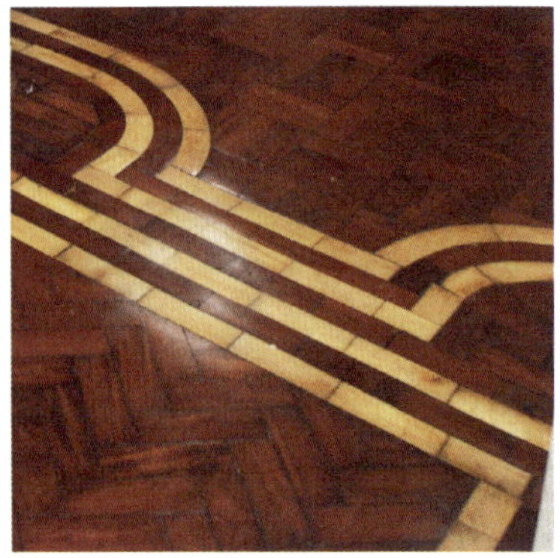

The fit and finish of the 1930s admissions hospital and TB sanatorium (above) were of the very highest quality. *Photographs by the author, 2014.*

The origin of the vast rococco mirror in the 'inspection lobby' is unknown, but its very scale and ostentation must have come as a shock to many patients. It has since succumbed to the vandals. *Photograph by the author, 2014.*

services to fill buildings, without regard to wider strategic objectives. The desire to retain local services for the benefit of local patients was doubtless sincere, but was also a natural response to the existential threat posed by the closure of the town's longest-standing industry.

It would take another 25 years for national strategy to achieve its final victory over local initiative. Even as the last patients departed the building, which since 1833 had been the epicentre of mental health services in the west of Ireland, battle lines continued to be drawn around the last acute wards in the 1930s admissions unit, which were 'expensively refurbished' despite having no definite future use.[7] At time of writing, a site that was home to over 1,600 patients at its peak retained just 14 beds falling under the inspection remit of the Mental Health Commission. The majority of the buildings stand empty, in varying stages of decay, with neither a clear future nor much hope of one. Walking the empty wards of St Brigid's Hospital to the sights and sounds of water trickling through fabric devastated by the theft of lead, copper pipes and electrical wiring, one's sense is not so much of an empty hospital, as of a post-industrial landscape of buildings and spaces rendered redundant by remote, faceless forces.

Further Reading

Oonagh Walsh, '"Tales from the Big House": The Connacht District Lunatic Asylum in the Late Nineteenth Century', in *History Ireland* 13:6 (Nov-Dec. 2005), pp 21–25.

'Landscape and the Irish Asylum' in Úna Ní Bhroiméil and Glenn Hooper (eds), *Land and Landscape in 19th Century Ireland* (Dublin: Four Courts Press, 2008) pp 156–70.

References

1. By way of comparison, the identical 150-bed asylum built at Limerick served a population of 880,000 and an area of 4,400 square miles. Population data, Census of Ireland 1841.
2. *Annual Asylum Report 1848*, HC 1849 [1054] xxiii, p. 5.
3. *Forty-Sixth Annual Asylum Report 1897*, HC 1897 [8639] xxxviii, pp 17–18.
4. The three-storey chronic block is a facsimile of Boyd Barrett's contemporary ward blocks at Castlerea and Mullingar. Eamon de Barra (ed.), *Irish hospitals 1956–1971* (Dublin, 1971), p. 58, p. 67.
5. *Report of the Inspector of Mental Hospitals 1942*, p. 16.
6. Total patient numbers through the 1950s generally exceeded 1,550 (discounting Ballinasloe patients lodged at other hospitals, which are sometimes erroneously included when this example is cited in other sources). Staff numbers in 1954 (the last year for which staff statistics were recorded by the Inspector of Mental Hospitals) was 434. Town population from Census of Ireland, 1961.
7. Mental Health Commission, 'Approved Centre Inspection Report, St Brigid's Hospital', Aug. 2012, p. 1.

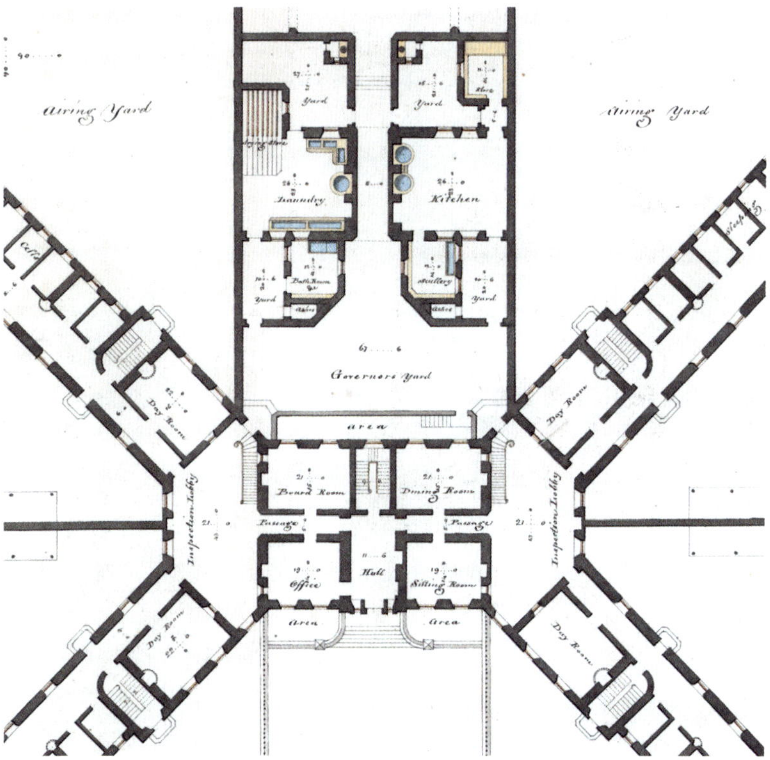

Detail of the Governor's House, 'Inspection Lobbies,' kitchen and laundry at the heart of the complex, 1830. *Image courtesy of the National Archives of Ireland (Office of Public Works Collection, OPW/5HC/4/883, 1)*

CASE STUDY 08

Years in operation
1833–Present

Original cost
£26,830

Capacity (min /max)
104 / 672

Architect(s)
Johnston & Murray,
John Sterling Butler,
Sir Thomas Drew,
P. J. Sheahan.

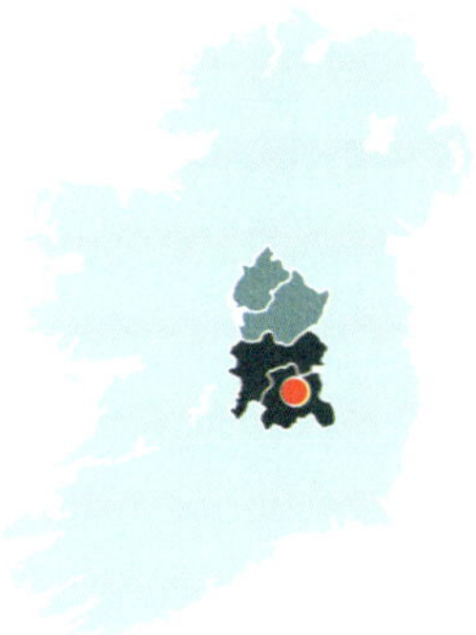

St Fintan's Hospital

(previously Maryborough District Lunatic Asylum)

From the flattest of midland fields whose topography offered nothing by way of picturesque effect, generations of staff and patients have created one of the finest asylum landscapes in the country. Within a few years of opening, the Maryborough District Lunatic Asylum already boasted formal pleasure grounds larger and more elaborate than any other asylum of the era, while the native and exotic trees planted at the time continue to enrich the site to this day.

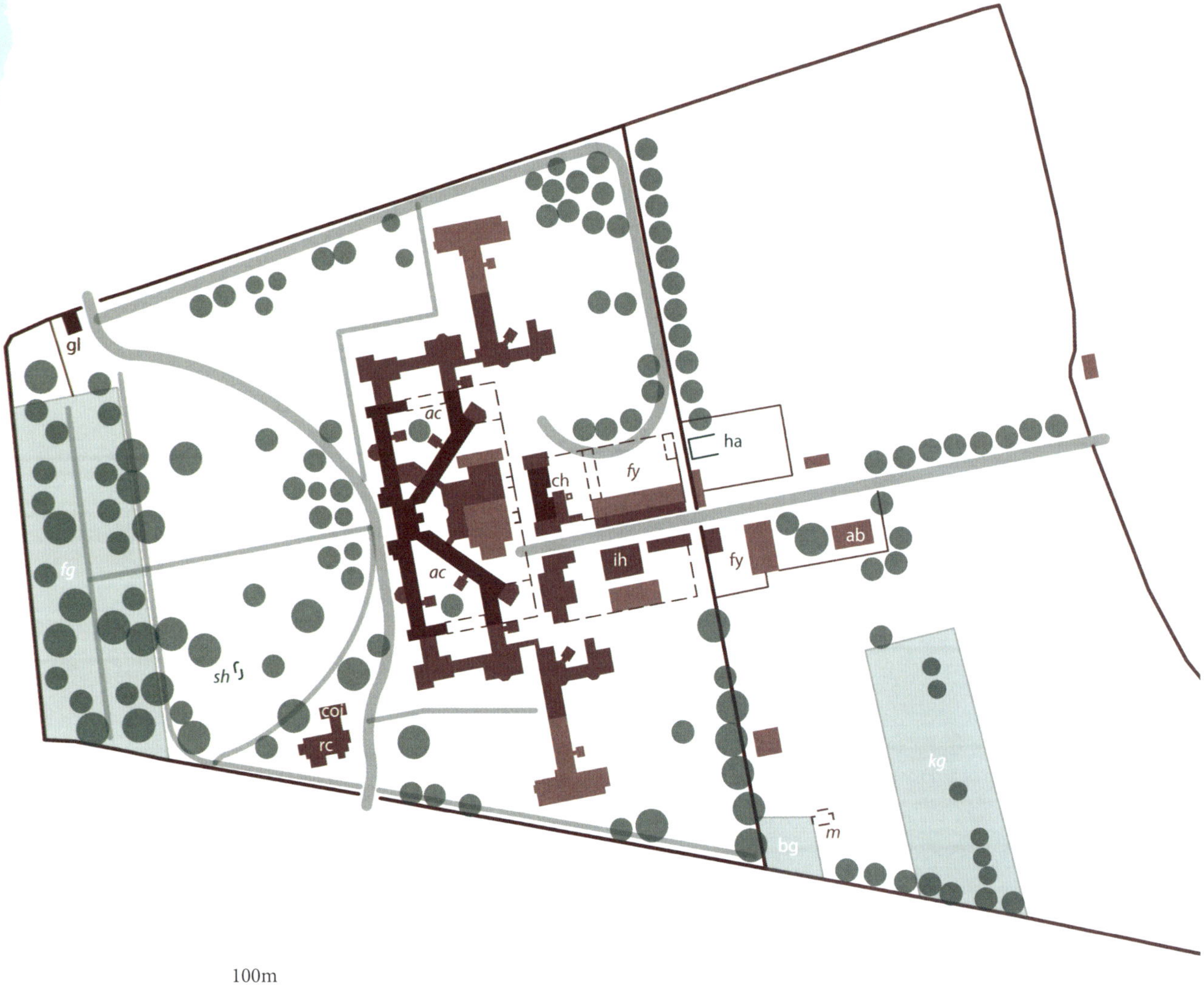

When the new asylum for the town of Maryborough was originally sanctioned by the Lord Lieutenant in Privy Council in 1828, it was intended to serve King's and Queen's Counties, Meath and Westmeath. An order dropping Meath and adding Tipperary and Longford was issued in 1830, but by the time the new 104-bed asylum actually received its first patients in April 1833, its catchment had been revised once more to serve Westmeath and Longford, with a combined population of over 539,500.[1] Patients of the latter two counties were transferred to the new Mullingar Asylum in 1855; thereafter changes would be in name rather than geography: the Maryborough District Lunatic Asylum, refuge for the afflicted subjects of King's and Queen's Counties, would be reinvented as the Portlaoi[gh]se Mental Hospital, home to half of a percent of the Free State citizenry of counties Offaly and Laois.[2]

The 22-acre site selected for the asylum may have been flat, but was not without its own complications. Comparison of two early site-layout drawings show that decisions were made to straighten the Dublin Road from its original meandering route to form a regular northern boundary, with a similar rationalisation of the Borris river along the western boundary.[3] The building itself was another of Johnston and Murray's standard second-class plans, completed in 1832 at a cost of £24,172, with a further £2,654 expended on fees, furnishings and the land itself.

The main building was subjected to three main phases of construction, in addition to countless minor alterations. The first major extensions, dating from the 1860s, presented as a pair of two-storey pedimented pavilions politely bookending the main building. Architect John Sterling Butler took care not only to execute these in high-quality limestone ashlar indistinguishable from the original, but also paid an unusual degree of deference to Johnston and Murray's composition by echoing many of its architectural mannerisms. Less care was evident in the clumsy bay-fronted extensions added later to create extra dayrooms, while the three-storey, red-brick ward blocks added by Sir Thomas Drew in 1898 – though not without merit in their own right – contrast starkly in scale, colour and style with the smooth, serene classicism of the original. A final pair of redbrick extensions opened in 1942, built on the strength of Sweepstakes funding of £70,834 during what was otherwise a lean period for hospital construction.[4] Designed by prolific hospital architect P. J. Sheahan, they take cues from the horizontal stone banding and articulated keystones of the 1898 extensions, while bearing more than a passing resemblance to Wright's almost-modernist Ardee Mental Hospital of 1933. (See Case Study 27). The collective effect is neither coherent nor beautiful – its kindest description may be as a legible architectural palimpsest of each generation's response to evolving institutional needs.

Water supply and effluent disposal arrangements were initially basic, with an intake from the Borris River near the Stradbally Road and untreated effluent discharged just 150 metres downstream, near the Dublin Road. It is a mark of the early importance afforded to the landscape setting that the unavoidable necessity of a pump house received full architectural treatment at the hands of William Murray, who enfolded it into an attractive colonnaded summer house that looked like it could have wandered in from the demesne of nearby Emo Court (see Chapter 2). As the asylum population grew from an initial 100 to over 480 by the end of the nineteenth century, the original water supply proved wholly inadequate. The asylum connected to the municipal water supply in 1898 and constructed its own 100,000-gallon reservoir in 1904. But just as the river proved inadequate for a near five-fold increase in population, so the effects of a similarly increased quantum of effluvia could not fail to offend downstream neighbours, especially the local prison authorities. After a decade of angst, agreement was reached in 1904 that the asylum would share the cost of culverting the now grossly polluted river through the prison grounds.[5]

A plain but pleasant pair of chapels in the parkland to the south of the site stand like older and younger siblings, joined at the hip by a later shared mortuary. Stepping inside, their interiors are as bare as most asylum chapels, but the chancel of the Catholic chapel reveals a dazzling surprise: a triptych of richly coloured figurative stained glass windows by Ireland's pre-eminent early twentieth-century stained-glass artist, Harry Clarke.

Quoted in the official history published to mark the hospital's sesquicentenary in 1983, the then RMS, Dr Liam Hanniffy, opined that the 'architecturally pleasing, structurally sound' old building could find new uses in rehabilitative medicine as its role in the delivery of acute psychiatric services inevitably diminished.[6] And so it has proven. A single ward stubbornly operating within the main building continues to deny the Mental Health Commission their coveted prize of announcing the final closure of all

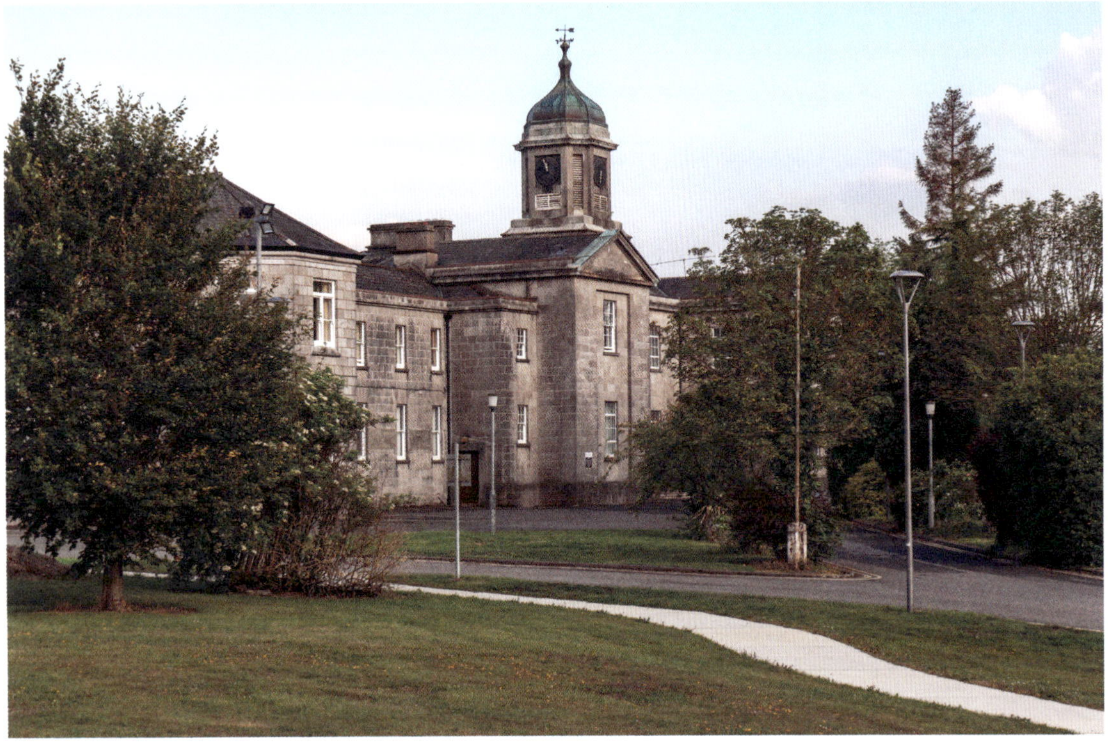

The mature asylum parkland is now a valued local amenity, even featuring on the marketing material of nearby housing developments. 'Irreedemably stigmatised,' indeed. *Photograph by David Killeen, 2019.*

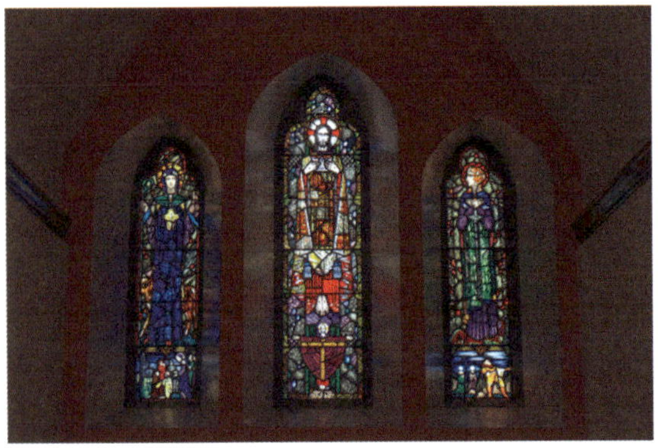

A triptych in the Catholic chapel by Ireland's pre-eminent stained glass artist, Harry Clarke, is an unexpected treat. *Photograph by David Killeen, 2019.*

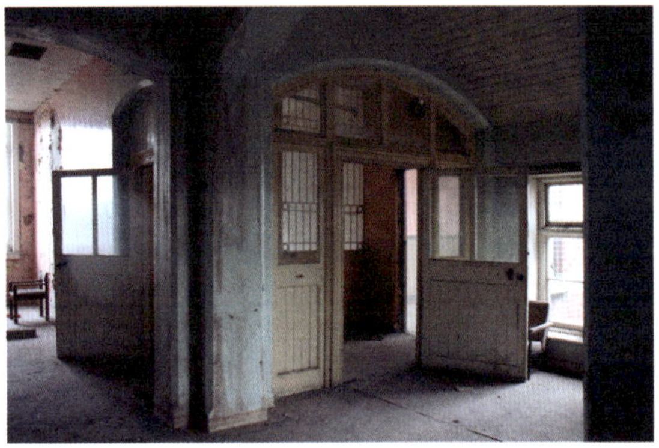

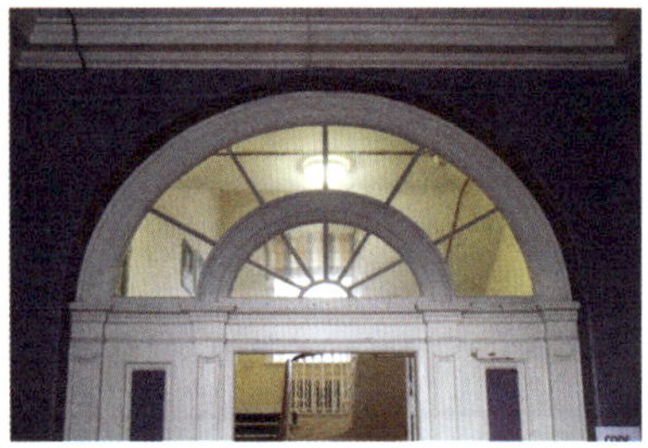

Original joinery details from 1833 (above) and 1898 (left). Photographs by the author, 2013.

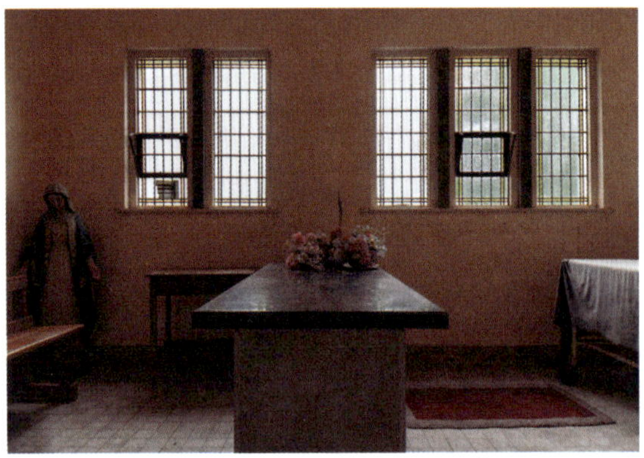

Hospital mortuaries allowed a more dignified departure for those who passed away within the walls. *Photograph by David Killeen, 2019.*

legacy asylum buildings, while the wider campus today is host to an impressive range of intensively used and continuously evolving public health services and clinics in a landscape setting that continues to be cherished and enhanced. Uniquely, almost every building and outbuilding on site is maintained in good repair; even the 1830s gate-lodge has been integrated into a new building housing a community addiction service. RMS Hanniffy's hope that 'St Fintan's will not be in ruins when its bicentenary comes to be celebrated in the year 2032' was certainly not misplaced.

Further Reading

Donal Murphy (ed.), *Tumbling Walls: The Evolution of a Community Institution, St Fintan's Hospital Portlaoise, 1833–1983* (Portlaoise: Midland Health Board, 1983)

References

1. Donal Murphy (ed.), *Tumbling Walls: The Evolution of a Community Institution, St Fintan's Hospital Portlaoise, 1833–1983* (Portlaoise, 1983), p. 16.
2. 530–550 patients resident during the 1920s; combined population of both counties 104,132. Census of Ireland, 1926.
3. Irish Architectural Archive, Workhouse Drawings Collection, 1830–31, Maryborough District Lunatic Asylum, 85/138, Sheet 116.
4. Eamon de Barra (ed.), *Irish Hospitals 1956–1971* (Dublin, 1971), p. 58.
5. Murphy, *Tumbling Walls*, pp 29–30.
6. Ibid., pp 83–4.

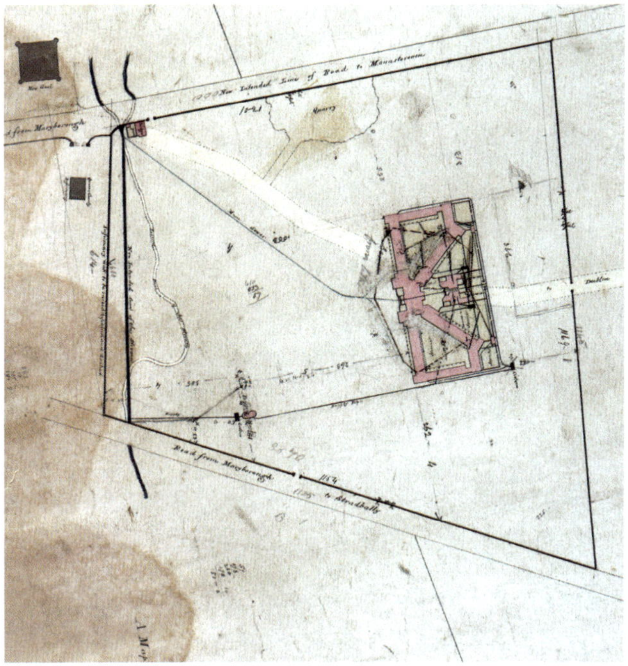

Major site works (above) were required to straighten both the stream and the Dublin Road. Note also proximity to the 'New Gaol' and County Infirmary, 1830. *Image courtesy of the Irish Architectural Archive (Workhouse Drawings Collection, 85/138: 116)*

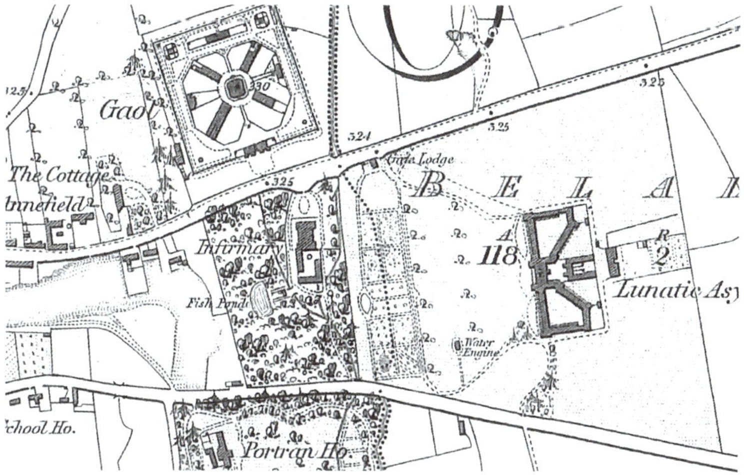

The asylum consolidated a new institutional quarter on the eastern edge of the town. *Reproduced courtesy of Trinity College Dublin (OS-Laois-10560-Sheet 13-1841)*

CASE STUDY 09

Years in operation
1833–2012

Original cost
£16,886

Capacity (min /max)
60 / 603

Architect(s)
Johnston & Murray,
James Otway

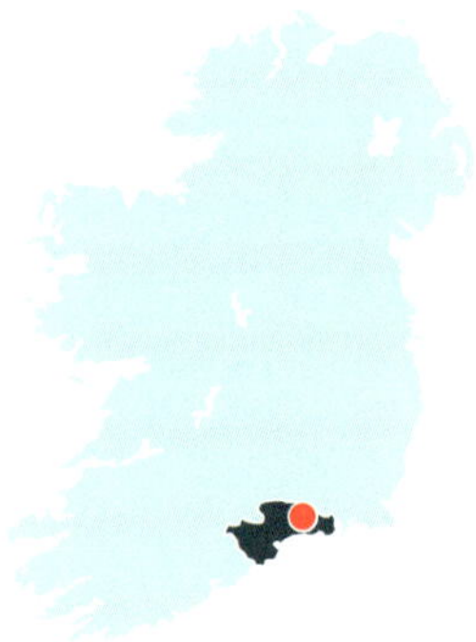

St Otteran's Hospital

(previously Waterford District Lunatic Asylum)

Even if every asylum tower did not actually contain a clock, the 'clocktower' would in time become one of the iconic images of asylumdom. At the time of writing, Waterford is unique not only in retaining its original clock mechanism from 1835, but in preserving the time-honoured horological tradition of manual winding – a task that has necessitated over 10,000 weekly ascents into the cupola in the intervening eighteen decades.

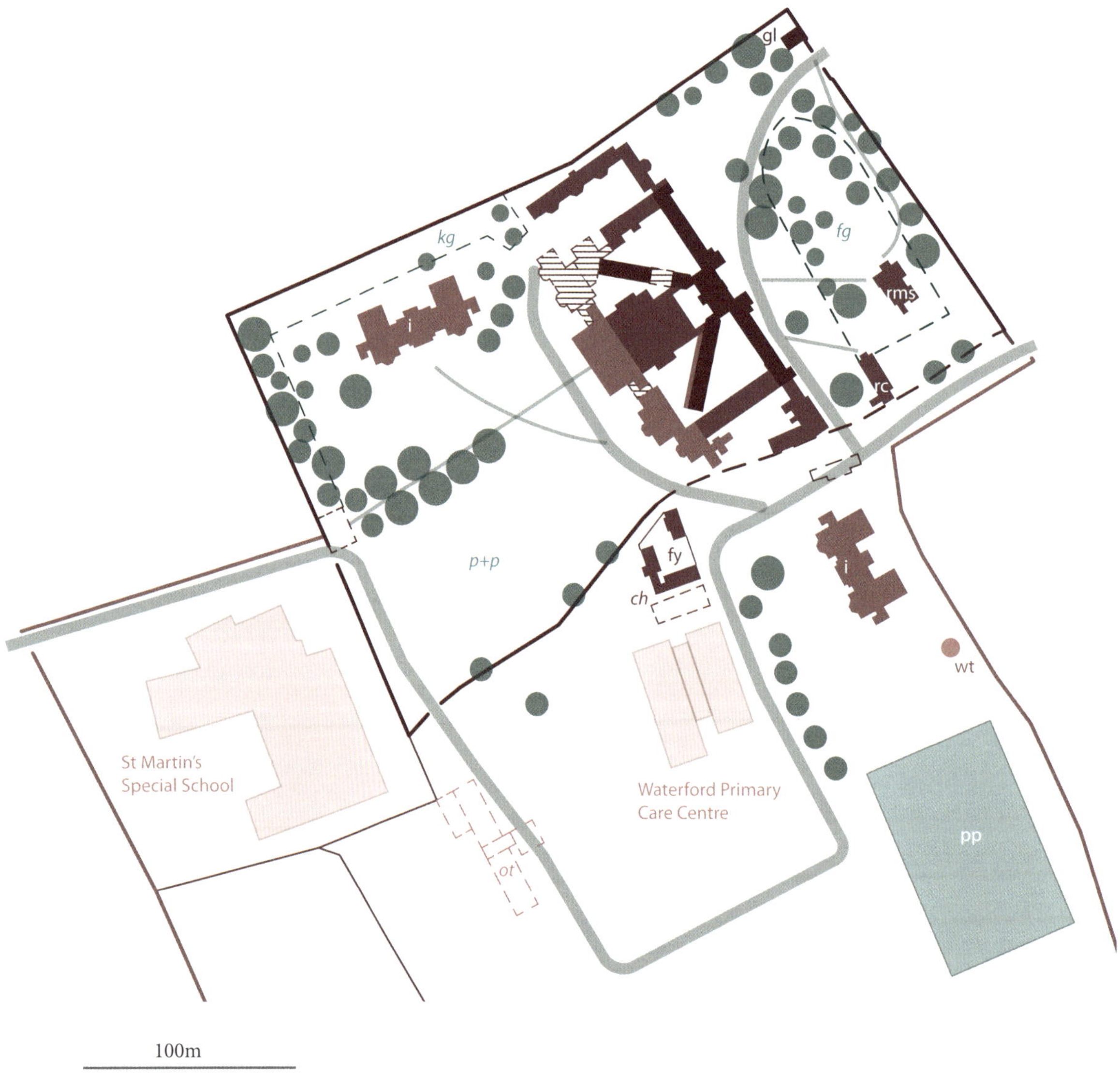

In his evidence to the 1817 Commission on the Lunatic Poor in Ireland, Thomas Spring Rice described the lunatic provision in Waterford as 'a few miserable cells attached to the House of Industry, resembling an ill-constructed gaol rather than a retreat for Lunatics'. He was, however, more impressed with the rigorous system of daily and weekly inspection that served to prevent abuses, supported by a tradition of local Quaker philanthropy that afforded the governors more financial latitude than most.[1] Waterford would be one of only two counties in the first phase of asylum construction where a new institution was sanctioned to serve a single county – by contrast most asylum districts comprised three, four or even five counties. Being justified neither by weight of population nor by any greater predisposition to madness on behalf of the Waterford citizenry, it seems reasonable to speculate that the Lord Lieutenant capitulated to representations by the grand juries of Waterford City and County, who regarded their existing provision as a proud expression of their civic credentials, the loss of which to another county would have been anathema.

Completed in 1835 at a cost of £16,887, the original building at Waterford generally followed Johnston and Murray's standard plan, albeit with the rear wings reduced to a single storey in height.[2] The growth in patient numbers over the first two decades was very modest when compared to many other institutions, easily accommodated by remodelling and reconfiguring existing spaces. As late as 1861, the Inspectors were able to describe Waterford as 'the only institution of the kind… adequate to meet the demands on it,' in no small part thanks to a local policy of 'drafting off' chronic cases to the nearby poor-house to make space for acute cases.[3] Yet by 1868 modest extensions were being erected to either end of the main building – finished in high-quality limestone ashlar to match the original – but their careless asymmetry unbalanced the formal architectural composition. Perpendicular wings of even less architectural distinction to the rear would follow in the subsequent decades.

A new Catholic chapel was added to the front of the asylum in 1878, but the biggest single phase of development would follow in 1895, comprising new two-storey-over-basement wings flanking a large dining hall, collectively creating a coherent new 'garden front' enjoying elevated views over the asylum landscape to the west. The red-brick construction, distinctive bay windows and decorative faience detailing were very much in keeping with institutional architecture of the period, albeit in stark contrast with the austere classicism and limestone detailing of the original. A side effect of this development was that access to the kitchen and service buildings was curtailed; the pragmatic solution was to further compromise the original façade by breaking an archway through the female wing to provide access for deliveries.

The first edition Ordnance Survey map depicts elaborate pleasure gardens in the grounds to the front of the asylum, and while these appear to have been simplified in favour of open parkland in the more detailed map of 1871, the landscape continued to provide the formal setting for the asylum, as conveyed most clearly in an iconic image captured by local photographer A. H. Poole, the sweeping avenue of neatly raked gravel evoking the sense of approaching a gentleman's seat (see Chapter Two). A male inmate – presumably not permitted to join his peers in the grounds for the photoshoot – nevertheless managed to sneak into frame and is evocatively captured peering from behind a barred window. Too busy composing the scene to have to have noticed the intrusion at the time, we can imagine the photographer's reaction when the image emerged from the glass plate negative in his darkroom. Poole also recorded a rare interior image of the asylum dining hall, featuring robust furniture, gasolier lighting, decorative stencilling, wall paintings, and even a token patient, all under the stern eye of the incumbent RMS, Dr Atkins.[4] (See Chapter Four)

Two freestanding single-storey villa infirmaries for 60 patients apiece were added in 1903, which, along with a new house for the RMS, cost in the region of £20,000.[5] This allowed the RMS's former lodgings within the central block of the original building to be repurposed as additional patient accommodation.

These would be the last significant building works at Waterford. Even when Irish Hospitals Sweepstakes capital funding became available from the 1930s, Waterford would draw down one of the smallest grant allocations of any mental hospital, sufficient only to renew the central kitchen and laundry. Instead, funds

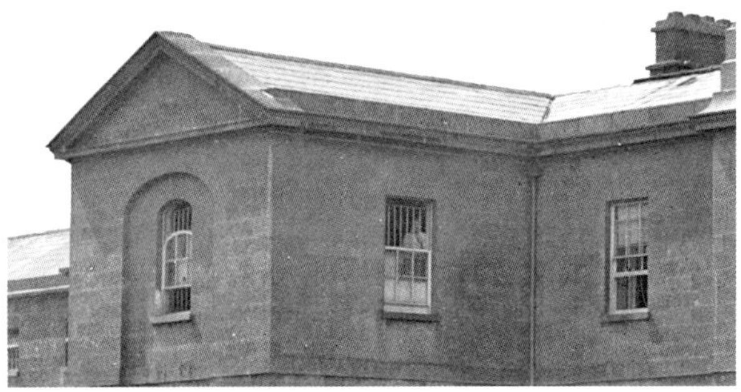

Image courtesy of the National Library of Ireland (POOLEWP 0131)

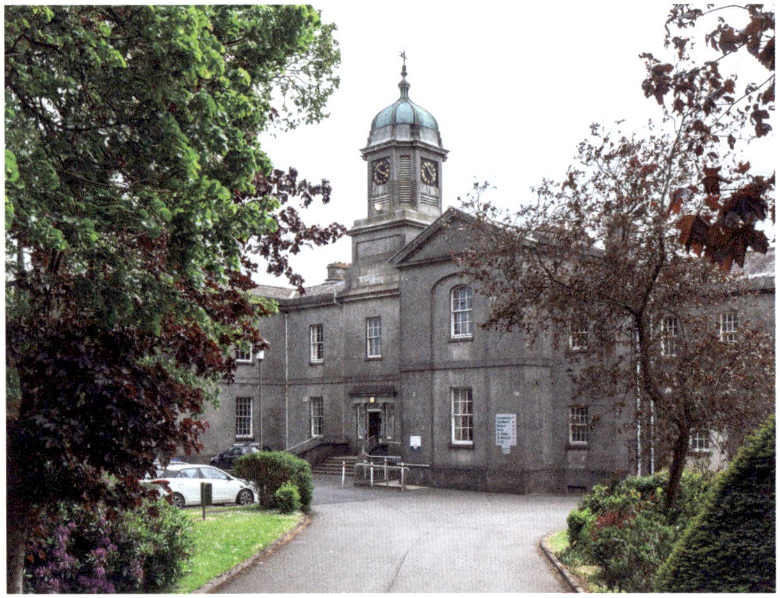

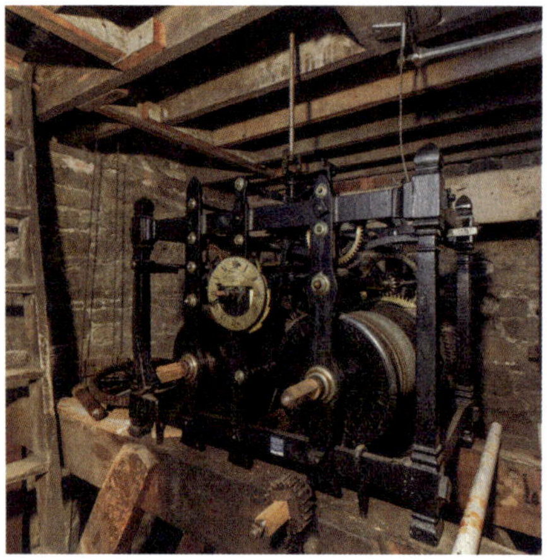

The cupola retains its original clock mechanism, which continues to be wound manually to this day. *Photograph by David Killeen, 2019.*

The classic set-piece (above) is little changed from when photographed by Poole, c. 1900. *Photograph by David Killeen, 2019.*

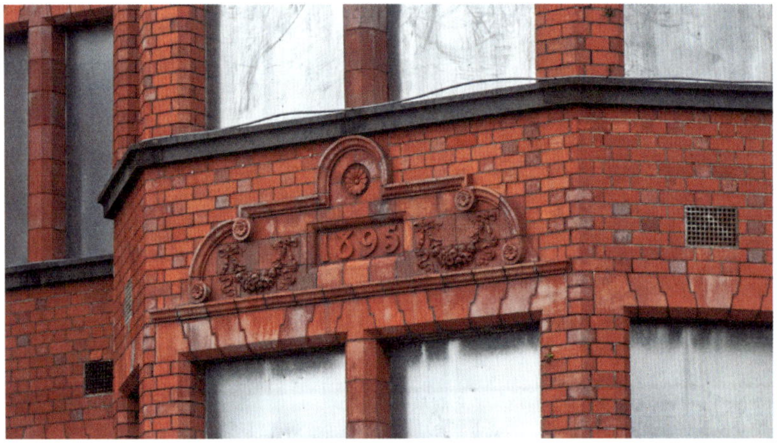

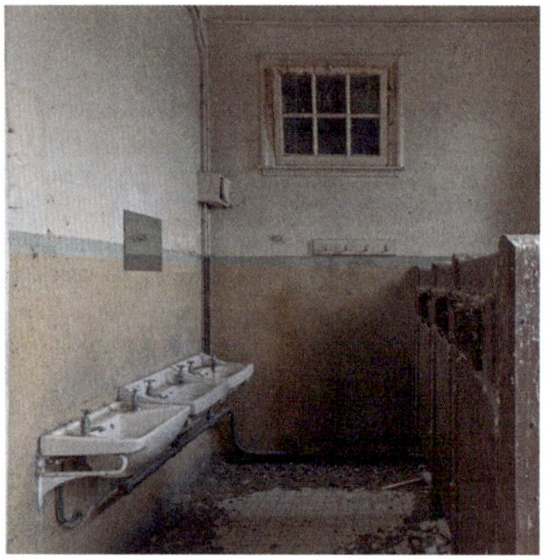

The expansion of 1895 (above and below) created a whole new 'garden front' overlooking the parkland to the rear. The modern conveniences of the day (right) have changed little in the intervening period. *Photographs by David Killeen, 2019.*

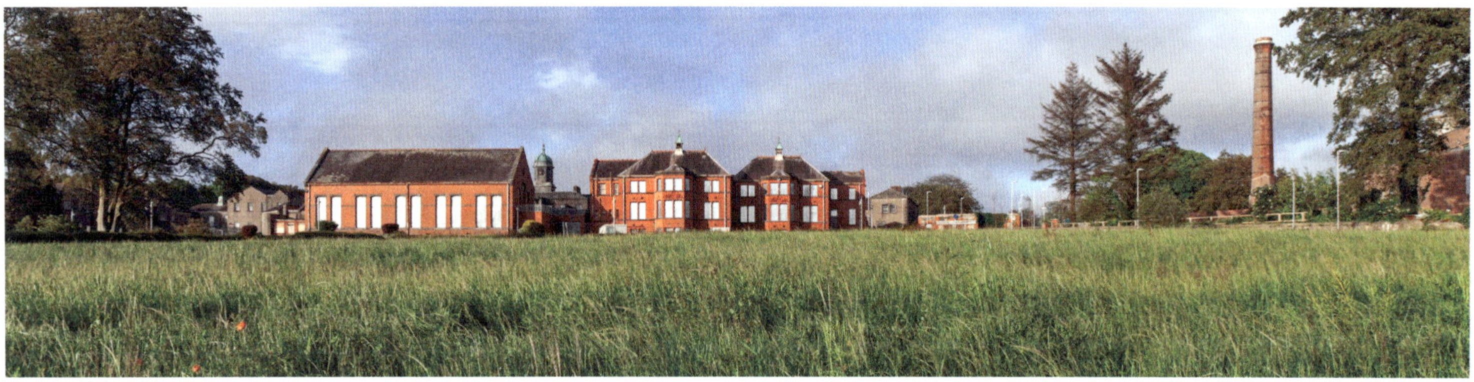

would be invested in expanding the hospital farm, which by the 1950s was almost 400 acres in extent. When it was later deemed inappropriate for patient labour to be used on the farm, an European Economic Community-funded industrial therapy unit – since demolished – was erected to provide occupational therapy for patients.

The shift to providing acute psychiatric care in the general hospital setting came early to Waterford with the opening of a new psychiatric unit at the nearby general hospital in 1965,[6] anticipating the recommendations of the 1966 Report of the Commission of Inquiry on Mental Illness. The population in the old hospital buildings declined slowly through the rest of the century, as one ward after another fell out of use. The female half of the 1895 extension was demolished after a fire and by the time the final patients departed the principal building in 2012, most of its remaining wings stood empty and decaying, with patients remaining in only a handful of smaller detached buildings on the grounds, including the RMS's house and one of the 1900s villas.

The hospital grounds – though now reduced and surrounded by suburbia on all sides – remain a very significant public landholding, but that alone is no guarantee of careful stewardship. In 2018 several acres of valuable residentially-zoned land were sterilised by the construction of a new primary care centre, despite numerous examples of such uses being successfully accommodated within redundant asylum buildings elsewhere. This unfortunate decision missed a rare opportunity to adapt the historic buildings to a compatible and sustainable new use, and diminished the financial value of the remainder of the holding. It remains to be seen who, if anybody, will ensure that the venerable asylum clock continues to chime the hours into the future.

Further Reading

Anthony Gyves, 'A History of St Otteran's Hospital' (unpublished MA thesis, University College Cork, 2010).

References

1. *Report from the Select Committee on the Lunatic Poor in Ireland*, HC 1817 [430] viii, , p. 13.
2. Despite references to the asylum being built for 100 patients, examination of the drawings and physical buildings imply that, like Clonmel, its design capacity was 60, before later modification of outbuildings to accommodate more patients. National Archives of Ireland, Office of Public Works Collection, 1836, Waterford District Lunatic Asylum, OPW/5/HC/4/882.
3. *Eleventh Annual Asylum Report 1861*, HC 1862 [2975] xxiii, p. 20.
4. National Library of Ireland, Poole Photographic Collection, c. 1905, Waterford District Lunatic Asylum, POOLEWP 0131, POOLEWP 0131a.
5. *The Irish Builder*, 26 Feb. 1903, p. 1614.
6. Brendan Kelly, *Hearing Voices: The History of Psychiatry in Ireland* (Dublin, 2014), p. 213.

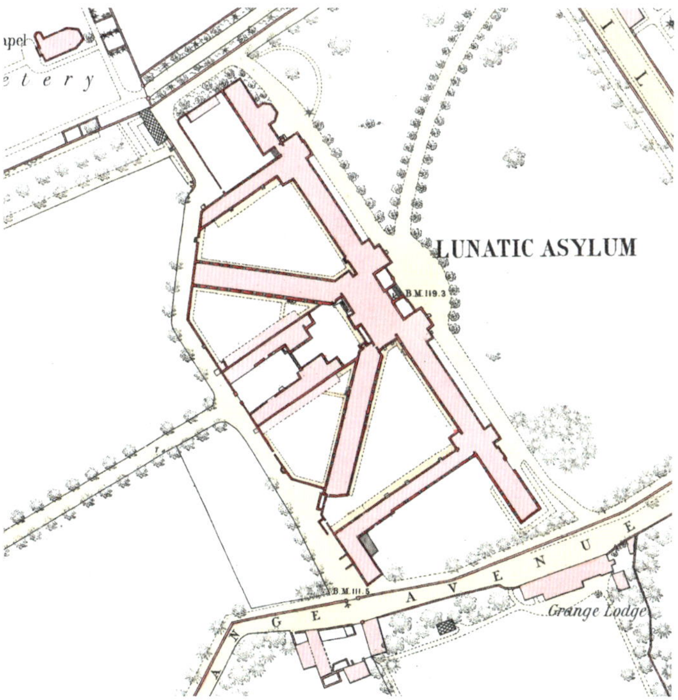

The asylum in its polite parkland landscape sat comfortably within Waterford's suburban-villa belt *Reproduced courtesy of Trinity College Dublin (OS-Waterford City-1056-Sheet 09:99-1872)*

CASE STUDY 10

St Luke's Hospital

(previously Clonmel District Lunatic Asylum)

Years in operation
1835–2012

Original cost
£16,586

Capacity (min /max)
60 / 863

Architect(s)
Johnston & Murray,
James F. Fuller,
McDonnell & Dixon

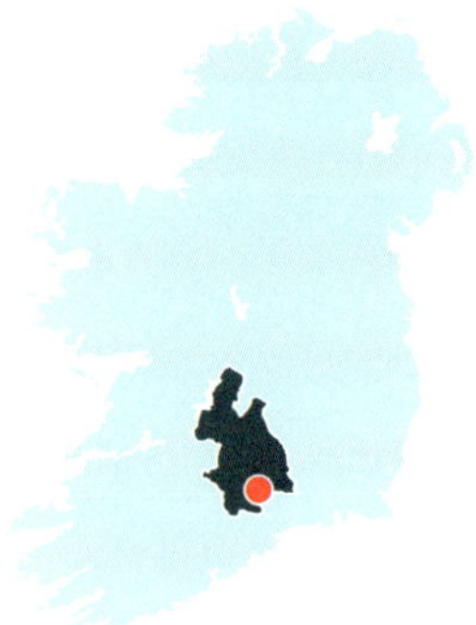

By repurposing not one, but two former workhouses during its existence, the leadership of the Clonmel asylum could rank amongst the least architecturally enlightened in the country. Yet at least one aspect of Clonmel's early twentieth-century evolution would anticipate more progressive trends: the informal dispersal of numerous 'villa style' ward buildings across the landscape. This ad-hoc accommodation policy preserved the principal building in something approaching its original form, but would also necessitate the construction of one bridge and two tunnels, and force the Resident Medical Superintendent to walk over a mile and a half daily just to complete his rounds.

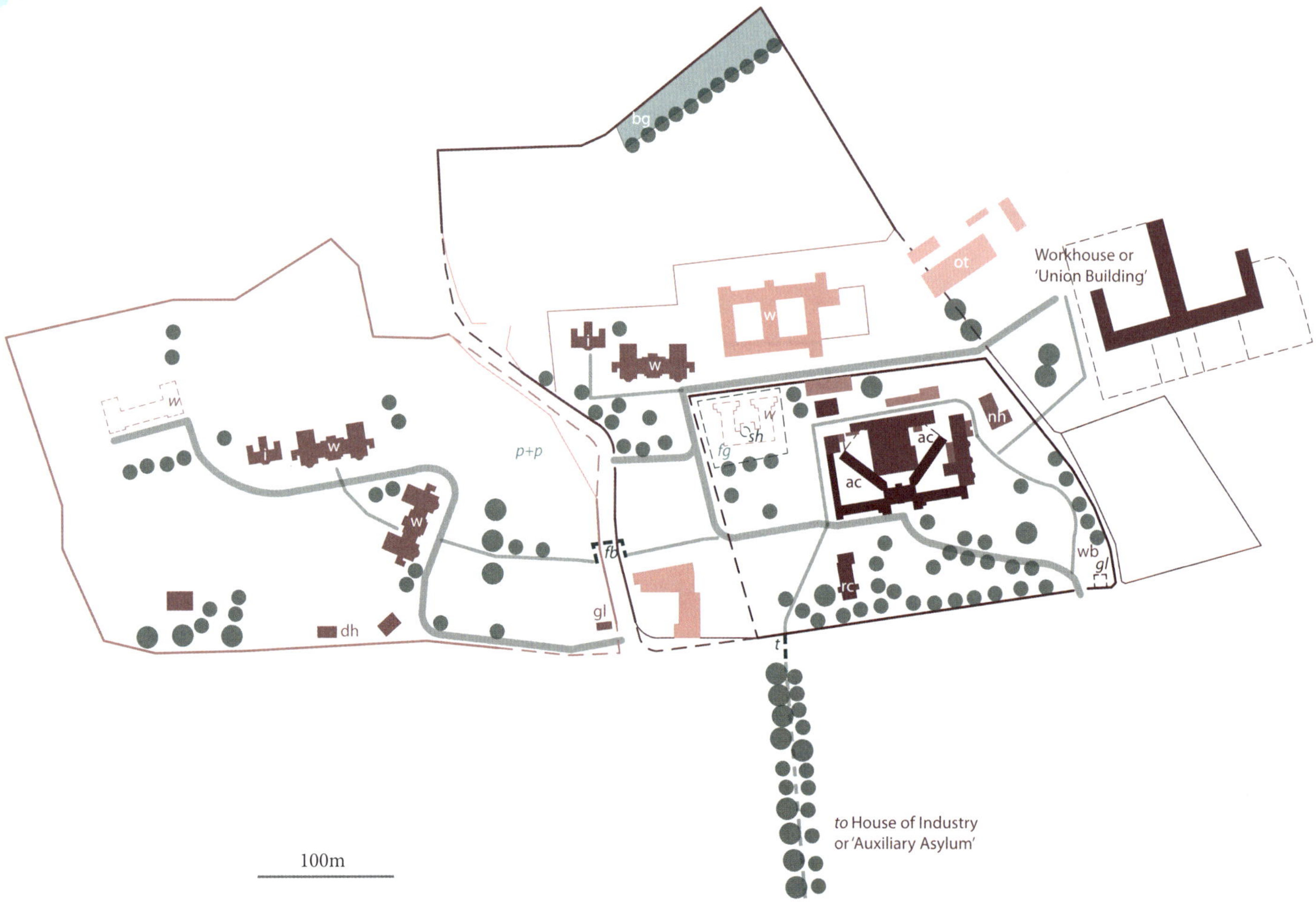

Outside of the major cities, Clonmel was one of a handful of urban centres to have made specific provision for the lunatic poor in the early nineteenth century. Founded in 1811, Clonmel's House of Industry featured a dedicated lunatic department, which in 1820 accommodated 39 patients. It may have been the prior existence of this facility that gave rise to such resentment when it was proposed that the future needs of Tipperary would be served by the new asylum in Maryborough. The governors of the Clonmel House of Industry wrote to the Lord Lieutenant to suggest the construction of an asylum in Clonmel to serve Tipperary and Waterford, an idea which presumably met with similar hostility in Waterford. Furious lobbying ensued, which abated only when the Lord Lieutenant sanctioned separate asylums for Clonmel and Waterford, as well as Maryborough.[1]

Completed in 1835 at a cost of £16,587, the original building at Clonmel was the smallest and cheapest of the first phase of asylums. Serving only a single county, Johnston and Murray's standard 100 bed plan was reduced to 60 beds by omitting the upper floor of the rear wings. And whereas most asylum buildings would be extended to labyrinthine complexity, the principal building at Clonmel remained relatively compact as most of the additional space required to accommodate a peak population in excess of 800 would be provided in separate buildings. Indeed, it is the only one of the early asylums whose original appearance has not been radically altered by later extensions, and which has also retained features such as airing yards and airing sheds which on most other sites have been lost .

The construction in 1853 of the new Union Workhouse – today's South Tipperary General Hospital - rendered the original House of Industry redundant. Already desperate for more space, the old building by the River Suir was purchased by the asylum governors and opened in 1862 as an auxiliary asylum to accommodate male patients, with the main asylum building reserved for females.[2] The building may have been bought cheaply, but expensive civil engineering was required to create a secure link to the main institution. In 1877, a connecting path was sunk into a deep cutting which passed beneath two public roads in tunnels, the route of which is still marked today by a parallel row of trees.[3] This security imperative would later lead to the construction of a fully enclosed footbridge to connect new lands acquired to the west of the Glenconnor Road, offering the populations within and without the walls rare glimpses of one another through the iron lattice.

The 1890s saw a burst of construction work at Clonmel, with the erection of a new east wing, a central dining hall which would later host the famous Mental Hospital dances of the 1960s, and a fine chapel in the parkland to the south of the main building. An architectural competition saw the latter commission awarded to Walter G. Doolin, an architect better known in Clonmel for his work at the Franciscan Friary with which it shares several architectural details. The last new building of the nineteenth century was less worthy – a timber and corrugated iron ward on the site of the former pleasure gardens, rather optimistically described at the time as 'enjoying sufficient sun and air to make it a perfect health resort.' In the time-honoured tradition of 'temporary' structures everywhere, it remained in use for most of the subsequent century.[4]

If a repurposed workhouse and a tin-roofed shed represented victories of economy over quality, things improved briefly in the first decade of the twentieth century. Five detached, single storey 'villas' of attractive and domestic scale and character were built across the grounds, anticipating a trend towards a less centralised, more informal model of asylum which would become popular across Europe in the following decades. Such dispersal presented significant administrative challenges, necessitating the purchase in 1932 of a motor-van to deliver meals to 14 far-flung wards while the Resident Medical Superintendent undertook his daily 1 ½ mile round by foot.[5]

The House of Industry auxiliary asylum was finally abandoned as unfit for human habitation in 1933, and only escaped demolition by being repurposed as an abattoir.[6] McDonnell and Dixon were commissioned to design its replacement, yet, unable to stomach the full cost of proper buildings, the hospital committee again resorted to type. One additional detached block was erected in the westernmost corner of the site, while to the east, the redundant infirmary of the former Union Workhouse was repurposed to create additional wards for mentally handicapped patients.[7] Substandard from the outset, the former deteriorated rapidly and was demolished in the 1990s, the latter would continue in service until eventually replaced by a new, if grimly utilitarian, 100 bed unit in 1985.[8]

The construction of a detached nurses home in 1913 – relatively early by Irish standards - was not sufficient to prevent a prolonged staff strike in 1919.[9] But while staff saw a gradual improvement in their pay and conditions through the twentieth century, patients were not equally empowered to improve their own lot.

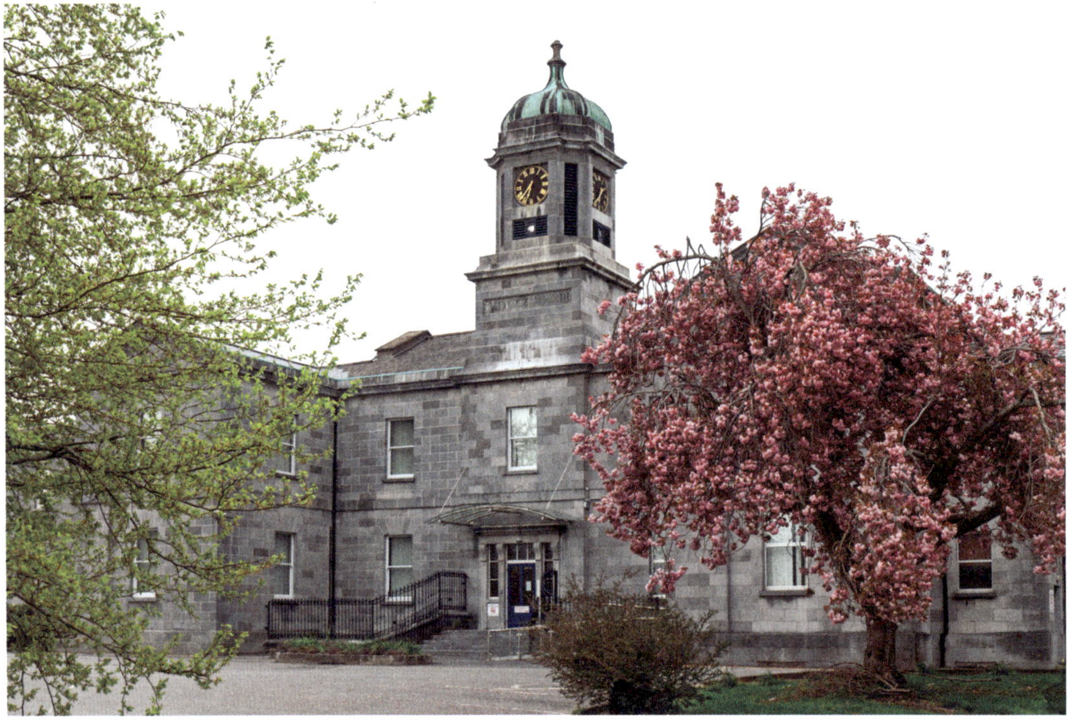

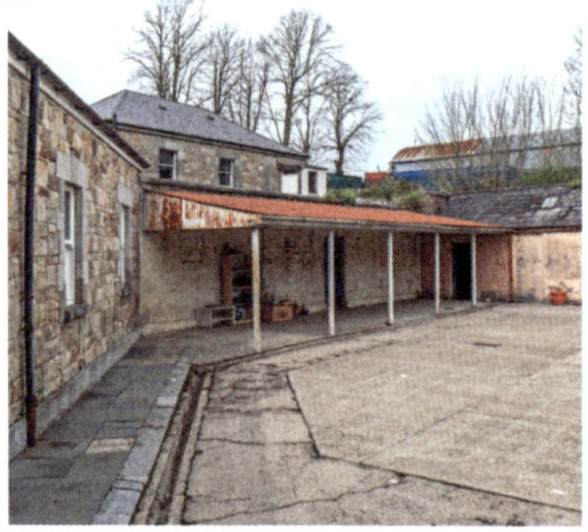

Spared the later accretions which disfigured most of its contemporaries, the asylum at Clonmel retains much of its original scale and character (above and below). *Photographs by David Killeen, 2019.*

Airing sheds (above) are a rare survival. *Photograph by David Killeen, 2019.*

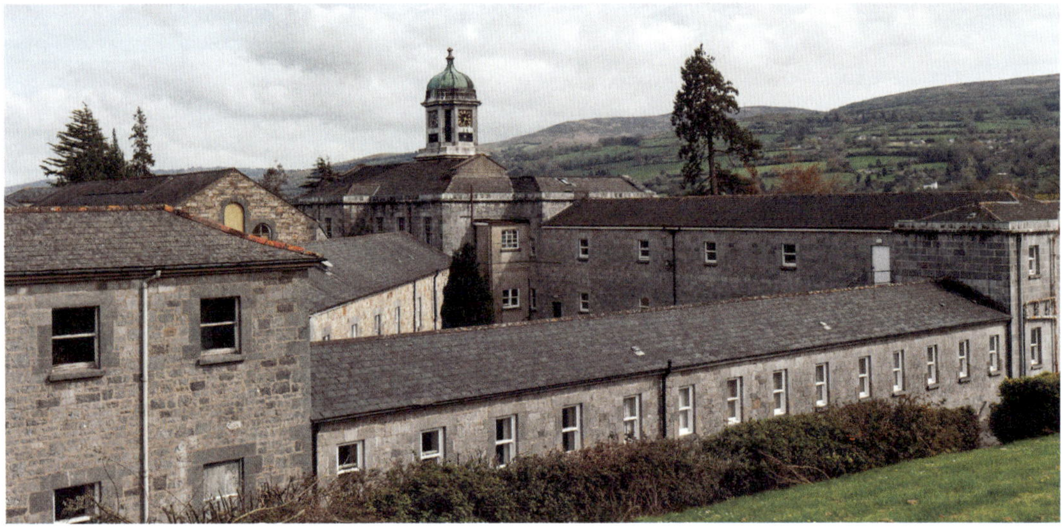

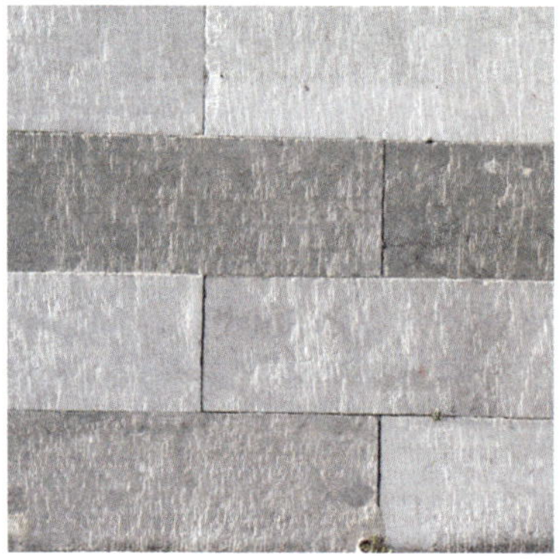

The fine limestone ashlar (above) looks as crisp as the day it was chiselled. *Photograph by the author, 2013.*

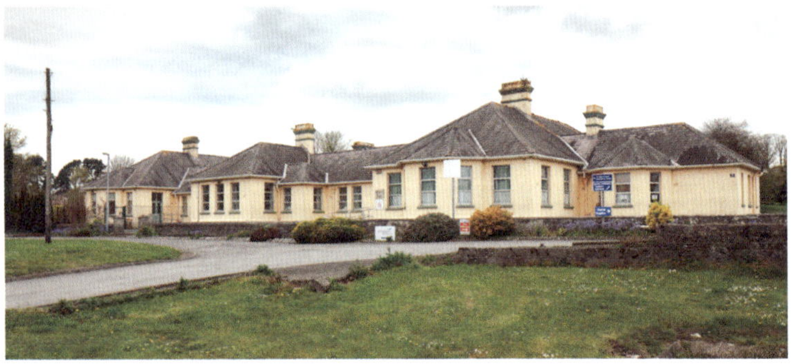

The domestic scale and character of the early twentieth-century villas (left) has allowed them to remain in use to this day. *Photograph by David Killeen, 2019*

A special report by the Inspector of Mental Hospitals in 1958 revealed conditions in Clonmel which were shocking even by the low standards of the era. Its findings remained secret to prevent 'great distress' to patients' relatives - the distress daily experienced by the patients themselves was seemingly of secondary importance (see Chapter Seven). Nevertheless, continuous investment in farmland saw the hospital estate expand from its original 11 acres to almost 350 acres by the 1950s. While much remains, several parcels have since been sold for local authority housing, leaving the original burial ground stranded incongruously in the middle of a housing estate. Happily, the parkland setting around the main building remains intact and boasts several fine specimen trees, which would have been more numerous still were it not for the ravages of Dutch Elm Disease.

The last residential patients departed the main building in 2012, parts of which have since been commendably refurbished to accommodate administration and other support services for the adjacent acute hospital. The dispersed 1900s villas continue to accommodate inpatient beds – their domestic scale and non-institutional setting allowing them to remain below the radar of contemporary closure campaigns. The solid boundary wall which for over a century separated the hospital from the community it served has been both celebrated and consciously punctured by the architects of a new day centre sited conspicuously at the most prominent corner of the site, as if to state that mental health services in the twenty-first century need neither to hide behind a wall, nor to prove a point by erasing all memory of its existence.

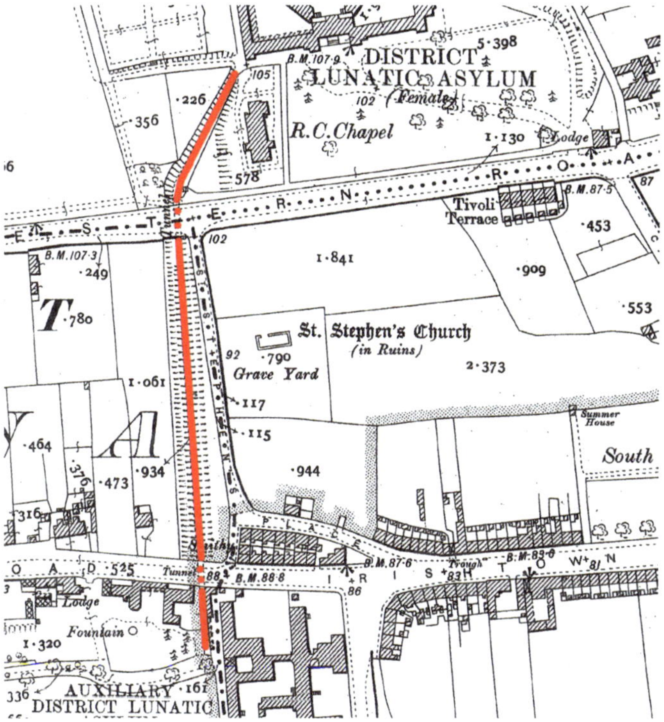

The old House of Industry was bought cheaply, but necessitated two tunnels to connect it to the main asylum. *Reproduced courtesy of Trinity College Dublin (OS-Tipperary-2500-Sheet 83:06-1906)*

Further Reading

Eamon Lonergan, *St Luke's Hospital Clonmel 1834–1984* (Thurles: Tipperary Star, 1984)

Eamon Lonergan, *The History of the South-Eastern Health Board, 1971–2004* (Kilkenny, South Eastern Health Board; 2004)

References

1. National Archives of Ireland, Chief Secretary's Office, 1831, *Various correspondence between the governors of the Clonmel House of Industry, the Lord Lieutenant, the Board of Control, and the Under Secretary for Ireland*, CSO/RP/1831/374, CSO/RP/1831/2684.
2. This is an interesting inversion of the trend witnessed in several county gaols, where the new 'reformed' buildings were allocated to male prisoners and the outdated old buildings were given over to females. See Richard J. Butler, *Building the Irish Courthouse and Prison: A Political History, 1750–1850* (Cork, 2019).
3. The building was bought for only £2,500, but the engineering works and land purchase cost £3,092. Eamon Lonergan, *St Luke's Hospital Clonmel 1834–1984* (Thurles, 1984), pp 30–03.
4. *Forty-Eighth Annual Asylum Report 1899*, HC 1899 [9479] xl, p. 28, and Lonergan, *St Luke's Hospital*, pp 37–8.
5. *Report of the Inspector of Mental Hospitals 1932*, p. 16.
6. And having survived unnoticed into its third century under a wrapping of later industrial cladding, it was finally demolished, unremarked, in 2019.
7. It came as some surprise to the author to discover that his great-grandfather chaired the meeting of the management committee at which this retrograde decision was taken. Lonergan, *St Luke's Hospital*, p. 60.
8. *Report of the Inspector of Mental Hospitals, 1988–89*, p. 122.
9. Lonergan, *St Luke's Hospital*, p. 45.

Years in operation
1850–2021

Original cost
£20,296

Capacity (min /max)
120 / 201

Architect(s)
Jacob Owen,
James F. Fuller.

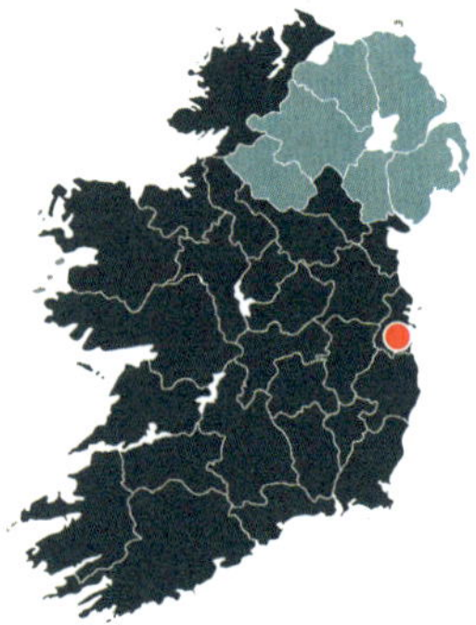

Central Mental Hospital

(previously Central Criminal Lunatic Asylum)

One by one, the high walls which bounded each asylum succumbed to the reforming zeal of mid twentieth-century psychiatry. But the most iconic asylum wall of all continued to serve its dual purpose – keeping patients within and the wider world out – right into the twenty-first century. Preserved within this hermetic perimeter stands Ireland's last living example of a large, publicly-funded, residential mental institution and a place which dares to suggest that the original conception of the asylum – for all its many irredeemable flaws – embodied therapeutic features which remain of value to this day.

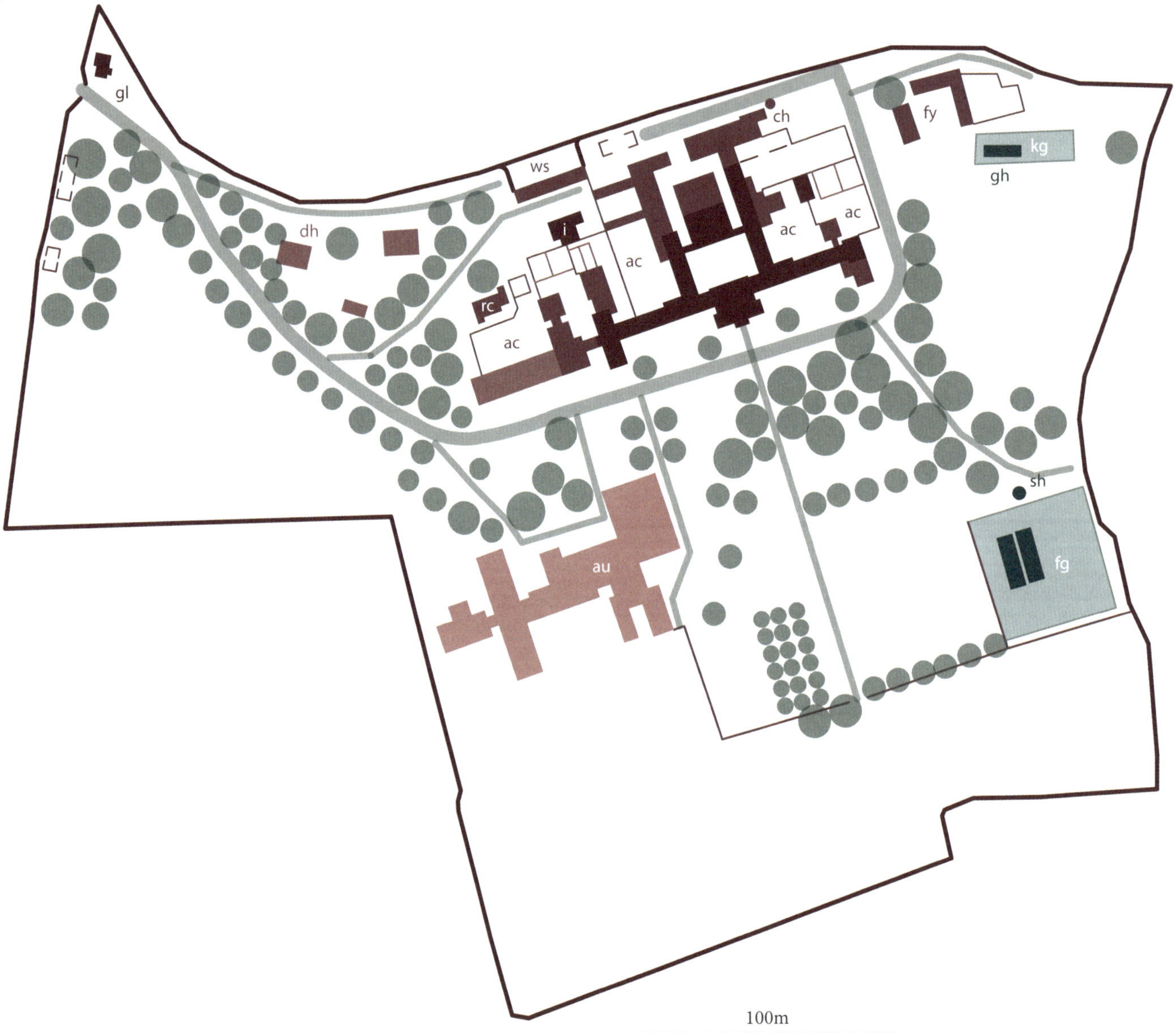

Before the eponymous 'Central Criminal Lunatic Asylum' legislation of 1845 had even passed parliament, the Board of Work's chairman and architect, Jacob Owen, was already at work designing the new asylum at Dundrum.[1] This asylum, latterly known as the Central Mental Hospital, opened in 1850 as perhaps the earliest purpose-built specialist facility of its type in the world,[2] a function it would continue to fulfil for another 170 years.

The selection of a site in a 'populous and highly respectable district' was not without controversy, exciting locally 'the greatest apprehensions… of all that fancy could combine in maniacs and murderers'. The Inspectors were eager to report that such unfounded fears were rapidly ameliorated by the reality of criminal lunatics who were 'as well conducted and tranquil' as any other – or perhaps more realistically, by the reassuring impregnability of the enclosing wall.[3]

The Inspectors' expressed the hope that the new criminal asylum, notwithstanding its unique status, would be organised 'on the same basis as a district asylum' and that those who designed and operated it would 'submerge as far as they could the prison elements of its role'.[4] The civic classicism and radial planning of Johnston's asylums were already tainted by association with prison architecture, so Owen opted instead for a collegiate Tudor Revival style, pointedly ranking the new asylum on a par with the Board's flagship projects – the three Queen's Colleges and the National Seminary at Maynooth. Of more practical consequence, this also heralded a move away from small cells and high windows, an increase in the quality and quantity of communal spaces, and the elimination of radial features in favour of a linear building with a sunny, southerly aspect. Upon completion, the Inspectors were full of praise for a building that they saw as '…characteristic of a private house, even more than of an ordinary asylum; the windows of ample size, and reaching along the corridors, dormitories and day rooms, within a couple of feet of the floor, are totally devoid of bars or grating…'[5]

The anti-carceral agenda was also reflected in the original design of the airing courts, whose enclosing walls were to be lowered locally and protected with sunken fences (ha-has) to afford patients a view of the wider landscape; their later subdivision into smaller yards of unmistakeably prison-like appearance sadly showed that the twentieth century could be less liberal than the nineteenth. The height of the outer boundary was likewise carefully disguised by another sunken fence, giving the landscape within the 'park-like appearance' of a genteel demesne with views to the Wicklow Mountains beyond.

Owen's approach embodied many principles that would go on to be codified in the Instructions to Architects issued to the private practitioners commissioned for the other new district asylums of the era. Rules governing its daily operation – aside from some financial and inspection requirements specific to the unique circumstances of a government-controlled Central Asylum – would also influence the rules by which all asylums came to be ordered.[6] Indeed the biggest practical difference between this asylum and its more conventional siblings arose not from the demeanour of its patients but from their gender: Owen had to work hard to maintain an impression of symmetry in an institution where - uniquely - the male side of the house was always much larger than the female.

The debacle around cost control during the second phase of asylum expansion saw the Board of Works relieved of most asylum-related duties, but they retained responsibility for the Central Asylum, bequeathing a complete drawing record for every subsequent phase of work at the site. By contrast with ever-increasing numbers crowding the district asylums, the numbers who warranted committal to the Central Criminal Asylum remained relatively low and stable throughout most of the period under question, meaning that the therapeutic potential of 'a more exact and intimate knowledge' of individual patients, already fading from view in the burgeoning district asylums, here remained viable.[7] Later extensions were therefore few in number and small in scale, and the buildings today look little different from Owen's original vision. But this seemingly modest insight reveals the absurd paradox underlying the exponential expansion of the wider asylum project: for almost a century, the majority of patients who swelled the ranks of the district asylums were legally branded as 'dangerous lunatics', yet the number of patients whose actions or behaviour actually warranted such a description has changed little from Owen's day to our own.

Generations of Dubliners have passed the great wall of Dundrum wise to its function, but blind to the appearance of what lay behind it. Gothic visions of a South Dublin outpost of Shutter Island are shattered upon entering what instead resembles a most improbable latter-day fragment of Eden. Permanent partition from the outside world has preserved, amidst the roads and terraces of twentieth-century suburbia, a 28-acre parkland landscape of tree-lined avenues, traditional hay meadows, formal parterres, kitchen gardens, an extant farmyard, a summer house and

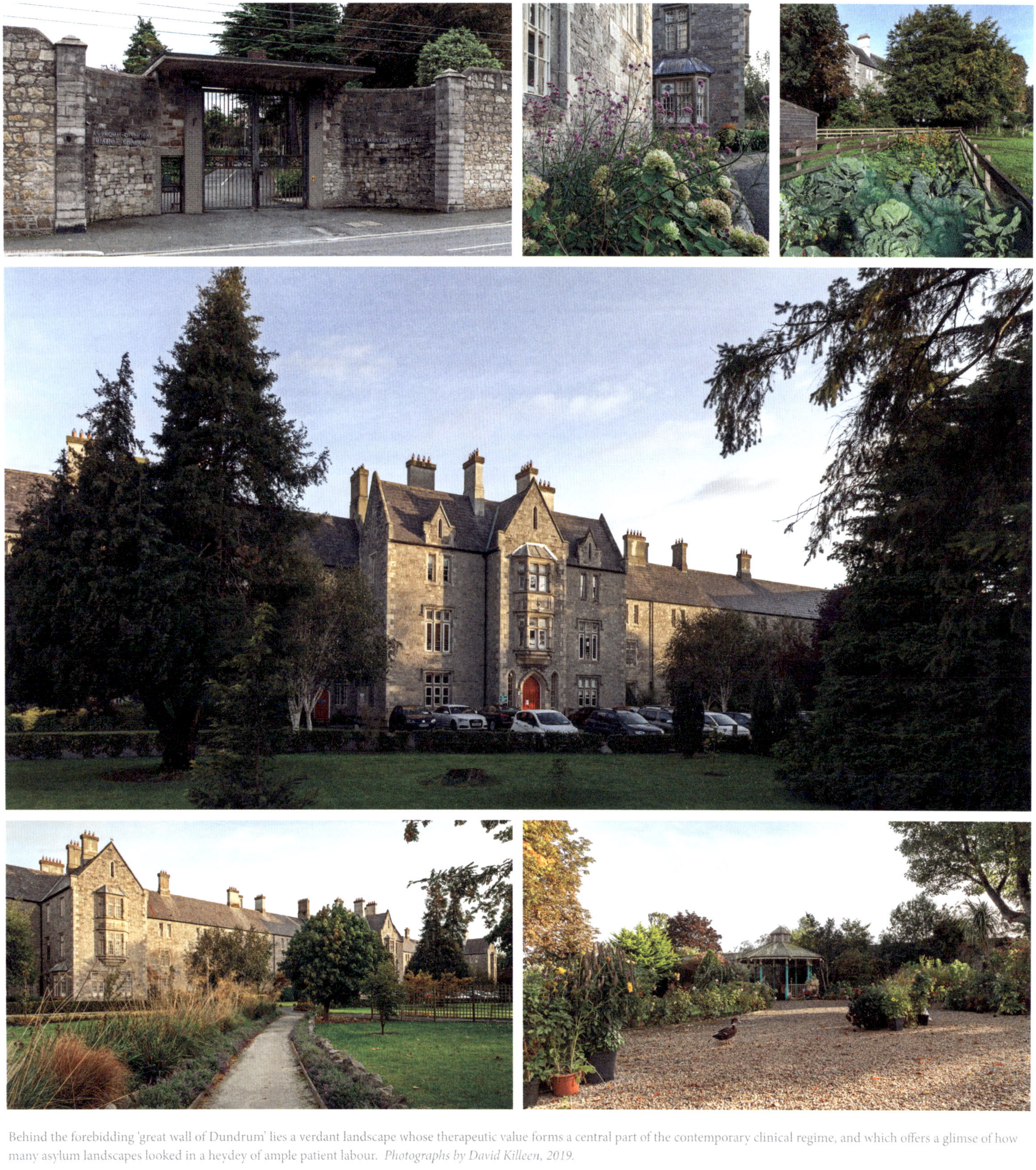

Behind the forebidding 'great wall of Dundrum' lies a verdant landscape whose therapeutic value forms a central part of the contemporary clinical regime, and which offers a glimse of how many asylum landscapes looked in a heydey of ample patient labour. *Photographs by David Killeen, 2019.*

beehives. Maintained entirely by the patients with the assistance of two professional gardeners, the grounds at Dundrum are living proof that historic approaches to landscape management can still play an important role in the modern therapeutic milieu, creating a virtuous circle that enhances both quality of life and quality of place. Dundrum's resident cohort is unique in the modern health service by virtue of their length of stay, but service-users elsewhere whose admission is measured in weeks rather than years could still benefit from muddying their fingers in the inherently optimistic activity that is gardening.

It is only a modest exaggeration to observe that the complex at Dundrum that greeted the twenty-first century hardly differed from that which bid farewell to the nineteenth. The main buildings saw little alteration beyond the usual sanitary annexes and the addition of a single-storey wing with a pleasant south-facing veranda, mildly evocative of an Edwardian billiards room or ballroom appended to an earlier country house. In the 1980s the bizarre decision was taken to erect a facility for disturbed children in the grounds – the building was complete before wiser heads comprehended the potential incompatibility of such a mix of cohorts on the site. The building – a joyless product of the straitened decade in which it was built – was later adapted as a unit to receive and stabilise acutely disturbed admissions, and its ultimate demolition will not be regretted.

At the time of writing, Dundrum is the last of Ireland's nineteenth-century asylums still occupied and used in a manner that would be familiar to those who conceived it. However, with the move to the replacement Forensic Mental Hospital at Portrane, this exceptional continuity of use will finally be broken. Dundrum's well-maintained buildings and valuable land bank will not remain empty for long – plans for sympathetic redevelopment are already in hand at the state's Land Development Agency. But having stood aloof for 170 years from the ever-changing world outside its walls, the day is coming when this most extraordinary place-out-of-time must re-join the daily fray of Irish society.

Further Reading

Pauline M. Prior, *Madness and Murder: Gender, Crime and Mental Disorder in Nineteenth-Century Ireland* (Dublin: Irish Academic Press, 2008)

References

1. *Annual Asylum Report 1848*, HC 1849 [1054] xxiii, p. 4.
2. Joseph Robins, *Fools and Mad: A History of the Insane in Ireland* (Dublin, 1986) p. 149. The equivalent English facility at Broadmoor was legislated for in 1857 and completed in 1863.
3. *Annual Asylum Report 1851*, HC 1851 [1387] xxiv, p. 13.
4. Robins, *Fools and Mad*, p. 100.
5. *Fifth Asylum Report 1851*, HC 1851 [1387] xxiv, p. 14.
6. Ibid., p. 32
7. *Eighth Asylum Report 1857*, HC 1857 session 2 [2253] xvii, p. 18.

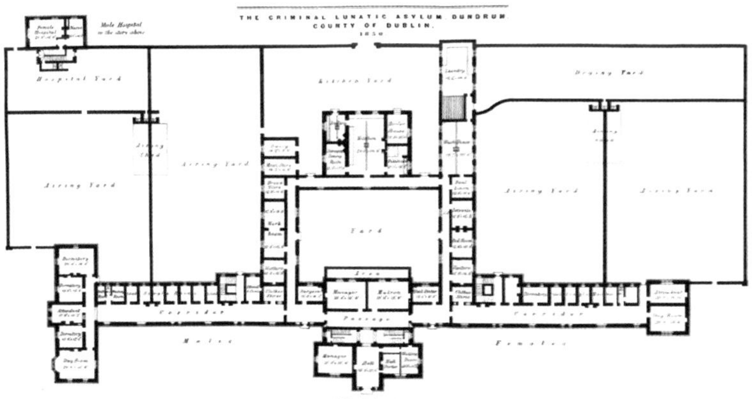

Owen's original design successfully downplayed the imbalance between male and female sides of the asylum. *(Civil Engineer and Architect, 22 Feb. 1851)*

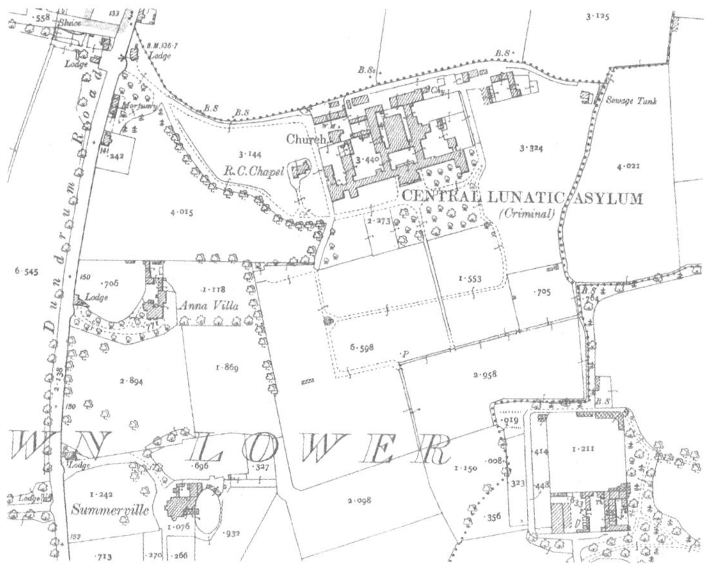

The asylum's position in the south Dublin 'villa belt' gave rise to local objections. *Reproduced courtesy of Trinity College Dublin (OS-Dublin-2500-Sheet 22:08-1910)*

CASE STUDY 12

Years in operation
1852–2006

Original cost
£24,919

Capacity (min /max)
150 / 510

Architect(s)
George Papworth, Richard Langrishe, Downes & Meehan

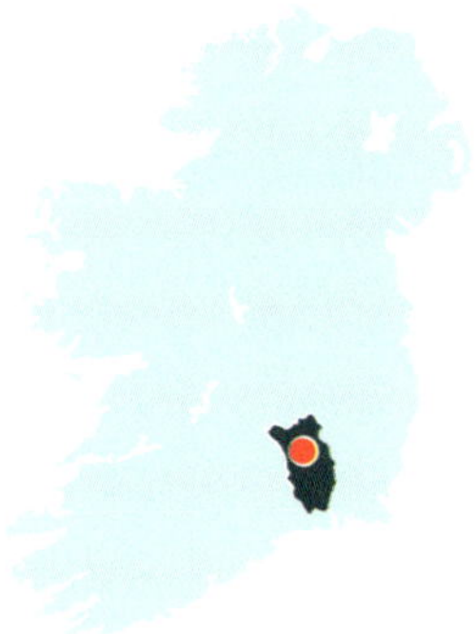

St Canice's Hospital

(previously Kilkenny District Lunatic Asylum)

The asylum at Kilkenny presents a dramatic silhouette, its array of Tudor Revival gables and chimneys bookended by a pair of five-storey towers with steeply pitched roofs. The monumental scale of these towers disguises the fact that Kilkenny, by the standards of Irish asylums, is actually not a very big building, and is the only one of the nineteenth-century district asylums where the patient population rarely exceeded 500.

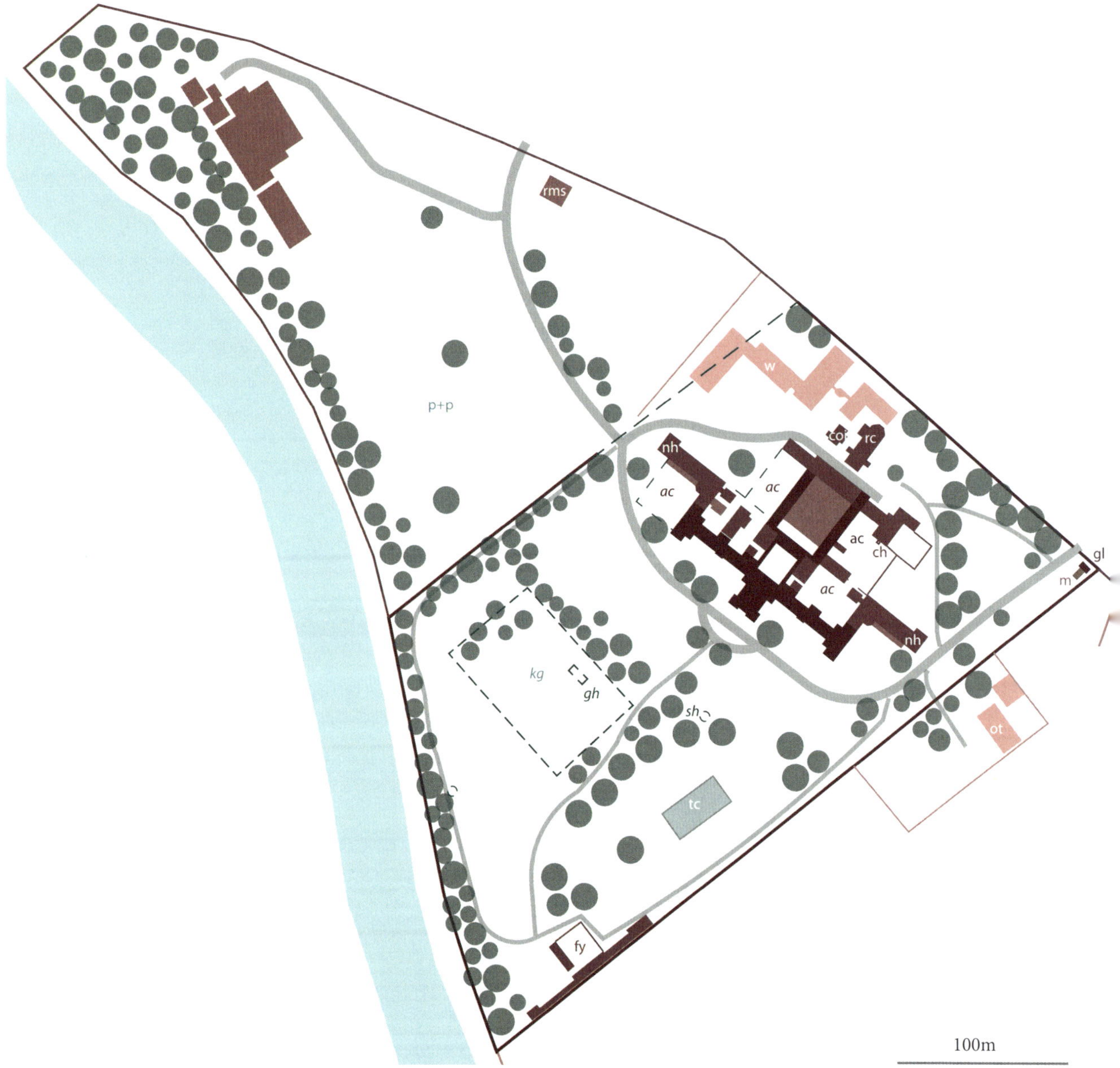

Even before the advent of the district asylum system, Kilkenny had its own 'Local Asylum' to serve the needs of the city and county. Located adjacent to the old Workhouse (latterly the House of Correction) on the Kells Road, the institution was sufficiently large to merit an independent governance and management structure (See Chapter One). A daily average of 50 inmates was recorded in 1844 – notwithstanding that Kilkenny had, since 1832, also been sending lunatics to the new district asylum at Carlow. The 1844 Report of the Inspector of Lunacy deplored the state of 'neglect, mismanagement, and discomfort' evident in the establishment and instructed that 'no new cases of insanity are taken in,'[1] a recommendation that would resonate over 150 years later as the Mental Health Commission in turn struggled to effect the final closure of institutions it deemed unfit for purpose.

As part of its 1845 report on additional asylum provision, the Inspectorate recommended that Kildare patients be transferred from Carlow to the Maryborough district and that the asylum at Carlow be expanded by 100 beds to meet the needs of Carlow, Kilkenny and Wexford.[2] Further correspondence and consultation over the following year, combined with the imperative to close 'this wretched institution' (the local asylum) instead convinced the Inspectors of the merits of establishing a new district asylum for 150 patients at Kilkenny, which opened in 1852.[3]

Designed by architect George Papworth towards the end of a long and prolific career, Kilkenny District Lunatic Asylum was an accomplished essay in the Elizabethan revival style. Its organisational layout adhered rigidly to the Instructions to Architects issued by the Board of Works, with the skill of the architect principally demonstrated in the massing, elevational treatment (including generously sized mullioned windows) and high-quality 'punched and drafted, or tooled and chiselled stone features'.[4] Papworth's task was easier than most, resulting in a building of manageable scale and pleasing proportions which, then as now, could easily be mistaken for an elite educational establishment. Like all asylums of the second phase, Kilkenny enjoys a broadly southerly orientation across a gently sloping site, but, unusually, the building is approached from north rather than from the south. This fact could have allowed Papworth to comply with the one 'Instruction' disregarded by all architects – that of providing south-facing airing courts – by flipping the formal 'entrance front' to the north. Papworth instead adhered to convention, necessitating a circuitous approach with dense planting to screen the rear of the building from the main avenue.

While demand increased at Kilkenny just as elsewhere, the absolute growth amounted to less than 400 additional patients over the course of a century – a quantum of increase that the likes of Cork, Ballinasloe and The Richmond each experienced in a single decade around 1900. As a result, later building works at Kilkenny tended to be modest in scale and arguably of better quality than was the case at the larger institutions.

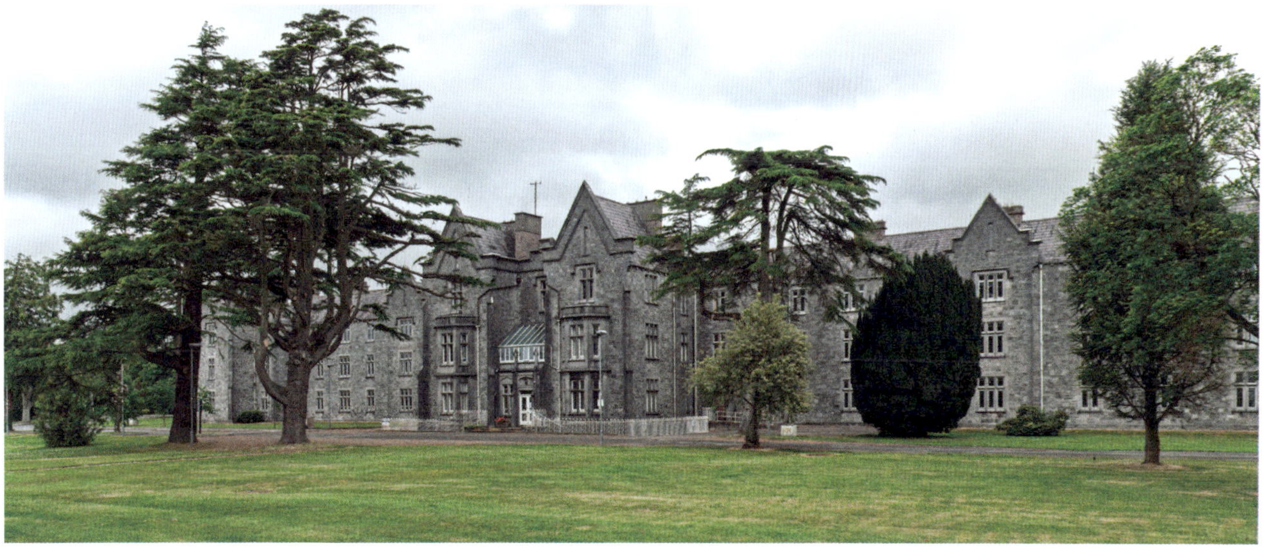

Its relatively modest scale, robust Tudor detailing and parkland setting make Kilkenny a posterchild for mid-nineteenth-century asylum architecture
Photograph by David Killeen, 2019.

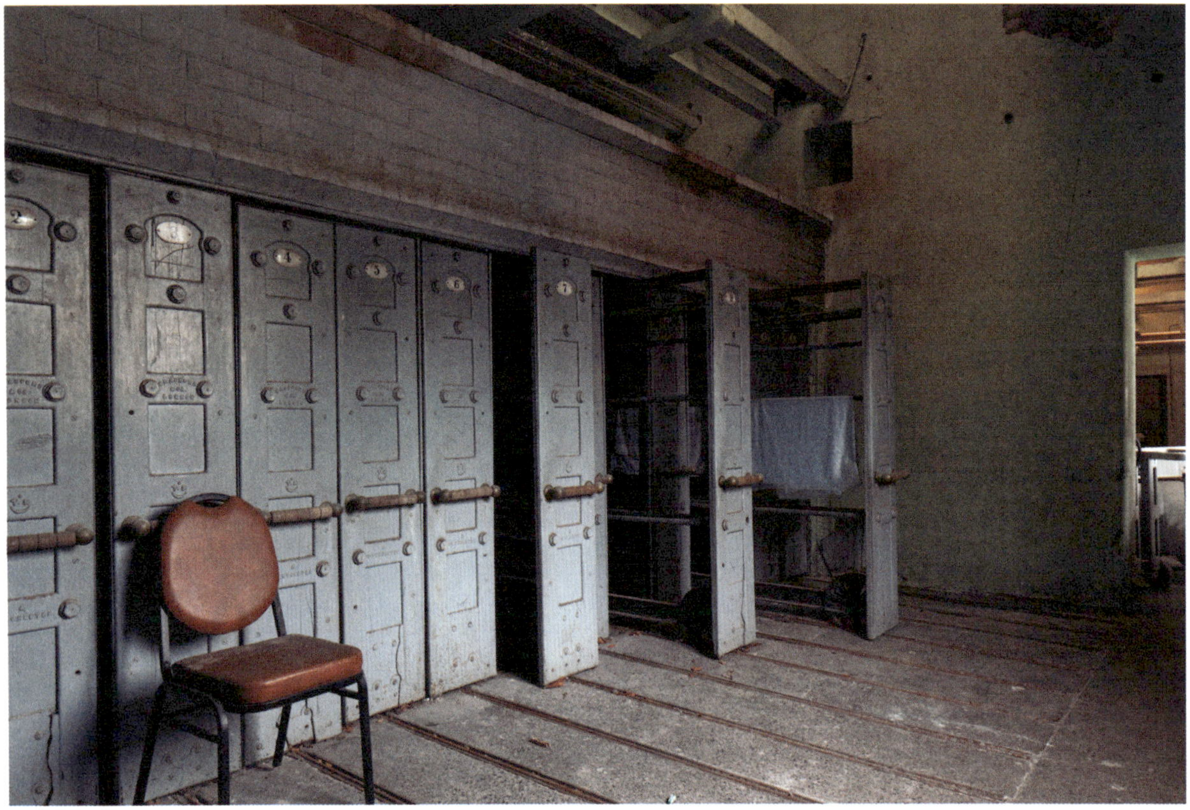

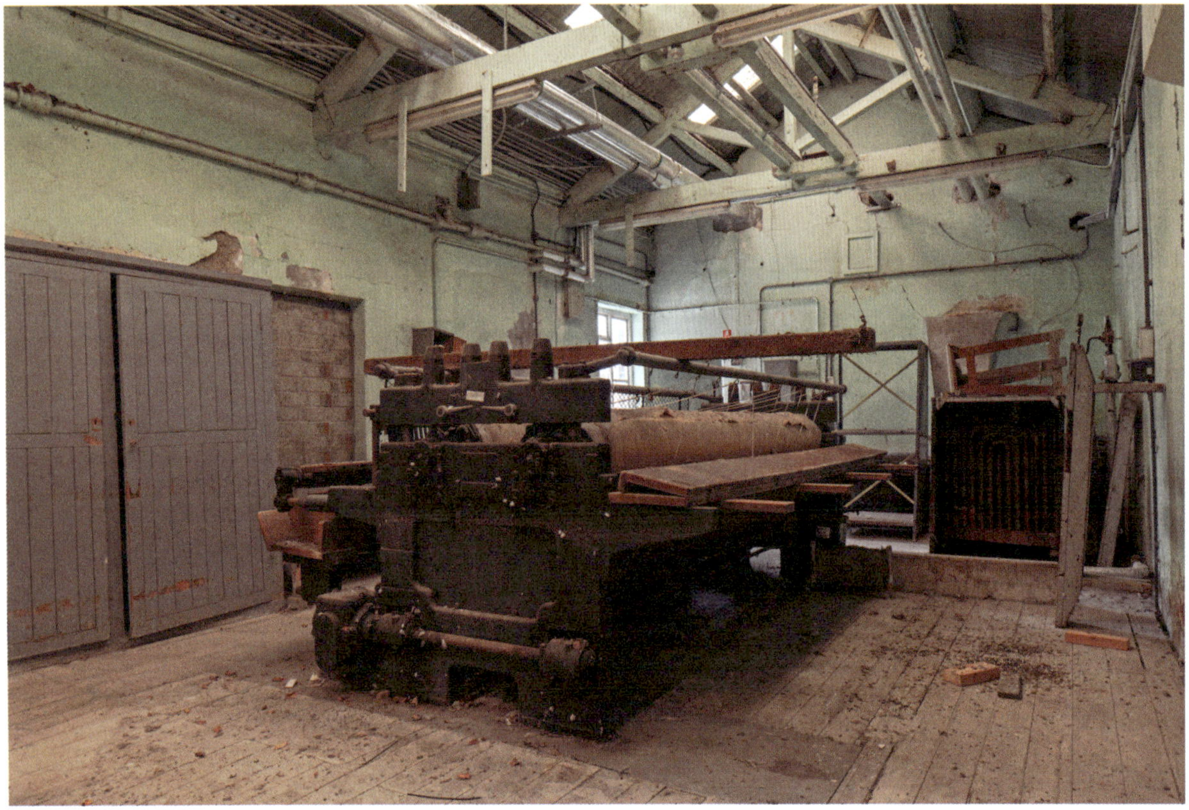

The laundry retains an impressive array of early equipment. *Photographs by David Killeen, 2019.*

Extensions completed in 1872, which increased capacity to 216 patients, were stylistically indistinguishable from the original,[5] while the 1890s would see the addition of the dramatic five-storey water towers at either extremity, which also included accommodation for male and female staff. The same architect, Richard Langrishe, was also responsible for the polychromatic Catholic chapel erected to the rear of the asylum in 1893, beside which stands a Protestant chapel like a younger sibling, similar in style though simpler in form.

The acquisition and conversion of the neighbouring Lacken House in 1906 provided additional patient accommodation and expanded the asylum grounds while avoiding the need for new buildings;[6] as such it was not until the 1930s that the tranquillity of the grounds would be disturbed again by construction of verandahs to the infirmaries at each side of the building. The 1950s saw the replacement of the central dining hall with a vast new barrel-vaulted dining and recreation hall, as well as a long overdue house for the RMS.

The major shift in the delivery of mental health services came in 2003 with the opening of the 45-bed Department of Psychiatry at St Luke's General Hospital, where thenceforth acute cases would be referred for admission and treatment. The last patients departed the principal building in 2006, but the HSE has repurposed many redundant ward spaces for administration uses, meaning that much of the building continues to be well used and maintained. The central hall still provides recreational and therapeutic opportunities for various service-users, while 20 older patients – including at time of writing one centenarian – remain in residence in a single-storey pre-fabricated building dating from 1971.[7]

The distinguished design and modest scale of the original building, the sensitivity of later extensions and an unspoilt parkland setting mean that Kilkenny today survives as an exemplar of the architectural and landscape aesthetic of nineteenth-century asylumdom. It equally serves as an example of a site that has made a graceful transition to new uses within the health service.

Further Reading

Eamon Lonergan, *The History of the South-Eastern Health Board, 1971–2004* (Kilkenny: South Eastern Health Board, 2004)

References

1. *Annual Asylum Report 1844*, HC 1845 [645] xxvi, p. 29.
2. *Annual Asylum Report 1845*, HC 1846 [736] xxii, p. 47.
3. *Annual Asylum Report 1846*, HC 1847 [820] xvii, p. 12, p. 52.
4. *The Dublin Builder*, 22 Jan. 1853, p. 60.
5. *Twenty-First Annual Asylum Report 1872*, HC 1872 [647] xxvii, p. 16.
6. Eamon Lonergan, *The History of the South-Eastern Health Board, 1971–2004* (Kilkenny, 2004), p. 95.
7. *Report of the Inspector of Mental Hospitals, 1977–79*, p. 10.

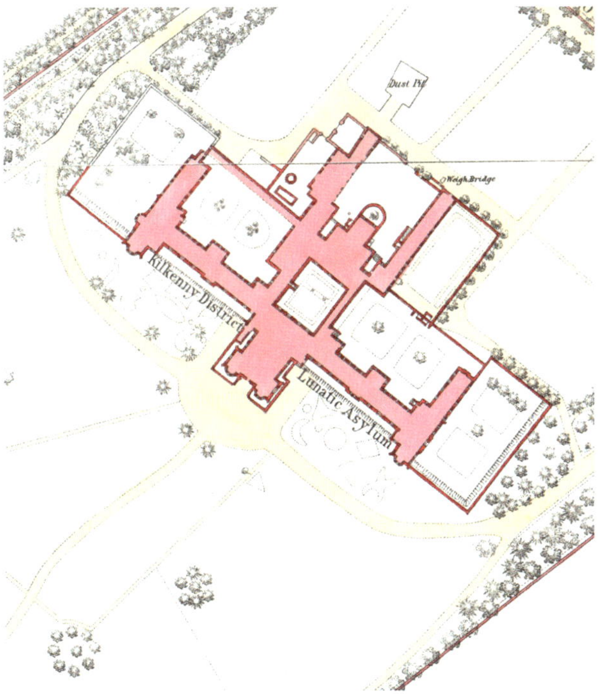

Walks meander through open parkland and belted woodland, puntuated by shady bowers. *Reproduced courtesy of Trinity College Dublin (OS-Kilkenny-1056-Sheet 18:48-1872)*

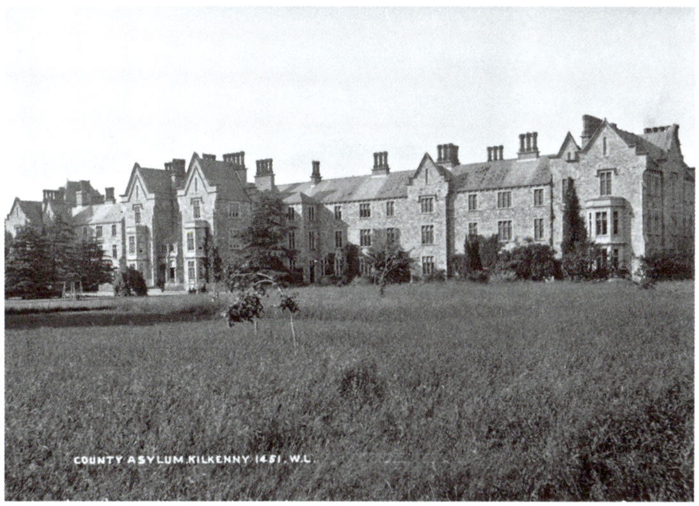

The set-piece has hardly changed in over a century. *Image courtesy of the National Library of Ireland (L_CAB_01451)*

CASE STUDY 13

Our Lady's Hospital

(previously Eglinton Lunatic Asylum, latterly Atkins Hall)

Years in operation
1852-1992 (main building)

Original cost
£86,339

Capacity (min /max)
500 / 2097

Architect(s)
William Atkins,
William Henry Hill
J. R. Boyd Barrett

If most stereotypes embody a kernel of truth, then it is entirely appropriate that for over 40 years, citizens of the southern capital revelled in the boast of having the both the longest and tallest building in Ireland. The latter crown has changed hands on several occasions since, but none have attempted the folly of challenging the building that has held the former title since the 1860s.

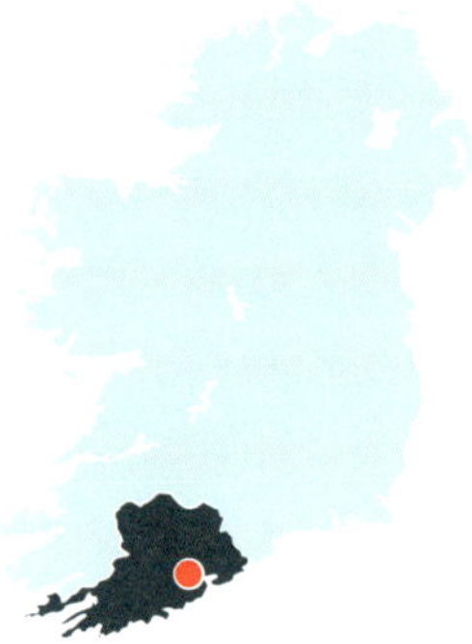

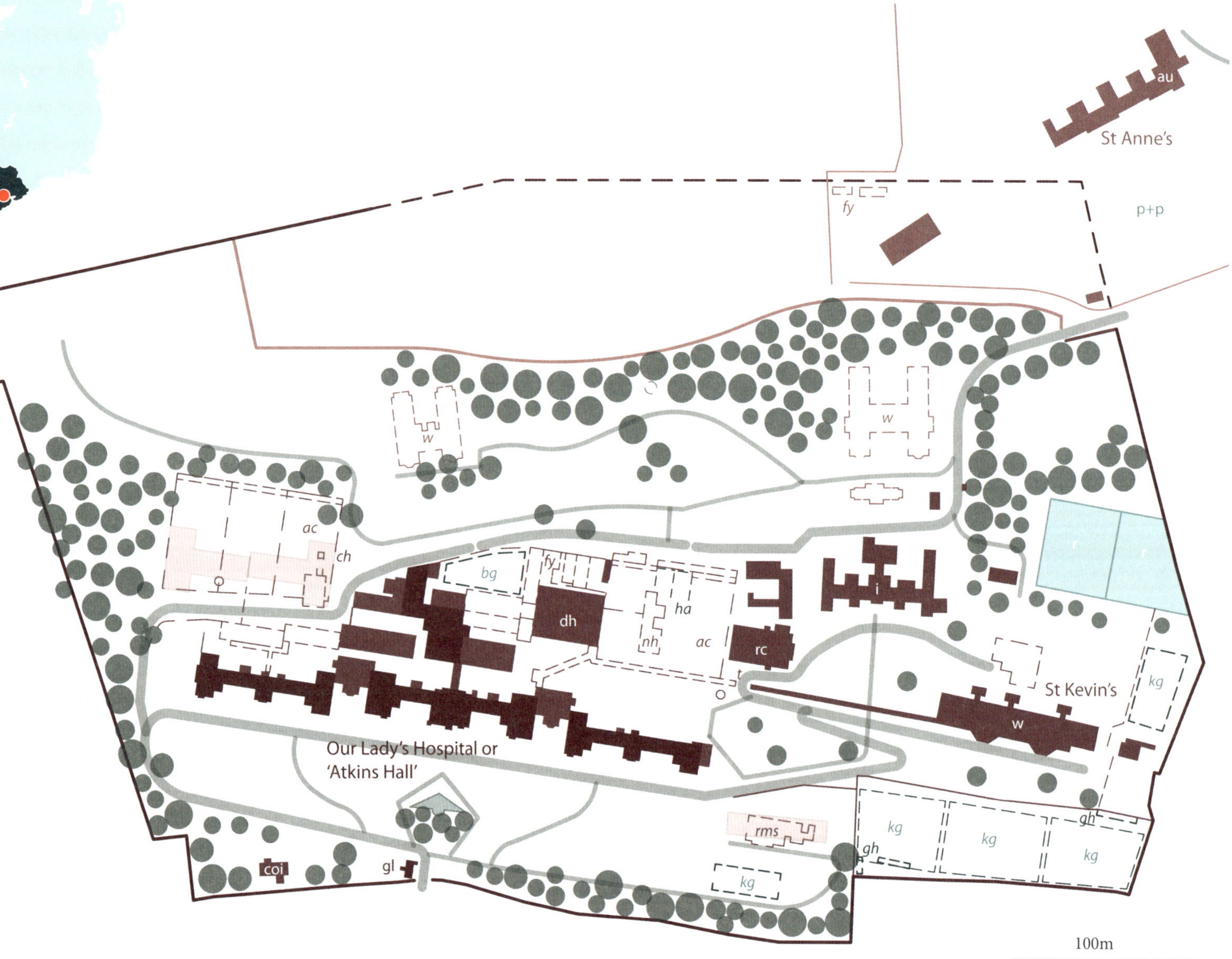

Cork's local elites were proud of their record in independently founding, funding and operating their own lunatic asylum for several decades before the nationally mandated system came into being. This independence was fiercely defended, but the Lee-siders were ultimately unable to resist the momentum of lunacy reform in the mid-nineteenth century. New legislation in 1845 saw the Cork institution re-designated as a district lunatic asylum, bringing it more firmly under the remit of the central administration in Dublin Castle and the Lunacy Inspectorate. Past glories were no defence against criticisms of an institution whose buildings had failed to keep up with evolving theories around treatment and care: 'defects in accommodation and structure' and a constrained city site would come to be seen as 'serious obstacles to the ...successful treatment of the insane'.[2] The Inspectors applied pressure to secure a replacement facility, eventually leading to the creation of new building that would ironically be named in honour of the Lord Lieutenant who had promoted the project in the face of local resistance.[3]

At 500 beds, the replacement building that was needed to remedy the 'many well-founded objections... both in a structural and sanitary point of view' of the old asylum would be largest proposed to date in Ireland, and large even by contemporary English standards.[4] Contrary to practice in other counties where the Inspectors selected the sites for the new asylums, the Cork governors stole a march on central authority and invited tenders for the purchase of 30–50 acres of land in the vicinity of Cork City, with 14 sealed offers received by the deadline.[5] Beyond details of acreage and price, many prospective vendors took the opportunity to extol the virtues of their particular site including fresh air, quietness, serenity, water supply and opportunities for occupation, some even displaying unexpected expertise in modern theories in the treatment of the insane:

> *it presents a remarkably extensive and delightful prospect, which is an adjunct to the curative treatment of the insane, deemed so indispensable by all who are skilled in the modern improvements in the management of the insane. The situation is particularly healthful...*[6]

A 37-acre site at Shanakiel was selected and a relatively low-profile local architect by the name of William Atkins was appointed to undertake the design. The decision to award the largest and most lucrative commission of the period to such a young and inexperienced practitioner was surprising, but Atkins rose to the challenge better than many of his peers. Daunted today by the building's sheer scale, it is easy to overlook the subtleties of Atkin's original design. His most significant decision was to disaggregate the accommodation into three separate blocks with a clear gap between each, to avoid creating an impenetrable wall of buildings along the Lee valley.[7] He likewise sought to avoid the dehumanising effect of a single long corridor running the length of the building; the three blocks were staggered and the original links between each were carefully offset so that the view along each shorter length of corridor could terminate in a window.

A four-storey central block, projecting single- and twin-gabled day rooms, tapering chimney stacks, six steeple-topped stair towers and three water towers of varying heights add considerable visual variety and create a most picturesque silhouette when viewed from the river valley below. Within the constraints of a symmetrical structure, Atkins playfully disposes a mixture of shouldered and gothic-arched single, bi- and tri-partite windows, arrayed between a selection of buttresses and decoratively executed bay- and oriel-windows. Not everybody was impressed: The Dublin Builder criticised the 'severe and forbidding character', of the exterior as being 'rather too expressive of its intended uses, which by some, no doubt, will be looked upon as an excellence but in this and like instances might judiciously be departed from'.[8]

But within less than a decade of opening, demand for increased space obliged Atkins to design infill extensions between the blocks, creating the improbably long (285 m) facade that he had originally striven to avoid. The Eglinton Asylum would thereafter rank amongst the three largest institutions in Ireland, and faced incessant demands for additional accommodation. With the building already impractically long and the steeply sloping site preventing perpendicular extension, most later developments would be separate structures, ranging in size from the pocket-sized Church of Ireland chapel near the gates (1884) to the four-storey, 33-bay, double-pile, red-brick edifice latterly known as St Kevin's (1894). Built to accommodate 434 male patients in enormous open-plan wards,[9] its unrepentantly institutional countenance, machined-brick finish and sheer scale make for a more domineering imposition on the city's skyline than its more picturesque predecessor. Its architect, William Henry Hill, seemed less perturbed than Atkins by long institutional corridors, constructing a 220-metre link to the main building.

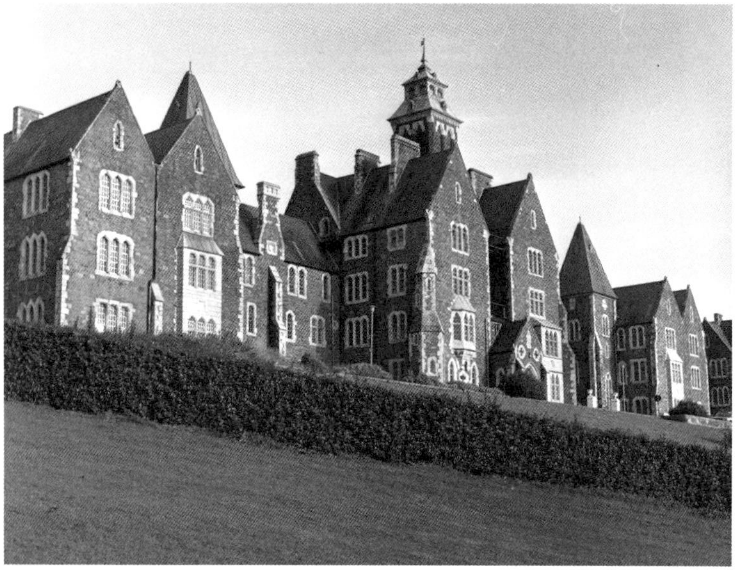

Central block of Atkin's 1852 building as it appeared upon closure in 1992. *Image courtesy of the Irish Architectural Archive (Photographic Collection, 075_088_CS_02_008)*

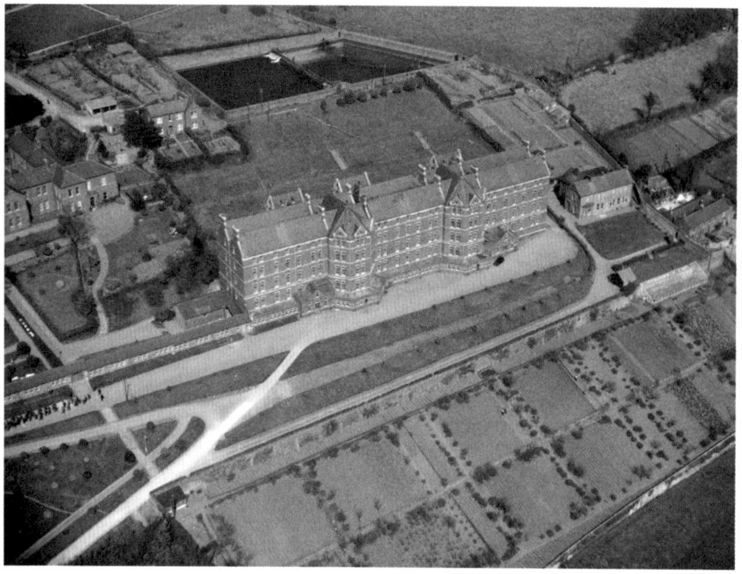

Aerial view of Hill's 1894 ward block, looming over the extensive walled gardens. *Image courtesy of the National Library of Ireland (NPA MOR979)*

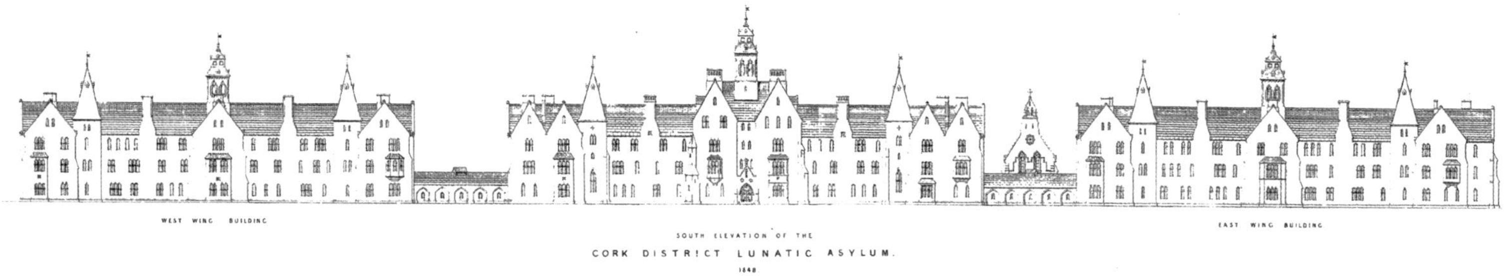

Elevation as designed by Atkins, before later infill blocks. *Image courtesy of ProQuest LLC (ProQuest House of Commons Parliamentary Papers, HC 1848 [983] xxxvii)*

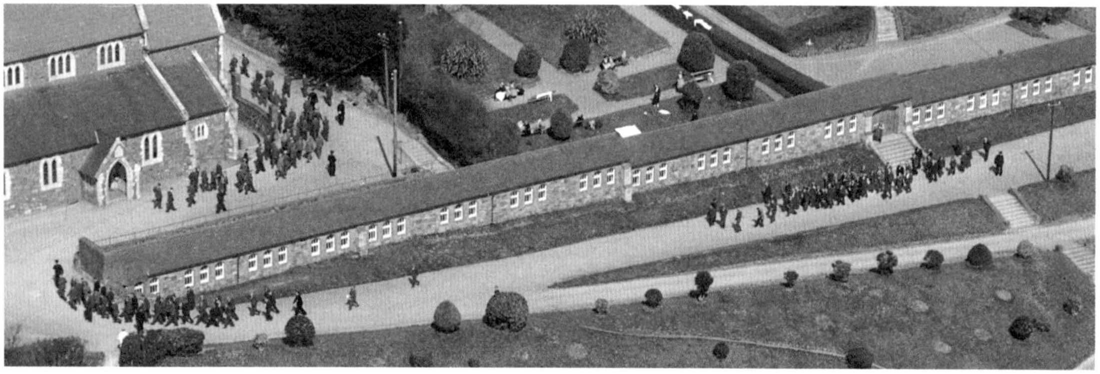

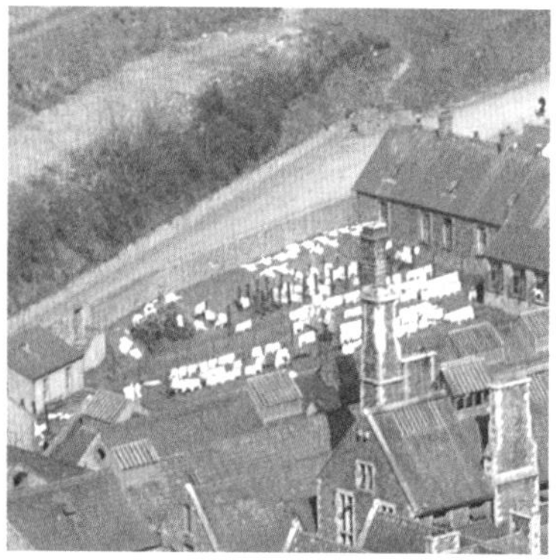

Rare glimpses of patient life when the institution was near its peak in 1955. *Images courtesy of the National Library of Ireland (NPA MOR980, 981)*

In the same decade the asylum would gain a Catholic chapel larger than most parish churches, and several rather less worthy 'temporary' tin buildings up the hill behind the main asylum. The steep topography may have increased the cost and difficulty of construction, but it did mean that most later buildings could enjoy sunlight and views beyond the shadow of the main building. A sequence of photographs taken on an ordinary April afternoon in 1955 provides an extraordinary insight into the daily lives of male and female patients, staff and officers of an institution at its operational peak.[10]

The grounds between the avenue and the front of the main building were landscaped with symmetrically arranged and impeccably maintained shrubberies and beds, giving a most favourable impression to any approaching visitor approaching. But this formal setting is entirely devoid of patients and peopled by only a handful of staff, one of whom may be the RMS striding purposefully back from lunch in his nearby house. Instead, the patients are found in the grounds to the rear. Five groups of 50–70 male patients – each likely representing a ward from St Kevin's – are being shepherded up the hill on their daily walk by uniformed attendants. A select handful of male patients are trusted to labour in the productive walled gardens below the institution, the heavy work of horticulture made harder by the steep slope. Their female counterparts have hung hundreds of sheets to dry in the bleaching green outside the laundry, but many other female patients appear to have little faith in the efficiency of that department, preferring to air their own laundry on the lawns and hedges. Another 300 or so are walking or lounging in enclosed spaces closer in character to large, verdant walled gardens than the cramped, bleak airing yards of old, but their activities all play out under the supervision of disturbingly prison-like sentry towers not found at any other asylum. And as a reminder of a time before the car was king, only three vehicles appear on the entire site, then home to over 2,000 patients and 350 staff.[11]

Of all of the institutions explored in this book, the later twentieth-century history of what came to be known as Our Lady's Hospital was amongst the least edifying. The Inspector in 1955 reported 'extremely difficult and frustrating conditions' where 'proper nursing of patients is rendered almost impossible';[12] by the late 1980s even nursing staff were prepared to describe conditions 'barely above lice level and difficult to maintain at that'.[13] Deteriorated beyond either physical or reputational redemption, the entirety of Atkin's 1852 building was closed to patients by 1992. University College Cork considered, but ultimately declined to adopt the building, which was instead sold to a private property developer. Decaying and derelict fabric and the difficulties of adapting the institutional layout for use as private residential apartments were but hiccoughs compared to the setback of a near decade-long property market crash, but works are again underway at time of writing and several of the other notable structures on the site have also been adapted to residential use.

Various other buildings on the Our Lady's site continued to be used for the delivery of mental health services for another two decades, with the last services finally transferred in 2009. Since then – and despite expensive security measures – the complex has been the subject of several arson attacks, most notably in 2017 when fire gutted two-thirds of St Kevin's. Ironically, all of the features that made this site appealing for asylum builders in the 1840s – its southerly aspect, elevated setting, spectacular views and proximity to the city – are equally coveted in today's property market. The State's Land Development Agency has recently received planning permission for a residential redevelopment of the rest of the site. The most prominent historic buildings are retained and reused; it remains to be seen how the more subtle features of this complex and challenging site will fare.

Further Reading

Hanora Henry, *Our Lady's Psychiatric Hospital Cork* (Cork: Haven Books, 1989)

References

1. Dublin's Royal Barracks (later Collins Barracks) had an unbroken frontage of over 300 metres when built in 1710. By the time the infill blocks at Cork were added in 1861, localised demolition had been carried out to break the barracks into several detached blocks, yielding to Cork the crown.
2. *Twenty-First Report of the Inspectors-General of Prisons*, HC 1843 [462] xxvii, pp 91–2;
3. Hanora Henry, *Our Lady's Psychiatric Hospital Cork* (Cork, 1989), pp 48–9; Frederick O'Dwyer, *The Architecture of Deane and Woodward* (Cork, 1997), pp 54–5.
4. *Seventh Annual Asylum Report 1855*, HC 1854-55 [1981] xvi, p. 12.
5. Henry, *Our Lady's Psychiatric Hospital*, pp 52–5.
6. Tender no. 4 received from Christopher Lloyd, cited in Henry, *Our Lady's Psychiatric Hospital*, p. 57.
7. Reuber regards Atkin's disaggregation of three detached blocks in Cork as the first 'pavilion' asylum, an interpretation the author struggles to share. It is a distinguishing feature of the pavilion model that the circulation routes are entirely separate from the patient blocks, whereas at Cork the ground floor wards remain principal thoroughfares. Markus Reuber, 'The architecture of psychological management: The Irish asylums, 1801–1922', in *Psychological Medicine* no. 26 (1996), pp 1179–89.
8. *The Dublin Builder*, 13 Dec. 1851, p. 790.
9. *Forty-Fourth Annual Asylum Report 1895*, HC 1895 [7804] liv, p. 109.
10. National Library of Ireland, Morgan Aerial Photographic Collection, ca. 1954, Our Lady's Hospital, Cork, NPA MOR 979, 980, 981.
11. Which most likely belonged to the RMS, the Protestant chaplain, and his Catholic counterpart. *Report of the Inspector of Mental Hospitals, 1955*, p. 48, p. 59.
12. Ibid., pp 21–2.
13. 'The scandal of the mental hospitals', *Magill*, 30 Oct. 1980.

CASE STUDY 14

St Finan's Hospital

(previously Killarney District Lunatic Asylum)

Years in operation
1852–2012

Original cost
£39,808

Capacity (min /max)
250 / 1,078

Architect(s)
Sir Thomas Deane,
James F. Fuller, .
J. R. Boyd Barrett

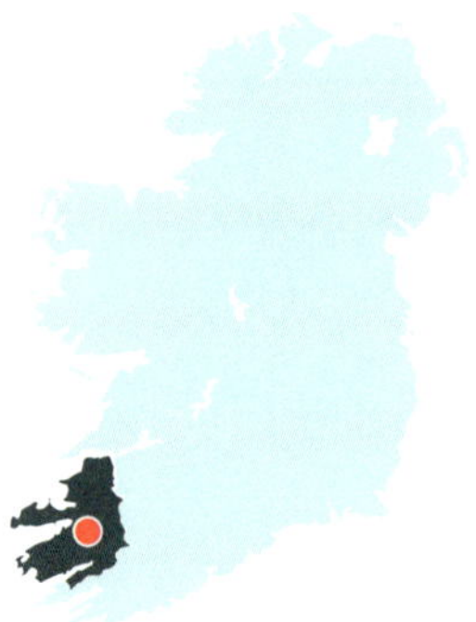

The asylum at Killarney is the most westerly of any such institution in Europe and with its spectacular views of the MacGillycuddy Reeks, enjoys one of the most sublime settings. However, its uniquely beautiful location also places it in the path of powerful Atlantic weather systems, such that during almost 170 years of its existence, this building has had to withstand stronger winds and heavier rainfall than any of its peers in Ireland, Britain, or possibly beyond.

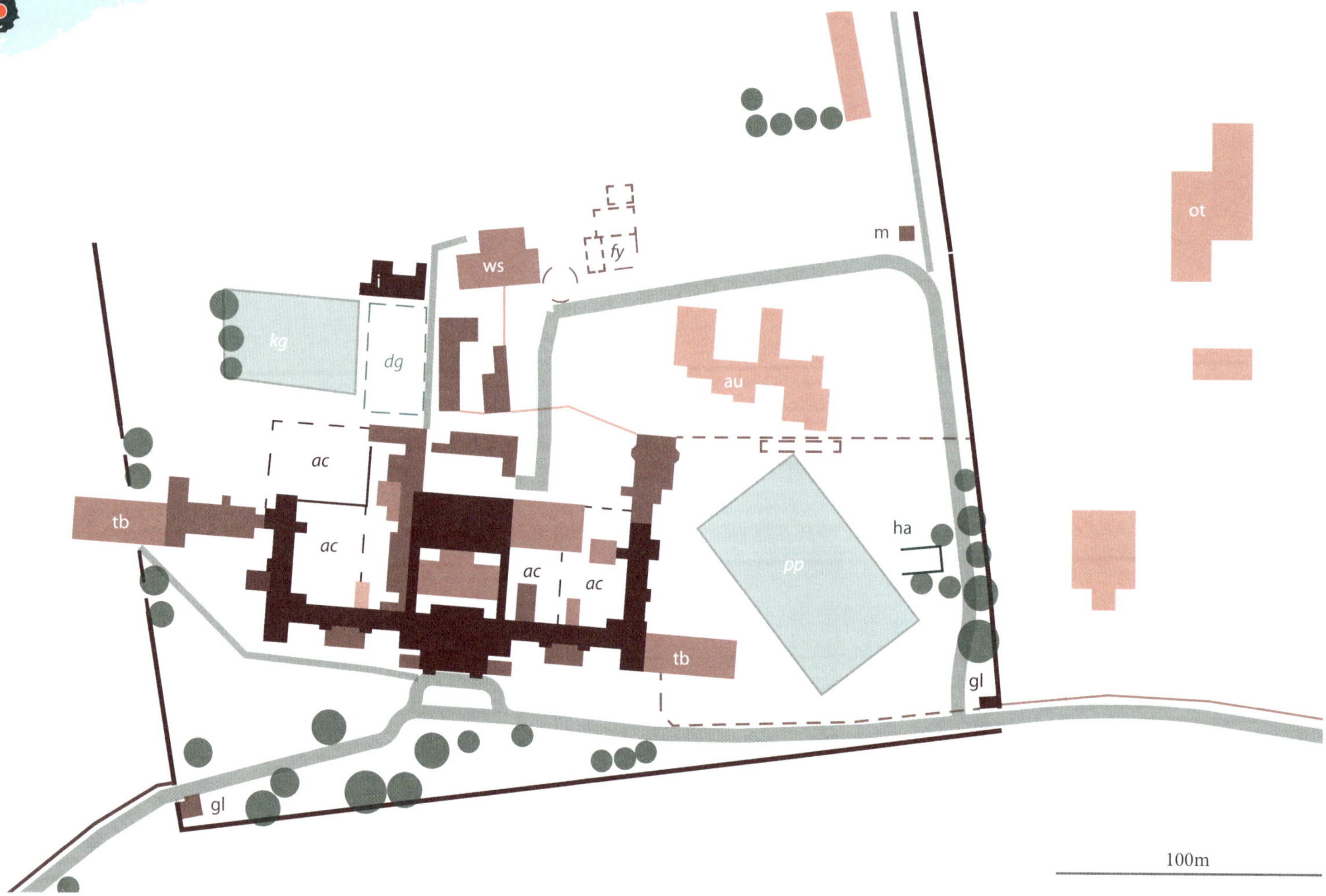

Kerry patients were originally provided for by the district asylum at Limerick, which opened in 1827. When consulted in 1844 on the possibility of erecting either a new provincial asylum for incurable patients, or a new district asylum to serve Kerry and the West Riding of Cork, the grand jury for County Kerry initially reported 'no opinion on the subject'. They may have been disappointed that the towns shortlisted for the prospective asylum – Millstreet, Mallow, Kanturk and Newmarket – were all in County Cork, but they equally passed up the opportunity to canvass for the new institution to be in their own bailiwick.[1] Ultimately faced with 'much difference of opinion' amongst the grand juries of Munster, the Lord Lieutenant concluded that a new district asylum should be erected at Cork, with one additional 'central repository' for incurable cases.[2]

Yet by the time the 1845 Act passed parliament and the next phase of asylum construction got underway, the dubious idea of consigning 'incurable' cases to a provincial asylum was dropped in preference of additional district asylums, including a separate institution for Kerry. The local grand jury finally deigned to express an opinion, recommending that the new asylum should be located not in the county town of Tralee, but in Killarney, and not so much for its sublime views as for the more pragmatic reasons of its 'centrality and a numerous resident gentry to superintend the general management of such an institution'.[3]

The architectural story of the Killarney asylum is initially one of opportunity lost. The well-established Cork architectural firm of Deane and Woodward, already appointed by the Board of Works to design the Queen's College in Cork, were awarded the Killarney commission. An early sketch by the (arguably) more talented partner, Benjamin Woodward, proposed a sculptural composition laid out on an H-plan, two storeys in height, dripping with architectural detail and comparable in aesthetic quality to the new Cork college, or indeed contemporary developments in Oxford or Cambridge.[4]

Alas, this design would not be realised. The Board of Works issued its Instructions to Architects, which significantly narrowed the scope for innovation and forced Deane and Woodward to fall into line with the other new asylums of the era. The resulting building, while less adventurous, still forms a highly picturesque addition to the skyline of the town. The usual array of Gothic architectural devices – bay- and oriel-windows, decorative buttresses, single-, paired- and triple-lancet windows – are here further refined with the addition of trefoil-headed arches, heraldic shields, and highly wrought chimneys that taper in multiple stages to terminate in distinctive lozenge-shaped stacks. The overall appearance is further enhanced by the contrast between brown-sandstone rubble-work and bright limestone dressings, while the steeply raked gables of the central block, stair towers and day rooms successfully counterbalance the overall width of the composition.

But the fine architectural treatment did not spare the building from serious defects from the moment it opened (see Chapter Four). The centrally ordained specification that external walls should be of un-plastered rubble masonry proved to be a poor decision in the context of Killarney's horizontal driving rain, further compounded by poor workmanship in execution. The grand jury were incensed at being burdened with the cost of constructing and then remediating a building that worked out to be 14 times more expensive per bed than the nearby workhouse.[5] At the subsequent parliamentary enquiry in Westminster, the views of Kerry delegation were made abundantly clear by local hereditary chieftain, The MacGillycuddy, who argued that 'you should not put your hand into a man's pocket and take out his purse without asking his leave.'[6] Their case was only partially vindicated, securing a government rebate of £1,455 as against a total project cost of £39,808.[7]

Whether in response to local climate or otherwise, the asylum at Killarney was one of only a handful in Ireland which eschewed the later trend towards detached buildings. Extensions to the male side in the 1870s carefully matched the original building, while on the main façade, twin-gabled day-room extensions likewise integrated quite successfully with Deane's original design. The extension to the female side in the 1890s presented a more utilitarian, institutional appearance externally and was unusual in featuring a double-loaded corridor layout internally. Patient spaces were also unusually well appointed internally with timber wainscoting and decorative ceiling linings – though these may have been a necessary fig-leaf for the persistent damp.

The chapel within the main building remained in use until the hospital finally closed, surviving complete with organ loft as the only unaltered example of its kind in Ireland. A diminutive Church of Ireland chapel – designed to seat a mere 16 patients and a possible contender for smallest place of worship in Ireland – hides in plain sight beside the main entrance.[8] By the early twentieth century, the overcrowded, under-heated and perpetually damp conditions prevailing at Killarney left

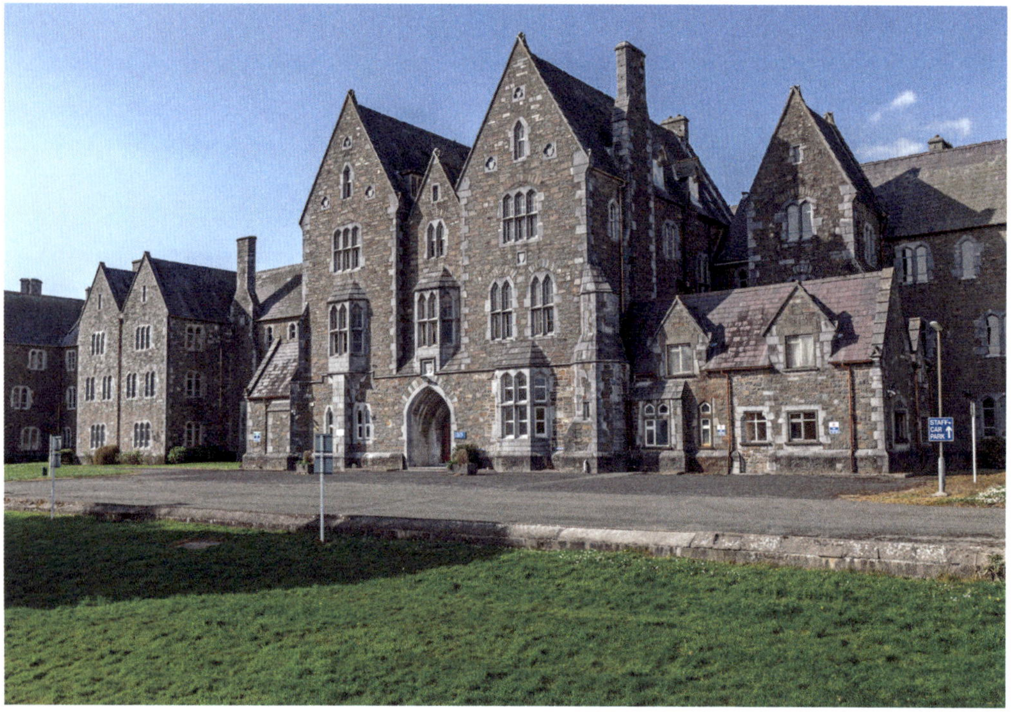

Deane may have had to tone down his partner's original design ambitions, but it remains an impressive edifice by any measure. *Photograph by David Killeen, 2019.*

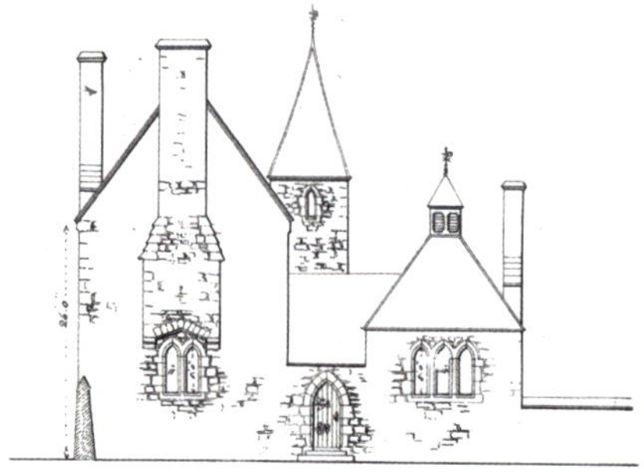

Even the modest detached infirmary (above and below) was to have enjoyed Deane and Woodward's elaborate treatment, but like the main building, was much simplified in execution. *Image courtesy of the Irish Architectural Archive (85/200: 002)*

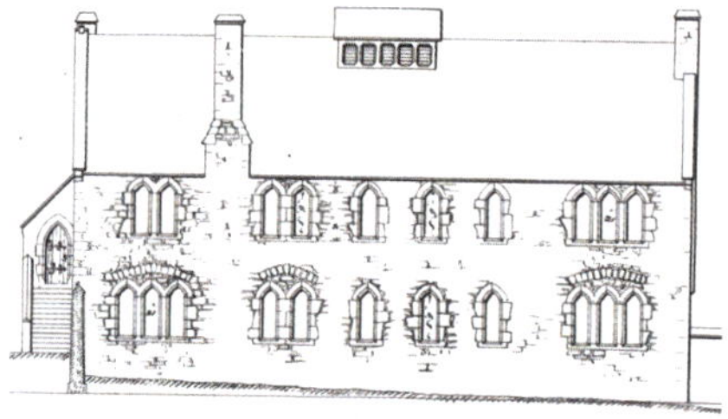

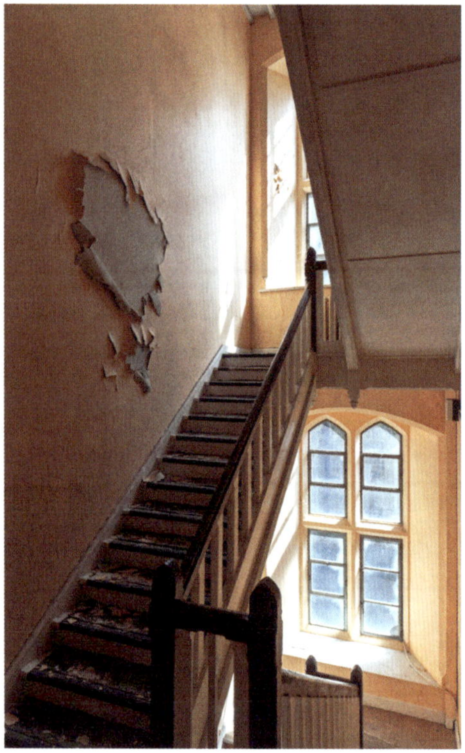

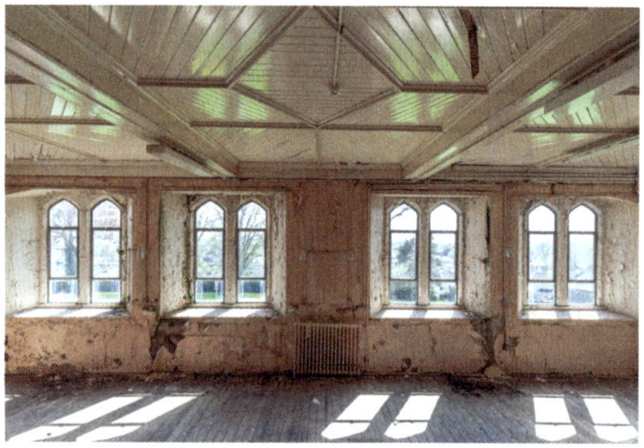

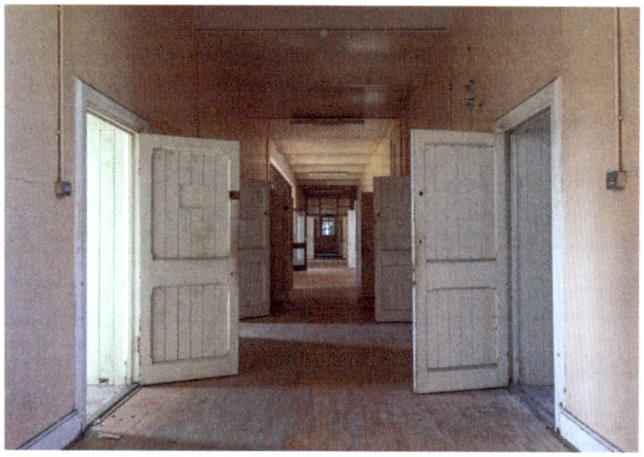

Many interiors retain good early joinery, as in the stair hall (above), day room (above right). *Photographs by David Killeen, 2019.*

Double-loaded corridors such as this - iconic interior of the American 'Kirkbride' asylum - are rarely encountered in Ireland. *Photograph by David Killeen, 2019.*

the institution highly prone to outbreaks of tuberculosis. In the 1930s, with assistance from the Sweepstakes, very fine isolation wards for tubercular patients were added at either end of the institution. Designed by James Boyd Barrett, the wards feature delightful verandahs at the first floor raised over open masonry arcades at ground level, all finished in his signature rock-faced ashlar. But even these healthy, light-filled spaces were insufficient to prevent the disease from taking its toll: mortality due to pulmonary TB remained high, accounting for almost a quarter of deaths in 1949. In the same paragraph as that grim statistic and with little apparent sense of irony, the Inspector was pleased to report good progress in tuberculin-testing the hospital's cattle herd.[9] And while the stereotype of the shrewd Kerry farmer is well worn, we can only speculate if the existence of three weighing machines in the store yard (where most other asylums made do with one) was in any way representative of the trustworthiness of local suppliers.

Today, the asylum and its handful of skeletal Scot's Pines make for a fairly stark silhouette over Killarney's northern suburbs, but its effect was originally softened by a heavily wooded setting. Dense planting on the female side of the asylum was seen to be reaching maturity in 1950s aerial photography, but the trees on the male side had already been cut – almost certainly at the request of male staff or patients desiring a clear view of the Sunday games in the adjacent Fitzgerald Park GAA Stadium. Much of that stadium was built by the labour of 60 patients in 1936, leading it to be described later as a 'bridgehead' between the hospital and the wider community;[10] a discreet door even linked the asylum and stadium grounds. And where other asylums featured enclosed airing yards, many of the male wards enjoyed direct access to a Gaelic football pitch and handball alley, albeit still securely fenced.

Tuberculosis wards apart, the twentieth century saw few other developments of note at Killarney. A breeze-block bunker containing two purpose-built admissions wards was opened in 1975, a move that ran contrary to prevailing mental health policy and whose existence would later frustrate efforts to transfer acute admissions to the psychiatric unit built as part of the new Tralee General Hospital, which as a result sat empty for several years in the late 1980s and early 1990s.[11] The hospital – rechristened as St Finan's in 1959 in honour of a local saint best known for running a leper hospital – continued to operate into the twenty-first century. Its doors finally closed in 2012, since which time it has stood empty.

As the town with Ireland's highest number of hotel beds per capita,[12] the best chance for saving the disused building at Killarney would appear to lie in a sympathetic adaptation as a distinctive addition to the town's tourism offer. Programmatically, asylum buildings can be very well-suited for re-use as hotels, offering a good combination of commodious central spaces, back-of-house facilities, and several floors of sleeping accommodation. However, the window of opportunity to achieve such a transformation is narrowing. The problems of penetrating damp and timber decay that afflicted the asylum in its early years returned with a vengeance once the central heating was turned off. While the building has been well secured against trespass and vandalism, it is harder to protect it against the insidious effects of a mild, wet and windy Atlantic climate seemingly optimised to accelerate decay.

Further Reading

Dermot Dwyer (ed.), *St. Finan's Hospital Killarney: A Medical, Social & Sporting History 1852–2002* (Killarney: St Finan's Historical Society, 2002)

Frederick O'Dwyer, *The Architecture of Deane and Woodward* (Cork: Cork University Press, 1997), pp 91–106

References

1. *Annual Asylum Report 1844*, HC 1845 [645] xxvi, p. 83.
2. *Annual Asylum Report 1844*, HC 1845 [645] xxvi, p. 79.
3. *Annual Asylum Report 1846*, HC 1847 [820] xvii, p. 52, pp 67–8.
4. For a detailed account of Deane and Woodward's execution of the Killarney commission, see Frederick O'Dwyer, *The Architecture of Deane and Woodward* (Cork, 1997), pp 91–106.
5. *1857 Commission Report*, HC 1857–58 [2436-II], p. 496.
6. Ibid., p. 493.
7. *1857 Commission Report*, HC 1857–58 [2436-I], p. 42; *1855 Commission Report*, HC 1856 [9] LIII.367, p. 30.
8. Dermot Dwyer (ed.), *St. Finian's Hospital Killarney: A Medical, Social & Sporting History 1852–2002* (Killarney, 2002), p. 81.
9. *Report of the Inspector of Mental Hospitals 1949*, p. 25.
10. Dwyer, 2002, pp 31–3.
11. *Report of the Inspector of Mental Hospitals 1988-89*, p. 173.
12. Approximately two beds for every three residents.

CASE STUDY 15

Years in operation
1853–present

Original cost
£41,405

Capacity (min /max)
300 / 1116

Architect(s)
William Farrell,
C. A. Owen

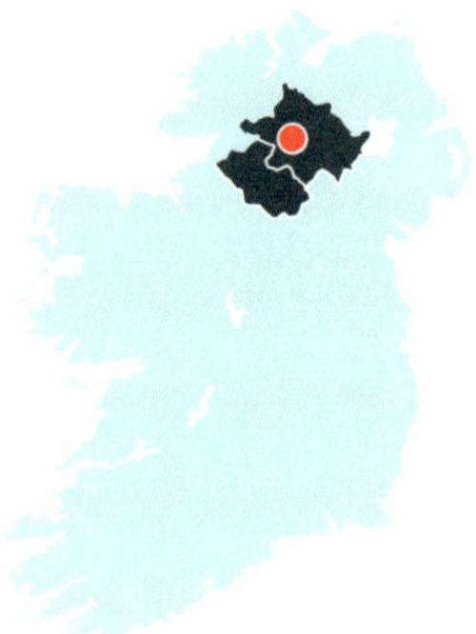

Tyrone and Fermanagh Hospital

(previously Omagh District Lunatic Asylum)

The 'Instructions' issued to designers of the second phase of Irish asylums stipulated that the buildings were not be 'not devoid of architectural character,' but of all of the asylums of this era, the main facade at Omagh comes closest to that undesired outcome. A meagre handful of bay- and oriel- windows are inadequate to relive a 62-bay facade characterised by barrack-like repetition of tall, narrow, unadorned, openings. The uninspiring elevation was in part driven by a layout which inverted the planning assumptions of other asylums of the era, albeit the benefits to the patients proved short-lived.

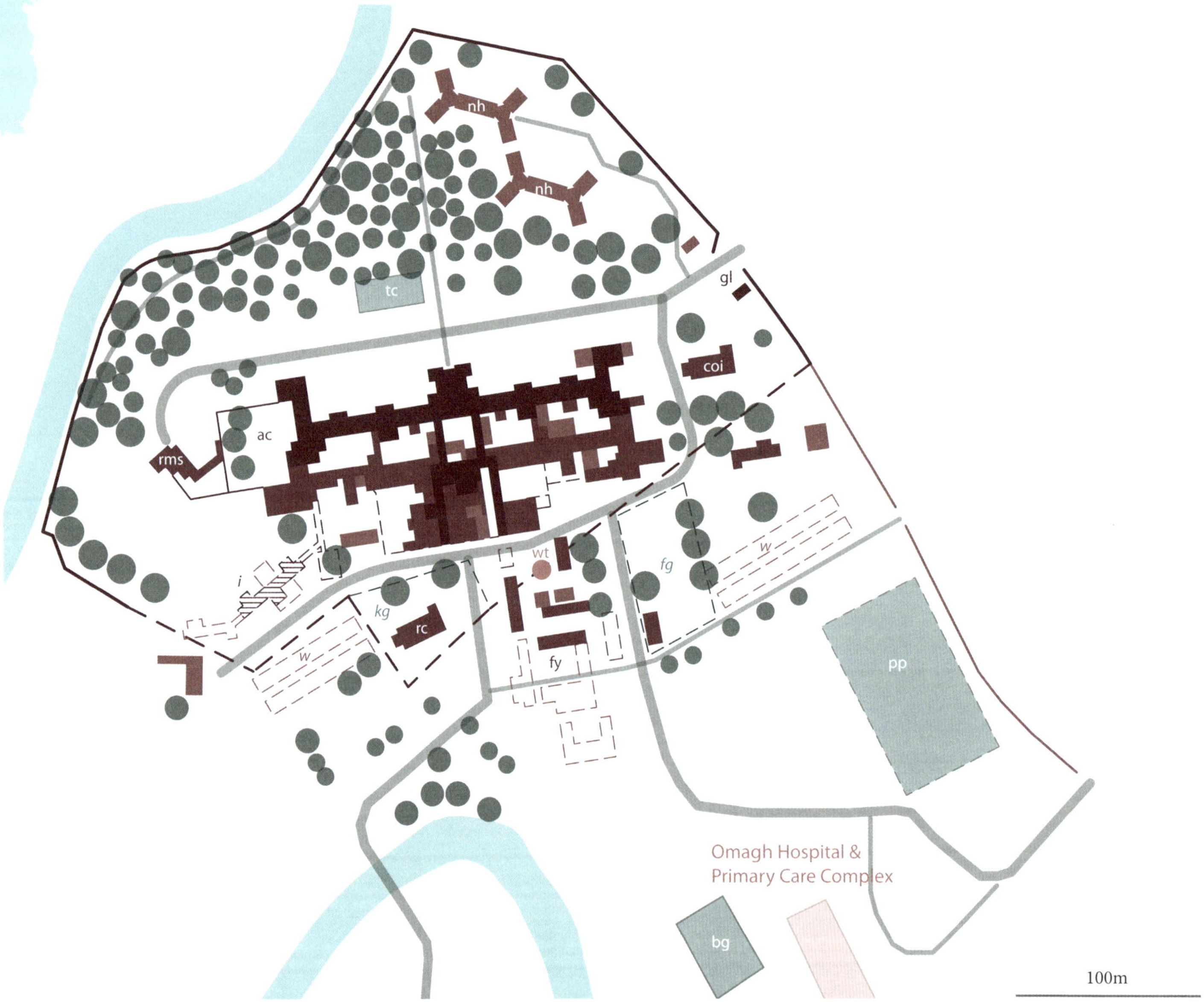

The Omagh District Lunatic Asylum was established to serve counties Tyrone and Fermanagh, whose patients had previously been assigned to the Derry and Armagh districts, respectively. Compared to the politicking that surrounded redistricting in the other provinces during 1846, the proposals in Ulster seem to have been relatively uncontroversial, the main change in execution being a reduction in Omagh's capacity from the originally proposed 500 beds to 300.[1] The asylum's catchment remained unchanged since its opening in 1853 and is reflected in the name by which the institution is known today: Tyrone and Fermanagh Hospital.

The site selected for the new asylum was a mile and a half from the town; a picturesque hill forming a miniature peninsula bounded by the Camowen River on three sides.[2] It may have been the specific characteristics of this setting that inspired architect William Farrell to deviate from conventional asylum planning of the era by facing the main entrance north rather than south. Today, thoroughly shrouded in mature woodland, Robert French's late-nineteenth-century photograph gives a sense of how dramatically this enormous edifice – half as long as Omagh's entire main street – once commanded the river valley when approached from the town it served.

Farrell's original design proposed day spaces on the front (north) elevation, but this was reversed after the main building contract was signed to bring the design into line with the brief provided by the Board of Works, which prioritised sunlight in the day-time spaces, with sleeping accommodation lying to the north. This explains the barrack-like appearance of the building's main (north) frontage: the internal division of cells and dormitories dictated a grid-like fenestration and prevented Farrell from indulging in the compositional creativity evident in most other asylums of the age. Moreover, the urgent imperative to implement such a major redesign while already in contract may have had more than a little bearing on the mediocrity of the façade design.[3]

Of greater significance to patients at Omagh was the fact that the airing yards – located as a rule to the rear of the main building – could enjoy a sunny southerly aspect in contrast to the gloomy north-facing yards so much criticised at other sites. However, the benefits of this approach would prove short-lived as the inevitable accretion of ancillary spaces – kitchens, laundries, his-and-hers' dining halls – that was needed to service the growing institution soon saw the airing yards hemmed in with buildings on all sides.

Even allowing for these unusual circumstances Farrell – in the twilight of an architectural career almost entirely devoted to ecclesiastical work – struggled to do justice to this largest of commissions. His sole ambitious gesture – a pair of octagonal turrets with sprocketed stone steeples – emerge awkwardly from square stair towers on which they sit and fail, in proportion and scale, to compensate for the overall monotony. By the same token, Omagh was at least spared from the criticisms of excessive expenditure on decorative stone levelled at other asylums, though not immune from similar charges of defective workmanship.[4]

Large wings were added to the rear in the 1890s, taking the total accommodation up to 700 and giving rise to a legal dispute with the building contractor that would drag on until 1902.[5] The first decade of the twentieth century also saw the erection of separate Protestant and Catholic chapels on the grounds – the former sited prominently near the main gate, the latter, larger and simpler, relegated to a more discreet site beside the farmyard to the rear. Uniquely amongst Irish asylums, a concrete landing stage was built on the river in 1914 to serve a ferry, a strange decision given the obvious impediments to navigability and where a siding from the adjacent Great Northern Railway might have better served.[6]

If the architecture of the building disappoints at close quarters, its landscaped grounds are some compensation. Facilities for cricket, football and tennis attest to an active sporting life for patients. The steeply sloping land between the asylum and the river was cut into a series of lawned terraces before giving way to a fine mixed woodland, sufficiently dense to screen a pair of nurses' homes that were injudiciously planted in the lower grounds in the 1960s. A plethora of other low-rise buildings mushroomed during the twentieth century only to fade away, leaving the landscape little worse off for their brief and unremarkable existence. The only regrettable loss is of the original detached 1850s infirmary, whose site today looks like a prehistoric cairn formed of the finest Victorian dressed stone. The roof of the main asylum building has been renewed in recent years at considerable cost, albeit many of the chimneys, which had enlivened the building's skyline, were lost in the process.

In an inversion of later twentieth-century policy south of the border – which moved acute mental healthcare services to general hospital settings – plans were prepared over several decades to re-locate the local general hospital to the Tyrone and Fermanagh

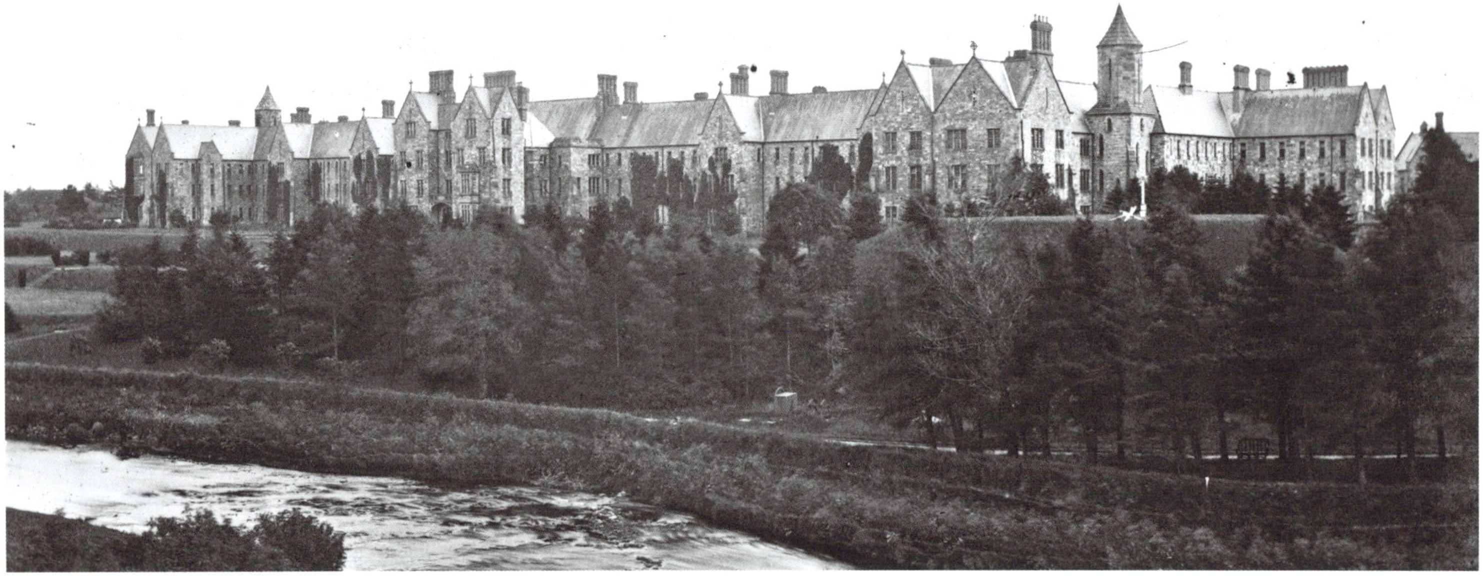

A dense roofscape of chimneystacks and a smattering of climbing ivy – both now gone – once softened the barrack-like monotony of Farrell's design. *Image courtesy of the National Library of Ireland (L_CAB_01980)*

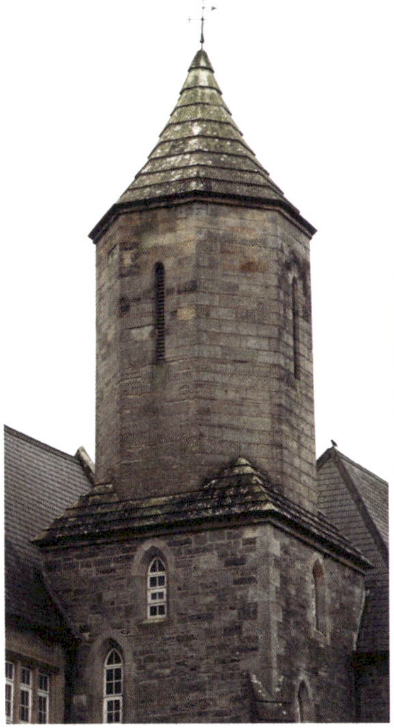

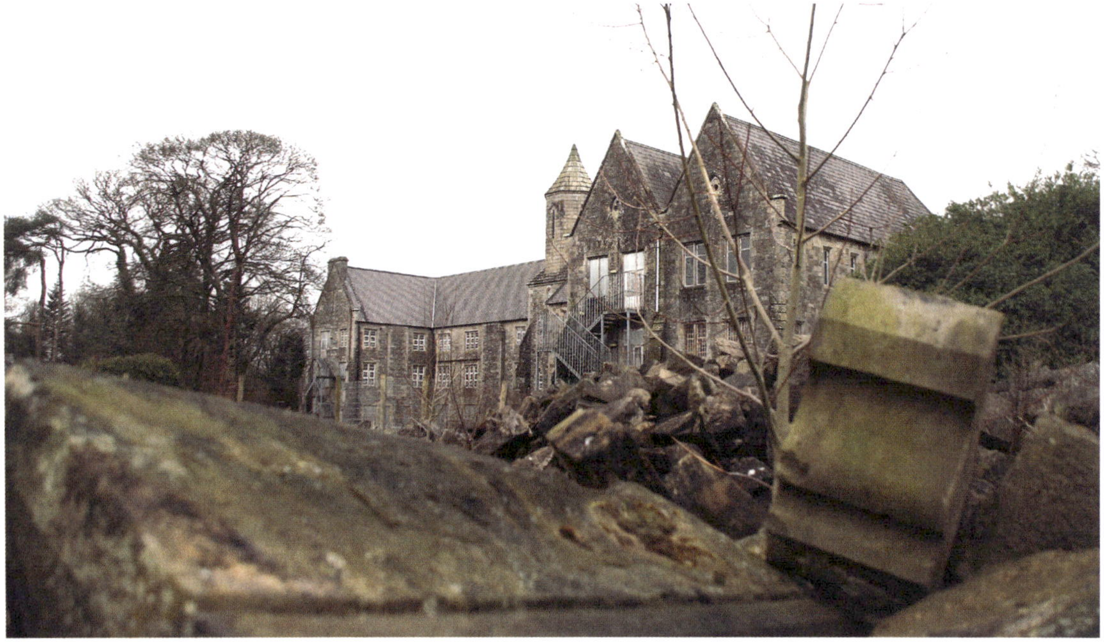

Farrell's sole architectural extravagance - a pair of octagonal turrets (above left), spring uncomfortably from square stair towers.
The detached infirmary was demolished and now reposes like a pre-historic cairn of the finest Victorian cut stone (above right). *Photographs by the author, 2020.*

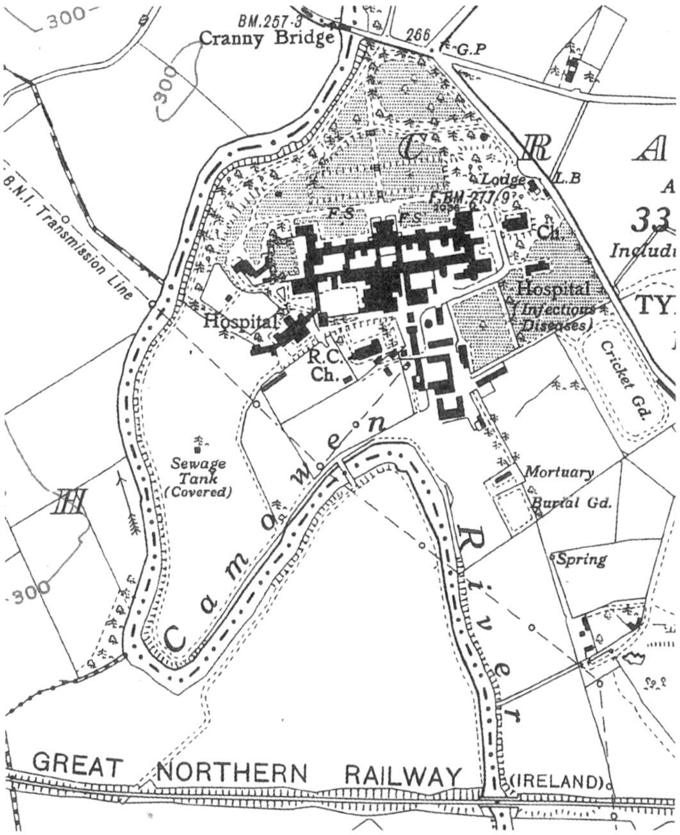

Map showing peninsula-like site. *Reproduced courtesy of Trinity College Dublin (OSNI-Tyrone-10560-Sheet 35-1948)*

Hospital site. While there is some irony in the fact that the old mental hospital was almost entirely wound down by the time the new hospital finally opened, the long-term future of healthcare activity on the wider campus implies that uses will eventually be found for those parts of the old asylum that currently lie vacant.

Further Reading

Robert McKinley, 'Tyrone and Fermanagh Hospital: A Chronological History' in Mitchell Haldane, ed. *Images of Omagh and District, Vol. 7.* (Omagh: Rotary Club of Omagh, 1999), pp 64-83.

Alistair Rowan, *Buildings of Ireland: North West Ulster* (London: Penguin, 1979) p. 447.

References

1. *Annual Asylum Report 1846*, HC 1847 [820] xvii, p. 53.
2. The local grand jury were offered the opportunity by the Board of Works to choose between two potential sites: one closer to town and further from the 'turf fields', the other the reverse. *1857 Commission Report*, HC 1857–58 [2436-II] p. 5
3. *1855 Commission Report*, HC 1856 [9] LIII.367, p. 6.
4. The inspectors found no excess of architectural embellishment on the building, but did report numerous defects associated with dampness and settlement that it recommended be rectified without recourse to the local ratepayers. *1855 Commission Report*, HC 1856 [9] LIII.367, p. 18, p. 20.
5. *The Irish Builder*, 13 Mar. 1902, p. 1074; Ibid., 3 July 1902, p. 1311.
6. Robert McKinley, 'Tyrone and Fermanagh Hospital: A Chronological History', in Mitchell Haldane (ed.), *Images of Omagh and District, Vol. 7* (Omagh, 1999), p. 71.

CASE STUDY 16

St Columba's Hospital

(formerly Sligo District Lunatic Asylum, latterly Clayton Hotel)

Years in operation
1855-1993 (main building)

Original cost
£40,271

Capacity (min /max)
250 / 1,012

Architect(s)
William Deane Butler,
Thomas N. Deane,
Thomas M. Deane,
McDonnell,
Dixon & Downes.

The spatial complexity of lunatic asylums makes them challenging to adapt. Modern hotels are amongst the very few uses whose accommodation needs prove reasonably compatible with the diversity of redundant spaces found in the typical asylum. So it is entirely appropriate that the institution once disparagingly referred to as 'The Leitrim Hotel' has confounded its sceptics and reinvented itself as just that. It still frequently plays host to hundreds of residents from the neighbouring county, but now in connection with its happier role as a popular wedding venue.

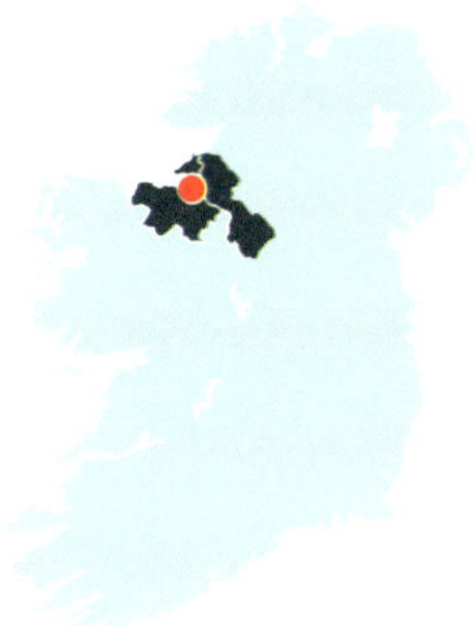

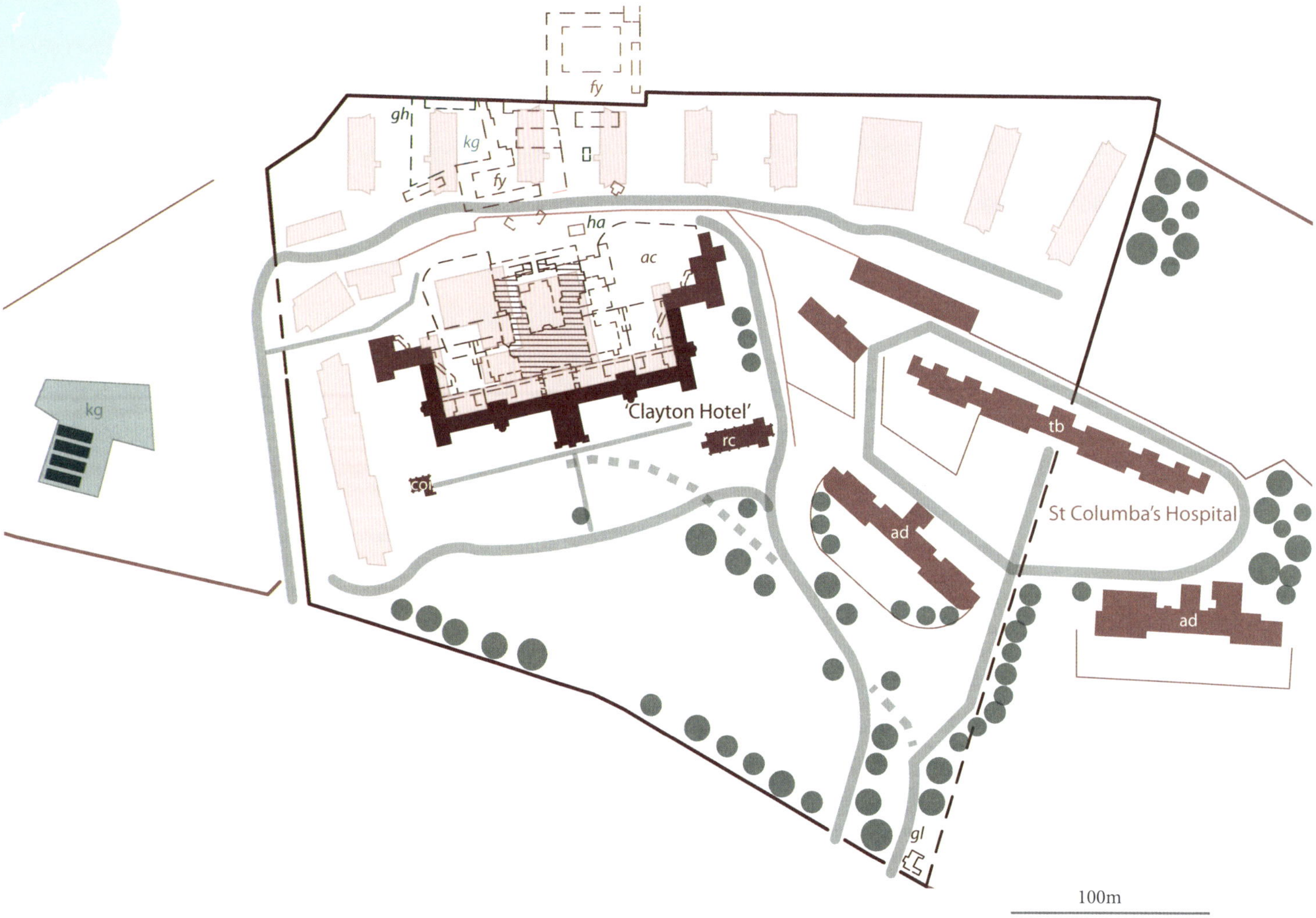

The location of the Connaught District Lunatic Asylum in Ballinasloe, on the eastern periphery of a large and poorly connected province, rendered it inaccessible to many who needed its services. Yet when the Ballinasloe governors were asked in 1844 to state their preferred option for expanding asylum accommodation in the province, their inclination was to defend their institution's status as the province's sole asylum. Uniquely amongst their peers, they also saw little difficulty with the continued detention of lunatics in workhouses and even prisons. Such antediluvian views were out of step with the times, and the Inspectors instead recommended to the Lord Lieutenant that a new asylum be provided at Sligo.[1]

The formation of a new asylum district comprising counties Sligo and Leitrim was approved in 1846, and the new asylum for 250 patients was opened in June 1855 on an elevated 30-acre site to the north of the town. The Board of Works entrusted the design to architect William Deane Butler, an experienced hand versant in both classical and Gothic idioms. Butler's superb Catholic seminary of St Kieran's in Kilkenny arguably ranks behind only Maynooth and the Queen's Colleges in Ireland's pantheon of Gothic-revival institutional architecture, which makes it all the more surprising that he chose to deviate from the Board of Works preferred Gothic by selecting an Elizabethan Revival style for Sligo.

The building at Sligo was the most expensive of the second phase of asylums on a per-patient basis, and it is easy to see why.[2] While the massing and roofscape of the building were simpler than the neo-Gothic asylums, Butler more than compensated in the detail. Finely articulated door- and window-surrounds, quoins, string courses and cornices, graciously balustraded entrance steps, curvilinear gables crowned by pinnacles, and bay windows with parapets of open-fretwork were present in both quality and quantity surpassed only by the best private mansions. His pièce de résistance was to have been a pair of towers crowned by bulbous spires and pinnacles, entirely of dressed stone, but this proved to be one extravagance too far: the towers were ultimately finished in a more rudimentary manner and today give the incongruous impression of having been transplanted from a provincial railway station.[3]

Butler's attention to detail went well beyond architectural trimmings. Unwilling to compromise either the location of fireplaces internally or the symmetry of his composition externally, he led chimney flues on tortuous journeys around windows and across rooms: a level of design egoism more common in buildings at the elite end of the architectural spectrum. Within, the spatial disposition, fit and finish of his interiors also demonstrated aspirations beyond the mundane. The central administration block featured a formal sequence of porches and halls separated by finely detailed glazed screens. Above was located a double-height recreation hall, galleried on four sides beneath a circular rooflight, echoing the top-lit bedroom landings of larger classical houses. By orientating the chapel perpendicular to the main building, windows could be provided above the altar and along both sides of the nave, more closely approximating the spatial sense of a real church than the other asylum chapels of the era. Most ingeniously of all, doors to the rear of the chapel's organ gallery could be opened to allow the instrument to serve the recreation hall. Even late changes were turned to advantage – the governors' request to add a separate dining hall was cleverly accommodated by infilling a previously open courtyard between the kitchens and the main building.

Less happily, Butler's strict adherence to the Instructions to Architects – in forming the day rooms as open-plan projections from the ward corridor with folding doors for winter use – proved to be less satisfactory in practice than the separate day rooms provided at some other asylums.[4] However, this paled into insignificance compared to the fallout from the cost of Butler's architectural self-indulgence. The total outlay of £40,271 was bitterly resented by the local governors who were now obliged to burden their ratepayers with annual repayments. The 1855 Commission of Inquiry concurred that the decorative stonework was 'effective in appearance, but expensive in execution' and 'too floridly carried out for such an institution'. This excess, together with an injudicious decision by the Board of Works to change the position of the building on the site, saw the Sligo governors secure a rebate of £3,000 to meet the 'useless and unnecessary expenditure in carrying out such a class of building'. The Board of Works were also obliged to remedy defects with water closets and dampness at no cost to the county.[5]

While relatively powerless to influence the design of the original asylum building, the local governors could at least shape the landscape that surrounded it: 'The grounds, too, are undergoing the necessary cultivation by direction of the Board of Governors, who have met on several occasions to make contracts…'[6] The parkland landscape they created still provides a fitting setting for the building, even within a wider context that is now radically altered.

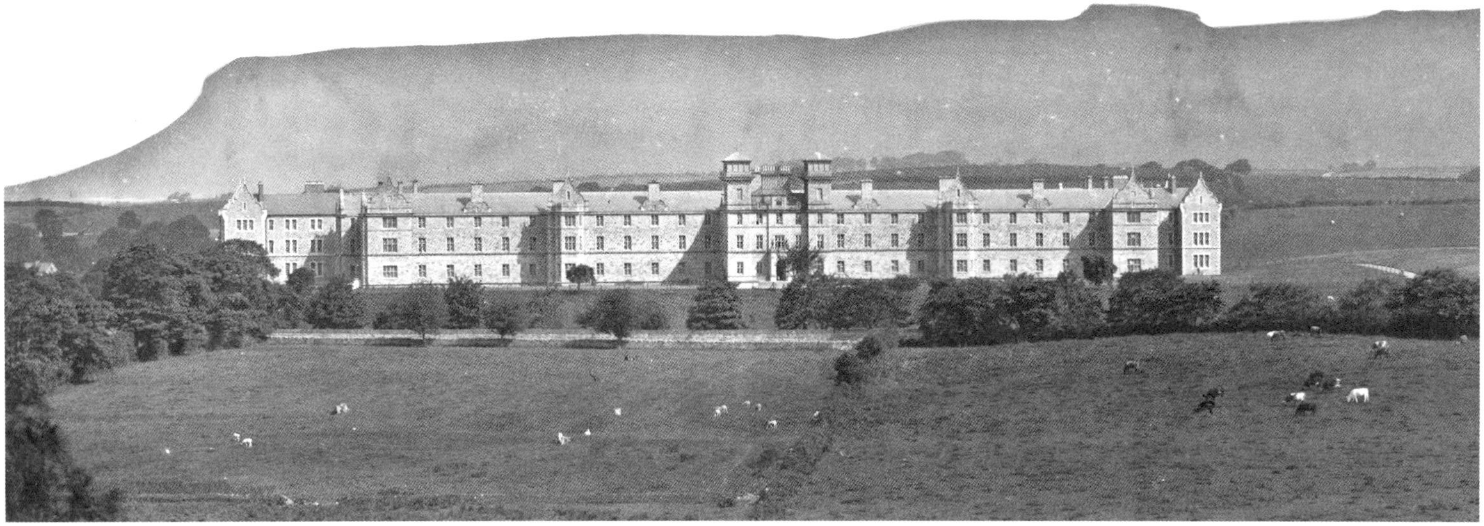

"Under bare Ben Bulben's head... an asylum stands near." *Image courtesy of the National Library of Ireland (L_CAB_05618)*

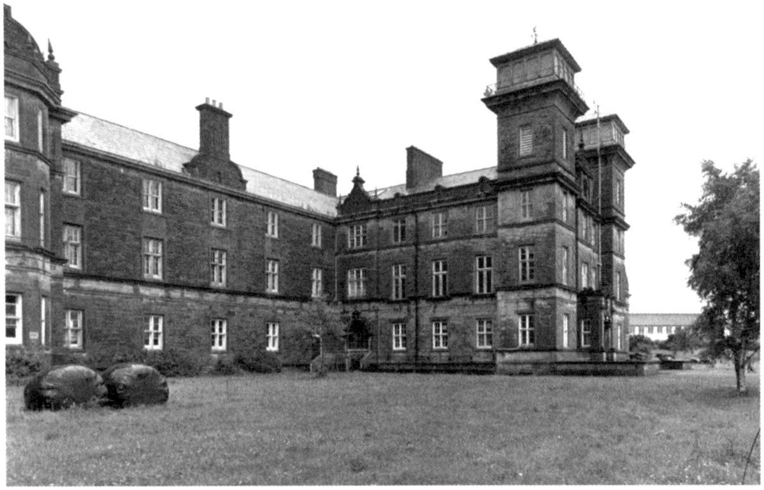

Windows stare blankly over lawns cut for silage, 1993 (above). The entire back-of-house area (below) was demolished when the asylum was redeveloped as a hotel. *Images courtesy of the Irish Architectural Archive (Photographic Collection, IAA: 072_035_CS_2_004 and 072_035_CS_3_006)*

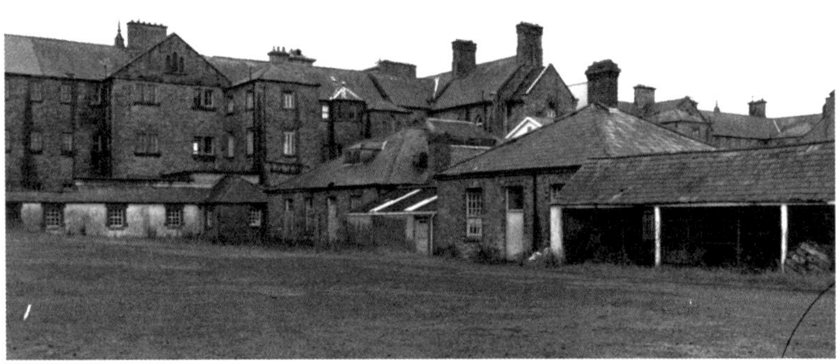

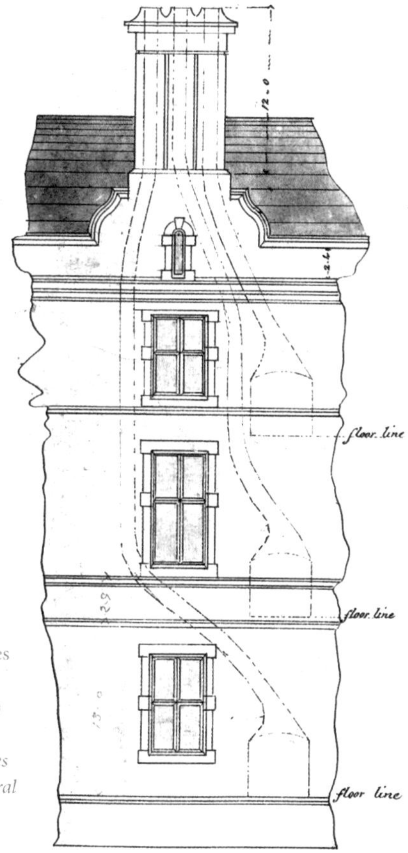

Butler's obsessive attention to architectural detail was at times counter-productive, as seen in the tortuous flue routes (right) required to achieve his facade composition (opposite). *Images courtesy of the Irish Architectural Archive (Sligo Lunatic Asylum Collection, 89/11)*

Architect Thomas Newenham Deane designed new wings for 300 patients at either end of the building, employing curvilinear gables in deference to the original design, but shunning the other embellishments that had caused so much controversy. Further improvements around the turn of the century drew lessons from the modern pavilion-echelon asylums of the era, including the addition of a ground-floor link corridor to the rear of the asylum to facilitate independent access to each ward without the need to pass through others. A pair of new chapels was completed in 1903, their symmetrical siting at opposite ends of the entrance front successfully downplaying their significant difference in scale.[7] The Catholic chapel, by Deane's son Thomas Manly Deane, is the more notable of the pair, echoing and reinterpreting many of architectural cues of the original building and crowned with a decorative flèche hardly less flamboyant than Butler's unexecuted stone spires. In a mark of the informal influence wielded by the Catholic clergy, the permission of the local bishop was originally sought in respect of its late addition to the design, albeit the local Canon eventually took the initiative and approved the change.[8]

In the early 1930s Sligo Mental Hospital would be a major beneficiary of the Irish Sweepstakes, drawing £105,215 in grants to fund a new infirmary and admissions units on the eastern portion of the site. These three buildings, designed by the partnership of McDonnell, Dixon and Downes, create a striking formal composition in their own right, a new axial approach terminating in a sheer limestone tower of strangely sinister proportions.[9] Tower aside, all three showcased the design features of contemporary sanatoria: copious areas of south-facing glazing, verandas and high-level windows to maximise cross-ventilation without exposing patients to draughts. These buildings remain in use within the mental health service at time of writing, albeit perhaps not for much longer.

In his 1990 report the Inspector of Mental Hospitals recommended the closure of the nineteenth-century building; over the course of the following year its patients transferred to the newer buildings on the site or onwards to community settings. In a series of photographs recorded in 1993, the old asylum already has the air of an abandoned country house whose once manicured lawns silently suffer the indignity of being mown for silage. Its future looked deeply uncertain, but having survived against the odds into the new millennium, the exuberance of a booming economy saw it converted into a hotel and the lands to the rear redeveloped for student apartments. Although most of Butler's more interesting interiors were lost and the entire back-of-house area was demolished, the conversion has preserved the building's most impressive external features and much of its structure while giving it a sustainable use for the foreseeable future.

References

1. *Annual Asylum Report 1844*, HC 1845 [645] xxvi, p. 78.
2. Construction cost at Sligo, excl. land and fitout: £148/patient. Strictly speaking, Dublin's New Richmond was costlier, but this reflects the consistently higher cost of construction in the capital city rather than the complexity of the building.
3. Irish Architectural Archive, Sligo Lunatic Asylum Collection, IAA: 89/11.
4. *1855 Commission Report*, HC 1856 [9] LIII.367, p. 10.
5. Ibid., pp 21–2.
6. *Seventh Annual Asylum Report 1855*, HC 1854–55 [1981] xvi, p. 15.
7. *Fifty-Second Annual Asylum Report 1902*, HC 1903 [1762] xxvii, p. 171.
8. *The Irish Builder*, 5 Jun. 1902, p. 1276.
9. *The Irish Builder*, 28 Jul 1934, p. 204; Eamon de Barra and John O'Sheehan (eds), *Oispidéil na hÉireann: Ireland's Hospitals 1933–1950* (Dublin, 1956), p. 58.

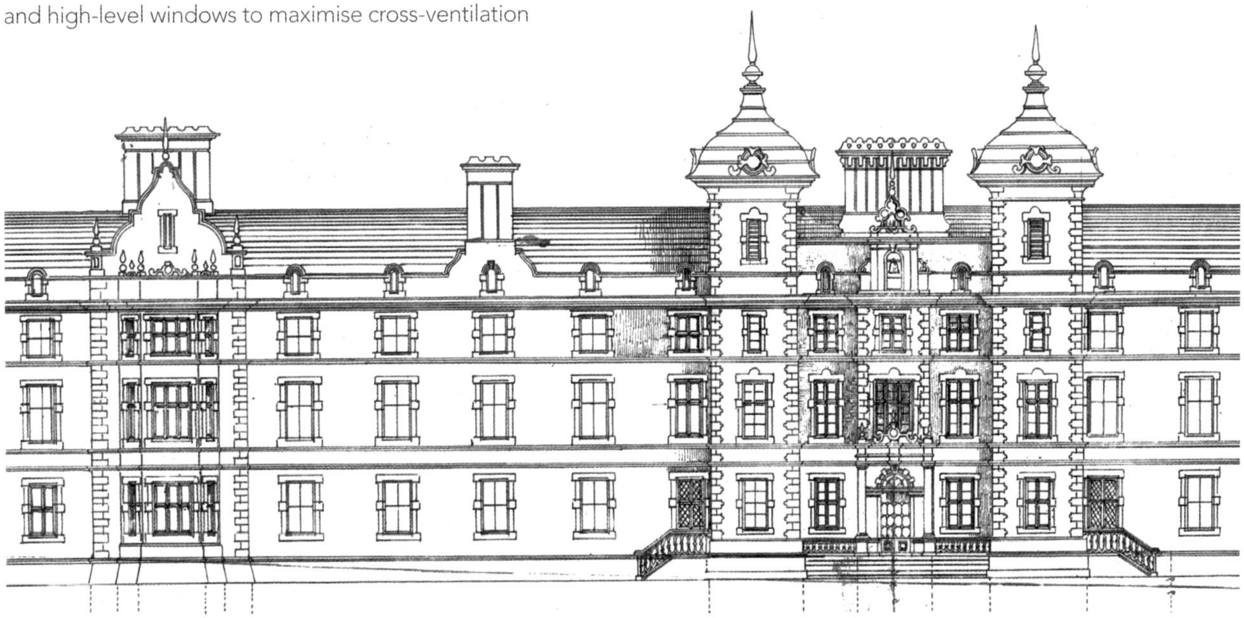

CASE STUDY 17

St Loman's Hospital

(previously Mullingar District Lunatic Asylum)

Years in operation
1855–2014

Original cost
£39,571

Capacity (min /max)
300 / 1,056

Architect(s)
John Skipton Mulvany,
William Kaye-Parry,
J. R. Boyd Barrett

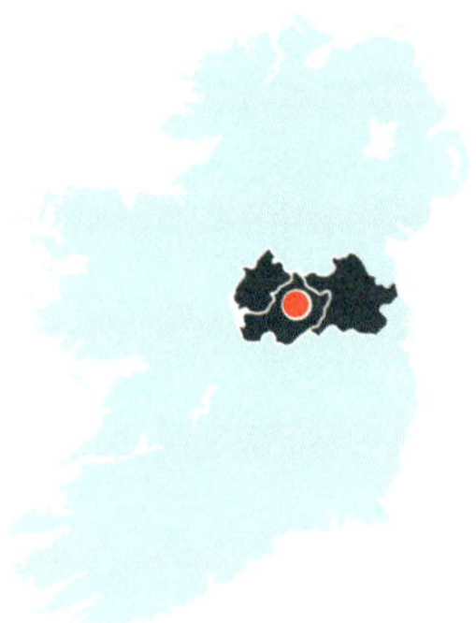

The district asylum system was a monumental bureaucracy which maintained impressive statistical records of its activities down to the most trifling detail. However, of the hundreds of thousands of people who passed through the Irish asylum system, only a tiny handful left behind any personal accounts of their experiences. Hannah Greally was one rare exception. Her story of two decades incarcerated in Mullingar still resonates powerfully down the now empty corridors of the wards she knew as 'Long Trench' and ' No Hope Hold,' depicting an institutional landscape which exercised complete control over those consigned to dwell therein.

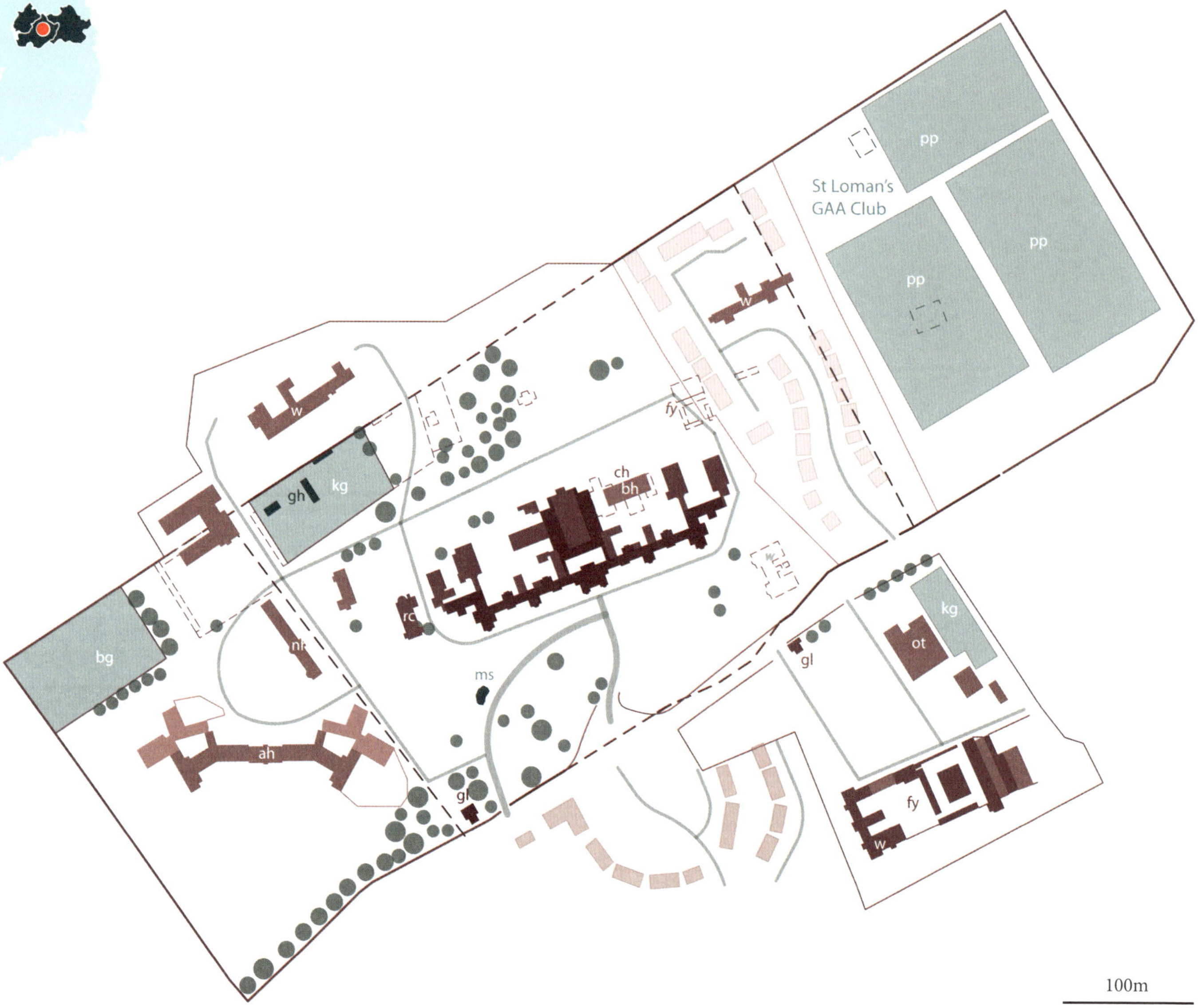

During the first phase of asylum construction, patients from Westmeath were catered for by the asylum at Maryborough. In December 1845 the Inspectors of Lunatics made recommendations for the reorganisation of asylum districts, proposing a new asylum for 500 patients at Mullingar to take patients from Westmeath, Longford, Louth and Meath – a catchment of 568,869 people – together with 50–100 acres of land to provide a 'model farm'.[1] In the event, Louth would remain part of the Richmond district and the Mullingar asylum was scaled back to 300 patients – still resulting in a building second only to Cork's Eglinton Asylum in scale. Architect John Skipton Mulvany's Tudor Revival composition represented a valiant attempt to address the design challenge of a 200-metre façade,[2] employing a variegated roofscape of gables and chimneys and a restrained application of architectural detailing including buttresses, bay windows, string courses and hood mouldings. Even so, it is the sheer scale of the building that today overwhelms all else: a gaunt cliff of dark-grey limestone not improved by a flat site and relatively meagre landscaping.

The building was completed in 1855 at a total cost of £39,571 or £132 per bed, making it the most economical of the second phase of asylums.[3] Happily for the patients, the relative parsimony did not prevent the interiors being finished to a reasonably high standard. Decorative plaster coving and attractive chimney pieces are found not only in the high-status spaces of the central block as may be expected, but throughout the bright, south-facing patient galleries and day rooms of the original building.

Mullingar's governors were relatively early to adopt the trend towards communal dining but – perhaps inhibited by horror at the impropriety of mingling of the sexes – insisted on two separate dining rooms. As mixed dining at other asylums did not presage a collapse of moral order, the governors within a decade authorised the construction of a single communal dining hall at the centre of the complex.

Roughly contemporary with the two dining halls of 1878, another pair of extensions were added to the north side of the building – large dormitories accommodating 40 beds in an open-plan layout around a central fireplace. 'Back-wards' by design, geography and perception, they stood in perpetual gloom, overshadowed by the main building and with narrow mesh-covered windows admitting 'only dim, fractional light'. It was almost certainly one of these spaces that was described by Hannah Greally as the infamous 'No Hope Hold':

> *'No Hope Hold', the chief security ward… was like the hold of a ship, with caged windows… The female padded cells were there, and other similar detention cells. The strait-jacket was used in the Hold and sedatives and other special drugs.*
>
> *You would meet there the cream of the Big House, the wild indomitable, the super eccentrics, the dreamers who no longer wanted reality. Strange, though, the pot did not call the kettle black there. It just nodded and said, 'Hello – you're sooty too'.*[4]

Liberal applications of sunshine-yellow paint and later privacy partitions utterly fail to mask the depressing character of these wards, which rank as the most inherently dismal spaces encountered by the author in any asylum in the country. In their defence, the same board of governors would go on to commission one of the brightest and most pleasant asylum chapels complete with a quirky rocket-like spire (1888), investing in electric light years earlier than most other asylums (1890) and even installing a Turkish Bath for the patients (1890). The tall chimneystack, which still dominates the bewilderingly complex back-of-house landscape, was also added around this time.

The scale of the main building having already exceeded all sensible limits, further expansion would take place in new freestanding structures. A standalone three-storey pavilion for working male patients was constructed across the road from the main holding, conveniently adjacent to the extensive asylum farmyard. Continued overcrowding in the institution – which by the turn of the century was home to 831 patients – also necessitated the erection of a 'temporary' ward building that, in common with similar buildings on other asylum sites, would become a depressingly permanent feature. On the eve of independence, Mullingar was one of four asylums in the new Free State to house over one thousand patients. The 1930s and 40s would see a sustained campaign of construction, mostly to designs of architect J. R. Boyd Barrett, including a new admissions unit inspired by the light and airy TB sanatoria of the age, and two bright new blocks for chronic patients almost identical to those designed by the same architect for Castlerea District Mental Hospital. A large, plain nurses' home completed the construction spree, whose significant costs were substantially offset by £139,310 in grants from the Irish Hospitals Sweepstakes.[5]

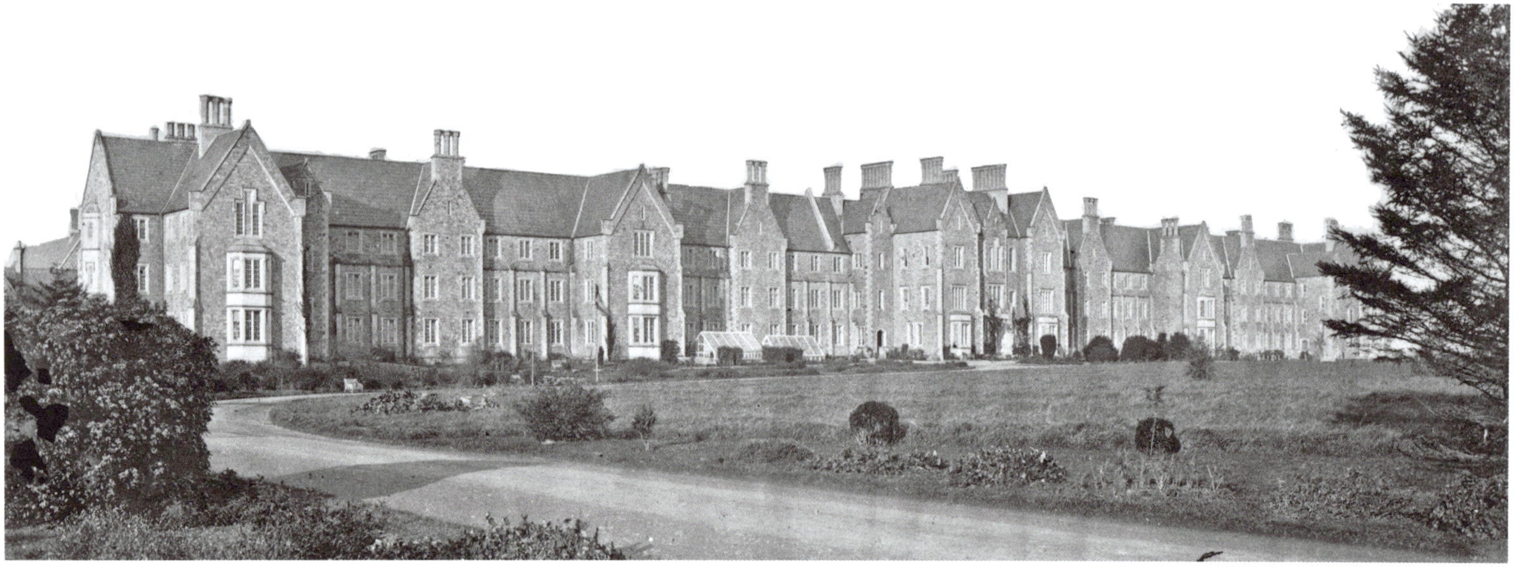

Multiple gabled breakfronts and elegant Tudor chimney stacks are insufficient to offset the scale of the Mulvany's 47 bay edifice. Also note the concentration of chimney stacks serving the administration block compared to the rest of the building. *Image courtesy of the National Library of Ireland (L_CAB_01593)*

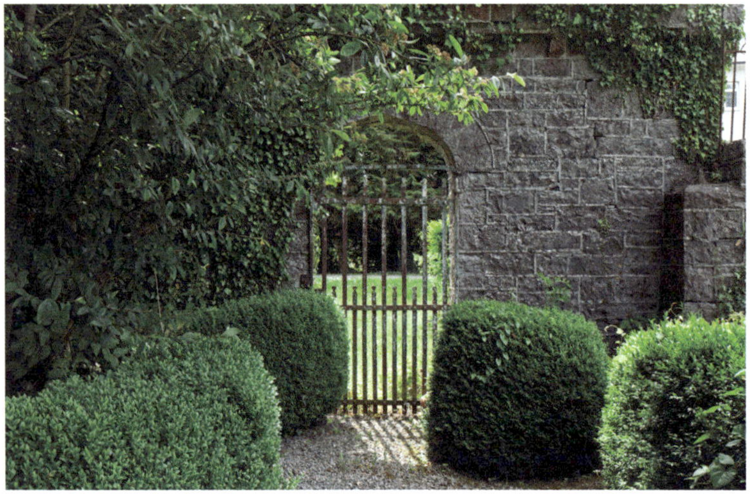

Castellated gateway to the walled garden.
Photograph by David Killeen, 2019.

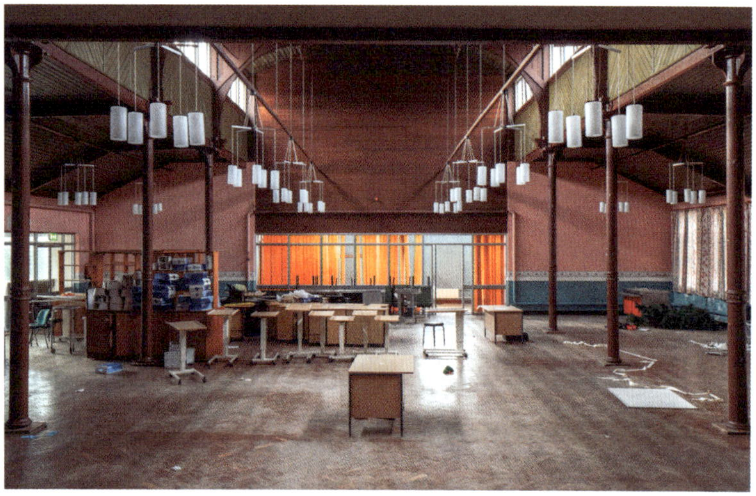

The vast central dining hall was commissioned once the governors overcame their dread of the sexes mingling at mealtimes. *Photograph by David Killeen, 2019.*

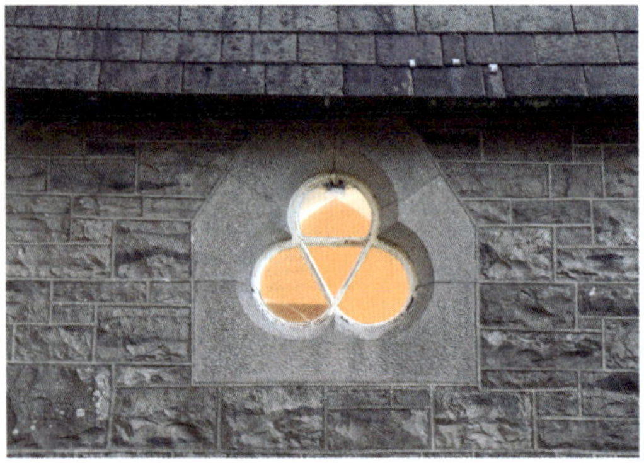

Mulvany's hand proved more adept in the finer details.
Photograph by the author, 2014.

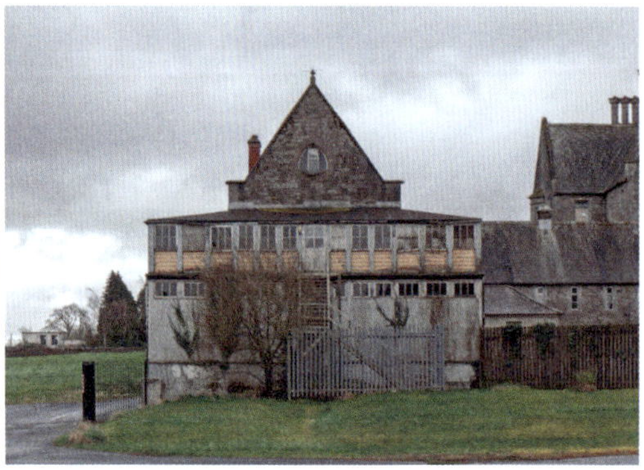

An early and rather home-made version of the TB verandah.
Photograph by David Killeen, 2019.

While the parkland landscape at Mullingar has some fine individual trees, it underwhelms compared to the scale and importance of the institution. A notable exception is the walled garden to the rear whose battlemented gateway and turrets would look more at home in the grounds of a Gothic-fantasy castle. Within the walls, glasshouses survive in a state of decay but the box hedging and paths are still maintained, offering a rare example of the sort of pleasure garden that once featured on almost every asylum site.

As wards once humming with daily life one-by-one fell silent through the later twentieth century, the enormous boiler at the heart of St Loman's Hospital continued to circulate warmth through the building's arteries, keeping the damp at bay and helping it to survive to the present day in reasonable condition. Since the departure of the last patients in December 2013 and their associated staff soon afterwards, the cavernous main building with its kilometre of corridors stands cold, empty and facing a deeply uncertain future. Hannah Greally may have felt a sense of vindication to see the end of an institution where she was involuntarily detained for almost 20 years, but the challenge of identifying and implementing sustainable and economic new uses for the building that affords us such a tangible connection with her testimony is daunting.[6]

Further Reading

Hanna Greally, *Bird's Nest Soup*, (Cork: Attic Press, 1987)

References

1. *Annual Asylum Report 1846*, HC 1847 [820] xvii, p. 52.
2. The total length comes to 230 metres, if the recessed single story infirmaries are included.
3. And the governors were awarded a further £1,715 rebate to defray the costs of excessive cut stone. *1855 Commission Report*, HC 1856 [9] LIII.367, p. 27, p. 29.
4. Hanna Greally, *Bird's Nest Soup* (Cork, 1987), p. 65, p. 79.
5. Eamon de Barra and John O'Sheehan (eds), *Oispidéil na hÉireann: Ireland's Hospitals 1933–1950* (Dublin, 1956), p. 58.
6. Unlike most other asylums, most of the valuable land in and around the hospital has already been developed for housing, alongside playing pitches for the eponymous St Loman's GAA club, which grew out of the hospital team, leaving a limited asset base from which to cross-subsidise any future regeneration.

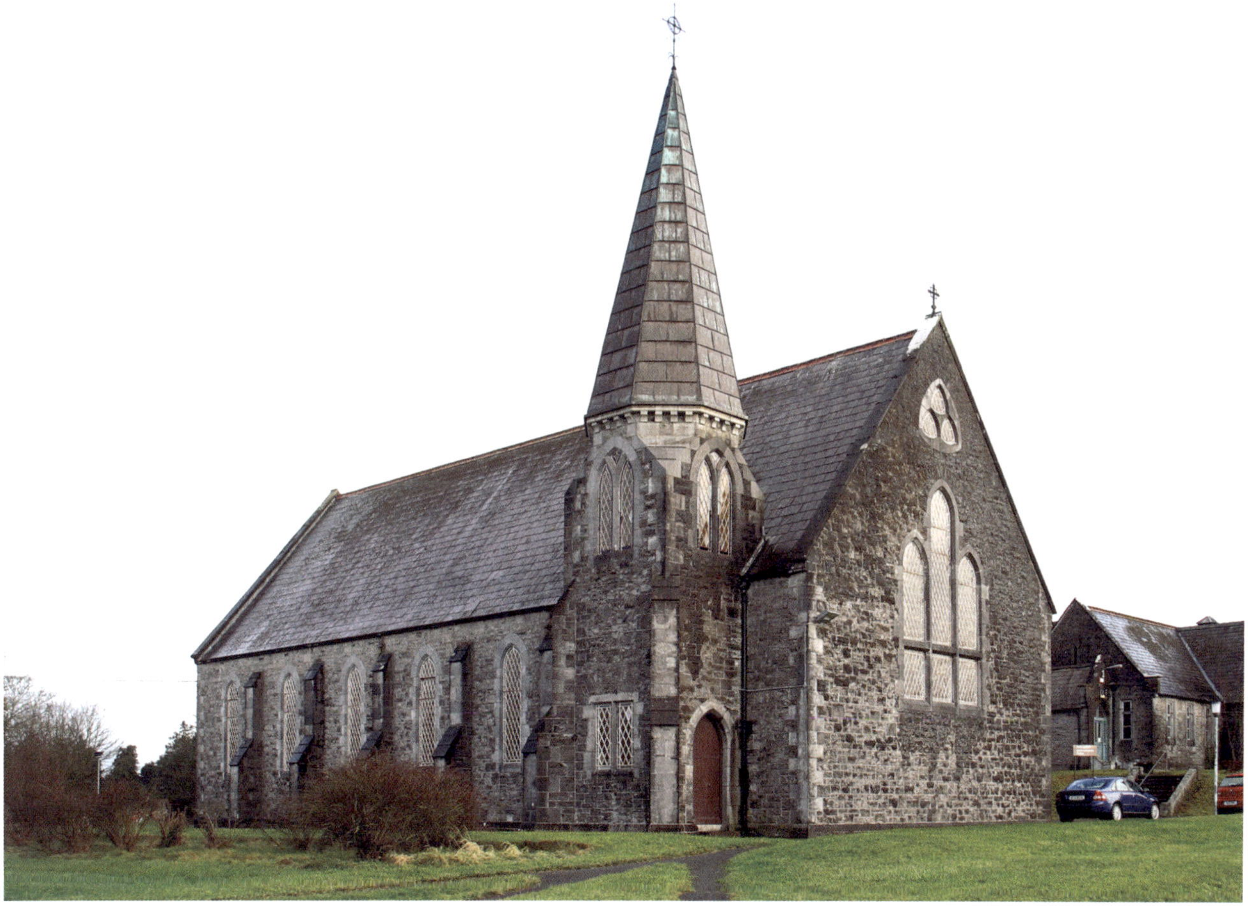

The asylum chapel was almost unique in featuring a tower and spire. *Photograph by the author, 2014.*

CASE STUDY 18

Years in operation
1865–2010

Original cost
£37,900

Capacity (min /max)
300 / 712

Architect(s)
George Wilkinson,
Charles McLaughlin

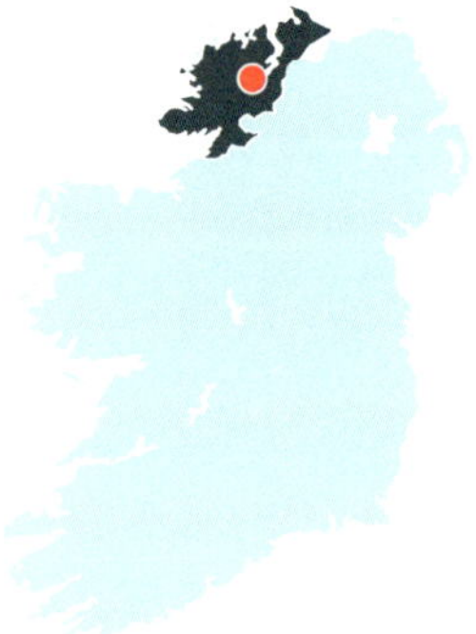

St Conal's Hospital

(previously Letterkenny District Lunatic Asylum / Tirconaill Mental Hospital)

The lunatic asylum was one of a handful of significant public buildings that acted as both an indicator and influencer of a town's relative vigour in the latter half of the nineteenth century. History shows that Letterkenny owes a double debt of gratitude to the Inspectors of Lunacy – firstly in being recommended in preference to the county town, and secondly in overcoming a grand jury sceptical about the very idea of a new Donegal asylum, despite the county 'furnish[ing] an extra average of the afflicted class for whom the Asylum is built'.[1]

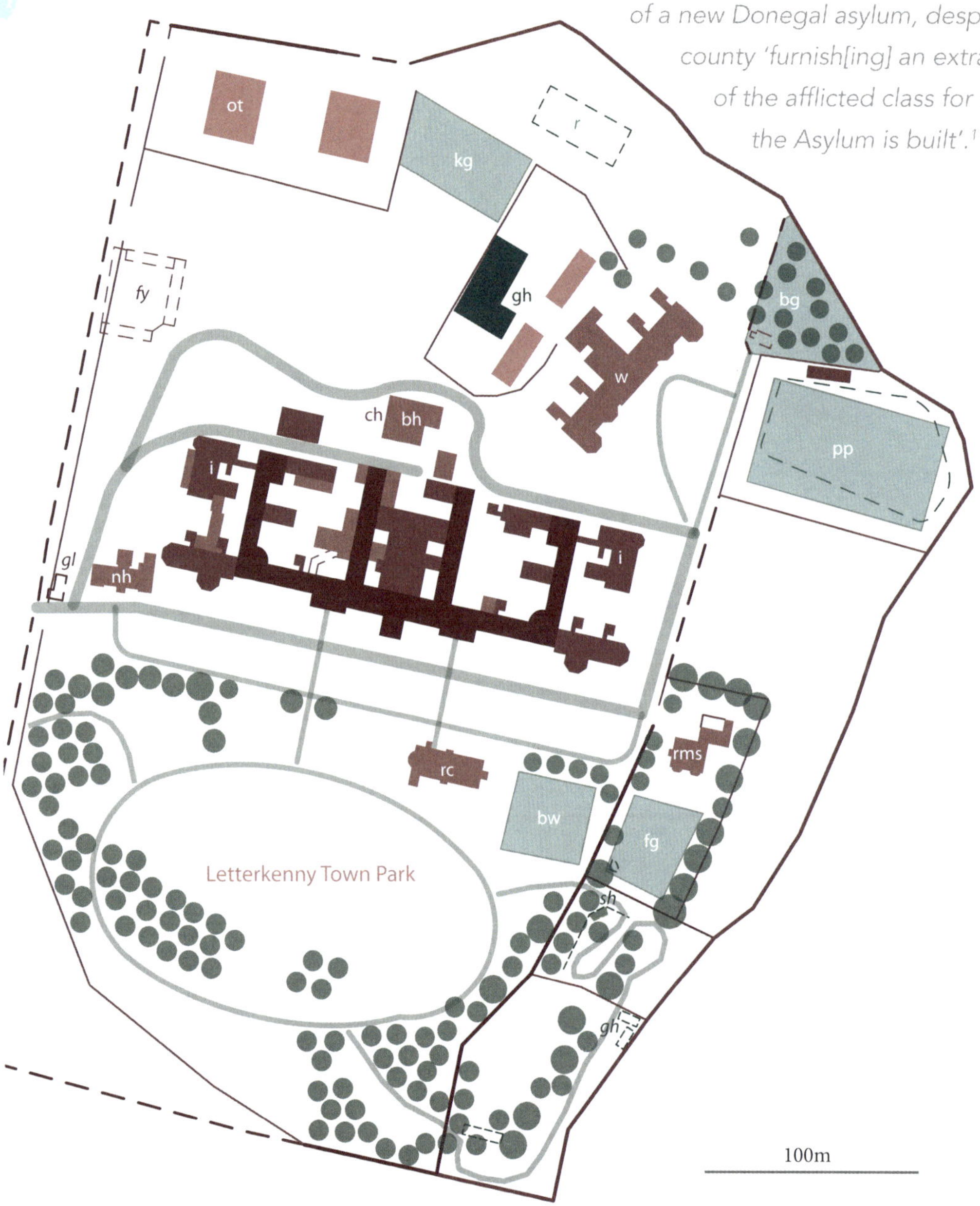

As a rare exception amongst the counties along Ireland's western seaboard, dedicated accommodation did exist for Donegal's pauper insane prior to the establishment of the district asylum system. However, the label of 'lunatic asylum' did not guarantee any particular standard of care, nor could much care be provided in eighteenth-century gaol cells in the basement of Lifford's county courthouse, which had been deemed unfit for habitation even by the prisoners for whom they were originally built.[2] The opening of the Londonderry asylum in 1829 brought Donegal patients into the new asylum system and would continue to serve the needs of the county until the 1857 Commission of Enquiry recommended the erection of a separate Donegal asylum 'at Letterkenny, or some other convenient place'.[3] With its union workhouse and fever hospital, Letterkenny was already staking its claim to urban primacy in the county. The erection of the asylum consolidated and reinforced a trend that saw the town later attract a Catholic cathedral and diocesan seminary, railway station, gasworks, and several banks and industries, while the county town of Lifford would lose its civic trappings of asylum, prison and courthouse in turn.[4]

But such benefits were as yet unforeseeable by the Donegal Grand Jury, who unusually joined their Derry colleagues in petitioning against the division of the district. Their argument was purely economic – the increased cost of sustaining two institutions in such close proximity was 'considered by the ratepayers … injurious to the interests of both counties'. Their petition to the Lord Lieutenant offered cheaper alternatives such as extending the existing Londonderry asylum or adapting workhouses to house incurables; both ideas were respectfully but firmly rubbished by the Inspectors, whose advice to the Lord Lieutenant carried the day.[5] Thus defeated, the county jurors then proceeded to battle one another over the financial settlement – the Donegal lobby seeking to 'participate… in the increased value of the site of the Derry Asylum… as building ground', the Derry brigade convincing George Wilkinson – in this instance acting as 'commissioner and valuator', that the argument was spurious as in order to realise its value as building ground 'it would be necessary to abandon the asylum and to build a new one elsewhere' at far greater cost.[6]

Notwithstanding Wilkinson's unfavourable adjudication, the reluctant Donegal jurors opted to retain his services for the design of their new asylum, perhaps unable to resist his appeal as a purveyor of no-frills buildings at cut-rate fees. Wilkinson rolled out a design almost identical to that at Castlebar (the architectural merits of which are discussed in more detail in Case Study 19, but with the rear wings raised to a third storey, which brought the total accommodation up to 300. With its rendered walls and brick dressings, Letterkenny looked more bleakly utilitarian than any asylum yet built in Ireland, but at a total cost of £37,900 for a 300-bed institution – which included the purchase of 40 acres of land – it also ranked as the cheapest on a cost-per-bed basis.[7] But internally at least, the asylum did not lack for modern conveniences. In addition to gas lighting provided by the Letterkenny Gas Company, the asylum featured a 'powerful steam engine and boiler, the operations of which pump cold and supply hot water to all parts of the building, fill the heating pipes, and give every facility for carrying out the cooking necessities'. Most impressive of all, in the eyes of the contemporary architectural press, was a warm air clothes drying closet, the likes of which 'we have never seen before.'[8]

Later extensions to the asylum closely matched the original in style and finish. The frontage was bookended by three-storey additions whose awkward mansard roofs likely concealed water tanks. Two-storey, bay-windowed additions beyond these muddled the composition further, so that when even more accommodation was needed in the opening decade of the twentieth century, it was wisely decided to start afresh by erecting a new detached block to the rear. Completed in 1906 to provide space for 200 'quiet and industrious' male patients at a time when the total number of patients topped 700, it was as large as an asylum in its own right, complete with dining hall and crowned with a cut stone cupola, the latter perhaps as a replacement for the earlier version removed from the centre of Wilkinson's building.[9]

While the Resident Medical Superintendents (RMS) who presided over the overcrowded asylums of the late nineteenth and early twentieth century may be criticised for surrendering to bleak resignation about the clinical futility of their cause, the skills they wielded to manage such highly complex organisations should not be underestimated. So when an RMS also failed in his administrative duties, the effects rippled through the institution. One of the first tasks that faced the Free State's new Inspector of Mental Hospitals was to investigate why Letterkenny's (recently renamed) Tirconaill Mental Hospital had the highest operating costs in the country – at £71 1s 2d per patient per annum, it was almost twice that of the cheapest, Castlebar, at £36 18s 2d per patient per annum.

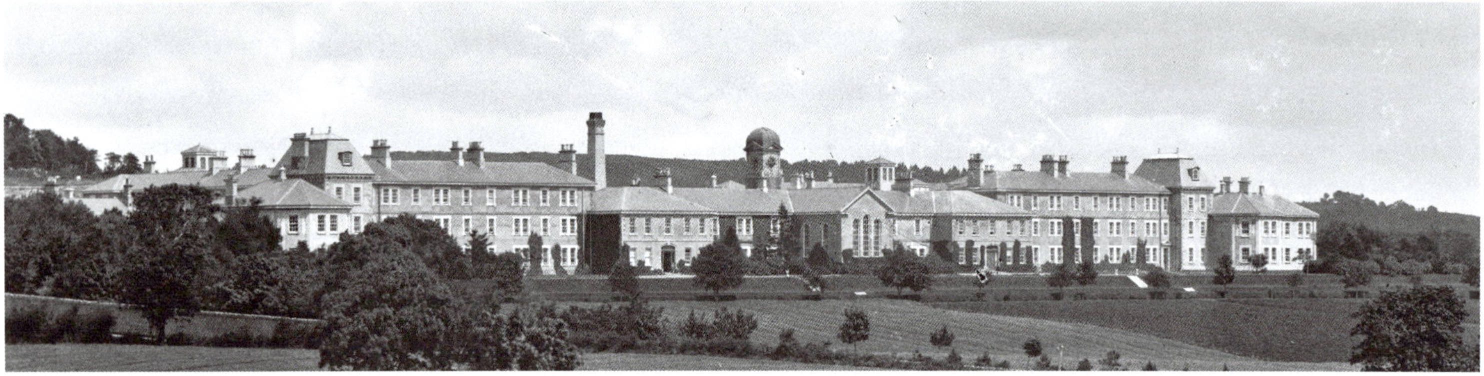

Detail of historic photograph, c. 1900, showing original disposition of central cupola over chapel. *Image courtesy of the National Library of Ireland (L_ROY_05892)*

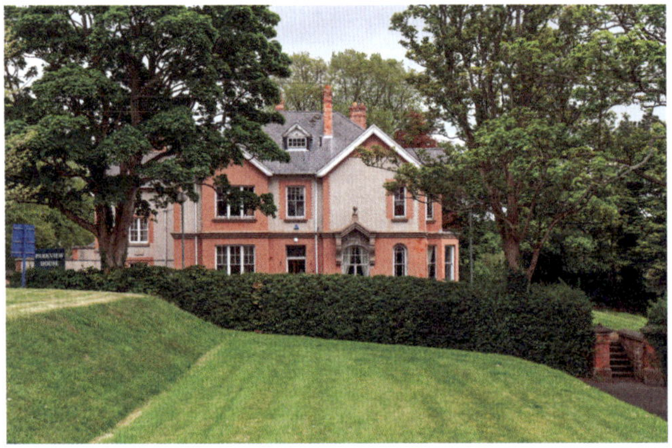

The fine residence for the RMS, like the remainder of the complex, has adapted to new uses *Photograph by David Killeen, 2019.*

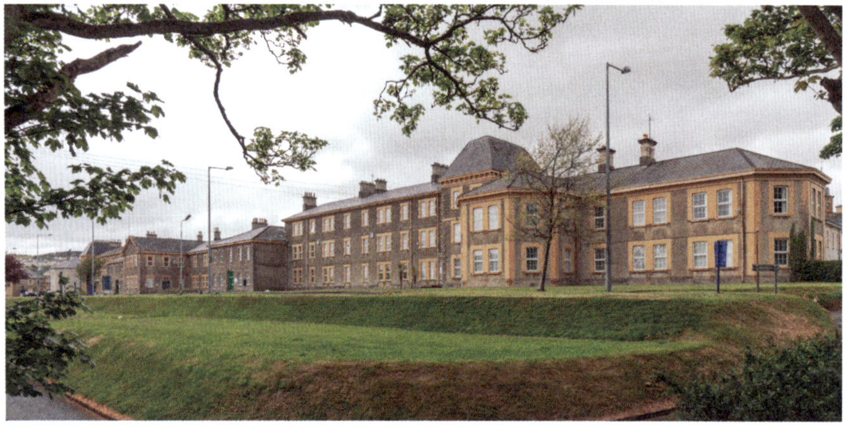

Multiple extensions in matching style make for a muddled frontage. *Photograph by David Killeen, 2019.*

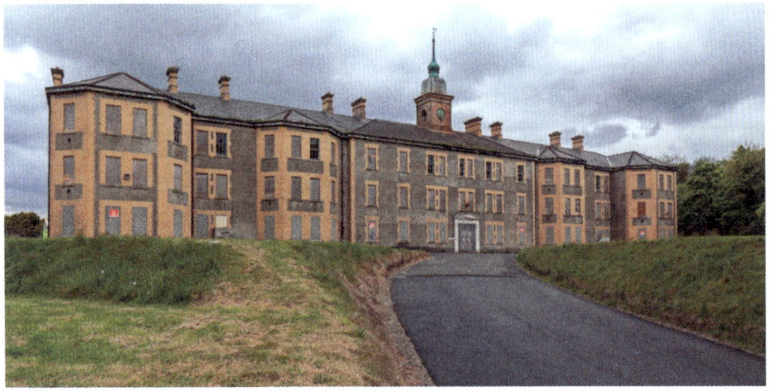

Only the detached 1906 block lies unused at time of writing. *Photograph by David Killeen, 2019.*

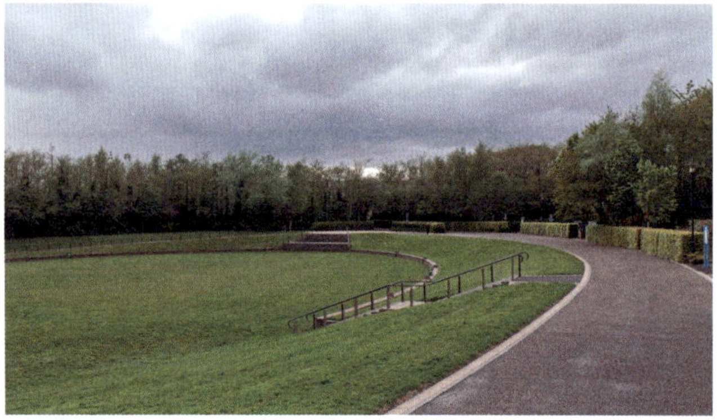

In another move worthy of wider emulation, the asylum landscape has been formally adoped as a town park. *Photograph by David Killeen, 2019.*

A sworn investigation in October 1923 revealed that 'the administration was slack to an extraordinary degree' and that the exorbitant costs in no way reflected 'a high standard of care and treatment'. The RMS and Matron duly resigned, wage cuts were sought, and despite a staff strike in April 1924, the institution slowly reverted to the mean by the end of the decade.[10]

The rest of the twentieth century saw relatively little new construction at Letterkenny as unusually, the patient population never much exceeded the 700 threshold it hit early in the century. Attention therefore shifted to staff accommodation: a new nurses' home in the 1930s and a dozen houses for married attendants in the 1940s. A Catholic chapel in the Romanesque style commandeered a prominent site in front of the asylum in the 1930s, allowing the old chapel at the centre of the main building to be converted to accommodation. The insertion of a mezzanine floor necessitated the removal of the double-height arched windows that had been the only other point of architectural interest in Wilkinson's main elevation, and there is a certain irony in the fact that the 1930s chapel, in turn, has been disfigured internally by the crude addition of a mezzanine.

That, however, is but a small criticism in the context of a place that has adapted gracefully to the changes wrought by deinstitutionalisation. As patient numbers dropped the hospital evolved to accommodate an impressive array of community and mental healthcare services. St Conal's Hospital lives on as an example of how such places can reinvent themselves to have a viable future within public health service. Meanwhile, in partnership with the local authority, the area in front of the asylum – known locally as the 'Showfield' for its historic use as a venue for the local horse show – has been reconfigured as a public park, combining the best aspects of the historic landscape with new public amenities. The residential institution may be consigned to history, but the Inspector's recommendation to locate it here, over 160 years before, continues to resonate to the benefit of the Letterkenny community.

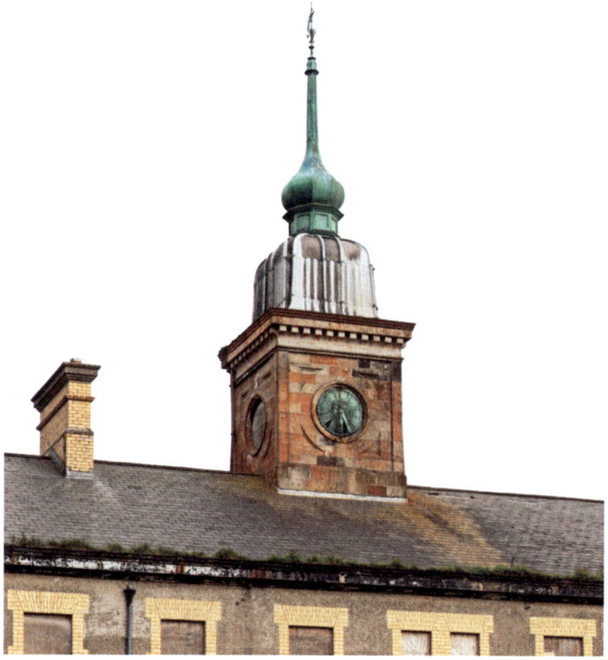

Cupola on the 1906 pavilion. Differences in detailing disprove the theory that Wilkinson's original cupola was physically disassembled and reconstructed. *Photograph by David Killeen, 2019.*

References

1. "County of Donegal Lunatic Asylum', *The Dublin Builder*, 1 Mar. 1865, p. 62.
2. *Fourth Report of the Inspectors-General of Prisons 1826*, HC 1826 [173] xxiii, p. 28.
3. The imperative for the new asylum to be located as close as possible to the geographic centre of the county also counted in Letterkenny's favour. *Tenth Annual Asylum Report 1860*, HC 1861 [2901] xxvii, p. 62.
4. Richard J. Butler, *Building the Irish Courthouse and Prison: A Political History, 1750–1850* (Cork, 2019), pp 4–8, p. 250, p. 392, pp 446–7.
5. *Tenth Annual Asylum Report 1861*, HC 1861 [2901] xxvii, pp 61–3.
6. *The Irish Builder*, 15 Nov. 1868, p. 285.
7. By way of comparison, at £126/bed (including land and fitout), this was almost half the £246/bed cost of the original Londonderry asylum. *Sixteenth Annual Asylum Report*, HC 1867 [3894] xviii, p. 22.
8. 'County of Donegal Lunatic Asylum', *The Dublin Builder*, 1 Mar. 1865, p. 62.
9. *Fifty-Fifth Annual Asylum Report 1905*, HC 1906 [3164] xxxix, p. 132.
10. *Report of the Inspector of Mental Hospitals, 1923*, p. 14; *Report of the Inspector of Mental Hospitals, 1924*, pp 16–17.

CASE STUDY 19

St Mary's Hospital

(previously Castlebar District Lunatic Asylum, latterly Galway Mayo Institute of Technology)

Years in operation
1866–2006

Original cost
£34,906

Capacity (min /max)
250 / 1,085

Architect(s)
George Wilkinson, P. J. Munden

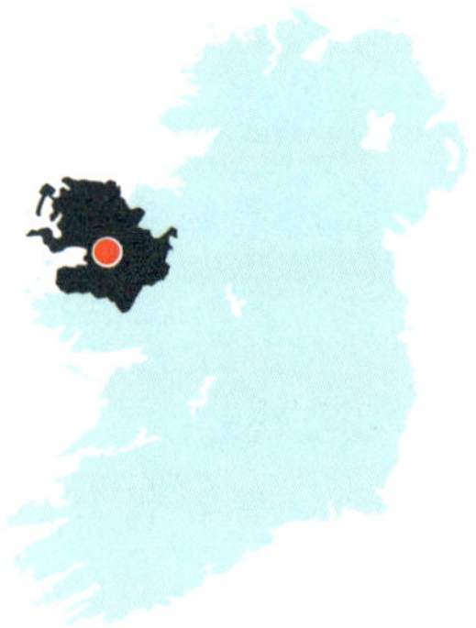

Even in their twilight years, Ireland's mental hospitals still seemed to have a life and momentum all of their own, making it hard for those who lived or worked a lifetime in them to imagine that they would one day cease to be. Today, former staff or patients who visit Castlebar must digest not only the demise of their institution, but also the startling transformation of the spaces they knew into a third-level campus that positively buzzes with life and promise.

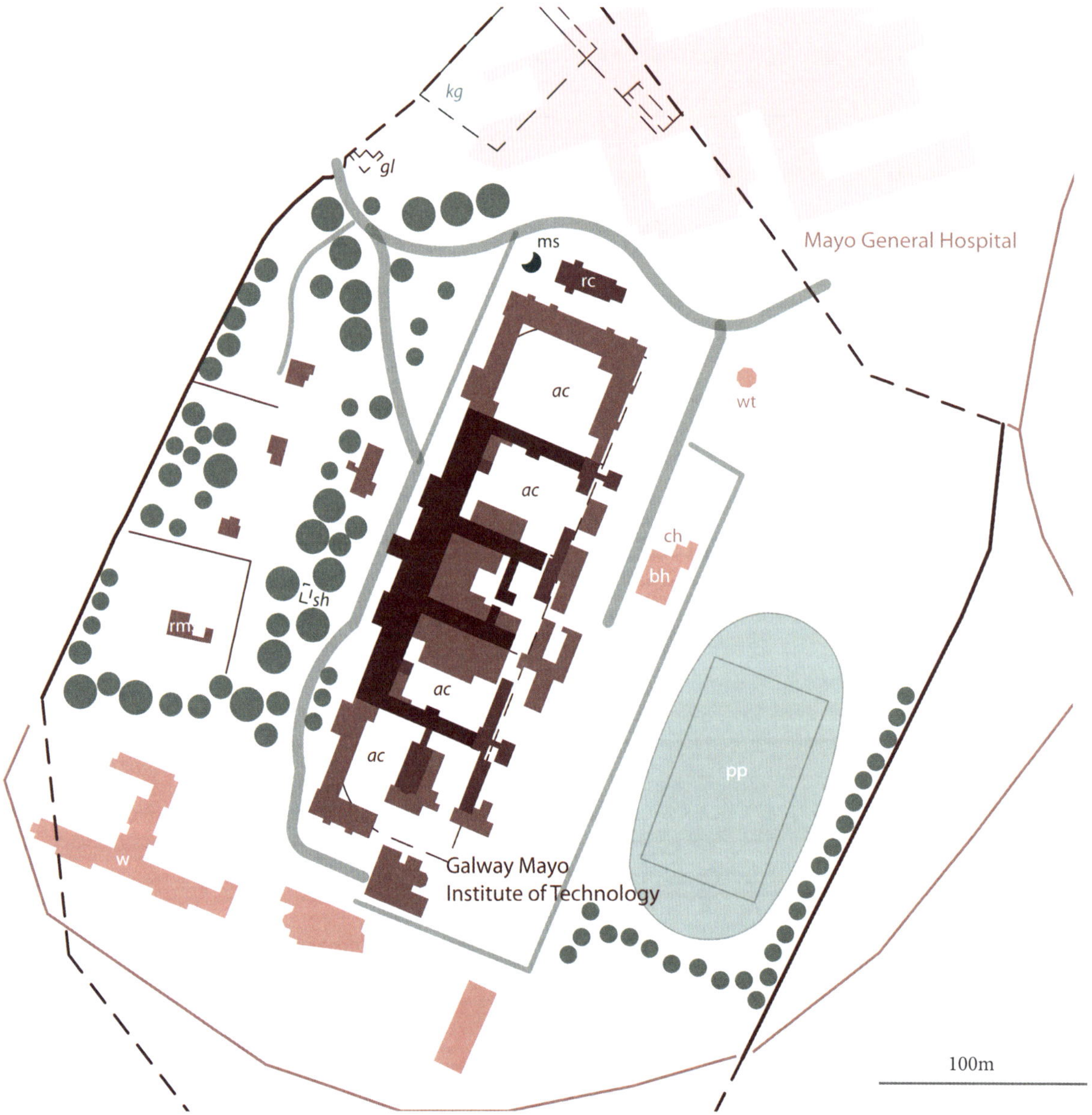

For the first two decades of the asylum system, the entire province of Connaught was served by a single asylum at Ballinasloe – necessitating a difficult journey of over 100 miles for some Mayo patients in an era when the rail network was still far from fully developed. In 1846 the Inspectors debated the merits of new asylums for both Mayo and Sligo, but while Sligo's new asylum was authorised in 1846 and opened in 1855, the Mayo proposal quietly languished.[1] It took the report of the 1858 Commission of Inquiry to resurrect the idea of providing a separate asylum for Mayo, to be located at Castlebar.[2]

In readiness for the predicted third phase of asylum expansion, the newly reconstituted Board of Control employed George Wilkinson – architect of Ireland's workhouse system – and offered local Grand Juries the option to retain his services for a fee. Mayo was one of only two counties to engage Wilkinson's services rather than select their own architect. The resulting building for 250 patients was completed in 1866 for a cost of £34,906, including land purchase, professional fees, furniture and fittings, and is essentially identical to Wilkinson's design for the asylum at Letterkenny – and almost as lacking in architectural distinction.

Wilkinson's main innovation was to provide a separate entrance for the male and female sides of the institution, with an understated chapel in the central position more typically occupied by the administration block and officers' quarters. Compositionally, the building is mediocre, with only the dressed limestone finish giving some sense of civic quality. But as seen by prospective patients, the domestic scale and informal character of Wilkinson's entrance blocks may have had the important benefit of making the admissions process a little less intimidating.

Within a decade of opening, the need for additional accommodation saw the Board of Governors approve the construction of a new infirmary and the conversion of part of the stables into a hospital for infectious diseases. Further works in the 1880s and 1890s included a boiler house and chimney, improved laundry and an observation ward. A detached Catholic chapel was added in 1903, a facsimile in blue limestone of the yellow sandstone version designed by W. G. Doolin for Clonmel Asylum in 1890, while the RMS was granted new detached lodgings around the same time. Plans for ambitious expansion were prepared by the architect R. M. Butler in 1914, but were thwarted by the upheaval of the subsequent decade. Later proposals to convert the adjacent disused prison to provide additional asylum accommodation were also fortunately shelved – that such an approach was even considered reflects how far the asylum system had fallen from the lofty ideals on which it was founded.[3] The old gaol – or at any rate its masonry – would ultimately be pressed into service, recycled into the long-awaited extensions designed

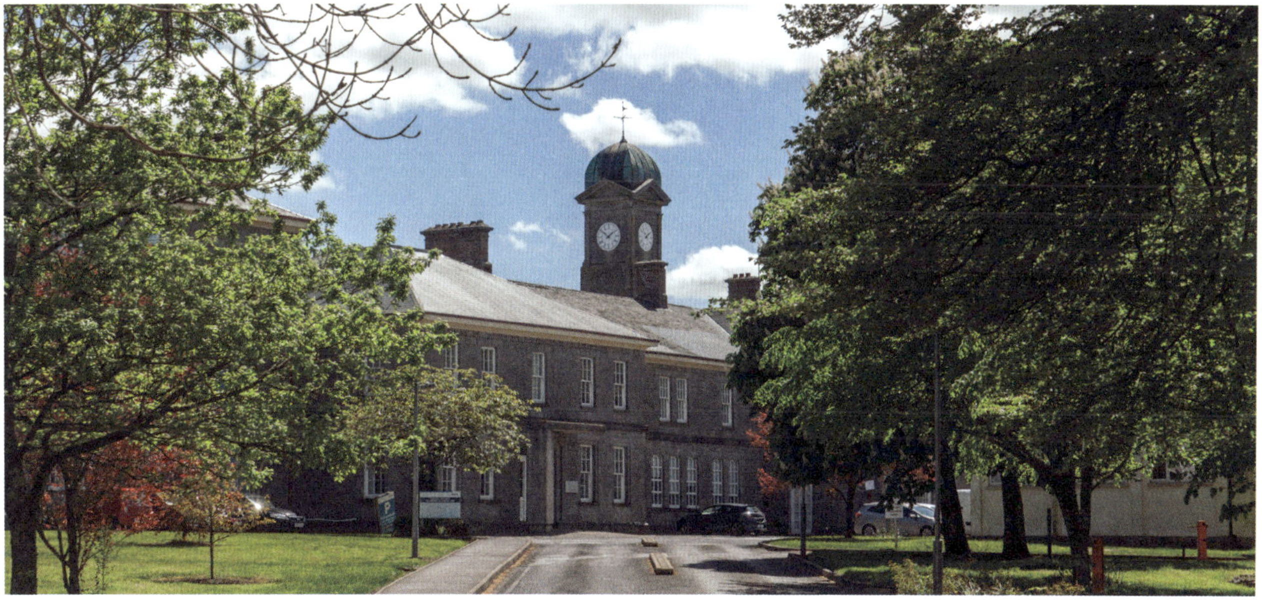

Attractive parkland, well worked limestone and the retention of the original cupola make Castlebar a far more appealing building than its twin at Letterkenny.
Photograph by David Killeen, 2019.

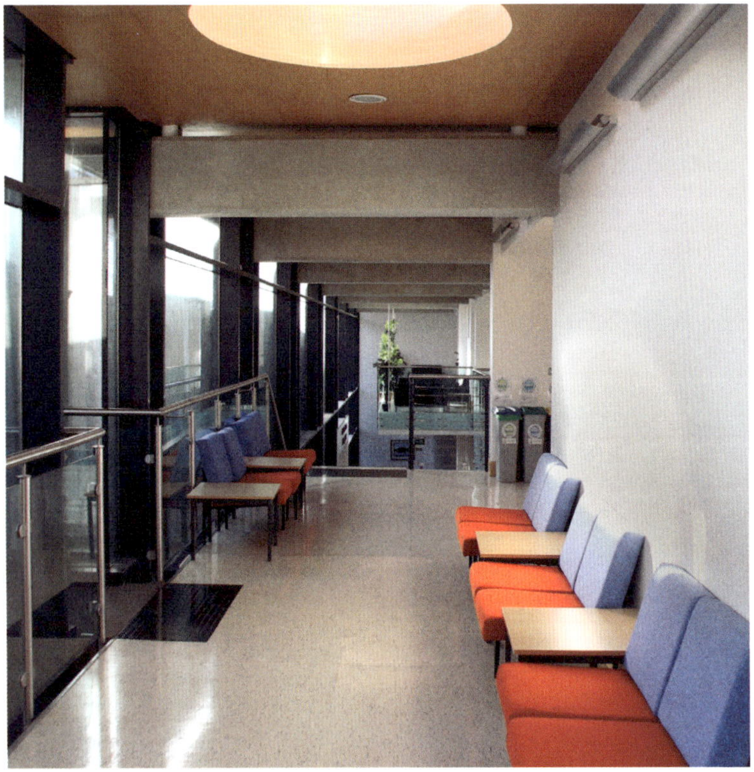

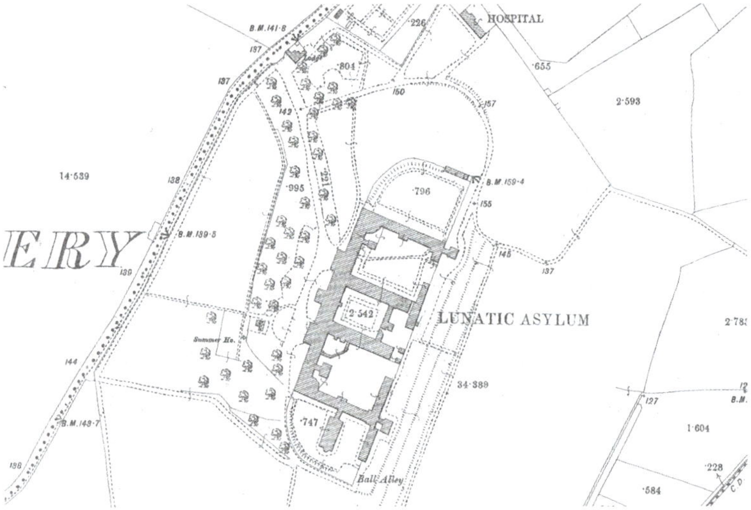

The asylum in its setting around the turn of the century (above).
Reproduced courtesy of Trinity College Dublin (OS-Mayo-2500-Sheet 78:13-1898)

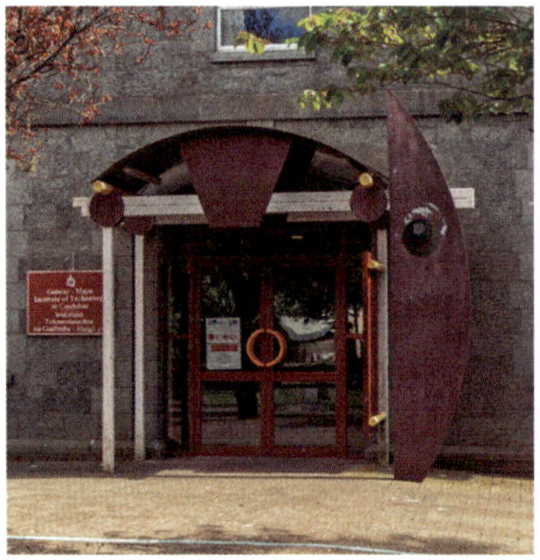

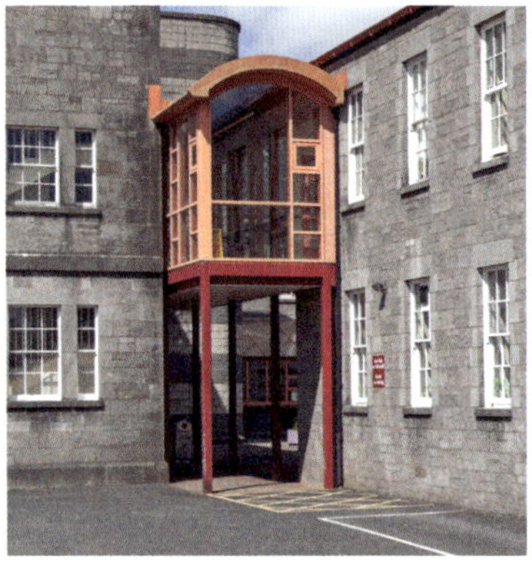

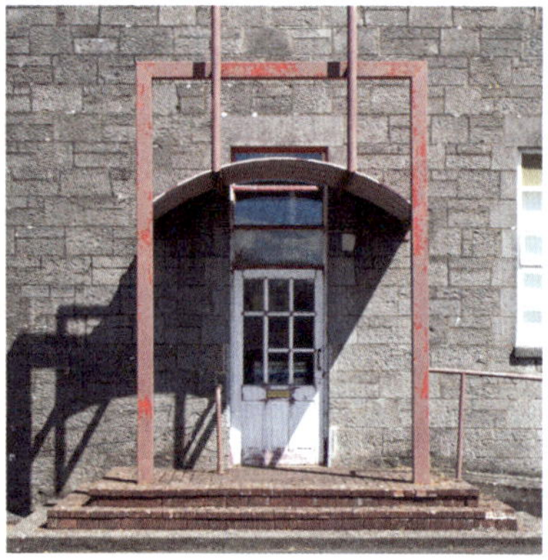

Modern interventions to serve new educational uses make a bold statement, but the historic buildings seem to wear them comfortably.
Photographs by David Killeen, 2019, and the author, 2014.

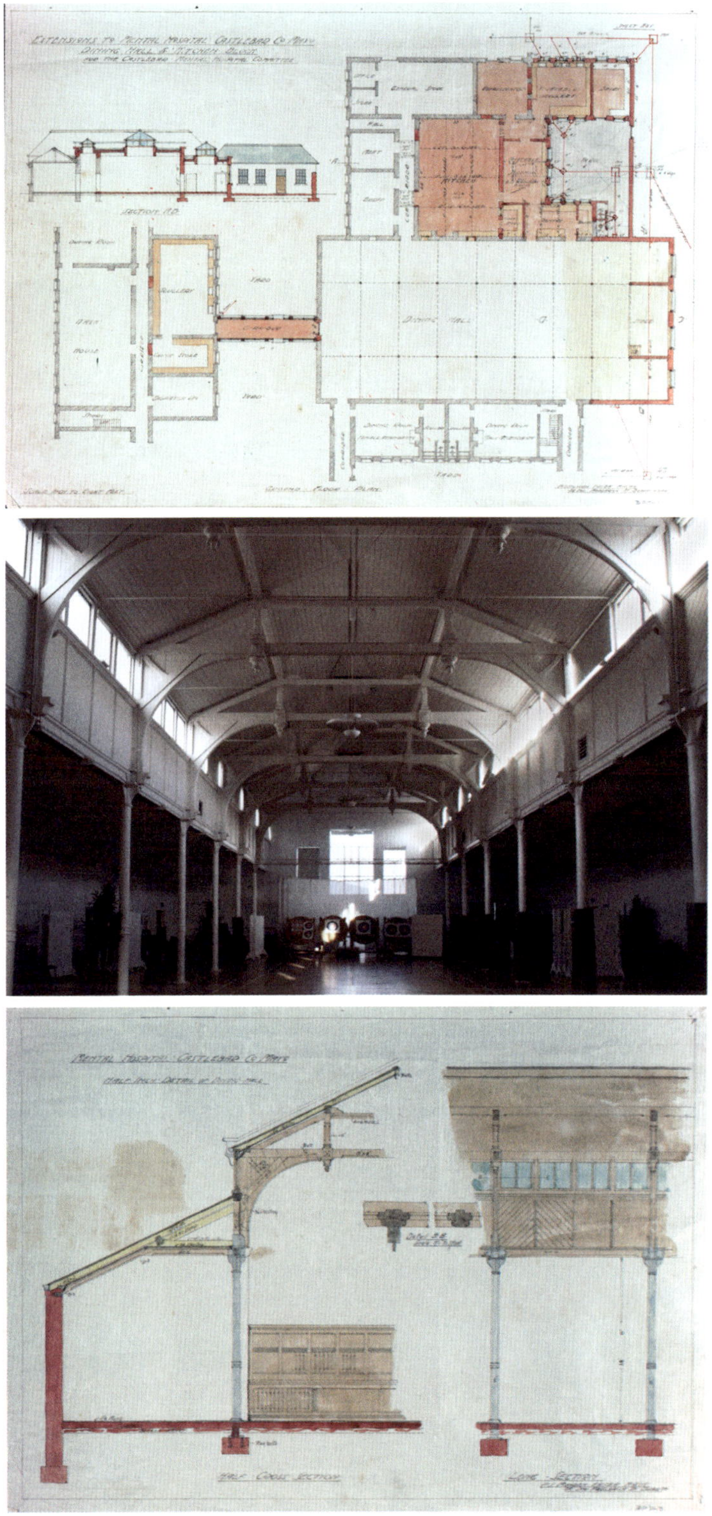

The main dining hall of the asylum was extended in the 1930s, and today hosts a far wider variety of functions than its designers could have imagined. *Images courtesy of the Irish Architectural Archive (2017/24: 01,03), photograph by the author, 2014.*

by architect P. J. Munden.[4] Completed in 1936 at a cost of £75,798, the three-storey wings at either end of the main frontage extended the total length of the building to over 250 m – longer than Mullingar and not much less than the record-holder, Cork. Two further wings extending perpendicularly to the rear resulted in a layout akin to a six-armed letter 'E'. The addition of a pair of two-storey pavilions identical to Wilkinson's original entrance blocks also complicated the legibility of the building, which now featured four identical 'front doors' with no obvious hierarchy between them. Indeed, it was a feature of this building that the style, material and detailing of each phase of expansion matched the original so closely that even the trained eye struggles to discern the phases.

As elsewhere, the demolition of the boundary walls was a seminal moment. This would be followed shortly thereafter by the construction of a new canteen in 1962 that was open to the public and which hosted a branch of the Mayo County Library until 1982.[5] In 1994 the south-west wing of the building was repurposed as a campus for the Galway Regional Technical College – latterly the Galway Mayo Institute of Technology – which has continued to expand into spaces vacated by the mental health service. The former dining and recreation hall can now add examinations and archery to its repertoire, while the buzzing student canteen occupies the old 'refractory' ward that was once home to the most disturbed patients – a transformation that remains remarkable to those who recall the equally cacophonous but far less joyous tumult of its former use. Those spaces not yet commandeered for education have served a variety of clinical functions associated with the adjacent general hospital, while the former chapel marries both uses in its recent adaptation as a medical education centre. Architecturally speaking, the buildings at Castlebar were never more than mediocre, but its recent history as one of Ireland's best examples of adaptive re-use makes it an exemplar to which other sites might aspire.

Further Reading

Joe McDermott, *St Mary's Hospital Castlebar: Serving Mayo Mental Health from 1866* (Castlebar, Western Health Board, 1999)

References

1. *Annual Asylum Report 1844*, HC 1845 [645] xxvi, p. 78.
2. *1858 Commission Report*, HC 1857–58 [2436-I] [2436-II], p. 24.
3. *The Irish Builder*, 5 Jan 1918, p. 5.
4. *The Irish Builder*, 18 Nov. 1933, p. 998; Joe McDermott, *St Mary's Hospital Castlebar: Serving Mayo Mental Health from 1866* (Castlebar, 1999) p. 33.
5. Ibid., p. 34.

CASE STUDY 20

Our Lady's Hospital

(previously Ennis District Lunatic Asylum)

Years in operation
1868–2002

Original cost
c. £35,000

Capacity (min /max)
260 / 674

Architect(s)
William Fogerty
with A. C. Adair,
P. J. Sheahan

By the third wave of asylum construction, architectural bravado had surrendered to technical pragmatism. This shift is evident at Ennis, where a central block dressed in outdated late-Georgian attire is flanked by patient wings of distinctly barrack-like appearance. But behind the unremarkable façade at Ennis stands a complex structure that employed some of the most modern technologies of its day to address the myriad challenges of accommodating ever-increasing numbers of patients under a single roof.

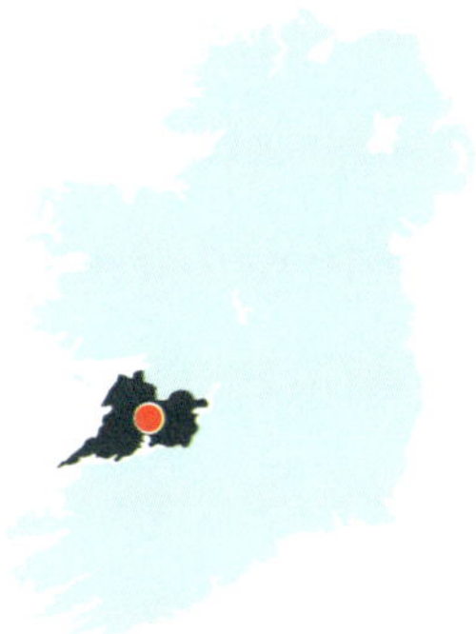

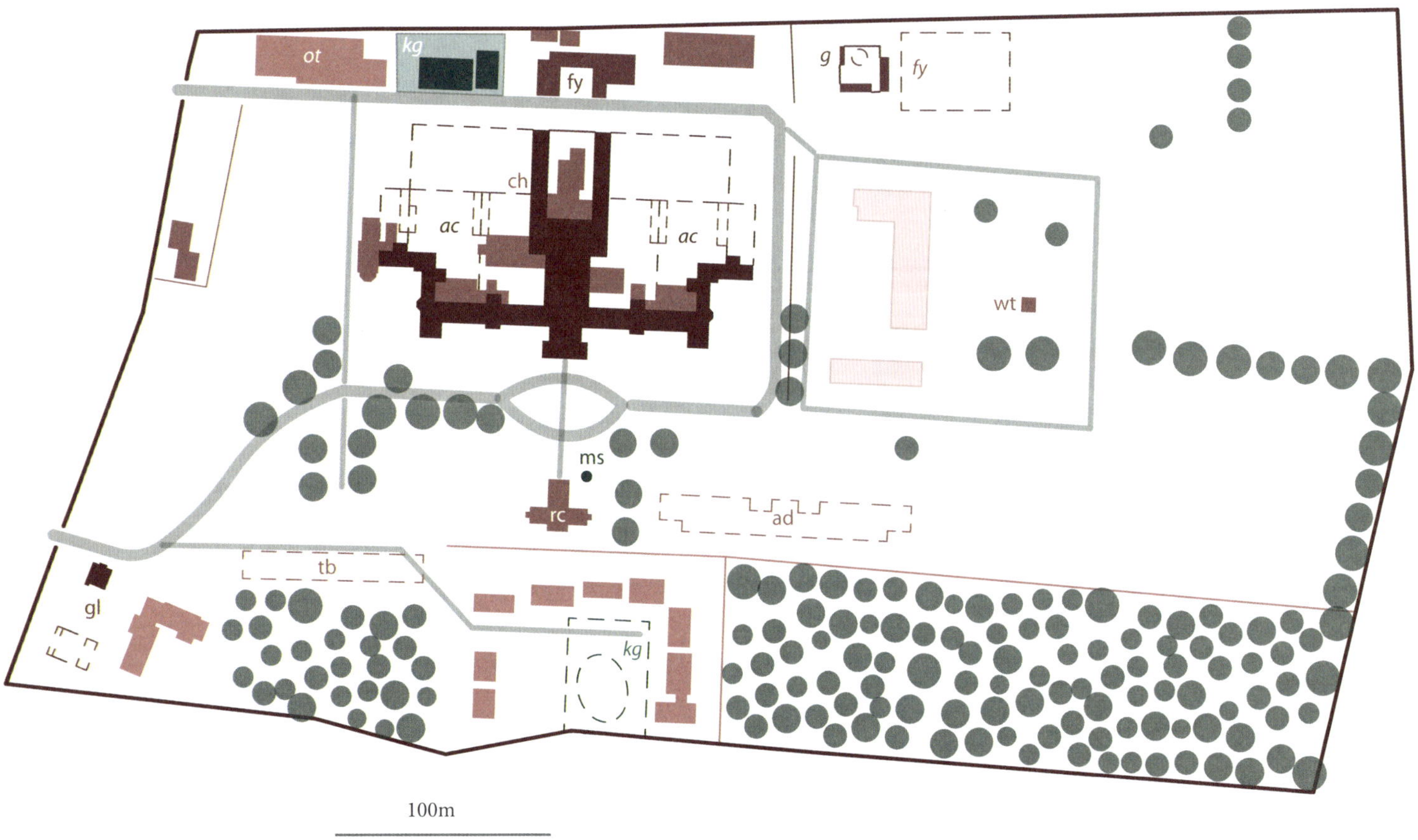

The report of the 1858 Commission recommended the separation of Counties Clare and Limerick into separate districts, facilitated by the construction of a new asylum at Ennis. A site north of the town was selected for 'its salubrity… its command of cheerful scenery, and its convenience to the main road of the county'. Proximity to a branch of the River Fergus was no small advantage, allowing a supply of water to be drawn, via steam-powered pump, to tanks atop the building's three water-towers.[1]

Opened to patients in 1868 at a cost in the region of £35,000, the list of pragmatic considerations to be addressed by architect William Fogerty was a long one, informed by a half-century of trial and error in asylum design and operation, as well as the pursuit of economies in construction and administration. The three floors of patient accommodation would thus be principally disposed as large dormitories and dayrooms. Shortcomings in thermal comfort and ventilation so common in older asylums were to be resolved by supplying warm air to each space from heating apparatuses in each wing, while stale air would be extracted via galvanised iron ducts driven by the up-draught from large fireplaces in the side-towers.[2] Whether either system proved effective in practice seems dubious; by at least one account open fires were still in use on wards into the 1980s.[3] A more resilient feature was the laundry drying closet, an innovation that would prove invaluable on a site subject to rainfall on more than 240 days every year.

Such ambitious mechanical systems needed a copious supply of fuel, so the plans included a yard for 500 tons of coal, to 'enable the Governors to obtain coal on much better terms, by taking the supply for the year at once'. Coal was also employed in the asylum's own gasworks, which allowed the entire building to be lit with gas manufactured on the premises and thus avoided the problems encountered elsewhere with unreliable town gas supplies.[4]

Other out-offices included a range of farm buildings, houses for the gardener and steward, and a dedicated 'stable for the board of visitors'. While the latter might initially seem like a self-serving extravagance, it was no less essential in an era of horse-powered transport than a visitor's car-parking space today.

Expectations for landscape design were also high. In their first inspection after opening, the Inspectors noted that five acres of potatoes and six acres of oats had been planted, but criticised the fact that 'no walks have yet been laid out through the grounds. The latter are still in a backward state as regards ornamental cultivation.' The following year they were pleased to report that £100 had been expended on ornamental plants – by way of context, such a sum equated to the annual maintenance costs for five patients.[5] The Ennis governors seem to have displayed a preference for imported evergreen species – still something of a horticultural novelty in the west of Ireland in the 1860s, but whose dense canopies today make for a rather gloomy setting.

In its day the character of the main building was described as 'simple and bold… [which] suits very well for works of the class'.[6] The emphasis on practicalities at the expense of architectural treatment was a sensible reversal of earlier priorities, but the dour architectural treatment did not go unnoticed. Author Kate Millett described her experience of involuntary confinement at the hospital in the 1980s thus:

> *'But when we get there, it is a barracks, a gaol. A gray Bastille lit by institutional police state lamps. My heart sinks… enter here and you are buried alive. The harsh light by the stone entranceway, the grey stretches of institutional pile… The malign intent of the place is clear; its detail is hazy.'*[7]

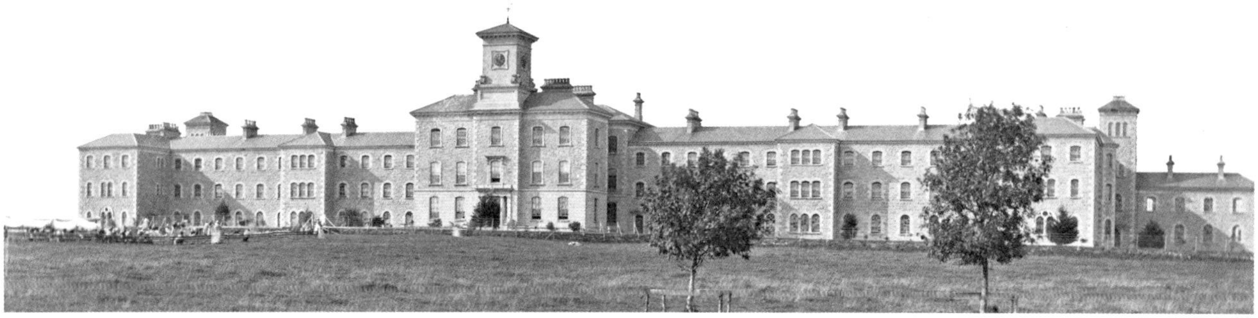

Image courtesy of the National Library of Ireland (L_ROY_04181)

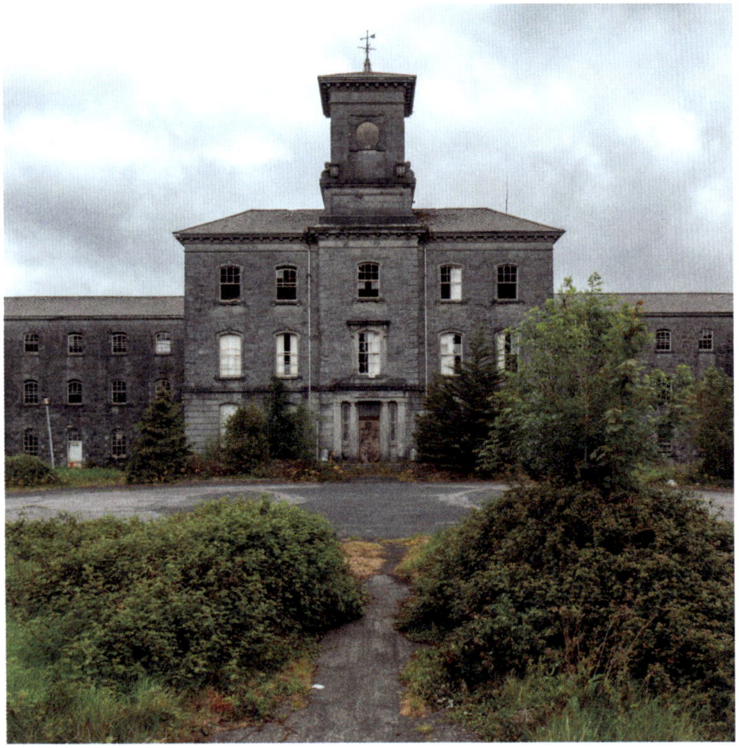

The asylum today stands as a monument to the failure of successive owners to secure a viable new use. *Photograph by David Killeen, 2019.*

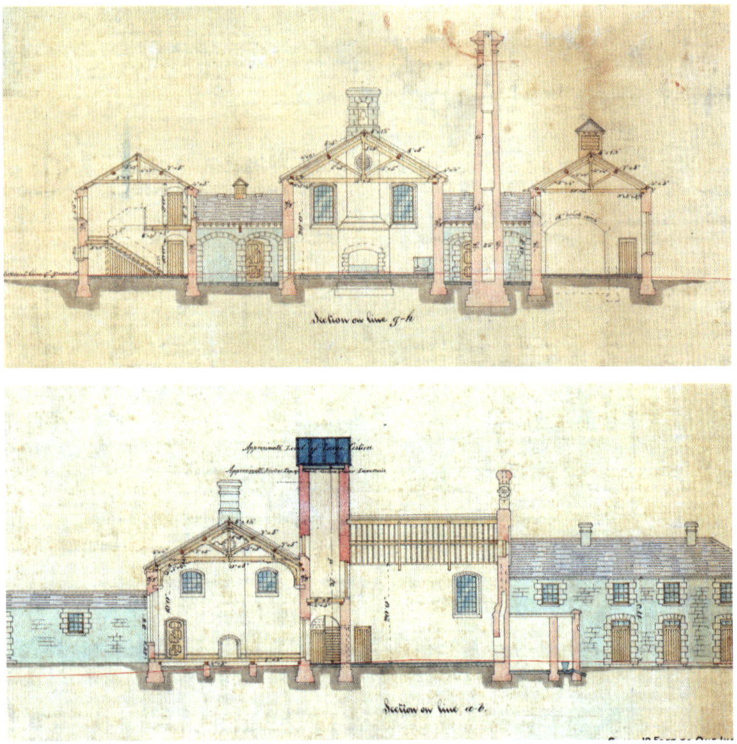

Behind an uninspired facade lay a complex of considerable technical innovation. *Images courtesy of the National Archives of Ireland (Office of Public Works Collection, OPW/5/HC/4/800, 14)*

Beyond a lopsided westerly extension and the addition of ungainly mansard roofs to the two-storey wings, the grey institutional pile would change relatively little throughout its existence. The most significant developments came in the early 1940s with the construction of a new cruciform chapel on axis with the main entrance, flanked by detached pavilions housing an infirmary, admissions unit and nurses' home.[8] Designed by architect P. J. Sheahan and substantially funded by the Sweepstakes, their useful life would be short: all but the chapel would be demolished as the hospital wound down towards final closure and eventual sale in 2002.

The peripheral lands passed to Shannon Development for the creation of a digital park for Ireland's designated 'Information Age' town. The main building languished for a decade before a private developer property secured planning permission to reuse the building as part of a private healthcare development in 2013.[9] A project that would have been ambitious even during the heady days of the Celtic Tiger was never realistic given the economic realities of the financial crisis and shifting government policies around private hospitals. Since then the building has continued to stand empty and successive owners have made little effort to secure it. With nothing more than the intercession of a forlorn statue of Our Lady standing between it and destruction at any time of the vandals' choosing, at the time of writing the building is once again on the market. Whether the future holds salvation or destruction remains to be seen.

Further Reading

Kate Millett, *The Loony-Bin Trip* (New York: Simon and Schuster, 1990)

References

1. 'Clare County Lunatic Asylum', *The Dublin Builder*, 15 Mar 1866 pp 71–2.
2. Ibid.
3. In her account of an involuntary stay at Ennis in the mid 1980s, author Kate Millett makes repeated references to gathering around an open fire in the dayroom, albeit in the context of a stream-of-consciousness narrative that is not always fully grounded in reality. Kate Millett, *The Loony-Bin Trip* (New York, 1990) pp 233-6.
4. *Seventeenth Annual Asylum Report 1868*, HC 1867–68 [4053] xxxi, pp 16–17.
5. Ibid., p.17; *Eighteenth Annual Asylum Report 1869*, H.C. 1868–69 [418] xxvii, pp 19–20.
6. 'Clare County Lunatic Asylum', *The Dublin Builder*, 15 Mar. 1866 pp 71–2.
7. Albeit Millett's life circumstances as an internationally famous and well-travelled academic, artist and feminist author, with past experience of admission to American asylums, mark her as quite unrepresentative of the average West of Ireland patient! Millett, *The Loony-Bin Trip*, p. 193.
8. *The Irish Builder*, 2 Oct. 1937, p. 882; *Report of the Inspector of Mental Hospitals, 1943*, p. 19.
9. Clare County Council planning reference no. 1221033, www.eplanning.ie/ClareCC/AppFileRefDetails/1221033/0, accessed on 6 Dec. 2020.

CASE STUDY 21

St Senan's Hospital

(previously Enniscorthy District Lunatic Asylum)

Years in operation
1868–2013

Original cost
c. £40,000

Capacity (min /max)
288 / 545

Architect(s)
James Bell with
James Barry Farrell,
C. A. Owen

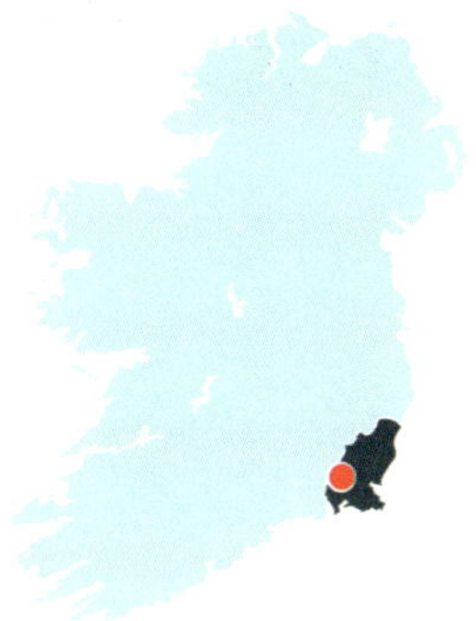

Sometimes, a building is so exceptional in its setting that local lore evolves a tale of designs being inadvertently swapped with those for those of another in a far-flung and suitably exotic part of the former British Empire. Enniscorthy is far from unique in Ireland in generating such a myth around a local landmark. What is more surprising is that this explanation for the extraordinary composition on the banks of the Slaney still has currency today, blind to the skill of the architect whose design very much sought to make the most of this spectacular site, and whose walls are built of bricks baked from the very clay of the site on which it stands.

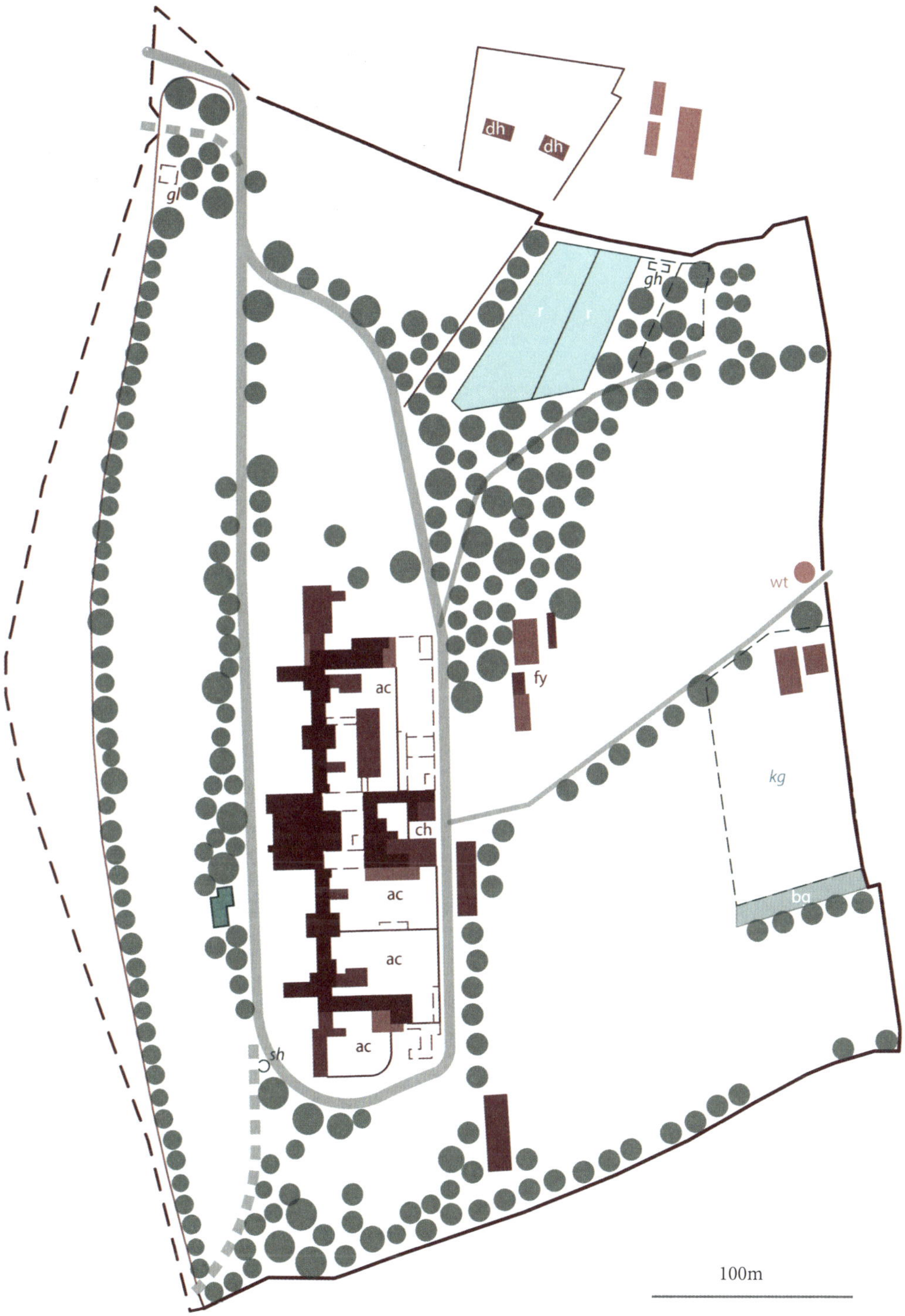

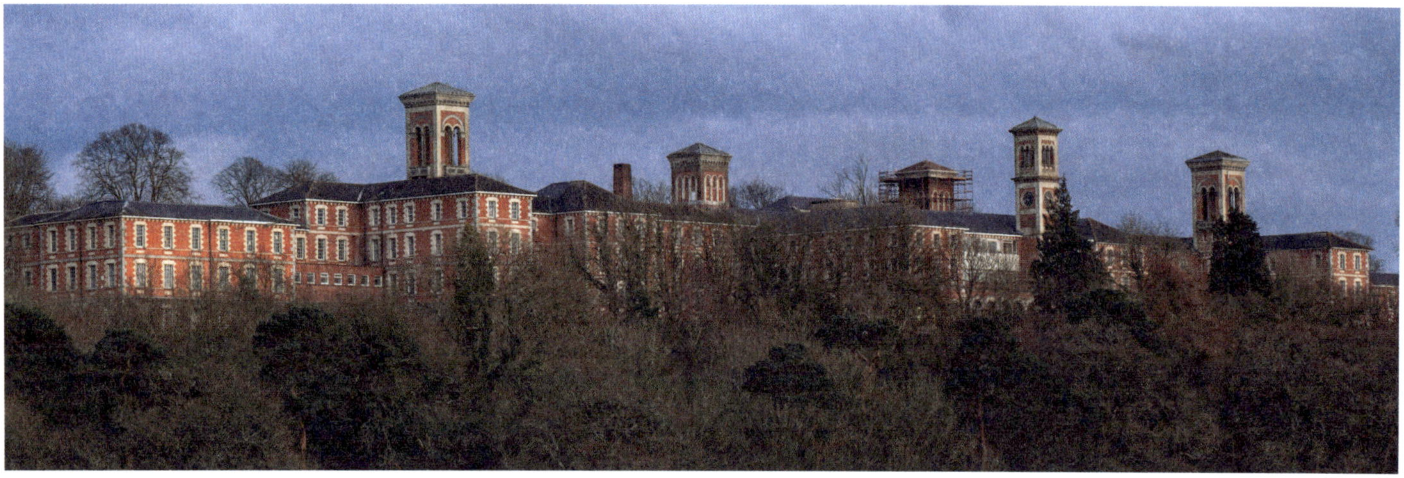

While a 'local asylum' had operated in Wexford town for several years, the county became part of a larger district with Carlow and Kilkenny after the opening of the Carlow District Lunatic Asylum in 1831. The provision of a separate asylum for Wexford was first suggested by the Inspectors of Lunacy in response to overcrowding at Carlow in 1847, but in the event Kilkenny would be the first county to achieve separation from Carlow. The 1855 Commission of Enquiry again recommended the provision of a separate asylum for Wexford and notwithstanding opposition from the grand juries of Carlow and Kildare concerned at the cost of maintaining their own institution without revenue from Wexford, the order for the construction of an asylum in or near Enniscorthy was signed in February 1860.

Architect and civil engineer James Bell, working alongside County Surveyor James Barry Farrell, produced a remarkable Italianate design for the new 288-bed asylum at Enniscorthy. In an era when economy of construction weighed more heavily on the minds of asylum commissioners than heretofore, Enniscorthy stands out from its contemporaries for its architecturally striking composition. The skyline is punctuated by no fewer than five campaniles between 90 and 112 feet in height, which, coupled with a steeply sloping and attractively wooded site, gives the impression of an Italian hill-town landed on the banks of the Slaney. Unlike the second generation of asylums, which as a rule faced south, the main façade of Enniscorthy faces west across the Slaney valley in response to the topography of the site. Obtaining a level ground floor required much of the building to be raised on a plinth of local Kilteely granite, and even so, level changes within the building remained inevitable.

The main structure is constructed predominantly of red brick that was baked on site from local clay, with contrasting white Paisley bricks used for detailing. The lively polychromatic brickwork and architectural detailing make for a striking building that belies the budgetary constraints of its construction. While acknowledging the success of the overall composition, an 1866 article in The Irish Builder sniffily observed of the decorative scheme that 'there is no timidity observable here; a little would have been salutary.' Internally, innovative developments included a system of ventilation whereby warm foul air from patient cells would rise via flues in the internal walls to a main duct running through the roof space, exhausting to the open air via the central towers.[1] Despite confidently predicting that the building would be open to patients in April 1866, it would be another two years before the first patients moved from Carlow into the as yet unfinished building, whose final cost was in excess of £40,000.[2]

Extensions in identical style were added at each end of the building between 1895 and 1900 to the designs of C. A. Owen, albeit of only two storeys over a full basement.[3] The northern extension was laid out as an open-plan, 40-bed dormitory on each floor; the extension to the south was only half as large, but with arches built into the rear wall to allow for a future extension which never materialised. Plans for new admissions units and a chapel drawn up in the 1930s by McDonnell, Dixon and Downes came to naught[4] – Enniscorthy would remain one of only three asylums in the country where a detached chapel was not constructed in the grounds. Indeed, all living and ancillary spaces for patients and staff would remain concentrated in the principal building or its extensions, with the result that the landscape setting remains remarkably intact.

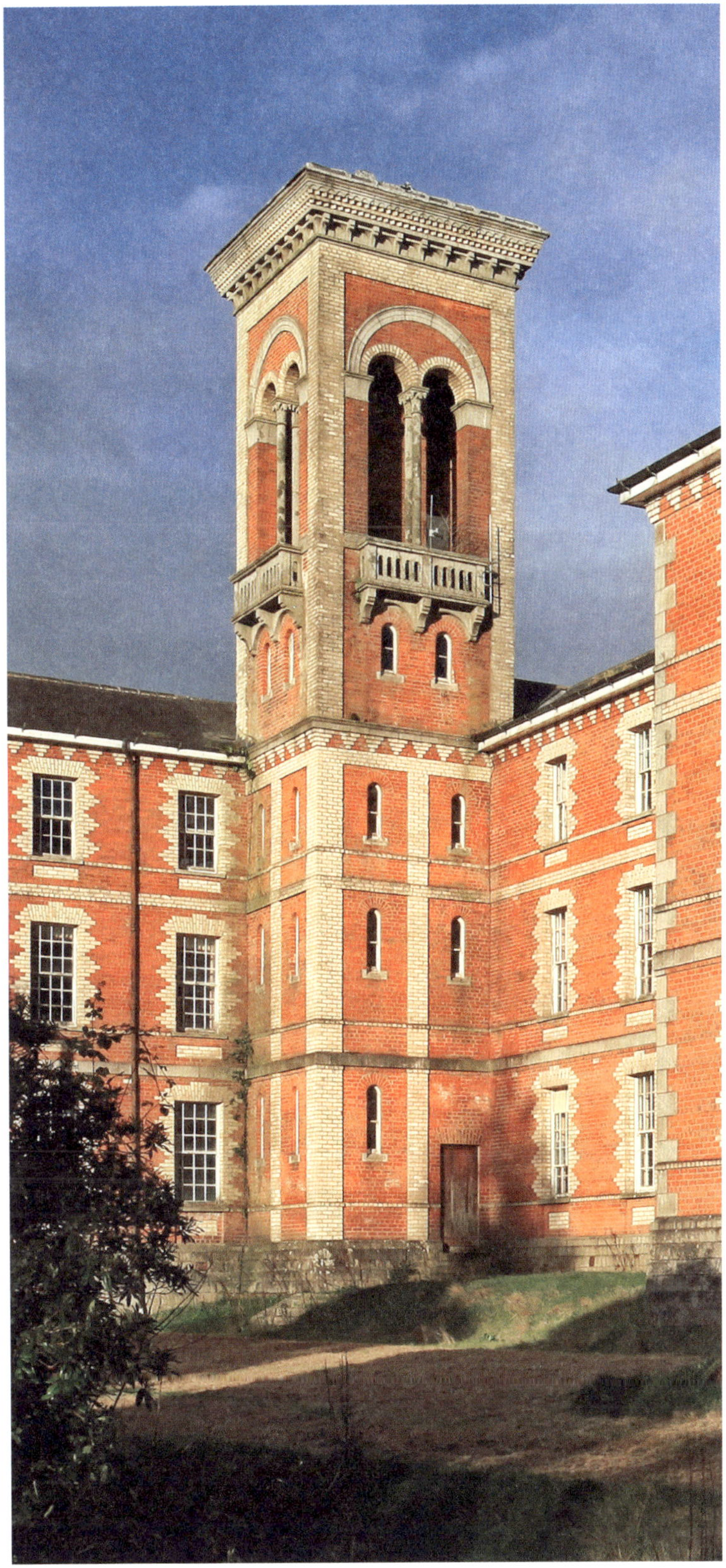

Enniscorthy's polychromatic brickwork and five Italianate campanile of various heights make for a spectacular addition to the local skyline (above and opposite). *Photographs by David Killeen, 2019.*

An open reservoir was constructed as part of the original works, to 'increase the storage in the case of a fire or lengthened drought',[5] from which the tanks 'at the top of each of five lofty towers will be kept constantly full, and will command any part of the building where water may be required'.[6] The wider landscape also features remnants of walled gardens, a discreetly located burial ground and a substantial farmyard that continued to be operated by the hospital on a commercial basis into at least the 1990s, providing fresh produce to St Senan's and other Health Board facilities long after most other hospitals ceased farming operations.

A major refurbishment programme in the 1960s saw the building's interior entirely reconstructed, with the insertion of concrete floors, modern partitions and services. The central administration block received a new façade reflective of the spirit of progress of the era, albeit destroying the effect of an Italian palazzo that had formed the centrepiece of the original design. While the 1960s refurbishment resulted in the loss of all historic interiors, it did render the building easier to physically adapt to new uses than almost any other in the country.

Yet as a very large building located well outside of a country town of 11,000 people, this was a site whose future after the last permanent residents departed in 2013 looked gravely uncertain. The hospital buildings on 45 acres, and a separate lot of 44 acres, were offered for sale on the open market, with a guide price of €780,000.[7] The buildings were purchased by a local consortium who has set out plans to redevelop them as a retirement living community, and who demonstrated their commitment to the building by undertaking extensive repairs to the historic structures even while these plans were still being finalised. As the first institution closed under A Vision for Change to be disposed of by the Health Service Executive, the success of this development will be seen as a portent for other sites that are deemed surplus to the future needs of the health service.

Further Reading

Hugh Kelly, *St Senan's Hospital, Enniscorthy: The History 1860–2011* (Enniscorthy, 2011)

References

1. "Lunatic Asylum, Enniscorthy', *The Irish Builder*, 15 Jan. 1866, p. 20.
2. Ibid.
3. *The Irish Builder*, 15 Sep. 1895, p. 218; 15 Aug. 1900, p. 451.
4. Frederick O'Dwyer, 'Architectural Heritage Impact Assessment Report, St Senan's Hospital Enniscorthy' (unpublished report, 2019), pp44-5.
5. *Seventeenth Annual Asylum Report 1868*, HC 1867–68 [4053] xxxi, p. 17.
6. 'Lunatic Asylum, Enniscorthy', *The Irish Builder*, 15 Jan. 1866, p. 20.
7. Helen McEntee TD, Dáil Éireann, 1 Feb. 2017, 937:1.

CASE STUDY 22

Downshire Hospital

(previously Downpatrick District Lunatic Asylum, latterly Downshire Civic Centre)

Years in operation
1869–present

Original cost
£60,599

Capacity (min /max)
300 / 1214

Architect(s)
Henry Smyth,
Watt & Tulloch

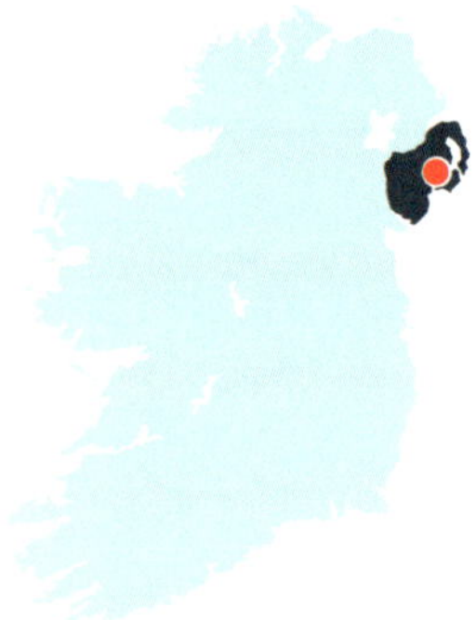

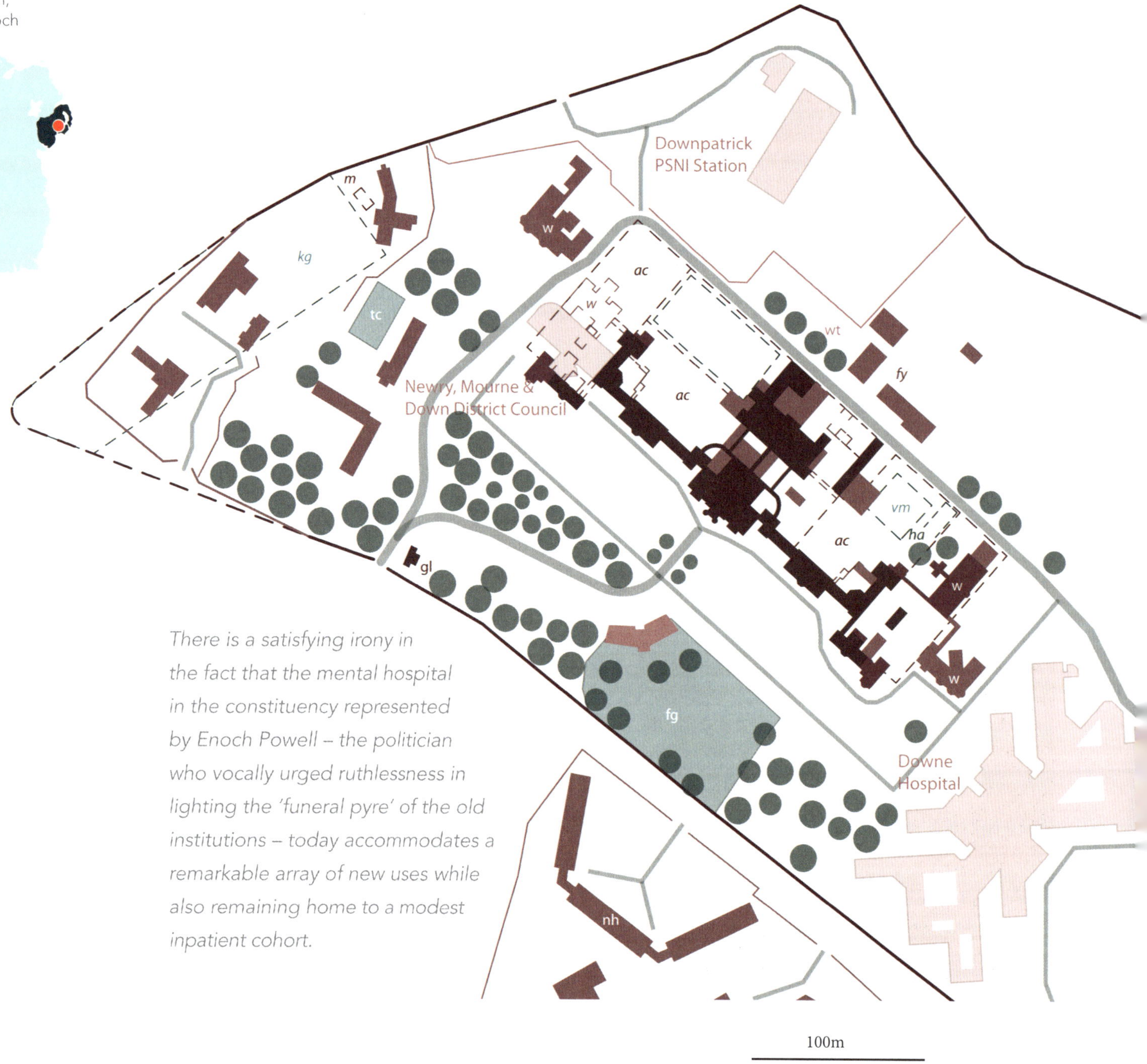

There is a satisfying irony in the fact that the mental hospital in the constituency represented by Enoch Powell – the politician who vocally urged ruthlessness in lighting the 'funeral pyre' of the old institutions – today accommodates a remarkable array of new uses while also remaining home to a modest inpatient cohort.

When the original Belfast District Lunatic Asylum opened in 1829, spaces were allocated in equal measure to patients from counties Antrim and Down.[1] The explosive growth of Belfast city upset this balance, such that a new asylum for county Down was recommended as part of the third phase of asylum expansion. Designed for a complement of 300, the new institution quickly filled with patients transferred from both Belfast asylum and the county goal, such that within three months of opening in 1869, there were already 222 patients in residence.[2]

The male and female sides of the asylum were provided with separate entrance blocks that doubled as residences for the RMS and Matron, not unlike Wilkinson's design for Castlebar and Letterkenny. But where the centrepiece of Wilkinson's composition was occupied by a chapel of diminutive scale and reticent detail, Smyth threw architectural caution to the wind. A 90-foot central dining and recreation hall of satisfying double-cube proportion stands behind a flamboyant clocktower 90 feet in height, flanked by circular turrets and surmounted by a steeply sprocketed roof and an orgy of High-Victorian decorative ironwork. As visually compelling as it is bizarre, the effect is further heightened by a carefully contrived approach sequence, whereby the main avenue suddenly turns to offer a dramatic axial vista of the tower in all its pomp. Smyth's wilful mixing of forms may have appalled his more stylistically literate contemporaries, but for sheer impact it is without peer. At a total project cost slightly over £60,000, this would also prove to be the most expensive asylum – measured on a cost-per-bed basis – since Johnston and Murray's ashlar-faced and masonry-vaulted edifices four decades earlier.

Beyond the extraordinary central set-piece, the building reverts to a more pedestrian institutional architecture, finished in machined-red brick with yellow brick dressings. While still in essence a corridor asylum, Smyth anticipates several tenets of the pavilion-echelon asylums of later decades, including a pair of detached infirmary pavilions linked by corridors, and a network of corridors bypassing the central block to facilitate independent circulation between patient wards and back-of-house areas.

But notwithstanding its well-resolved plan, the building fell short in other respects. In particular, the Inspectors rued the fact that despite enjoying the services of three chaplains, the asylum had no chapel, and they urged the governors to rectify the situation 'as the necessity for it is too apparent to require any argument in its support'.[3] The necessity was seemingly not at all apparent to the governors, and Downpatrick would remain a rare outlier amongst Ireland's asylums in never erecting separate chapels for the various denominations it accommodated.

The first major expansion of the asylum took place in 1882, when a large block for 120 male patients was erected, unusual only for the absence of any equivalent on the female side. Additions in the 1890s and 1900s by Watt & Tulloch were more conventionally planned as matching pairs, and in each case as detached blocks

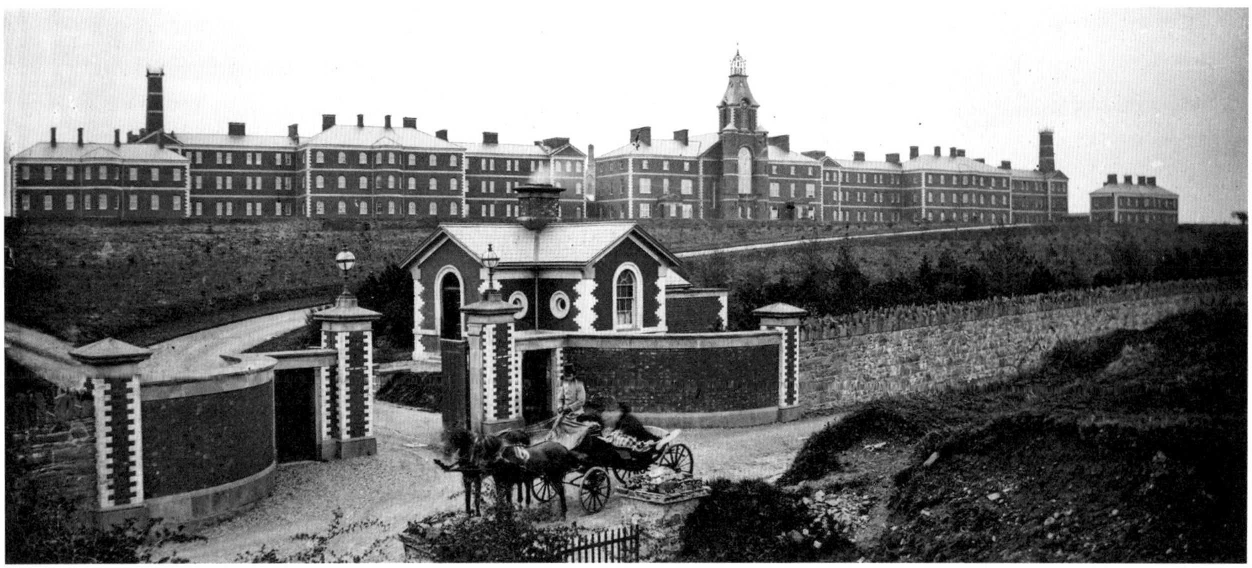

The arrival of such a large structure in the local landscape must have had a dramatic impact. Historic photograph, c.1870. *Image courtesy of the National Library of Ireland (EB_0663)*

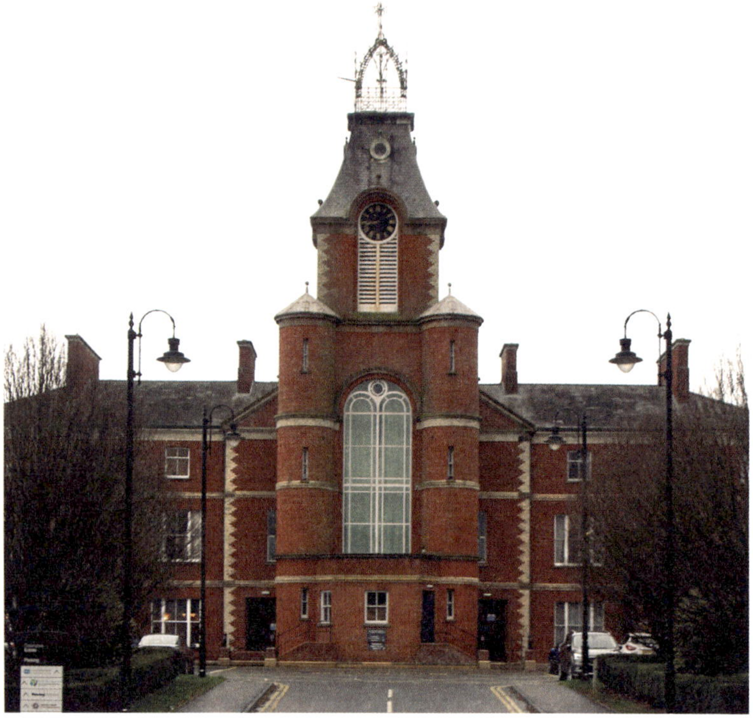

Smyth's spectacular tower is a victory of exuberance over taste, but nonetheless dominates the approach to the asylum. *Photograph by the author, 2020.*

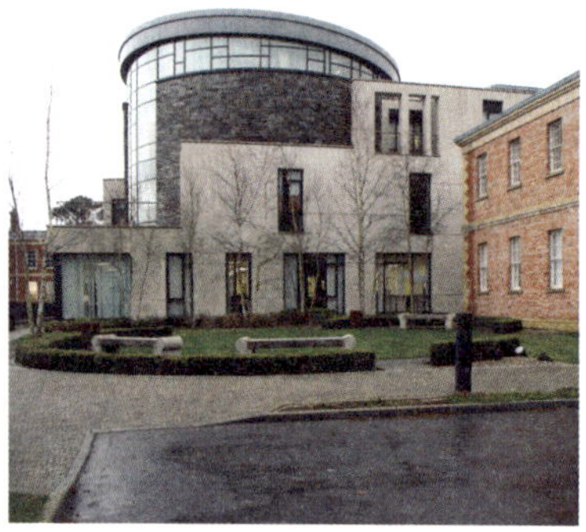

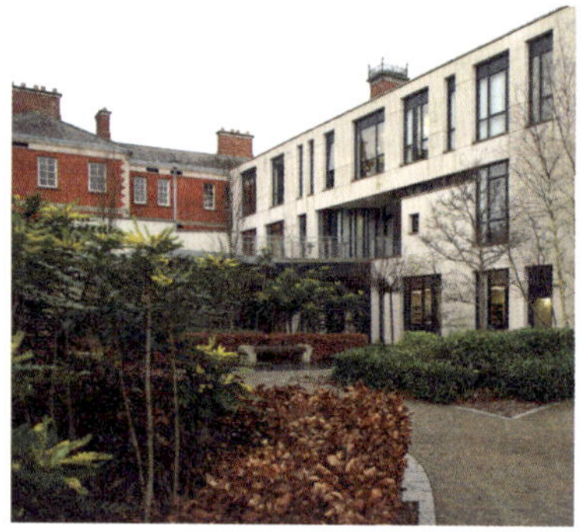

Modern additions alongside the historic buildings facilitate the transformation of the complex into a vibrant civic centre. *Photographs by the author, 2020.*

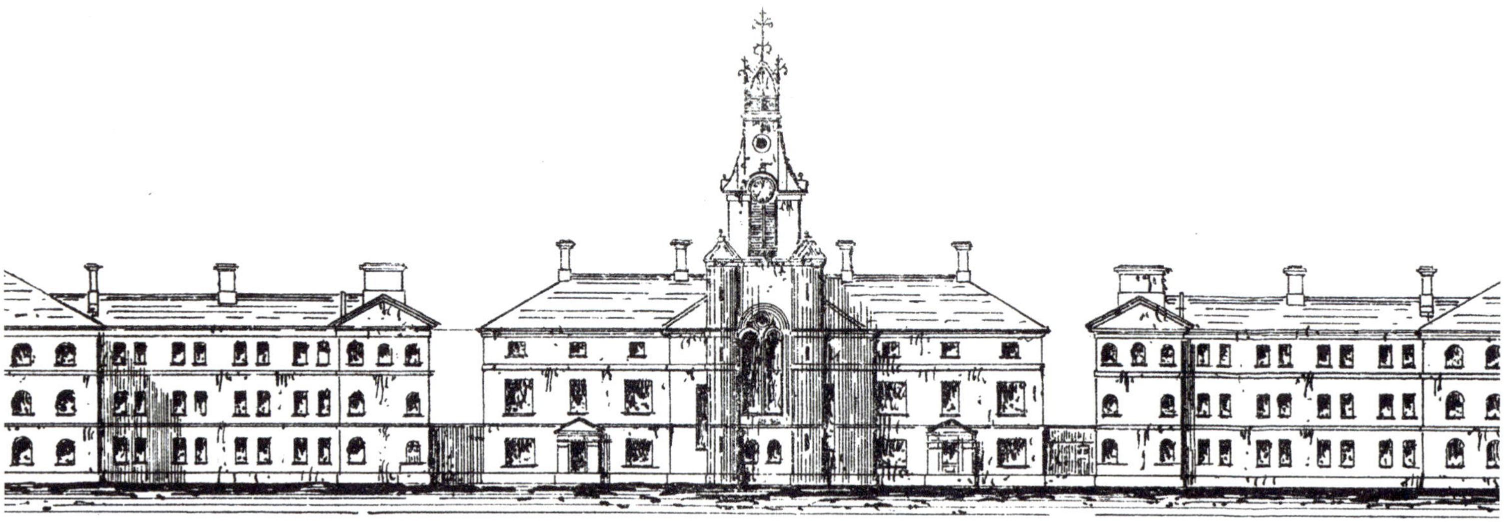

Elevation (above), plan and site layout drawing (opposite) by Henry Smyth, Architect, 1883. *Images courtesy of the National Archives of Ireland (Office of Public Works Collection, OPW/5HC/4/944)*

connected to the main building by a corridor. Smyth's original plan thus proved quite adaptable, evolving over time into something not dissimilar from the standard pavilion-echelon planform of the late nineteenth century. The original 50-acre holding soon doubled in size with the purchase of adjacent farmland, while male patients were also employed in the kitchen gardens, in 'making walks and laying down the pleasure grounds', the latter benefiting from a creative restoration in recent years.[4] Other notable landscape features included a viewing mound in the male airing courts alongside an unusually early ball alley; structured outdoor occupation for females here, as elsewhere, was seemingly limited to hanging out the laundry on the bleaching green.

The peak and decline of what was latterly known as Downshire Hospital played out later than at equivalent institutions in the Republic and mainland Britain, only reaching its zenith of 1,214 patients in 1967. This may help to explain why a large new nurses' home was constructed as late as 1961, at a time when few other hospitals countenanced major building projects.[5] Patient numbers did inevitably decline and while the male wing of 1882 remains in use as an inpatient mental health facility to this day, the remainder of the site has been repurposed to suit a remarkable range of uses. Lands to the south of the main asylum became the site of a large general hospital, while a new police station and fire station were constructed to the north. The Great Hall at the heart of the main asylum building was significantly upgraded in 1998 to create an intensively used venue for local performing arts and voluntary groups, alongside its continuing role of hosting medical conferences. The old female side has been expensively refurbished to provide stunning offices for the Newry, Mourne and Down District Council and the Northern Ireland Housing Executive. Bare granite staircases, once criticised for their cold, institutional countenance, are reinvented as cherished historic features bathed in soft feature lighting. Those who knew the place in its former incarnation must look on in disbelief, those responsible for similar buildings elsewhere should take note.

Further Reading

Sean Kelly, *A Grand Old Lady, A history of the Downshire Hospital, 1869-2014.* (Dundonald: South Eastern Health and Social Care Trust, 2012)

References

1. *Eighth Annual Prison Report 1829*, HC 1830 [48] xxiv, p. 18.
2. *Nineteenth Annual Asylum Report 1870*, HC 1870 [202] xxxiv, p. 17.
3. *Twentieth Annual Asylum Report 1871*, HC 1871 [440] xxvi, p. 15.
4. *Twenty-Third Annual Asylum Report 1874*, HC 1874 [1004] xxvii, p. 40.
5. Sean Kelly, *A Grand Old Lady: A History of the Downshire Hospital, 1869-2014* (Dundonald, 2012), Chapter 7 (no pagination)

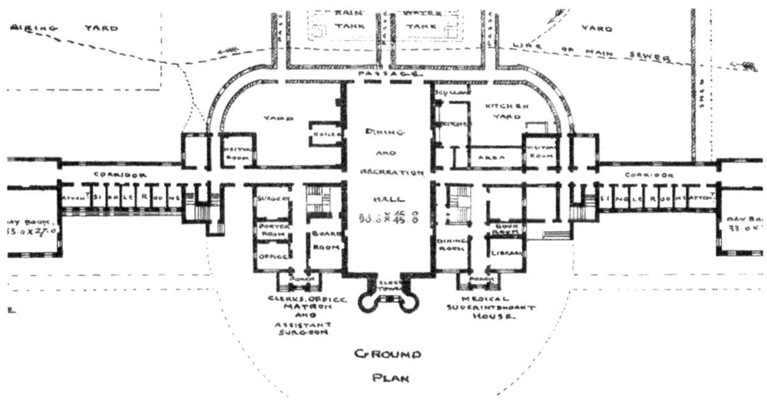

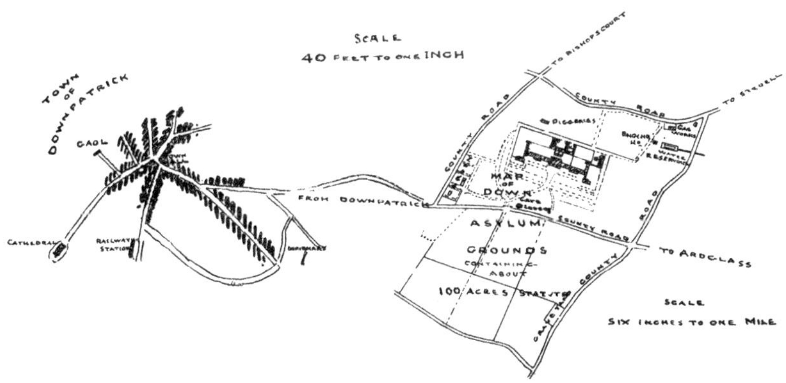

CASE STUDY 23

Years in operation
1869–2020

Original cost
£57,662

Capacity (min /max)
340 / 839

Architect(s)
John McCurdy,
Cormac MacLynn,
Arthur Lardner.

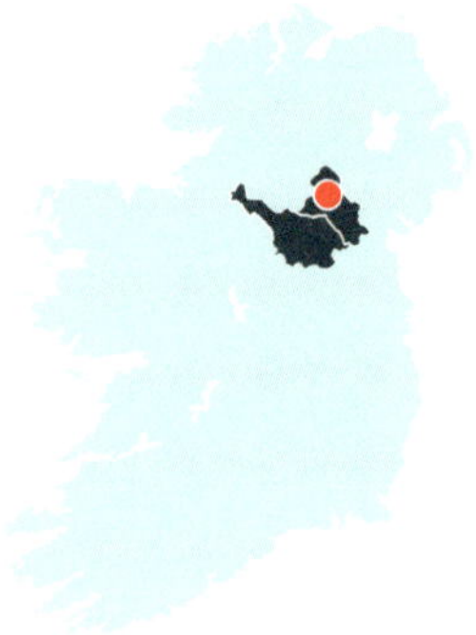

St Davnet's Hospital

(previously Monaghan District Lunatic Asylum)

Great buildings start with great clients. The modest character and disjointed nature of the structures that survive on site belie the fact that Monaghan District Lunatic Asylum was a building decades ahead of its time. This feat owes no less to the creativity of its architect than to the diligence with which its local client researched the best international precedents, and then strove to do even better.

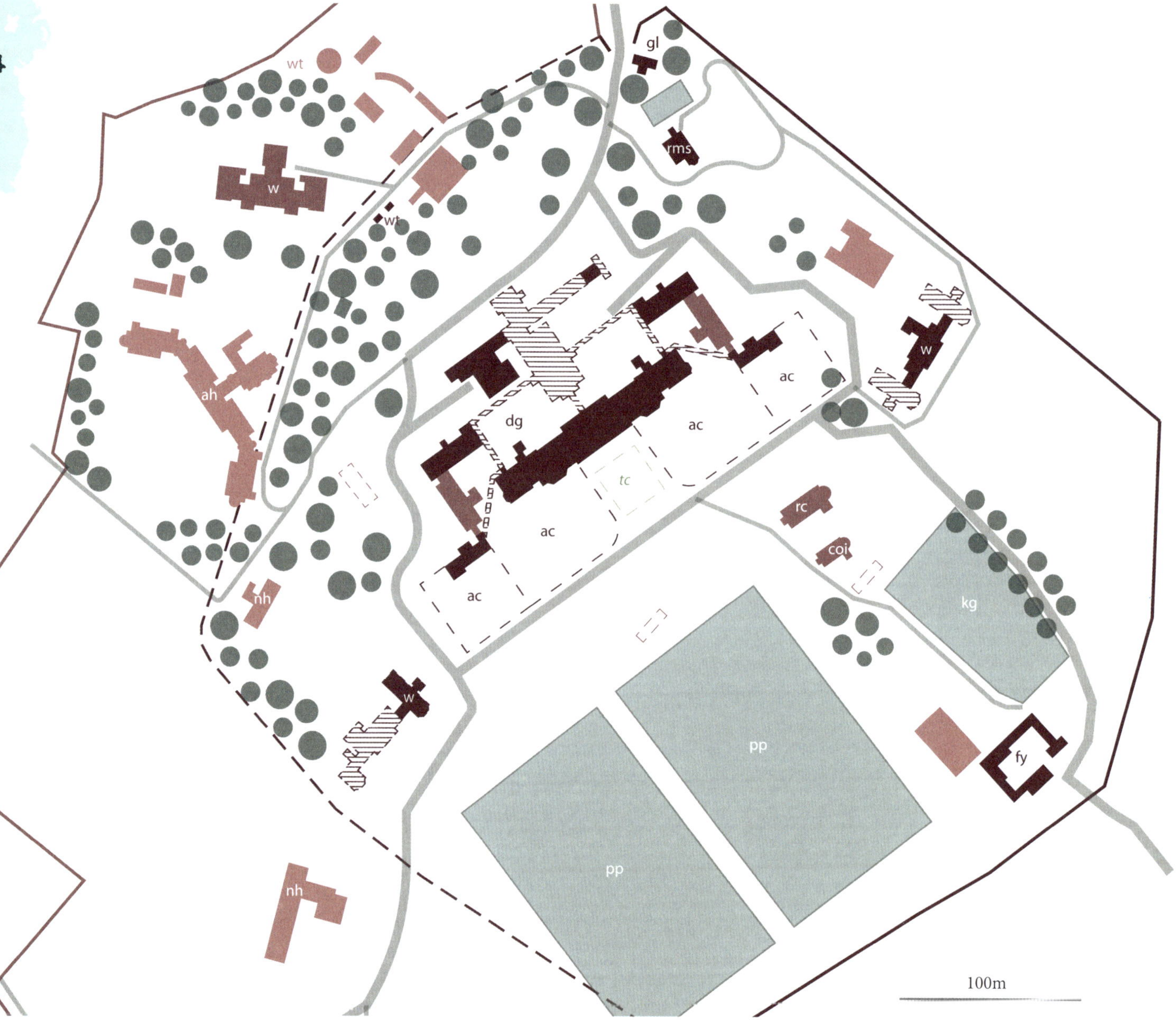

When the Armagh District Lunatic Asylum opened in 1825, its catchment included patients from counties Monaghan and Cavan. The 1858 Commission of Inquiry recommended that Cavan be detached to form its own district,[1] but an order was instead issued in 1861 to erect a 160-bed asylum for Monaghan. A few months later, this order was rescinded in favour of a new asylum for 300 patients serving both Counties Monaghan and Cavan – a decision doubtless the result of much politicking at the time, and one that also fortuitously aligned the asylum districts with a future international border that none of its protagonists could have foreseen.[2]

By March 1862 the grand juries of both counties had appointed a Joint Lunatic Asylum Committee who undertook responsibility for identifying a site, procuring an architect and delivering the project, under the supervision of the Board of Control. This committee took its responsibilities very seriously and were clearly determined to procure the best building possible. They invested considerable time and effort in researching the best English precedents, and were sufficiently confident in the veracity of their own findings as to face down the central powers in the Board of Control on matters of design.

The fruit of their labours was an extraordinarily detailed design competition brief that – notwithstanding concerns in the industry around the terms of architectural appointments for the five other asylums then underway – attracted a quality field of 19 competitors who demonstrated 'an uncommon amount of ability'. The result was announced in favour of architect John McCurdy of Dublin, whose design for an asylum for 300 patients represented a synthesis of dozens of recommendations drawn from eight different reference sites, and resulted in a building that at least equalled, if not surpassed, the very best asylums of the era.[3]

The significance of McCurdy's design lay not in its aesthetics – the humble rubblestone walls with brick dressings adhere strictly to the requirement for a building 'as plain as may be consistent with a slightly appearance' – but in its spatial organisation and layout. The first notable feature is that the main entrance was located to the north, thus allowing patient spaces to span the entire south of the building with direct access to sunny airing courts. The separation of 'entrance front' from 'garden front' was a longstanding device in country-house design and had been employed in some English asylums, but prior to McCurdy, Irish asylum architects almost without exception prioritised the aesthetics of the set piece entrance above the experience of the patient. At the centre of the complex lay a large dining and recreation hall with an orchestra gallery, beyond which the male and female wards and infirmaries were disaggregated into several detached blocks, connected by over 1,000 yards of link corridors.[4] In this, Monaghan offered a vision of the future 'pavilion-echelon' type of asylum, a decade before the first major asylum would be constructed to such a plan (Gloucester 1881), and three decades before it would become the dominant model for new asylums across Britain.

McCurdy's architectural vision also embraced a wide range of auxiliary buildings and ancillary structures constructed contemporaneously across the site, from water towers to gate lodges and farm buildings. Most significantly, these included freestanding wards in detached pavilions, 'now so much advocated by the highest [international] authorities on insanity', but again three decades before this approach would be popularly employed at other Irish asylums.[5] A very fine detached house was provided for the Resident Medical Superintendent (RMS) – a break from conventional practice whereby the RMS was traditionally obliged to live within the main building. The local Board of Governors believed that a superior detached dwelling would allow them to attract a 'more than ordinarily efficient' candidate for the role, and more importantly allowed the prime southerly aspect in the main building to be prioritised for patient accommodation.[6]

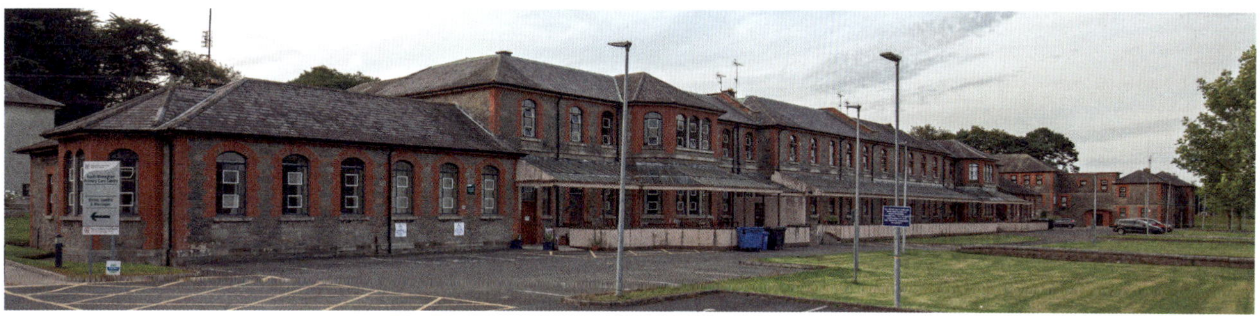

McCurdy's inversion of conventional asylum planning allowed the entire southern frontage (above) to be dedicated to patient spaces. *Photograph by David Killeen, 2019.*

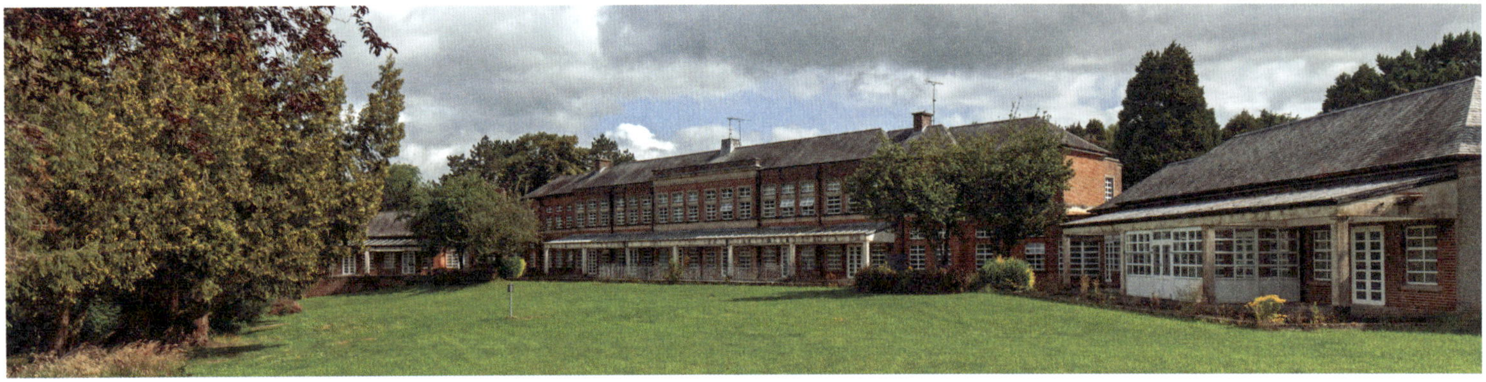

MacLynn returned Monaghan to the architectural vanguard 80 years later with his light-filled admissions unit. *Photograph by David Killeen, 2019.*

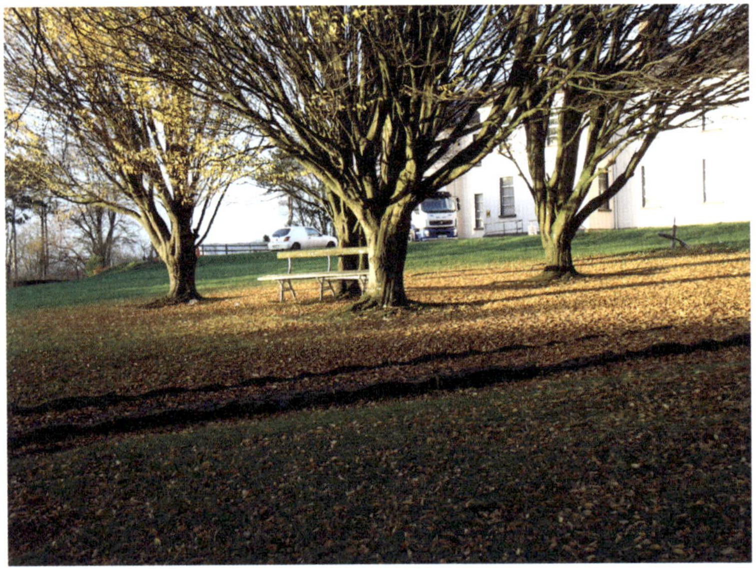

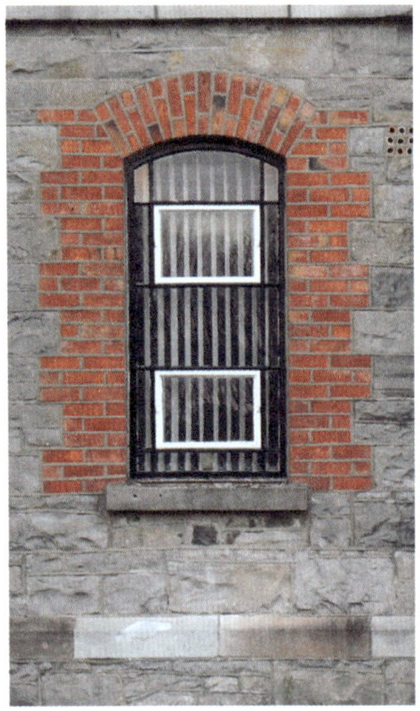

'*As plain as may be consistent with a sightly appearance*': rubble-stone walls, brick dressings, and distinctive 1950s steel windows. *Photograph by the author, 2014.*

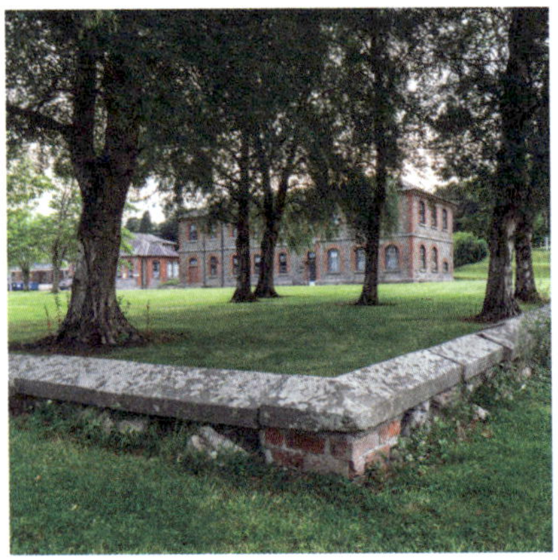

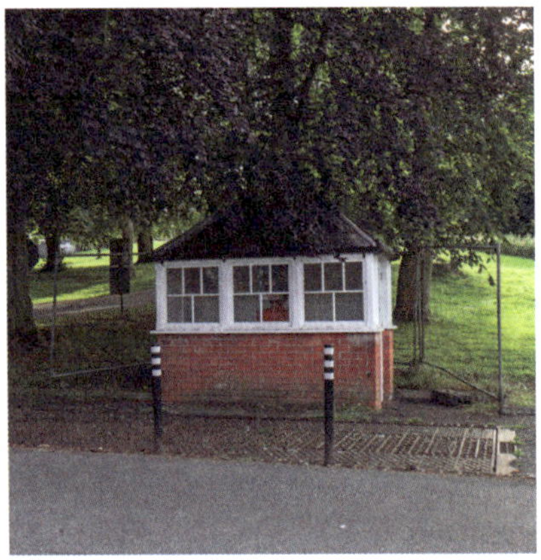

Subtle details of the earlier landscape endure, including the ha-ha walls to the former airing court (above left) and the recently restored Avery weighbridge (above right). *Photographs by David Killeen, 2019.*

So visionary was McCurdy's design that nearly three decades later the Inspectors of Lunacy would still describe the building thus: '…unlike the other Irish asylums built at this time, the original plan would appear to have been an excellent one – answering in many of its details the requirements of modern asylum architecture.'[7] But notwithstanding the many merits of its original design, Monaghan was not immune to the extreme overcrowding experienced all across Ireland at the close of the nineteenth century, and later governors resorted to less satisfactory solutions. New extensions added in 1889 increased total capacity to 520, but by infilling the space between the formerly detached pavilions, they had the regrettable effect of wholly enclosing some of the airing courts. The former County Infirmary was refitted to provide 40 beds and the possibility of repurposing the nearby workhouse was discussed. Reluctant to commit to yet more major capital expenditure at a time when major legislative change was anticipated, the governors in 1898 erected temporary wooden buildings for another 122 patients, but it was still not enough.[8] Yet during the same period, money was found to erect two very fine new chapels for Roman Catholic and Anglican worship in the grounds to the south of the asylum. A large, if architecturally mediocre, new ward pavilion was finally completed in 1907 at a cost of approximately £10,000, situated on additional lands acquired to the north.

The 1930s would see Monaghan return to the vanguard of best practice in hospital architecture. In 1933 the hospital committee instructed the preparation of plans with a view to seeking funding from the Hospital Sweepstakes Fund.[9] Five years later work started on a new infirmary, admission hospital and nurses' home to the design of Belfast architect Cormac MacLynn. The design reflected the very best of hospital and sanatorium design of the era, with wards orientated to maximise exposure to natural light and ventilation through large windows and glazed verandahs, book-ended by semi-circular day rooms capturing all-day sunlight, and finished throughout in high-quality materials with attractive Art Deco flourishes.[10]

It was an inauspicious time to commence such an ambitious project – material and labour shortages arising from the outbreak of World War II prolonged the contract by at least two years, delaying completion until 1943. Worse was to come as the Joint Management Committee, under duress from the County Council and burdened by debts incurred to meet the final bill - which exceeded the tender of £93,942 by 25 per cent and the initial project estimate by some 40 per cent – leased the buildings to the local authority for use as a tuberculosis sanatorium.[11] By the time these exemplary new buildings were returned to the mental hospital after 1958, the Committee had already commenced a series of major alterations to the old asylum buildings and erected another nurses' home to a low-key modern design by Arthur H. Lardner.[12]

Visiting the St Davnet's Campus today, it is hard to orientate oneself around a large and disparate complex of buildings with no obvious front door. McCurdy's original entrance block, kitchen, dining hall and connecting corridors were all swept away, to be replaced by a new central kitchen and canteen for the entire campus, which opened in 1961.[13] The original spatial hierarchy and organisational logic of the site has thus been erased, albeit the remaining buildings stand in an excellent state of repair. Rare survivals include the original asylum farmyard and an Avery weighbridge with its recently restored weigh-room: all encouraging indicators that even the subtle historic features of this site continue to be appreciated and cared for.

St Davnet's is of interest today not just for its architectural history, but as a site where a very diverse range of former asylum buildings have successfully transitioned into modern, community healthcare uses, within a wider landscape which is home to numerous other voluntary and sporting organisations. The main building of 1869 would continue to accommodate patients until 2020, and even then they did not move far, for the replacement facility actually comprises an extension to one of McCurdy's original freestanding pavilions; against all the odds, the visionary Victorian asylum lives on.

Further Reading

Anne McLellan, Niamh Nic Ghabhann and Fiona Byrne, *World Within Walls: From Asylum to Contemporary Mental Health Services* (Monaghan: Health Service Executive, 2015)

References

1. *1858 Commission Report*, HC 1857-58 [2436-I] p. 24.
2. Anne McLellan, Niamh Nic Ghabhann and Fiona Byrne, *World Within Walls: From Asylum to Contemporary Mental Health Services* (Monaghan, 2015), p. 4.
3. 'The Proposed New Lunatic Asylum for Monaghan', *The Dublin Builder*, 1 May 1863, p. 77.
4. 'Monaghan and Cavan New Lunatic Asylum', *The Irish Builder*, 1 June 1869, p. 135.
5. Ibid.
6. McLellan, *World Within Walls*, p. 4.
7. *Forty-Fifth Annual Asylum Report 1896*, HC 1896 [8251] xxxix Pt.II.1, p. 18.
8. McLellan, *World Within Walls*, p. 37.
9. *The Irish Builder*, 2 Dec 1933, p. 1043.
10. 'Mental Hospital at Monaghan: A worthy addition to Ireland's modern hospital buildings,' *Irish Builder and Engineer*, 10 April 1943, pp 141–2.
11. *The Irish Builder*, 27 Nov 1937, p. 1058; 8 Jan 1938, p. 31.
12. Niamh NicGhabhann, '…all the most approved modern arrangements: Building for Mental Health Care at Monaghan, 1886–1950s', in McLellan, *World Within Walls*, p. 169.
13. Timeline included in preface to McLellan, *World Within Walls*, no pagination.

CASE STUDY 24

Years in operation
1898-present

Original cost
£111,157

Capacity (min /max)
400 / 827

Architect(s)
John Lanyon

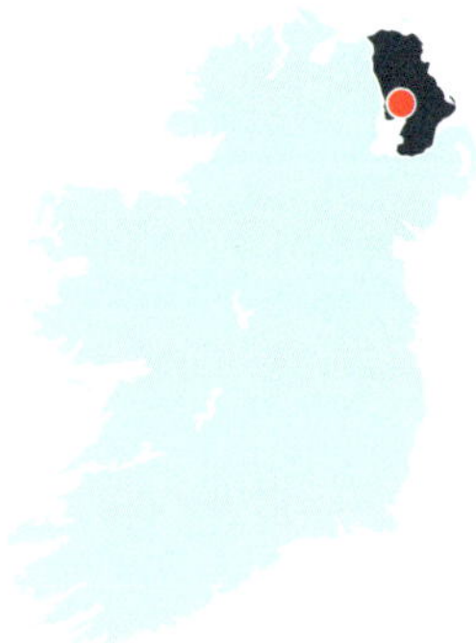

Holywell Hospital

(previously Antrim District Lunatic Asylum)

By the close of the nineteenth century, the standard requirements for new asylums across the United Kingdom almost inevitably resulted in institutional complexes of vast scale but scant aesthetic appeal, beyond the set piece of the central administration block. At Holywell, architect John Lanyon satisfied the myriad technical demands of a pavilion-echelon asylum, but also managed to include sufficient architectural embellishment that the rambling complex could almost be described as picturesque.

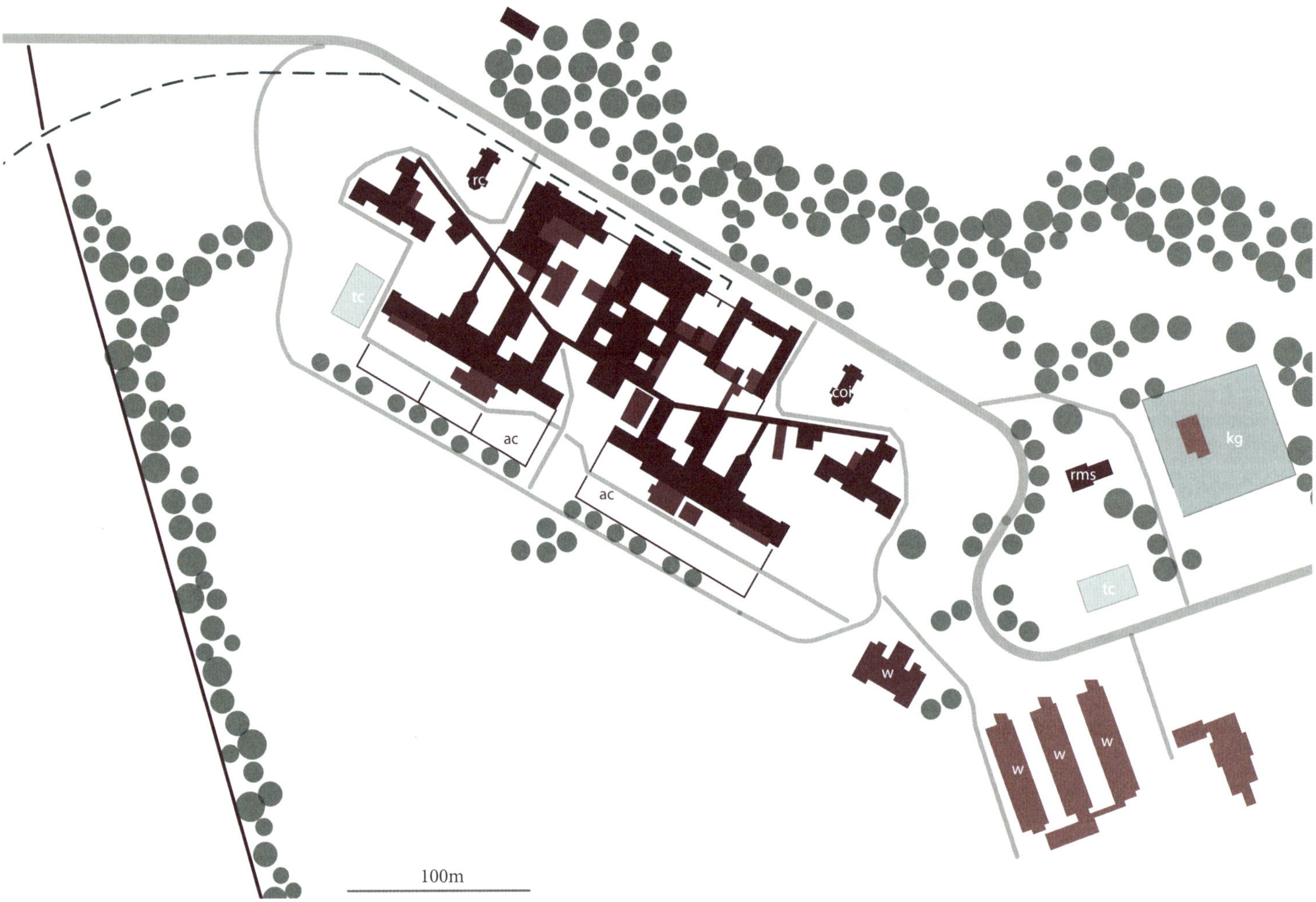

When the Belfast asylum opened in 1829, its district included patients from County Antrim, and it would continue to serve the needs of the county until the opening of the new asylum for 400 patients at Holywell. The first patients transferred to the new building in April 1899, [1] but by 1901 it was already 48 patients over capacity, with the same number again temporarily lodged in the Ballymena workhouse.[2]

John Lanyon's layout adheres to the standard pavilion-echelon plan: a central spine containing spaces for administration, kitchen, stores, dining and recreation, flanked by laundry, workshop and plant areas along the northern façade. Patient pavilions were laid out to maximise southerly exposure, all linked by a network of single-storey corridors. Holywell is actually a small version of the type, having only two detached pavilions on each side, albeit original drawings confirm the unrealised expectation that an additional pavilion would be added on each side at a later date to bring the total capacity up to 600 patients.

The (relatively) smaller scale of the complex makes for a less daunting edifice than Portrane, but credit must also go to Lanyon for his application of architectural elements to improve the attractiveness of the whole. In addition to the obligatory clock-cum-water-tower whose Italianate campanile marks the main entrance, a series of lesser towers, roof ventilators, chimneys, rooflights and dormer windows, many crowned with decorative ironwork, create a skyline full of incident and variety, while the selective introduction of unusually low, single-storey eaves achieves a human scale in a building typology that is usually the antithesis of homely.

The infirmary blocks to the southern front feature attractive brick arcades, some with glazed verandah-style roofs. These blocks open onto a pair of walled airing courts that unusually still survive, including the system of ha-ha-style earthen banks and dykes, which concealed the boundary wall from view. The three-storey blocks for chronic patients are the least successful, where relatively mean windows make for gloomy interiors and a barrack-like exterior.

The pair of chapels – here unusually of equal size as dictated by local denominational demographics – are presented as freestanding buildings set in open green space, enhancing the appeal of the entrance front. An unusual feature of the plan – at least in the Irish context – is the stacking of the central recreation hall over the dining hall. This clever spatial solution affords greater flexibility of use for the former, unconstrained by the interruption of thrice-daily meal sittings in the latter.

While the architecture may have been pleasing, the mechanical services for such a large institution proved troublesome from the outset. The on-site water supply drawn from the eponymous 'Holy Well' – which had previously been deemed potable and of adequate pressure – was found to be deficient on both counts. Meanwhile, the governors' decision to opt for a technically advanced plenum heating system in preference to a simpler option of radiators and open fires was suspected to be the cause of excessive coal consumption – estimated at 3,000 tonnes for a full year.[3] The handling of such large quantities of coal was at least made easier by the fact that the asylum was connected directly to the rail network. Although common in England, Holywell was one of only two asylums in Ireland to have its own railway siding, and the only one to boast a tramway that conveyed goods the final stretch from the siding into the store yard.

The asylum at Holywell was Lanyon's last major work, and he died just as the project was nearing completion. Had he lived just a few years longer, he would have experienced the frustration of seeing a newly installed asylum committee ignore his carefully considered blueprint for future expansion and instead commission a mediocre ward block, which stands awkwardly to one side of the main complex. But apart from that and some modest single-storey blocks from the mid-twentieth century, the complex otherwise remains almost exactly as Lanyon designed it.

The hospital population peaked in 1958 at 827; the following year, as part of a drive by the RMS to create a 'therapeutic community', publication commenced of a new hospital magazine, Speedwell. Neither the existence of such a magazine, nor its contents, were especially unusual, but in publishing material penned by patients themselves, it does offer an alternative insight into hospital life during a period of considerable change and even hope. Alongside news of the diverse range of social and therapeutic activities, several budding poets offered witty views of the patient experience, ranging from the gastronomically upbeat:

Wardsmaids with the dinner
Wardsmaids with the tea
Keep our tummies happy
Until the day we're free

To the thirst-slakingly cynical:

Ah! What is that I hear? – 'tis the final blast of the ref's whistle, and behold! a bespectacled gent on the touchline yelling – 'Paraldehyde all round – free drinks on the house!'[4]

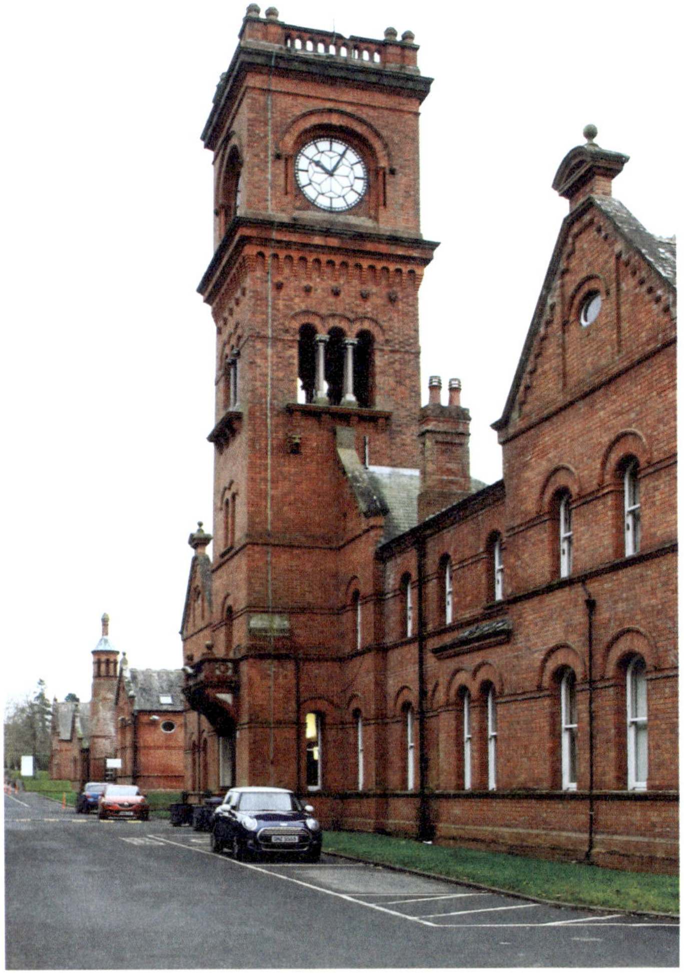

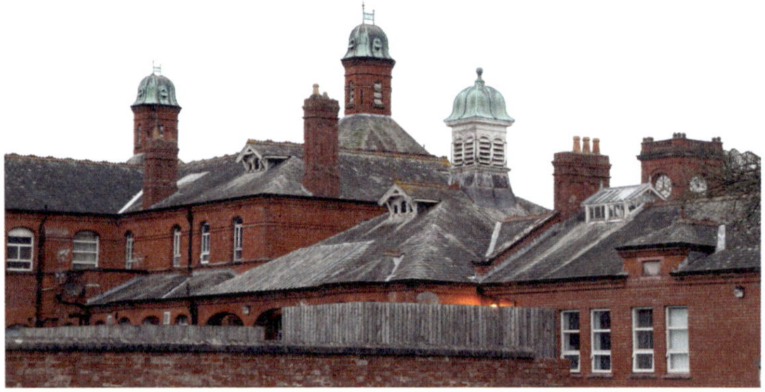

Lanyon transformed the functional necessities of water storage (left) and ventilation (above) into picturesque additions to the asylum roofscape.
Only his three storey chronic block (below) disappoints. *Photographs by the author, 2020*

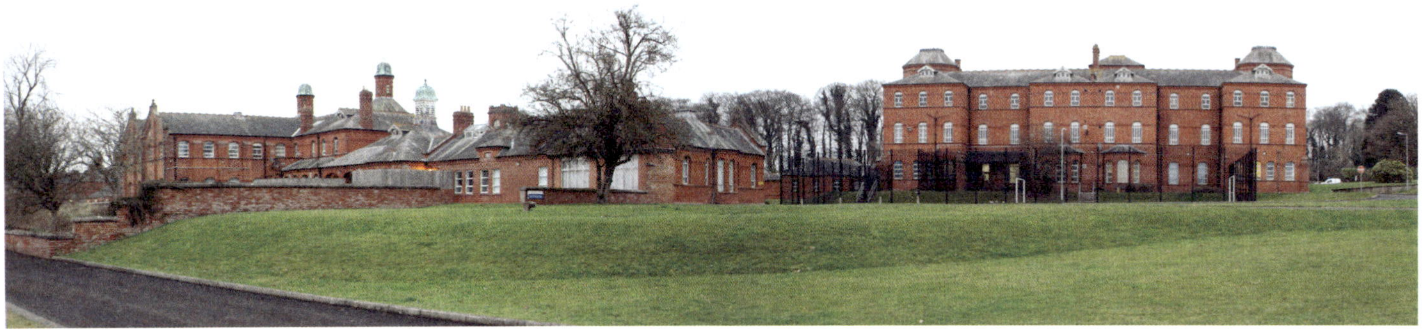

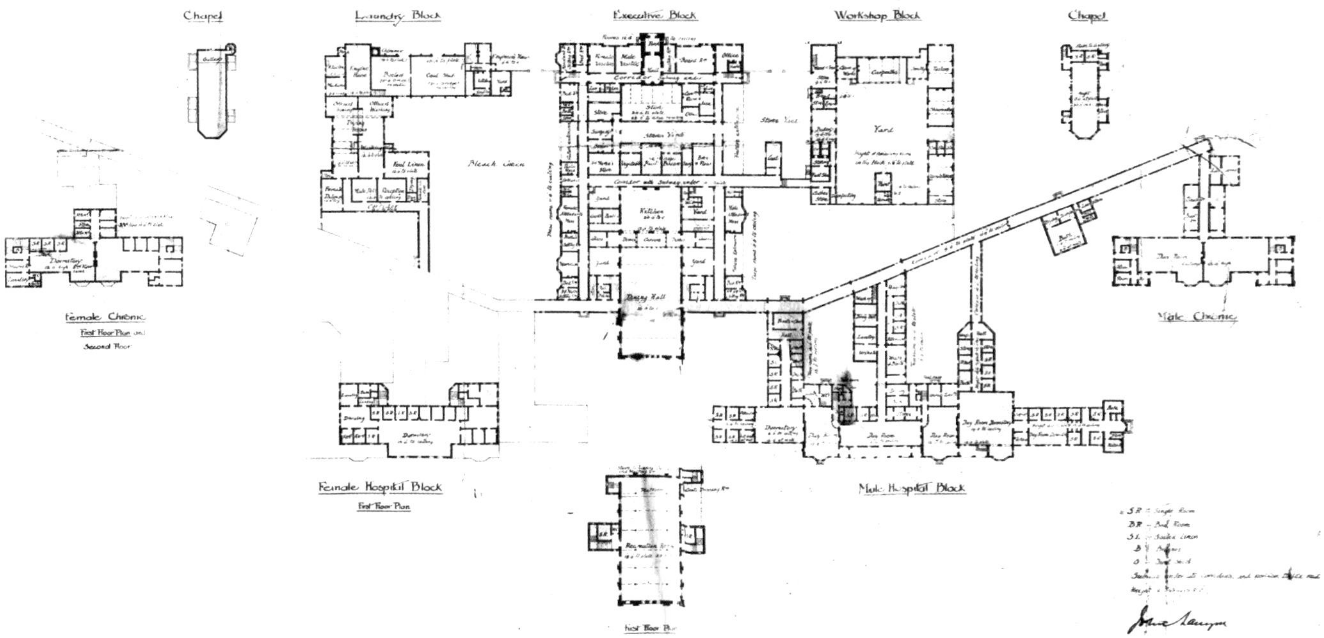

The asylum was built for only one-third as many patients as Portrane, but its architectural programme was hardly less complex. *Image courtesy of the Irish Architectural Archive (Workhouse Drawings Collection, 85/138: 082)*

At the time of writing, Holywell is one of the last nineteenth-century asylums in Ireland where patients remain resident in several parts of the original building, although discussions are ongoing around the construction of replacement facilities at the nearby Antrim Area Hospital. While the complex has survived to the present in a reasonable state of repair, it remains to be seen what the future holds if and when the last patients do finally depart.

Further Reading

Marc Mulholland, *To Comfort Always: 100 Years of Holywell Hospital, Antrim, 1898–1998* (Antrim: Homefirst Community Trust, 1999)

References

1. *Forty-Ninth Annual Asylum Report 1899*, HC 1900 [312] xxxvii, p. 96.
2. *Fifty-First Annual Asylum Report 1901*, HC 1902 [1265] xl, p. 72.
3. Ibid, p. 71; *Fifty-Second Annual Asylum Report 1902*, HC 1903 [1762] xxvii, p. 73.
4. Patient poems cited in Gillian McClelland, 'Speedwell Magazine: An insider view of Holywell Psychiatric Hospital, 1959–1973,' in Pauline M. Prior (ed.), *Asylums, Mental Health Care and the Irish 180 –2010* (Dublin, 2012), p. 57, p. 59. Paraldehyde was routinely used in mental hospitals as a universally administered bed-time sedative.

St Ita's Hospital

(previously Portrane Auxiliary Asylum)

Years in operation
1901–2013

Original cost
£378,100

Capacity (min /max)
1,200 / 1,647

Architect(s)
George Ashlin,
Vincent Kelly

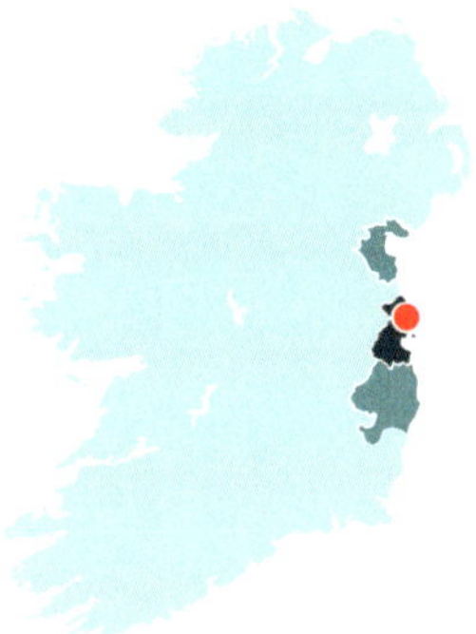

Early pioneers of the asylum frequently described their work in almost utopian terms. Their idealism soon faded, but medical and architectural professionals continued to collaborate in the creation of building types ever more finely attuned to the organisational needs of the institution. The pavilion-echelon asylum represented the zenith of this endeavour – vast complexes within whose bewildering web of corridors could be found every requisite for a thousand or more patients, located in rural settings far removed from the perceived stresses of urban life..

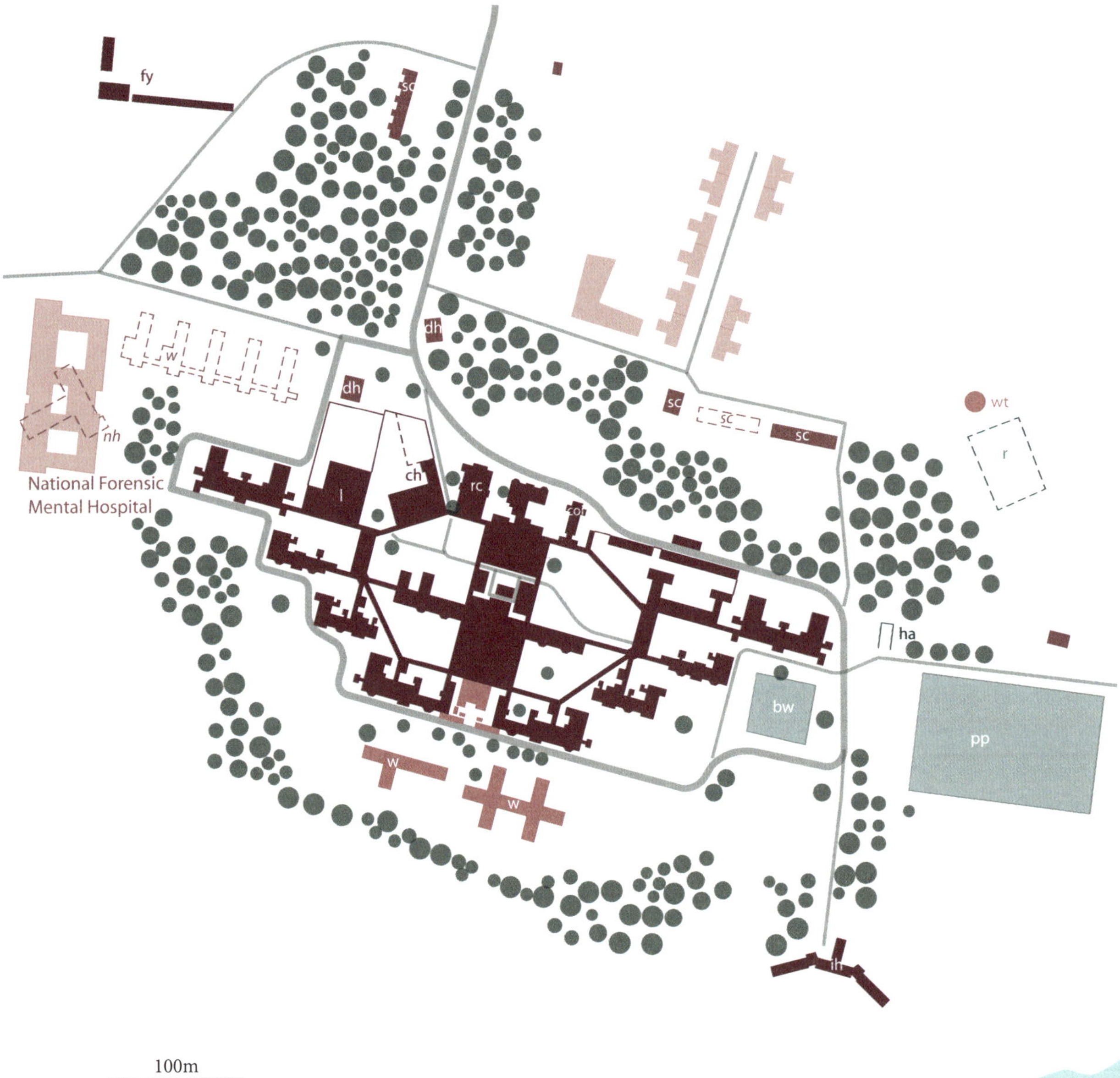

Even by its own abject standards, the overcrowding at Dublin's Richmond Asylum in the 1890s had deteriorated past the point of crisis. An entirely new building was needed, and it was imperative that its site would remedy the perceived ills of the original setting at Grangegorman, whose grounds were now hemmed in by suburban expansion and whose very soil was contaminated by years of defective drainage. The decision in 1891 to purchase Portrane Demesne comprehensively addressed both critiques – a large agricultural estate of 469 acres on the Donabate peninsula, some 13 miles distant from the parent institution and permanently aired by healthy breezes blowing off the Irish Sea.[1] This 'escape to the country' was just what the asylum doctors ordered, but whether by virtue of accident, design or blunt economics, the governors could hardly have identified a site anywhere within a similar radius of the capital that conveyed a greater sense of physical and psychological isolation from the wider world.[2]

The architectural competition administered by the governors to award the commission for the country's largest civilian building project was not without controversy, even if the shortlisted designs all conformed to the same underlying principle: the 'pavilion-echelon' model.[3] The pavilion-echelon could be seen as a precursor to urban land-use zoning, where every function would be housed in a separate, purpose-designed building, all connected by a mesh of communication corridors through which patients, staff and supplies could circulate without ever setting foot out of doors, and beneath which ran the many utilities needed to sustain modern levels of comfort. At Portrane, eight separate pavilions were provided for male and female patients categorised according to degree of insanity – acute, semi-acute, chronic and infirm – all enjoying a southerly aspect to maximise sunlight and ventilation. These pavilions were arrayed symmetrically in a 'broad-arrow' formation about a central core of shared facilities and ancillary areas, including administration department, dispensary, kitchens, bakery, stores, and a dining-cum-recreation hall with an orchestra gallery and a stage – a space large enough to hold the entire 1,200 patient complement and comparable in scale to the National Concert Hall at Earlsfort Terrace.

The man ultimately charged with the task of pulling these elements into a coherent whole was George Ashlin, better known as one of Ireland's most prolific church architects. During his career to date, Ashlin had not built so much a sanitary annexe to a lunatic asylum,

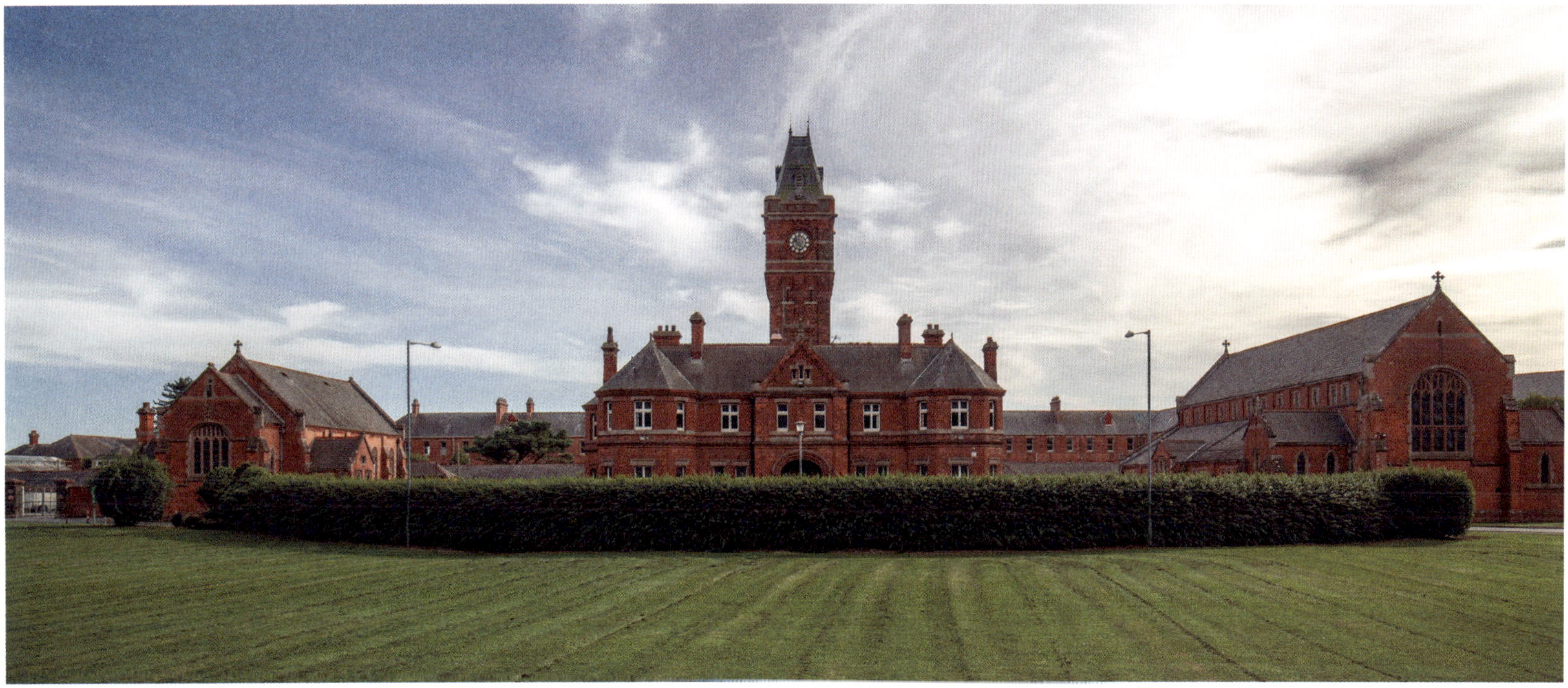

Entrance front comprising administration block flanked by Church of Ireland and Roman Catholic chapels and presided over by the iconic clocktower. Photograph by David Killeen, 2019.

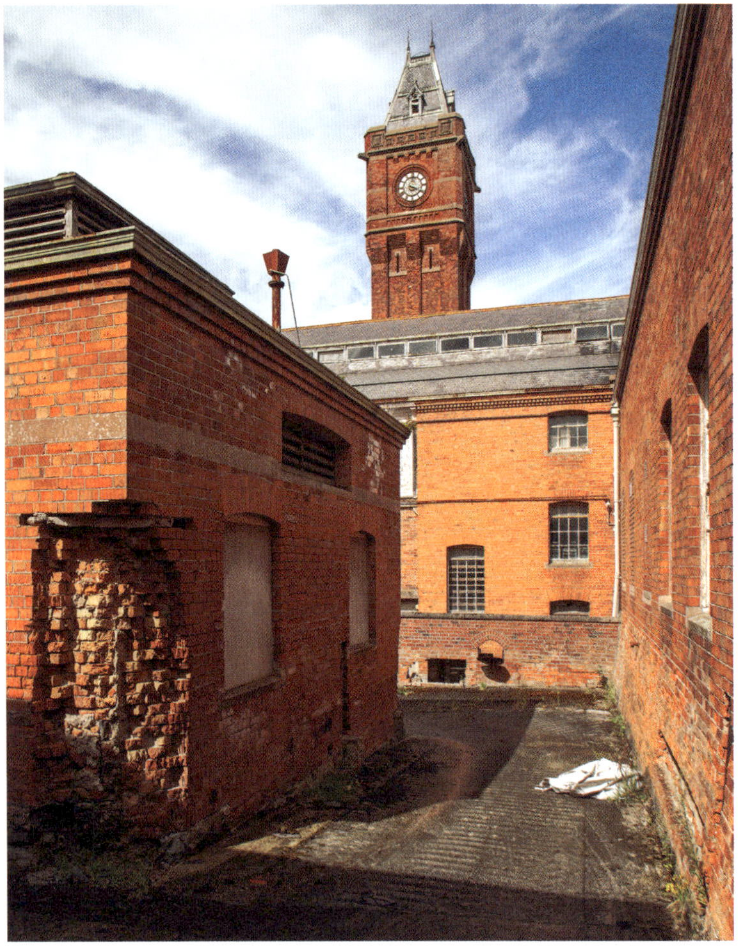

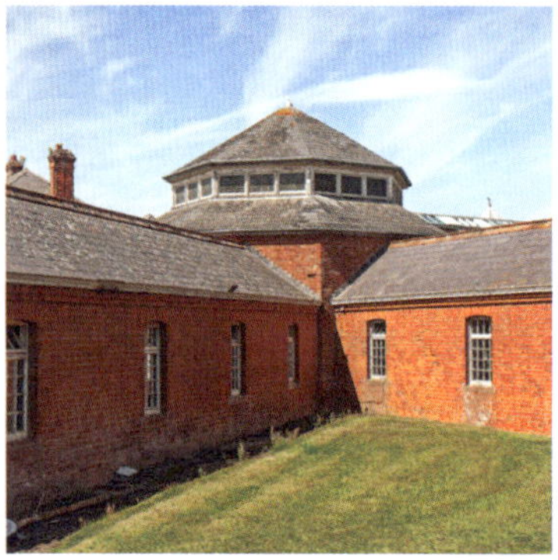

The web of corridors is punctuated by toplit lobbies. *Photograph by David Killeen, 2019.*

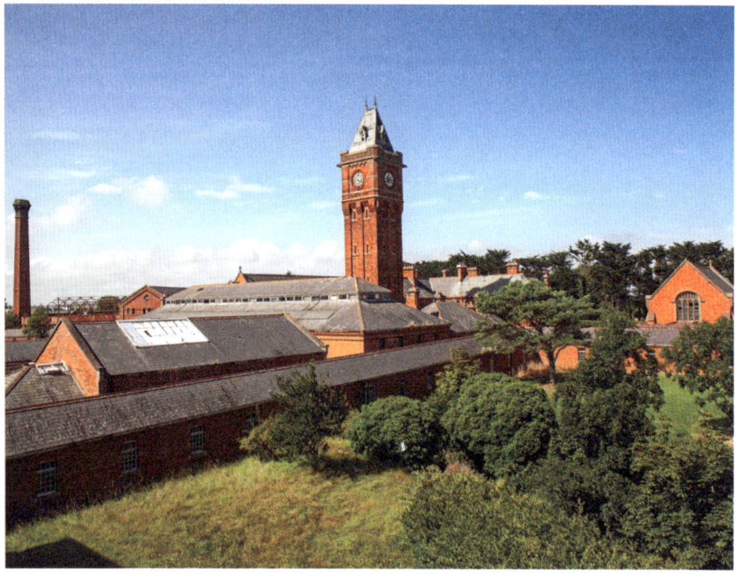

The tower dominates the entire complex, including delivery area (above) and airing courts (above, right). *Photographs by David Killeen, 2019.*

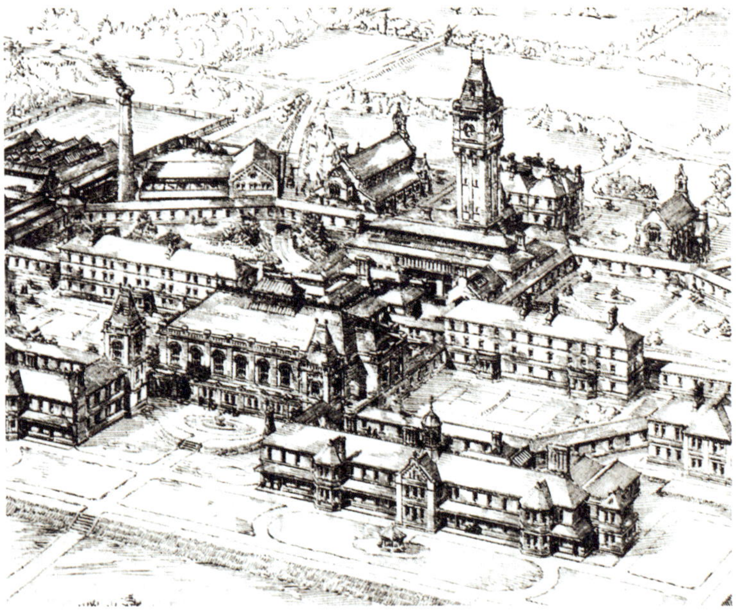

Ashlin's competition winning entry from published in the Irish Builder, 1900. *Image courtesy of the Irish Architectural Archive (Ashlin and Coleman Collection, 76/1:144)*

but his high standing in the ecclesiastical world and connections with almost every major religious order in the land had seen him complete a veritable catalogue of purpose-built institutions to cater to every imaginable social need and moral failing.[4] The Portrane commission would draw upon both sides of his professional experience. Formal, ceremonial and other 'landmark' structures throughout the complex are adorned with late Victorian detailing clearly drawn from ecclesiastical precedents, most notably high-quality internal joinery, stained glass and decorative ironwork. The more numerous spaces for patients and subordinate staff are inevitably more pragmatic exercises in 'institutional vernacular', raised just above the level of the banal or the barracks through the economic application of limited decorative flourishes.

Unsurprisingly given Ashlin's career, the most architecturally distinguished space is the Roman Catholic chapel, but this is not where Portrane makes its most powerful impression. The generously top-lit kitchen and laundry, the galleried central stores reminiscent of a grand train station, its cavernous undercroft whose walls are lined with the thousands of meticulously labelled spare parts and materials needed to maintain this machine of a building: all are strikingly memorable. But neither these – nor even that vast dining hall whose barrel-vaulted ceiling of decorative plasterwork is slowly crumbling onto the floor beneath – represent the abiding image of the place. Rather, it is the corridors – nigh on a mile by measure but seemingly infinite to walk, running north-to-south and east-to-west, setting off on diagonal trajectories and reconvening at top-lit hexagonal and octagonal lobbies designed to orientate but destined to confuse – this otherworld of corridors is what no visitor to Portane can forget.

Venturing upon a building project of a scale and complexity beyond anything the domestic construction industry had achieved before was not without risk – as any observer of Ireland's contemporary struggle to deliver a new National Children's Hospital can attest. Contracts for the new complex were signed with Collen Brothers contractors in August 1896, at which time it was anticipated that the total cost of the project would be somewhere in the region of £240,000.[5] However, by 1902 the spend stood at £317,280,[6] and by the time additional works at the site were complete in 1906, the total cost, including an arbitrator's award of £10,500 in favour of the contractor, amounted to some £378,100.[7] An abrupt change of client governance mid-contract in the wake of local government reform of 1898 cannot have helped, but changes by the client must also have played a part, as the true scope of constructing what was in essence a brand-new town for close to 2,000 people gradually became apparent.[8]

While the great 'mothership' at the heart of the complex would change relatively little once complete, construction never truly stops across an estate that peaked in excess of 1,100 acres. Patient labour transformed the cratered moonscape left behind by the contractors into something approaching a landscape, albeit never close to the quality of those that so enhanced the earliest asylums.[9] New cottages for married attendants were added incrementally along both sides of the main avenue, much like the ribbon development that straggles along the approaches to any ordinary town. In 1917 a new isolation ward for infectious diseases was constructed in the healthiest spot imaginable – just a hundred metres from the shoreline – employing an early version of the cranked plan that would become de rigeur in the TB sanatoria of later decades. Other notable projects included Vincent Kelly's pair of flat-roofed, single-storey and starkly minimal wards of 1955 and a substantial five-storey nurses' home a decade later – all made possible with Sweepstakes money and all now demolished. As the twentieth century drew to a close and the doctrine of moving patients into more home-like surroundings gained traction, a plethora of single-storey units sprung up around the estate – ostensibly in the 'community' but still within eyeshot of the domineering water-tower.

The build quality of some later twentieth-century units may prove questionable, but they at least held the promise of not needing major maintenance within the working lives of those who commissioned them. As for the 'mothership', the burden of maintaining such a complex structure began to crystallise long before the loans that funded it were paid off. In 1921 the Inspectors thought it worthy of note that the task of repainting the windows was underway, a thousand done but nearly as many more to go.[10] But what was feasible in an era when a large able-bodied patient population could undertake such work would become a growing challenge as the buildings advanced in years and the cohorts being cared for within them declined in capability.[11] In 1982 the hospital was left entirely without power for 31 hours during a snow blizzard – an occurrence that surely would not have been tolerated at any other healthcare facility in the state, but which reflected mechanical and electrical systems that had limped along for years on a policy of make-do-and-

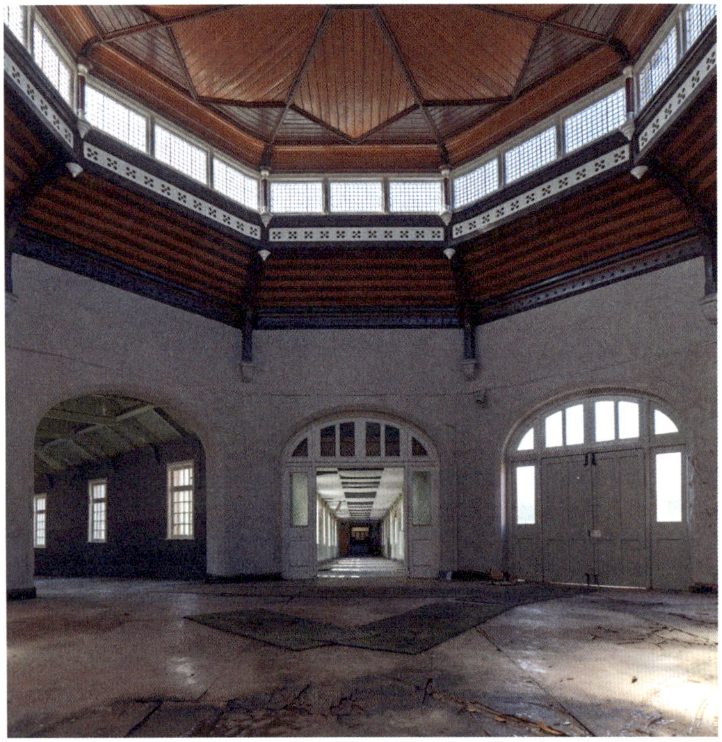

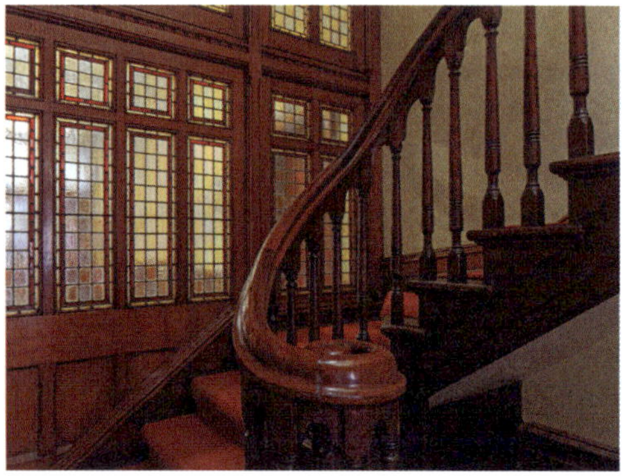

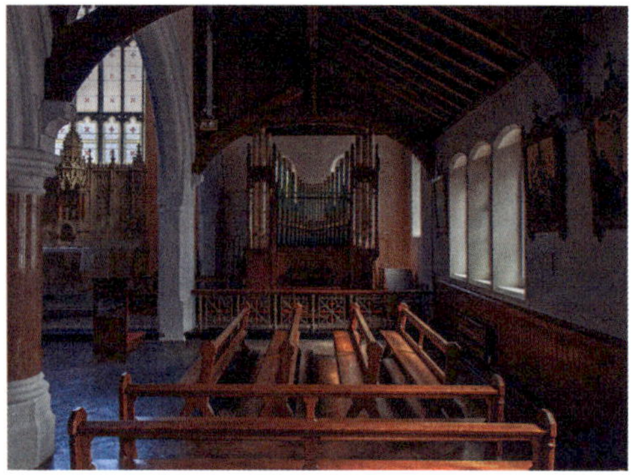

Beyond the obvious set-pieces of the asylum chapels (right), Ashlin's experience as a church architect found its expression in finely detailed internal joinery, as in the corridor lobbies (above) and administration block (top right) *Photographs by David Killeen, 2019.*

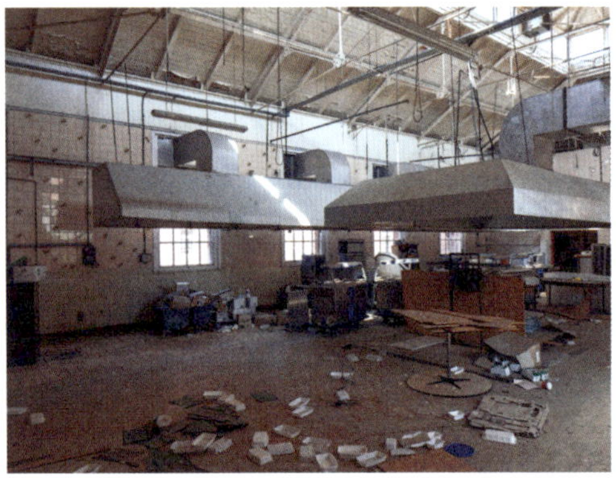

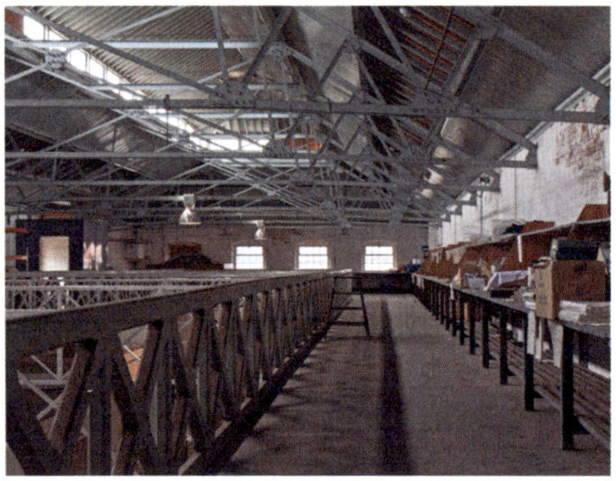

The more utilitarian spaces of kitchen (left), central stores (middle) enjoyed ample daylight from large roof lantern-lights. *Photographs by David Killeen, 2019.*

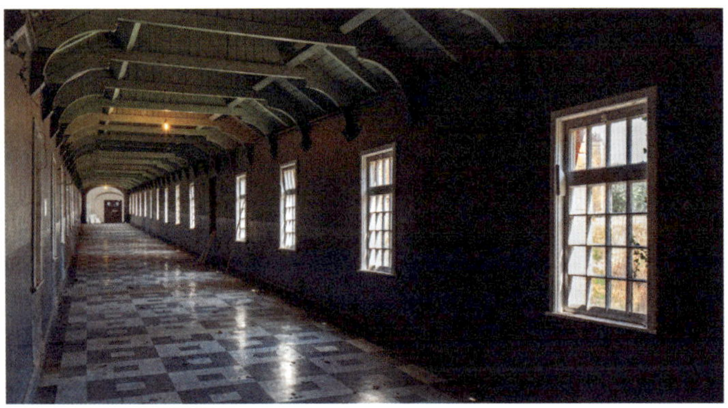

Portrane's labyrinthine corridors have more recently formed the backdrop for films such as The Secret Scripture, 2016. *Photograph by David Killeen, 2019.*

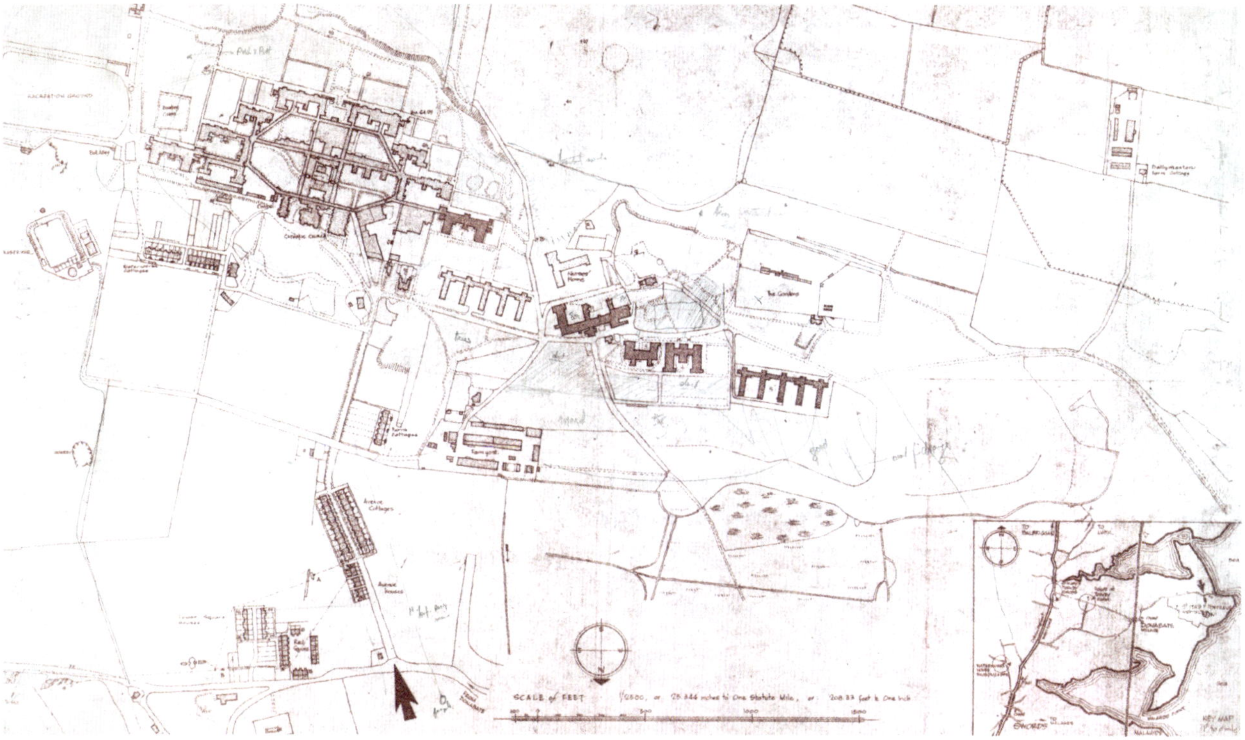

Vincent Kelly's drawing of 1953 shows the complex near its maximum extent. *Image courtesy of the National Archives of Ireland (Office of Public Works Collection, OPW/5HC/4/974, 1)*

mend.[12] The central kitchens, built to prepare 6,000 meals per day, continued to serve HSE facilities across the wider region, but the unpalatable costs of upgrading their bright, top-lit spaces saw the chefs deported to a grim porta-cabin encampment tacked onto the south of the building. Today, clearing autumn leaves from five miles of rainwater gutters and valleys seems like a task of Herculean magnitude, before even attempting to keep abreast of the repairs needed to prevent local leaks from turning once habitable spaces into derelict ones.

Thus stands Portrane today: majestic, brooding and imperious, but also anachronistic, melancholic and slowly deteriorating. Proximity to a commuter railway station may ultimately see the buildings transformed, like many of their English counterparts, into a residential development for those whose escape from the madding crowds of the capital city is now a voluntary decision. But in being selected as the site for the new National Forensic Mental Hospital, which provides secure and therapeutic sanctuary for some of our most troubled citizens, Portrane will continue to function as a place of 'asylum' for generations to come.

Further Reading

Annie Ryan, *Walls of Silence* (Callan: Red Lion Press, 1999)

References

1. *Forty-Third Annual Asylum Report 1894*, HC 1894 [7466] xliii, p. 152.
2. A second estate in the locality – Seamount to the south of Malahide – was also considered. Perhaps more so even than the healthy sea air, the opportunity to discharge sewage directly to the sea rather than a local watercourse (with the potential to contaminate drinking-water supplies) would also have been seen as a major benefit for such a large project.
3. Showing a cavalier attitude towards the competition procedures, the governors put the entries on public display before adjudicating a winner, declared three designs to be of co-equal merit, but then permitted only one of these three to rework their design to bring it in line with budget, much to the chagrin of runner-up, William Kaye-Parry. 'The Portrane Asylum Competition', *The Irish Builder*, 15 Apr. 1895, p. 99. The matter was also raised in parliament: Horace Plunkett MP, House of Commons, 16 May 1895, 4.33, cc. 1329.
4. Dictionary of Irish Architects: George Coppinger Ashlin, www.dia.ie/architects/view/72/ASHLIN-GEORGECOPPINGER, accessed on 28 Nov. 2020.
5. *Forty-Eighth Annual Asylum Report 1899*, HC 1899 [9479] xl, p. 34.
6. George Wyndham MP, House of Commons, 30 Jan. 1902, 4:101, cc. 1341.
7. Like any 'mega-project', the final cost of the Portrane project is difficult to define with certainty. Wyndham in 1902 noted a spend to date of £317,280 and anticipated a further spend of £45,350, giving a total of £362,630. The loans itemised in the Annual Reports of the Local Government Board, 1902–1906 broadly align with this estimate, with the late addition of £3,000 for unforeseen works to the water supply, and the £10,500 arbiters award.
8. To the design capacity of 1,200 of the main building must be added patients in the existing Portrane House, the 'temporary' wooden buildings, the full retinue of staff and, in some cases, their families.
9. The incumbent RMS, Connolly Norman, acidly observing of the therapeutic value of such work: 'Even the demented can wheel a barrow.' *Richmond District Asylum, Dublin: Annual Report of the Medical Superintendent to Joint Committee of Management for the year 1905*, p. 22.
10. *Sixty-Ninth Annual Asylum Report 1919*, HC 1921 [1127] xv, p. 23.
11. With an increasing bias towards intellectually disabled adults and children, which represented half of the patient population by the early 1980s.
12. Annie Ryan, *Walls of Silence* (Callan, 1999), pp 33–4, p. 91, p. 98, p. 102.

CASE STUDY 26

Years in operation
1906–present

Original cost
£168,112

Capacity (min /max)
650 / 2200

Architect(s)
Jackson & Tilley,
Watt (Graeme) and Tulloch,
G. T. Hine.

Purdysburn Hospital

(previously Purdsyburn Villa Colony, latterly Knockbracken Healthcare Park)

For a local authority still swelling with pride from its elevation to the status of a city, a lavish new city hall was an obvious expression of civic ambition and self-esteem. But Belfast's simultaneous investment in not one, not two, but three major healthcare projects in the first decade of the twentieth century made it clear that the fruits of burgeoning capitalism were also there to be harnessed for the benefit of its citizens.[1]

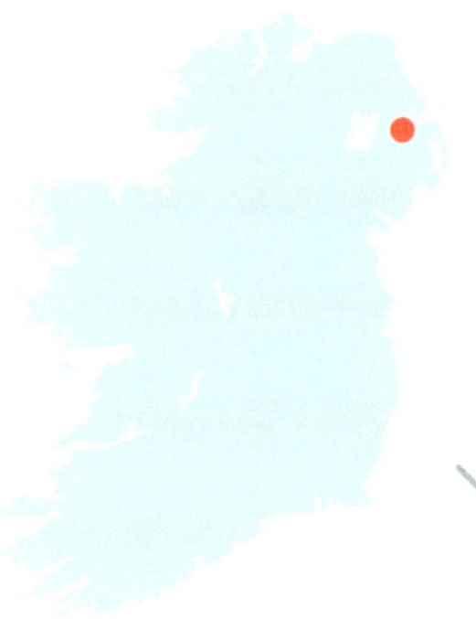

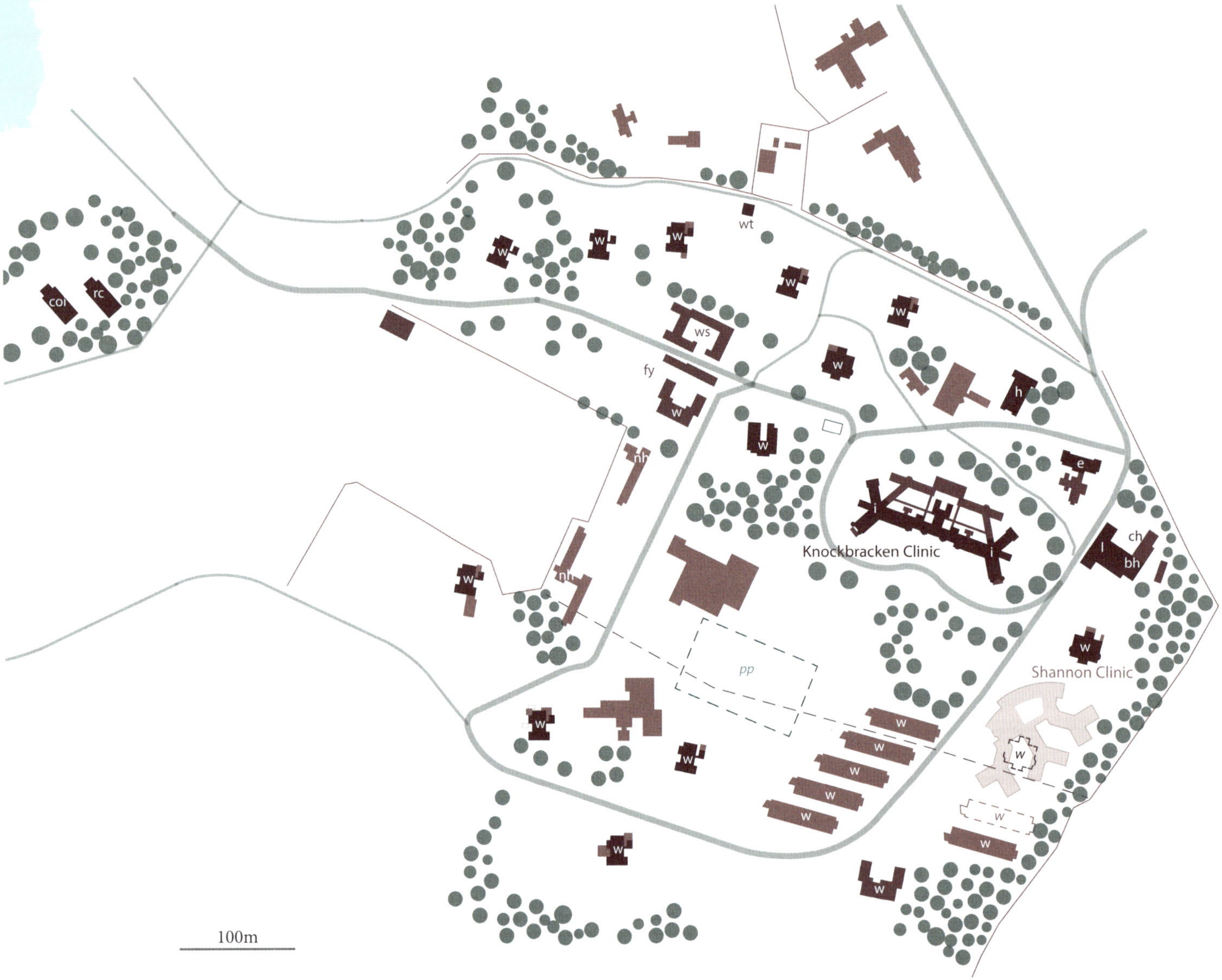

The story of Belfast District Lunatic Asylum begins in 1829 with the opening of a standard Johnston and Murray asylum on a rural site between what would later become the Grosvenor and Falls Roads. (see Case Study 4). Constructed at a time when the built-up area of Belfast was about two-thirds that of Cork, by the close of the century the city looked like it may soon challenge Dublin for the title of Ireland's largest city. This rapid urban growth not only increased the demands placed upon the asylum, but also constrained it from expanding further on its existing site. Decanting patients to new district asylums in Downpatrick (1865) and Antrim (1898) temporarily relieved some pressure, but could not prevent patient numbers climbing inexorably past the 1,000 mark by the close of the century.

In 1894 the Inspectors excitedly reported that 'The Governors have, with a liberality creditable alike to their intelligence and humanity, agreed to the purchase of one of the most beautiful estates in the neighbourhood of Belfast with a view to the erection thereon of a new and modern asylum.'[2] An architectural competition for a new hospital for 800 patients resulted in the appointment of the local firm of Jackson and Tilley in 1897.[3] Tender drawings for the first phase – a block for 360 chronic patients - were already underway when the 1898 Local Government Act gave rise to a change of client, as the old board of governors was replaced by a newly constituted asylum committee. The incoming committee reappraised the project, and in 1901 determined that their new institution would be designed as a 'villa colony'. The villa colony concept was growing in popularity on mainland Europe, but the committee's decision at Purdysburn would mark out Belfast as a pioneer on these islands at a time when conventional pavilion-echelon asylums were mushrooming by the dozen in the hinterlands of Britain's large industrial cities.[4]

Proponents of the villa colony system sought to remedy the demoralising institutional environments of the old corridor asylums by affording patients the greatest possible degree of freedom commensurate with their condition, in a physical setting supposed to emulate a 'normal' village community and devoid of any visible evidence of enclosure. At Purdysburn the 'villas' that lend the system its name comprised ten detached blocks accommodating around 50 patients each, whose external appearance and internal layout and furnishings were designed to resemble, as much as possible, a comfortable if rather bloated middle-class home.[5] The asylum was built in two main phases – four villas between 1902 and 1906 to the designs of Watt (Graeme) and Tulloch, with the remainder of the complex being completed between 1909 and 1913 to designs of renowned English asylum architect, G. T. Hine – allowing the old city asylum to be finally vacated in 1915.[6]

The villas were supposed to replicate a sense of normal life, to the extent that staff cooked separately for patients in each villa and the RMS even encouraged the keeping of pets.[7] But not all central services necessary for the smooth running of a large asylum could be devolved or dispensed with. Ancillary structures familiar from the traditional asylum - including an administration block, laundry and recreation hall - would still be provided, but as detached buildings. The biggest building on the site was the infirmary, but even this was smaller than any asylum building seen since Johnston and Murray's earliest asylums, and much more convincingly domestic. It is also an interesting building in its own right – not least for the innovative layout of the flanking convalescent wings, each centred around a pair of top-lit, hexagonal winter gardens.[8]

If the clock-cum-water tower came to be seen as a physical expression of the dictatorial asylum regime of old, then designers of this 'free' asylum could be expected to avoid any such negative associations. The pragmatic functions of elevated water storage and a large clock for outdoor workers remained necessary, but were provided for in a structure with few architectural trappings, located far from the administrative heart of the complex. The power-laden 'trust and obey' messaging of traditional asylum architecture was turned on its head: here, the institution trusted the patients. More surprising is that the obligatory duo of chapels was also relegated from sight to a remote woodland clearing, whereas they might have been expected to play a more prominent role in the visual choreography of a model settlement. But on the whole, the Inspectors were impressed:

> *These villas provide accommodation of an entirely novel character, and carry out, in the fullest sense, the liberal and unrestrained treatment of the insane. No buildings could give a greater idea of freedom. There is not a bolt or a bar to be seen. Every door is open, and every window is provided with full-sized panes of glass, and opens to the fullest. The rooms are bright and cheerful, and are comfortably and tastefully furnished, and supplied with books, papers, plants, and other objects of interest.*[9]

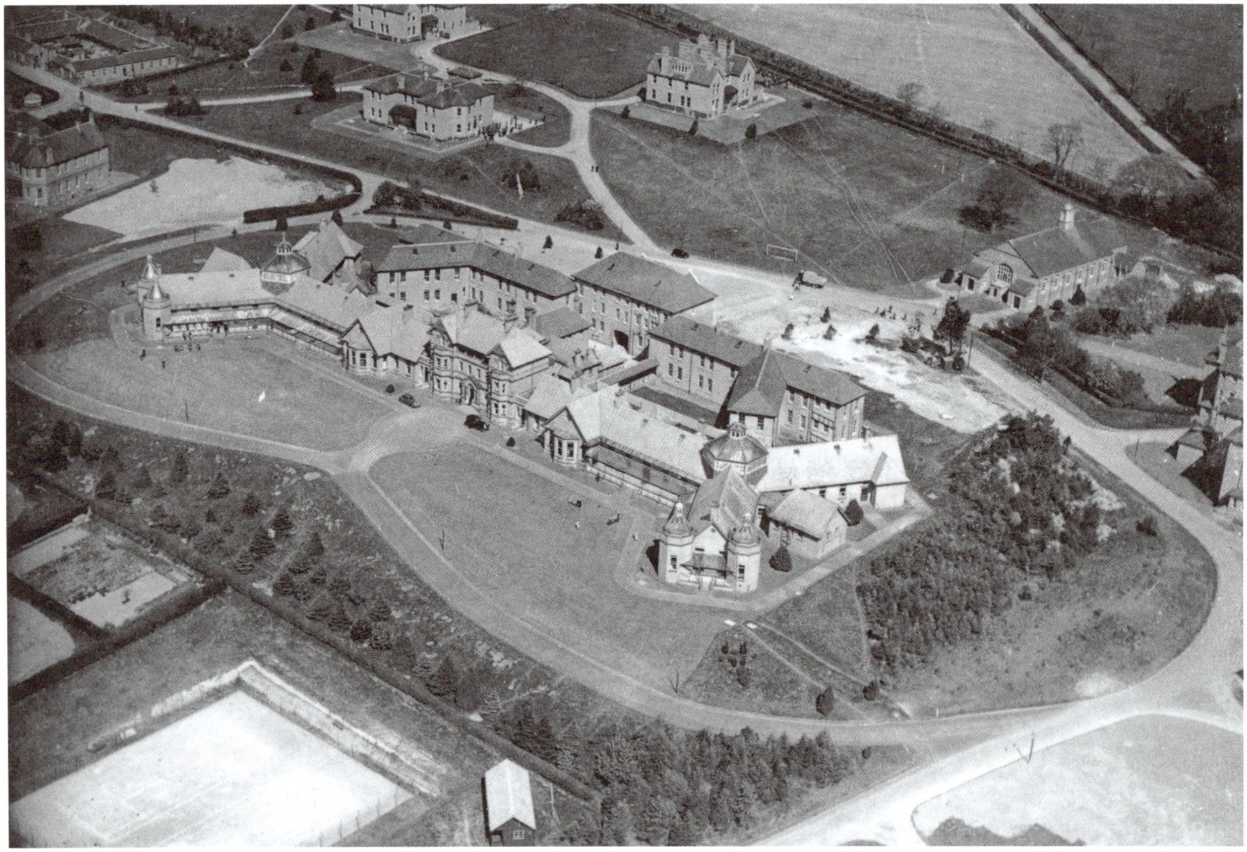

Aerial photgraph, c.1940s, showing the centrally located infirmary and recreation hall amidst a wider landscape of freestanding villas. *Image courtesy of National Museums Northern Ireland (Belfast Telegraph, HOYFM.BT.22)*

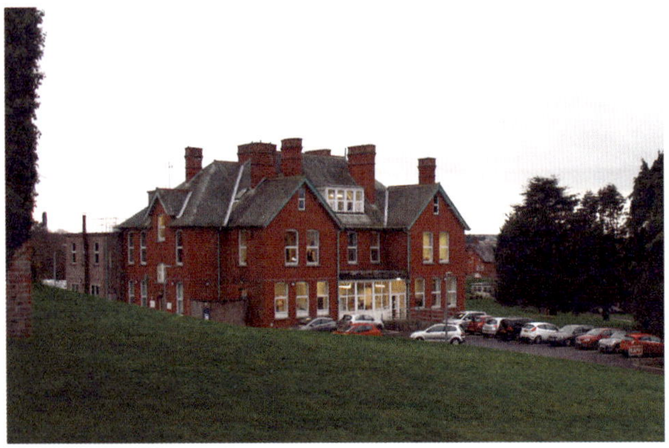

The detached villas were of appealing, domestic character.
Photograph by the author, 2020

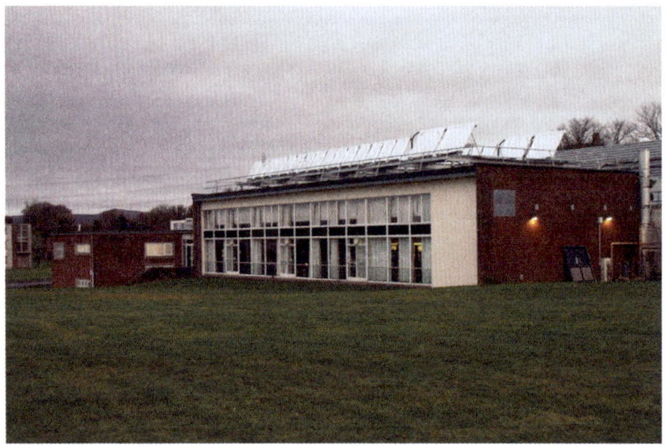

A new canteen built in the 1950s reinforced the sense of hospital-as-campus.
Photograph by the author, 2020

Indeed the Inspectors had been fairly enthusiastic cheerleaders for the venture throughout, flagging as early as 1899 the possibility of adopting the villa model for at least part of the new asylum[10] encouraging the asylum committee in 1903 to prepare a holistic masterplan for the site instead of building villas ad hoc[11] and upon completion lauding:

> *the great and beneficent enterprise upon which they embarked when it was decided to abandon the old and outworn building in the city, and to provide for the insane poor of Belfast an institution which in many respects sets an example to the country, not least in the combination of economy with efficiency which characterises it.*[12]

It is a bitter irony – and a subject worthy of research beyond the scope of this book – that this exemplary new asylum went on to experience a mortality rate far higher than was ever witnessed in the cramped city-centre site, being consistently higher than the national average through the 1910s and often the highest in the country, even before reaching a tragic peak during the influenza pandemic of 1918 when just shy of one fifth of its patients died in a single year.[13] Infectious disease would sadly prove more effective at reducing asylum populations than the most curative architectural solutions.

No less important than the innovative architecture, the enormous landholding at Purdysburn was seen as an opportunity to grant patients a larger measure of (controlled) freedom than was possible within the cramped confines of the old city asylum. There, '…no patients are taken beyond the grounds. At Purdysburn the demesne is so extensive as to render this unnecessary, while at Grosvenor Road it would not be possible.'[14] The combination at Purdysburn of a gently rolling landscape, mature woodland and the intentionally informal disposition of buildings made for a scenic and naturalistic setting, but one that could still in no way be mistaken for a 'real' suburb or village. Even today, a walk around what is now known as the Knockbracken Healthcare Park is a somewhat disorientating experience, having neither the predictable spatial hierarchy of a traditional asylum, nor the internal boundaries and enclosed private gardens of the middle-class suburb to which its villa architecture seemingly aspires.

The villa-colony system would prove no less prone than any other to continued overcrowding during the first half of the twentieth century, and hence equally in need of drastic deinstitutionalisation in the second. However, the inherently flexible nature of a system of detached buildings in a spacious setting has allowed the site to evolve to meet new needs. No less than 50 individual buildings now populate the campus, including a 1950s canteen, a centre for nursing education, and a pair of utilitarian 1960s nurses' homes (now derelict). Today, the campus is host to a truly bewildering array of community, learning disability and mental health services and associated charitable and voluntary organisations. Even if some individual buildings stand derelict, it is heartening to see how a site borne of civic desire to create the best possible environment for its patients in the early-twentieth century continues to serve the diverse needs of the community in the twenty-first.

Further Reading

Stephen Hamilton and David Martin, *The Burn, The Fever and Beyond* (Belfast, 2016).

Stephen Hamilton and Hugh O'Donnell, *Purdysburn Hospital: The Legacy of a Villa Colony,* (Belfast, 2013).

References

1. The year 1906 was an auspicious one for Belfast, witnessing the opening of the new City Hall, a new Fever Hospital at Purdysburn, the new Royal Victoria (general) Hospital and the first phase of the Purdysburn Villa Colony.
2. *Forty-Fourth Annual Asylum Report 1894*, HC 1895 [7804] liv, p. 96.
3. Forty-Sixth Annual Asylum Report 1897, HC 1897 [8639] xxxviii, p. 18.
4. A new asylum entirely along villa-colony lines, as distinct from the addition of a few satellite villas orbiting a mighty mothership, as at the London pavilion-echelon asylums of Bexley, Horton and Long Grove. The specialist epileptic colony at Ewell, Epsom, is of similar date but represented a typology that was beginning to diverge from the classic general purpose asylum.
5. Gillian Allmond, 'Light and Darkness in an Edwardian Institution for the Insane Poor: Illuminating the Material Practices of the Asylum age,' in *International Journal of Historical Archaeology* 20:1 (2016), pp 15–17.
6. *Sixty-Seventh Annual Asylum Report 1917*, HC 1919 [32] xxv, p. 19.
7. *Sixty-Third Annual Asylum Report 1913*, HC 1914 [7527] xli, p. 78.
8. Gillian Allmond, '"The outer darkness of madness": The Edwardian Winter Garden at Purdysburn public asylum for the insane', in *The Archaeology of Darkness* (Oxford,2016) pp 120–4.
9. *Fifty-Fifth Annual Asylum Report 1905*, HC 1906 [3164] xxxix, p. 80.
10. *Forty-Eighth Annual Asylum Report 1898*, HC 1899 [9479] xl, p.131.
11. *Fifty-Second Annual Asylum Report 1902*, HC 1903 [1762] xxvii, p. 83.
12. *Sixty-Third Annual Asylum Report 1913*, HC 1914 [7527] xli, pp 76–7.
13. From an average annual mortality rate that hovered in mid-single digits in the 1890s, the rate shot up to 13.1 per cent in 1915 and 19.7 per cent in 1918 before dropping slightly to 14.8 per cent in 1919, consistently between 5 and 10 percentage points higher than the national average.
14. *Sixty-First Annual Asylum Report 1911*, HC 1912–13 [6386] xxxix, p. 79.

CASE STUDY 27

St Brigid's Hospital

(previously Ardee Mental Hospital)

Years in operation
1933–present

Original cost
c. £138,000

Capacity (min /max)
370 / 419

Architect(s)
H. T. Wright

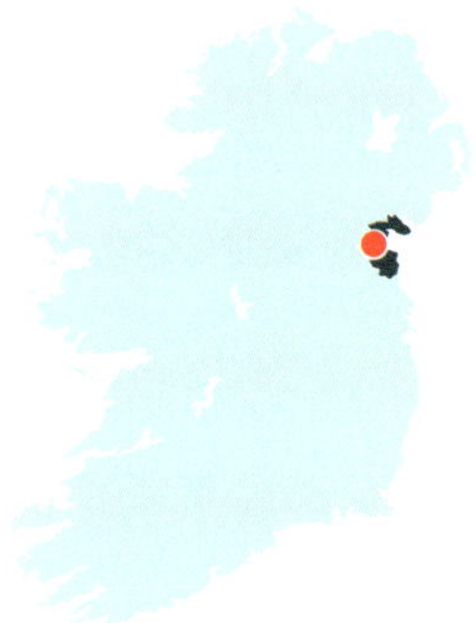

The new mental hospital that opened in Ardee in 1933 would be the first of its type never to bear the moniker 'asylum'. A world away from the overcrowded Dublin institutions to which patients from county Louth had previously been consigned, the architect of this thoroughly modern structure nevertheless felt himself bound by many of the trappings of traditional asylumdom, most notably the domineering presence of a central clocktower.

The boundaries of Ireland's asylum catchments were continuously redrawn throughout the nineteenth century as large districts were gradually divided along individual county lines. However, even as the neighbouring county of Meath was reallocated to the new Mullingar asylum in 1855, patients from Ireland's smallest county would continue to be sent to the country's largest asylum – the Richmond in Dublin. The early establishment of rail links between county Louth and the capital meant that patient transfers were actually less onerous than those experienced by patients travelling within larger, less developed counties. But as the nineteenth century rolled into the twentieth, the challenges of meeting the needs of the capital's burgeoning patient population eclipsed the minority interests of counties Wicklow and Louth with whom it shared a district.

In terms of representation on the board of 33 governors, Louth was even more disadvantaged than its relative proportion of the patient cohort would suggest. The new county council established after the local government reforms of 1898 took a more active interest in the question of separating their district from the Richmond, culminating in a deputation to the new Minister for Local Government and Public Health in 1924 to make their case. Their request for a separation was sanctioned in principle, but their original proposal to adapt the former Ardee workhouse for use as an asylum was rejected, leading to the ultimate decision to construct an entirely new facility on part of the former Ruxton estate outside the town.[2]

Despite Louth County Council's attempts to retain local architect John McGahon to design the new hospital, the Department of Local Government insisted

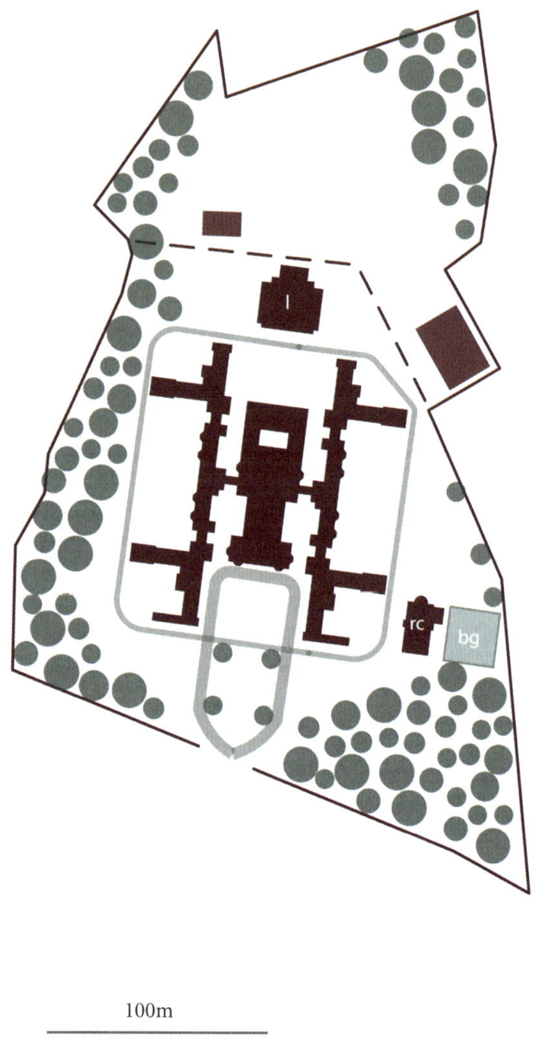

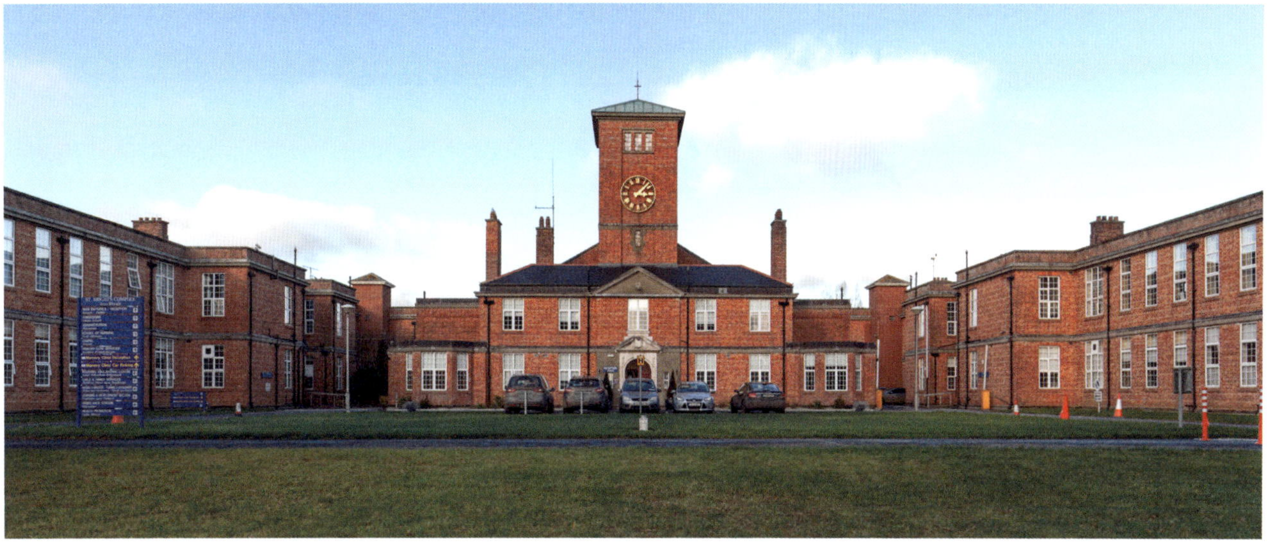

Modern, classical, mannerist - Wright put multiple styles to work in his competition winning design for Ardee. *Photograph by David Killeen, 2019.*

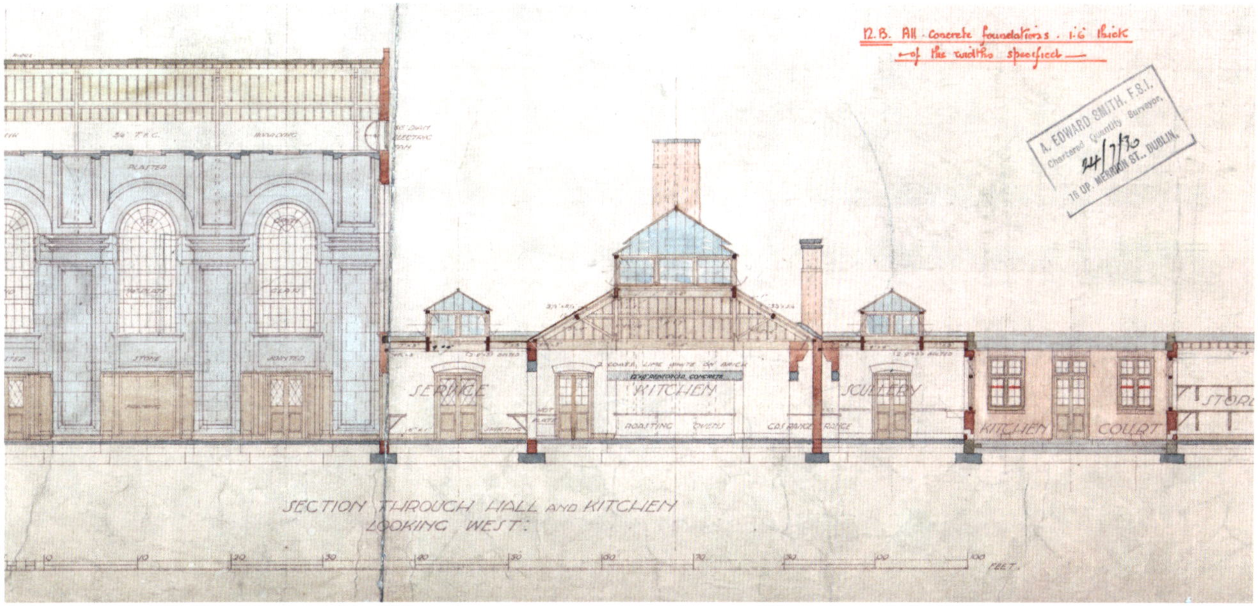

Cross section through dining hall, servery, kitchen and stores. *Image courtesy of the National Archives of Ireland (Office of Public Works Collection, OPW/5HC/4/974, 3)*

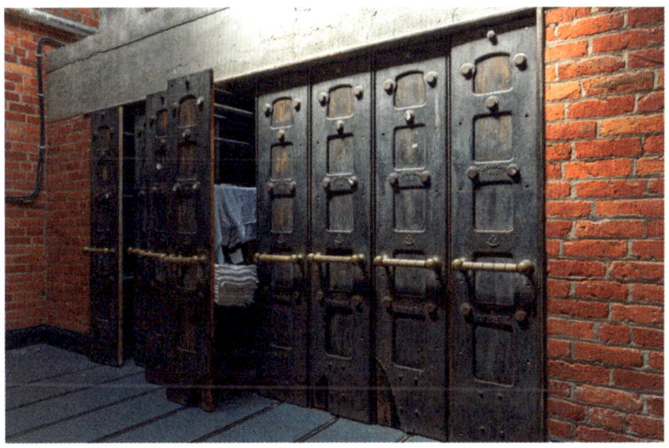

Laundry drying racks: high technology in a building where patient wards were still heated by open fires. *Photograph by David Killeen, 2019.*

on a properly administered architectural competition.[3] Thirty-four entries were received from across the British Isles, with a little-known Scottish architect, Henry Thomas Wright, selected as the winner. The Department refused to sanction payment of fees to McGahon for his early work, but he later received a small consolation prize in the form of a commission to design the freestanding chapel to the east of the main hospital.[4]

Stylistically, Wright's winning design was a curious hybrid. The simple volumes, strongly horizontal massing, flat roofs and continuous parapet lines of the ward blocks hint at the influence of international Modernism, but any such impression is submerged beneath Wright's conservative devotion to symmetry and eclectic approach to detailing. Three of the building's four sides are composed as symmetrical facades, but the unifying effect of his continuous string course and cornice is somewhat undermined by a strange medley of slender sliding-sash windows, wider casements and canted bays. Internally, the recreation hall features classically derived plasterwork which, observed alongside the high-quality joinery throughout the remaining 'public' areas, suggests that Wright – for all of his dalliances with earlier and later styles – was at heart an Edwardian. The central administration block – the traditional set piece of every formally planned institution – is modest in scale and domestic in character, enlivened only by a Mannerist doorcase to the main entrance. It could be that Wright wished to downplay the building's institutional nature, but if so, his inclusion of a central clocktower of unabashedly muscular proportions had decidedly the opposite effect. The building may have been a modern psychiatric hospital in name, but it still struggled to shake off the century-old architectural marker of the asylum.

In plan, Wright's design was also a mix of precedent and progress. At a time when England's only new mental hospitals – Runwell in Essex and the fourth iteration of Bethlem in the south-London suburb of Beckenham – were planned as 'villa colonies' comprising dozens of smaller buildings dispersed across a parkland setting, Wright's design for Ardee consolidated all but the laundry and boiler house into a single structure. A central spine comprising administration block, recreation hall and kitchens was flanked on either side by four almost identical two-storey ward blocks for male and female patients – a form whose basic principles would not have been unfamiliar to the architects of the London Metropolitan Asylum Commission's 'economic' asylums, over 50 years earlier.

However, the internal layout shows that Wright was keenly aware of the twin imperatives of efficiency of use and ease of superintendence. The wards themselves comprised L-shaped, open-plan dormitories for 44 patients apiece, with some single rooms opening off, all designed to be supervised by a single attendant. Separate day rooms for each ward, denoted externally by bay-windows, occupy the position between the dormitories and the shared facilities – an eminently efficient arrangement that saw patients naturally migrate towards the centre of the building by day and retreat to the extremities by night. Together with a decent level of sanitary provision, well-equipped kitchen and state-of-the-art disinfecting laundry, this building was by most measures a thoroughly modern hospital.[5] Indeed, in describing Wright's design as a 'masterly plan', The Irish Builder was especially pleased to observe that Ardee had been recommended as a worthy exemplar to architects competing to design a new mental hospital in Surbiton, Surrey.[6]

Completed in 1933 at a time when the national mental hospital population was already close to its all-time peak, Ardee largely escaped the chronic overcrowding that had afflicted its Dublin predecessor for generations, and hence never needed to be extended. Indeed, this is the only instance that the reader will encounter between these pages where the footprint of the principal building remains unaltered since the day it was built. And while the last occupied ward is now in the process of being wound down, the hospital unexpectedly found itself once again in the frontline of the public health service in late 2020, as a Covid-19 test centre for counties Louth and Meath.[7]

References

1. The tender was awarded at a cost of £79,987, but the final cost was later stated by the Minister for Local Government as being around £138,000. Seán T O'Ceallaigh TD, Dáil Éireann, 28 Apr. 1936, 61:12. This cost was offset by a rebate of £32,660 from counties Dublin and Wicklow, and a grant of £45,976 from the Sweepstakes.
2. Lisa Butterley, 'Institutional reform in mental healthcare in Ireland: The establishment of the Ardee Mental Hospital, 1933, in its historical context' (unpublished PhD thesis, NUI Maynooth, 2014), pp 85–6, 123–4.
3. *Report of the Inspector of Mental Hospitals, 1929*, p. 22.
4. Butterley, 'Institutional reform in mental healthcare in Ireland,' pp 163–4, p. 177.
5. *Report of the Inspector of Mental Hospitals, 1929*, p. 23;
6. The Irish Builder, 1 Jul. 1933, p. 541.
7. Drogheda Independent, 3 Oct. 2020, www.independent.ie/regionals/droghedaindependent/news/ardee-service-will-be-able-to-test-up-to-3500-39569126.html, accessed 23 Jan. 2021.

CASE STUDY 28

St Patrick's Hospital

(previously Castlerea Mental Hospital, latterly Castlerea Prison)

Years in operation
1939–1994

Original cost
£163,509

Capacity (min /max)
400 / 493

Architect(s)
J. R. Boyd Barrett

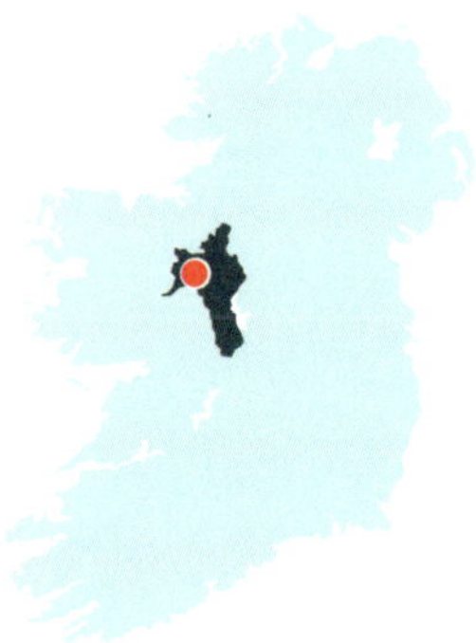

Castlerea may have the shortest history of any of the institutions featured in this book, but it has also witnessed more change than most sites twice its age. Its design was a curious hybrid, melding the formalistic layout of the traditional asylum with the architectural expression of the modern hospital, as if anticipating the fact that its first use would be as a tuberculosis sanatorium. After a mere 40 years serving the purpose for which it was actually built, a community anxious to secure local employment would succeed in having the site transformed into a prison, a facility with which the town's name is now nationally synonymous.

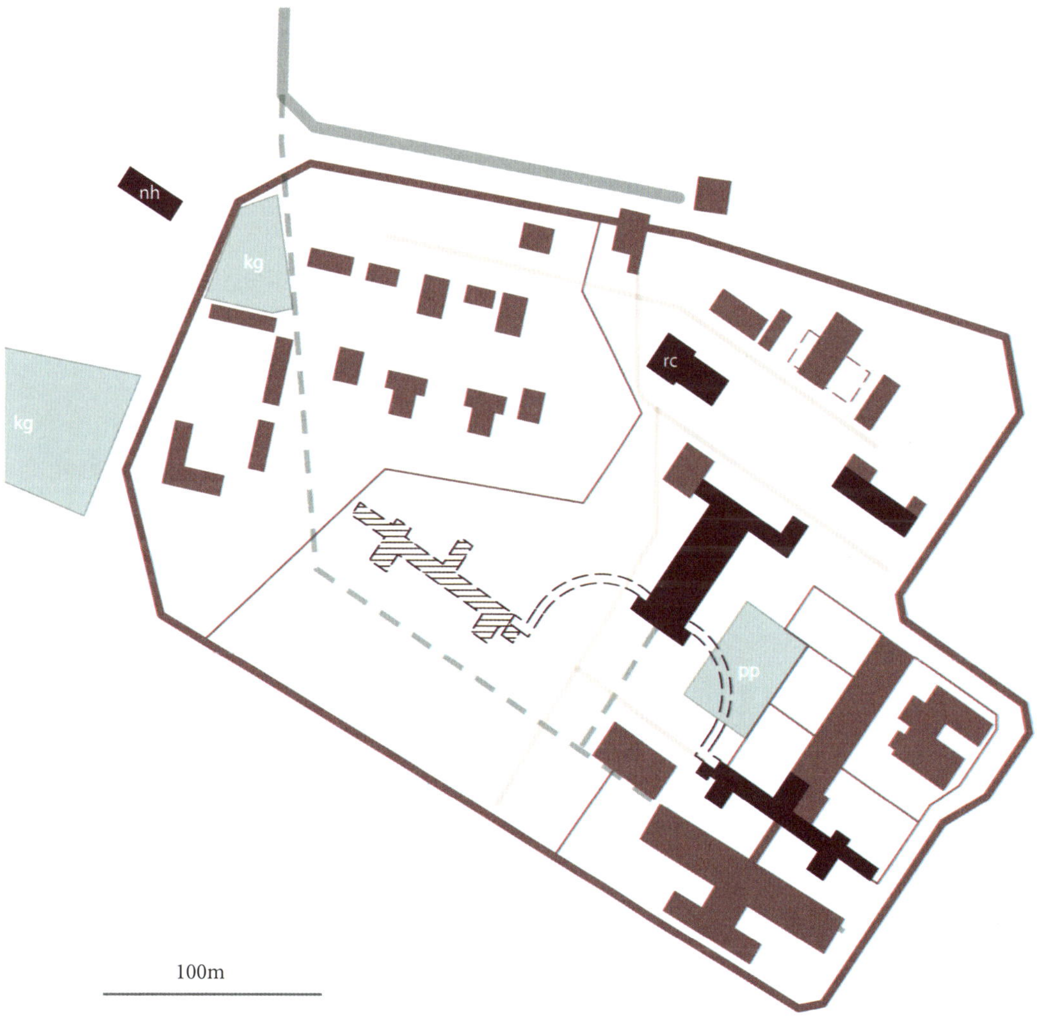

That Roscommon was so late in being provided with a dedicated county institution is perhaps unsurprising, given that the main asylum at Ballinasloe was originally sited within Roscommon county bounds, and indeed was more accessible for prospective Roscommon patients than many Galway residents. But in response to chronic overcrowding in the main institution in Ballinasloe, the Joint Mental Hospital Committee in 1932 authorised a subcommittee with 'the widest possible powers' to prepare a report on the options for an auxiliary facility.[1] Within a year, the committee had completed the purchase of Harristown House and its 320-acre demesne, outside Castlerea, as the site for a new District Mental Hospital. Architect J. R. Boyd Barrett was engaged for the design, in parallel with a new Admissions Hospital and detached infirmary on the Ballinasloe site.[2] Boyd Barrett had also been engaged by the County Board of Health to design the new County Hospital at Roscommon, making for a family of four architecturally distinguished healthcare buildings in this corner of Connaught that share a common architectural language, detailing and finishes.

Despite its conception as a 'District Mental Hospital', Castlerea may be considered as the last institution in Ireland to be constructed along the lines of the traditional self-sufficient asylum – a standalone complex located deep within a large agricultural landholding. Tenders for the new hospital for 400 patients were invited in June 1934, in parallel with the new buildings at Ballinasloe. Fortuitously, John Sisk and Co. completed the works in 1939, just before the Emergency gave rise to crippling shortages of essential building materials. It is recounted locally that the hospital committee, on hearing that the Irish Army was to requisition the new building as a barracks, moved in the first dozen patients and staff under cover of darkness to stake their claim to the building. However, the committee ultimately lost control of the building as it was instead commandeered for use as a tuberculosis sanatorium in 1948. A warren of single-storey, flat-roofed buildings were added during this time, such as were common in the green-field sanatoria of the day.[3]

The architectural layout derives from the pavilion-asylum designs of the early twentieth century. At the core of the complex stands a central administration block, recreation hall and ancillary spaces. Link corridors – unusual in being curved, colonnaded, and open air – connect the core to symmetrical flanking ward pavilions for male and female patients, complete with glazed south-facing verandahs. The overall arrangement was highly reminiscent of a Palladian country house, albeit with the traditional hierarchy inverted as the large, flanking, three-storey ward blocks dwarf the modest two-storey administration block, whose sole claim to architectural prominence was a central cupola – the classic signifier of traditional asylum design for over a century.

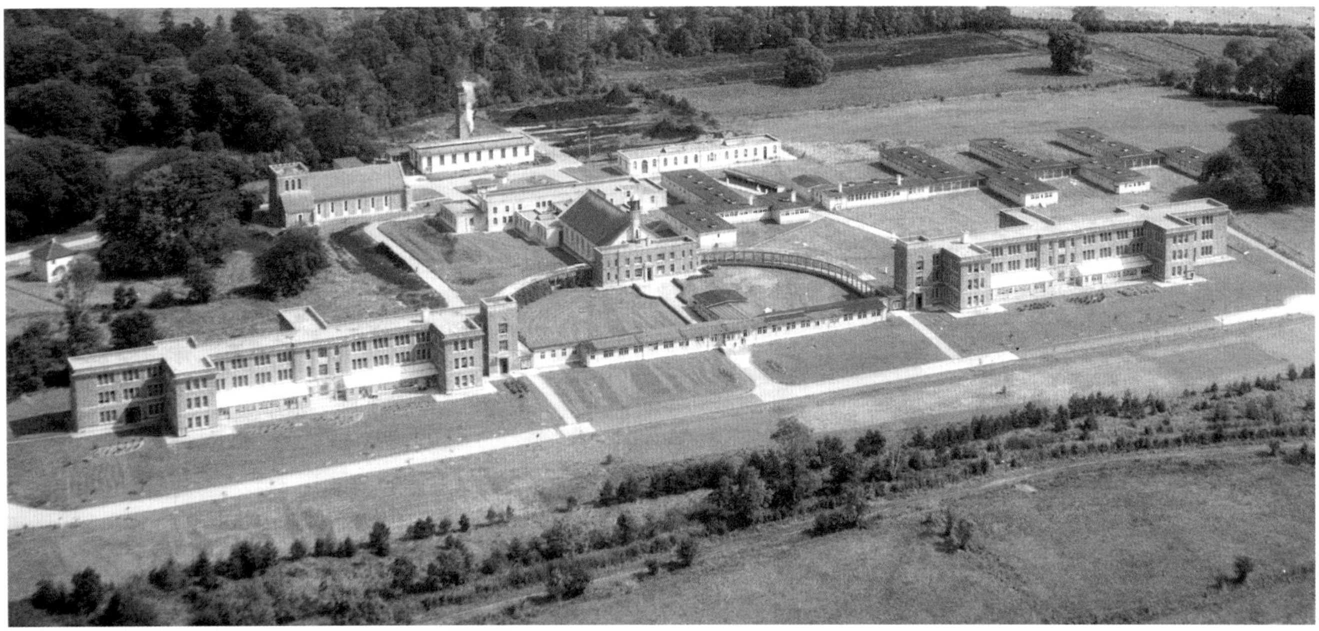

Aerial photograph, 1954, with additional buildings added during period of use as TB sanatorium. *Image courtesy of the National Library of Ireland (NPA MOR433).*

Local Ballinasloe limestone was used throughout, cut into regular ashlar blocks with a rock-faced finish distinctive of Boyd Barrett's 1930s general healthcare buildings. Large, tripartite sliding sash windows flooded the interiors of the modern ward blocks with daylight, while interior finishes included high-quality wood block and terrazzo flooring. Somewhat counter-intuitively for a wholly stone-faced building, window sills and surrounds were changed to concrete as a cost-saving exercise, The Irish Builder noting 'it appears strange that so large a saving can be effected by using concrete in the window sills alone in a district where some of the finest limestone in Ireland is quarried.'[4] The value-engineering measures did not extend to the chapel, which, unusually for an asylum/hospital chapel, was adorned with a rather inelegant and bizarrely battlemented tower.

The abatement of the tuberculosis epidemic allowed the hospital buildings to revert to mental health use in 1955, albeit with 100 beds dedicated to the treatment of mental patients with TB.[5] The facility continued to serve Roscommon patients for over 40 years, until the shock announcement by the Minister for Finance in his 1986 budget speech that the institution, by now known as St Patrick's Hospital, would close. A concerted community campaign failed to save the hospital and its 262 employees, but by the time of its final closure in 1994, political pressure had succeeded in designating the Castlerea campus as the location for a new prison for the west of Ireland. By 1995 a secure perimeter wall was constructed around the entire complex, and the first group of prisoners entered the facility in December 1996.

Castlerea now operates as a committal prison for remand and sentenced male prisoners from Cavan, Donegal, Longford and the five counties of Connaught, with an operating capacity of 340.[6] The central block and recreation hall of the original hospital remain in administrative use, while the former east wing houses the prison kitchen, library and education centre. All prisoner cells are located in purpose-built, top-lit galleried wings added since the 1990s. The practical difficulties of upgrading the 1930s east wing to meet the security standards of even ancillary uses led to the decision to demolish its long-disused western counterpart.[7] The entrance sequence to the facility is also radically altered, such that the architectural logic of the original hospital complex is almost illegible. The complex looks set to remain in use by the prison service for the foreseeable future, although the architectural legacy of the former mental hospital will inevitably fade further over time.

References

1. *The Irish Builder*, 23 Apr. 1932, p. 390.
2. *Report of the Inspector of Mental Hospitals, 1933*, p. 25.
3. National Library of Ireland, Morgan Aerial Photographic Collection, NPA MOR 432–435.
4. *The Irish Builder*, 2 Jun. 1934, p. 453.
5. *Report of the Inspector of Mental Hospitals, 1955*, p. 10.
6. Irish Prison Service, Castlerea Prison, www.irishprisons.ie/prison/castlerea-prison/, accessed 22 Jan. 2021.
7. Martin Reilly, Governor, Castlerea Prison, conversation with the author, 7 Jul. 2020.

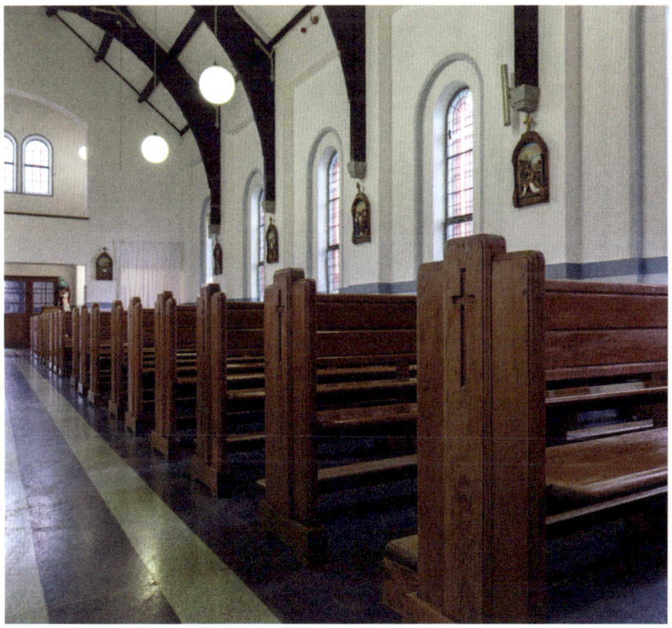

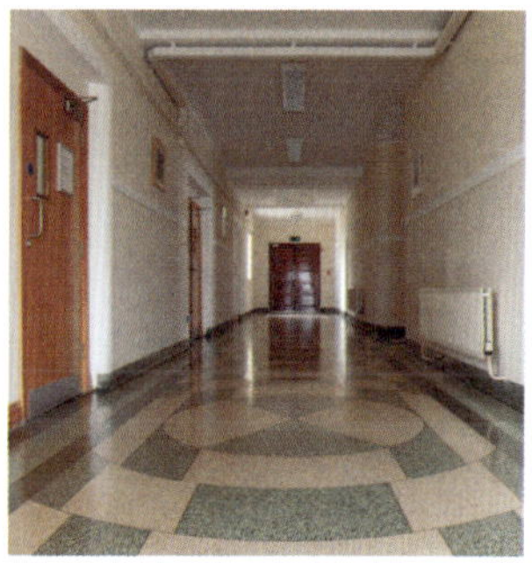

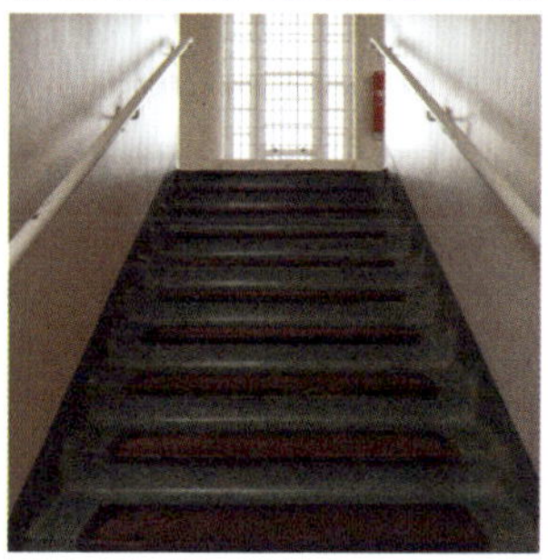

The new prison was actively welcomed as an alternative source of employment. *Photograph by the author, 2020.*

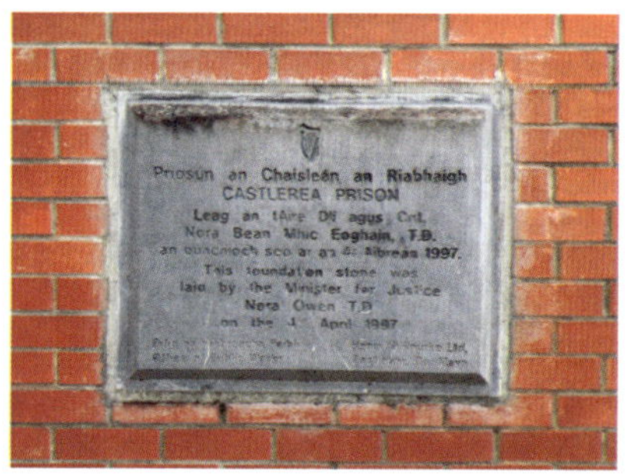

High quality finishes and detailing in evidence throughout, with bespoke pews in the chapel and fine terrazo floors throughout. *Photographs by David Kileen, 2019.*

CASE STUDY 29

Gransha Hospital

(incorporating Stradreagh Hospital, Lakeview Hospital, Grangewood Unit)

Years in operation
1960–present

Original cost
c.£2,000,000

Capacity (min /max)
800

Architect(s)
Matthew A. Robinson

The last purpose-built mental hospital on the island of Ireland was almost a century in gestation, such that by the time it eventually opened, the doctrine of standalone green-field institutions for the mentally ill was already passé. Many of the buildings that opened to such acclaim in 1960 would themselves remain in service for little more than 50 years before being relegated to redundancy.

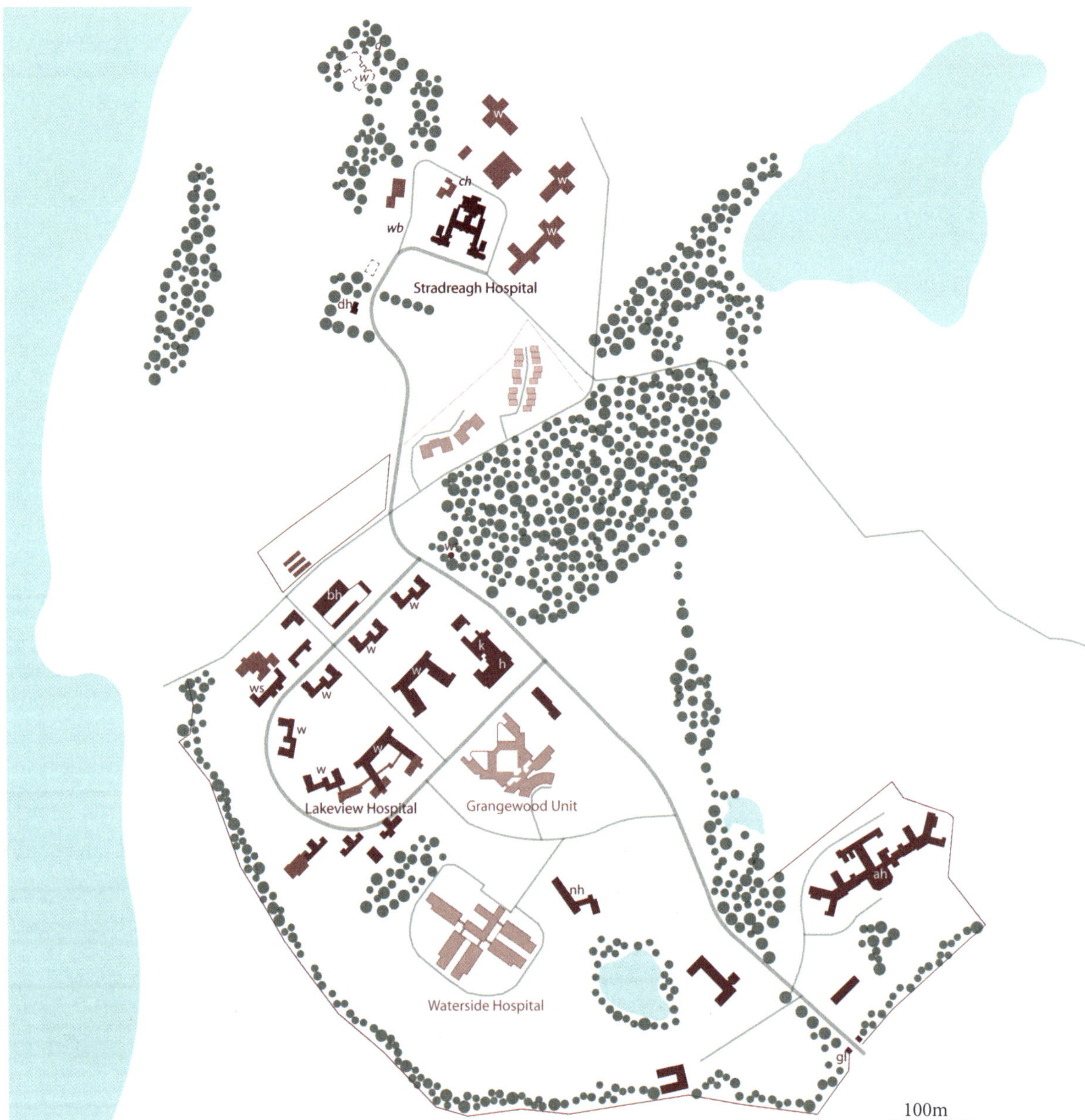

The Londonderry District Lunatic Asylum was one of the earliest of Johnston and Murray's new asylums, opening in 1829 on a site not far north of the city walls. Rapid urban growth soon engulfed the old asylum, constricting its future expansion (See Case Study 5). As early as 1862 the Inspectors spied opportunity in this challenge, observing how the 'great advance in the value of land' could be capitalised upon to fund a new asylum 'in a more rural and retired location'.[1] The board of governors soon agreed on the principle of this proposal, but 'when the immediate locality came to be selected, differences of opinion arose between former advocates… ending in a do-nothing policy' that stymied progress for a generation.[2]

In September 1893 the board of governors once more resolved to build, and even secured approval from the Board of Control for the project before again collapsing into internal dissent, with local interests promoting competing sites across the county at Limavady, Coleraine and Dungiven.[3] In the end the city faction won the tussle, resulting in the purchase of lands at Gransha, some three miles upriver on the east bank of the River Foyle.

The site may finally have been secured, but the governors proved unwilling to follow with the requisite buildings. While their Belfast counterparts were pioneering their new villa colony at Purdysburn, the first 60 male 'working patients' who moved to Gransha in 1898 had to make do with a tin-and-timber ward.[4] The first permanent building on the site, to designs of local architect Matthew Alexander Robinson, opened in 1905. It is an astylar, generic institutional pile of machined-red brick, entered via a three-sided forecourt and linked via glazed corridors to a dining hall and ancillary spaces to the rear. Less obvious today is the fact that the building was 'of a complex and ornate design, constructed of stronger and better materials; and supplied with internal fittings of a much more costly character' to serve a cohort of 'acutely insane' patients.[5] Containing only 100 beds, the building fell far short of what was needed to fully replace the old asylum in the city, which was still struggling to accommodate over 420 patients.[6] Despite the Inspectors advocating that the asylum committee should 'take time by the forelock' and expedite design of subsequent blocks, progress again stalled. With the exception of staff housing and some farm buildings, another half century would pass before Gransha would reverberate to the sounds of major construction.

In 1956 plans based on the 'villa system' were drawn up for the new Gransha Mental Hospital. With an ultimate capacity of 800 patients, it would include an admissions unit, separate villas for acute and convalescent cases, and buildings for administration, indoor recreation, occupational therapy and nurses' accommodation.[7] When the initial phase opened in 1960, it was lauded as the first new mental hospital erected in the United Kingdom after the second world war – its cheerleaders were not to know that it would also be amongst the very last purpose-built institutions of its type. The clinical model was based on the wholly open-door approach pioneered by Dr Macmillan at Mapperley Hospital in Nottingham, and promoted in a specially produced film, The Open Door, written and directed by the late John Hume. The new institution was intended to signify 'a total change in attitude' – both clinically and spatially – from the grim regime that pertained in the old city centre asylum.[8] Hume and the others involved could not have imagined that they would live to hear their sincere endeavours derided as 'without a doubt an institution designed to make people ill'.[9]

The dispersal of some 20 detached buildings along an internal road was an explicit break with nineteenth-century asylum design, but the end result sadly had all the charm of an industrial estate. Aside from some modest trappings of mid-century style on the recreation and administration blocks, the buildings were for the most part bland and joyless. The admissions unit was arguably the best of them, perhaps because its cranked plan and copious glazing harked back to the bright and airy TB sanatoria of earlier years. More surprisingly, it was the occupational therapy workshops that came closest to capturing the pioneering optimism of the project, their bluntly functional but highly glazed façades revealing and reflecting the renewed importance of structured therapeutic activities as part of a reformed clinical regime.

If Robinson's 1905 building – known in its latter years as Stradreagh Hospital – was architecturally unremarkable, its commanding site on the highest part of the estate, with fine views over the Foyle, offered some compensation.[10] Alas, the same cannot be said of the new 1950s hospital. Where contemporary commentators described the complex as having an atmosphere of 'fresh air, freedom and openness',[11] one might equally substitute 'windswept, barren and bleak'. Beyond the symmetrically placed modern gate-lodges flanking the main entrance, the buildings were marooned in a monotonous sea of roads and grass, unrelieved by any new planting and ignoring the potential of the estate's existing lakes, woodland and

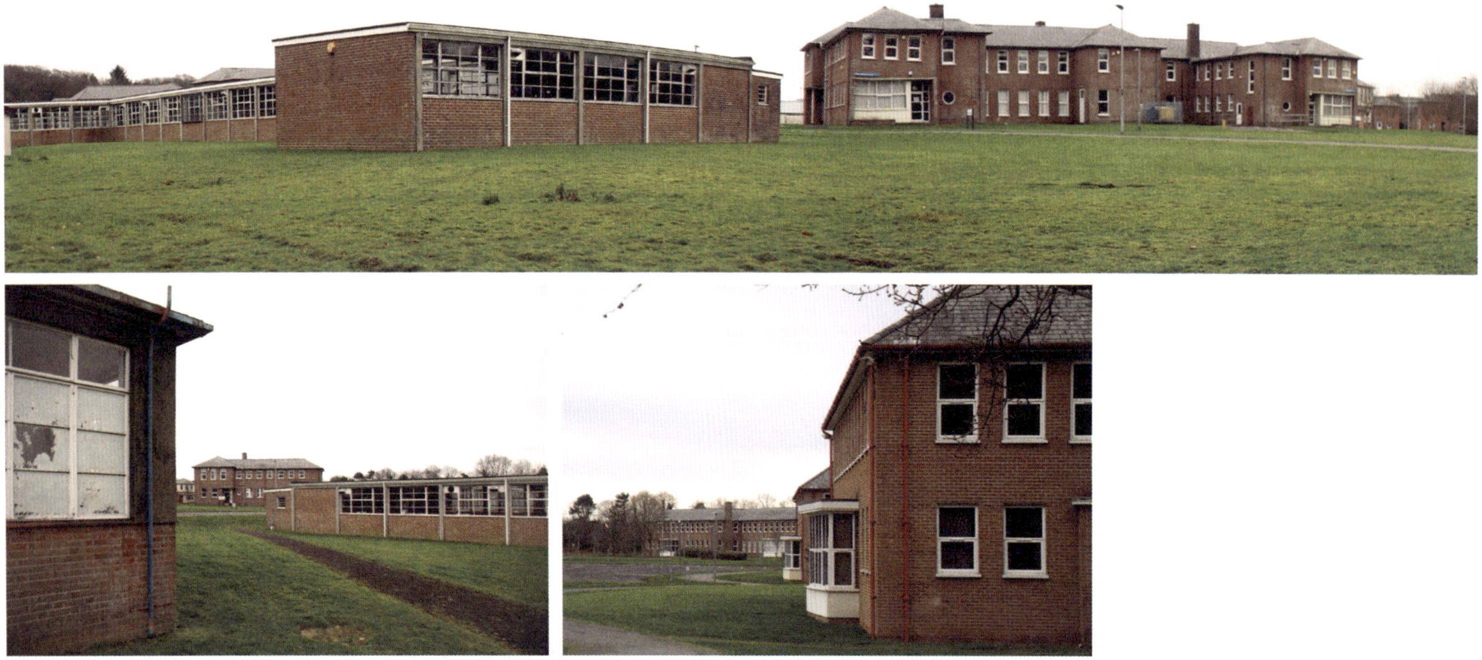

The buildings of the new 1950s hospital were laid out as dispersed villas across a windswept landscape. *Photographs by the author, 2020.*

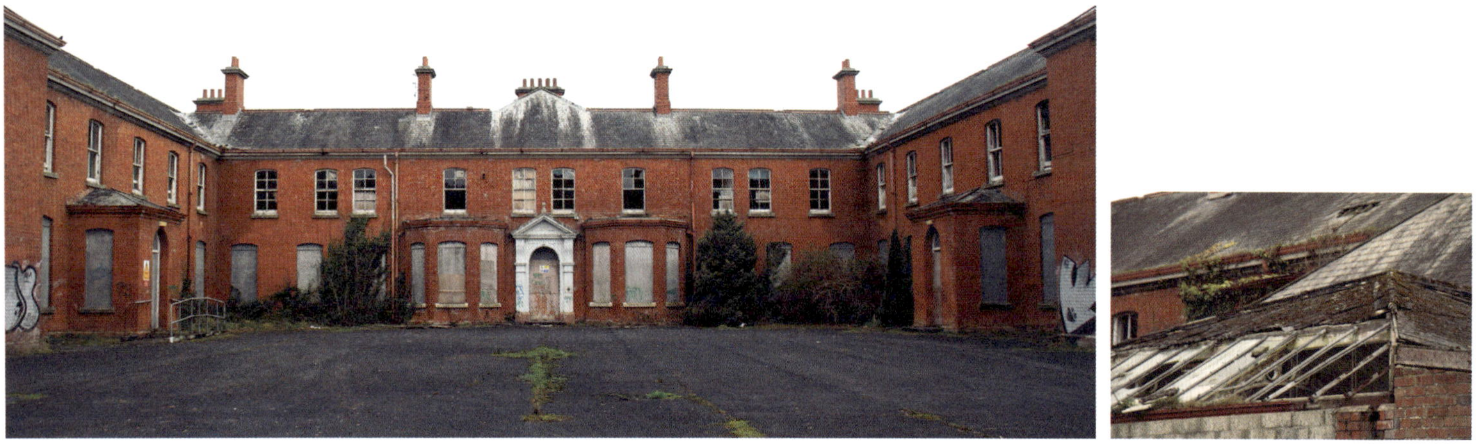

The 'stronger and better materials' of Robinson's 1905 block proved equal to the turmoil of 'acutely insane' patients, the hustle and bustle of secondary school students, but not the depredations of nocturnal salvage operations. *Photographs by the author, 2020*

riverside setting. For the designers of this pioneering new hospital, landscape had ceased to be valued either as an aesthetic setting for buildings or as a therapeutic resource for patients; and the intervening decades have improved matters only slightly.

The 1970s and 80s saw the addition of several new single-storey units; cheaply built, they are already disused and shuttered, like many of their 1950s and 60s counterparts. The 1905 building – despite enjoying a second life as an integrated secondary school, succumbed to arson in 2016, while the lead of the once sun-soaked admissions unit has proven more appealing for reuse than the building itself. The patient services they once housed have moved to new buildings on the same site: the 1990s Waterside Hospital, several streetscape-style units for supported living, and the Grangewood acute admissions unit, which opened in 2012. The latter in particular is a rare deviation from six decades of received wisdom around the benefits of co-locating acute mental health facilities on general hospital sites; the local health trust is either remarkably outdated, or quietly confident that all things ultimately come full circle.

Few institutions in Ireland can claim to have commissioned and decommissioned quite as many buildings in a 50-year period as Gransha Hospital, with even relatively young buildings abandoned in response to changing healthcare practices or, daresay, as a convenient, if expensive, remedy for negative perceptions and accumulated prejudices. After stubbornly resisting the urgent demands for new buildings for more than a century, it is as if the local authorities adopted Enoch Powell's conception of the hospital as a disposable 'shell to contain certain processes' with all the zeal of the converted. The taxpayers who fund such wasteful largesse can at least console themselves with the thought that the site at Gransha is big enough to accommodate the next generation of buildings when the latest additions fall from grace, c. 2035.

References

1. *Eleventh Annual Asylum Report 1861*, HC 1862 [2975] xxiii, p. 15.
2. *Forty-Eighth Annual Asylum Report 1899*, HC 1899 [9479] xl, p. 182.
3. Ibid., p. 184.
4. Ibid., p. 185.
5. *Fifty-Third Annual Asylum Report 1903*, HC 1905 [2262] xxxv, p. 133; *Fifty-Fifth Annual Asylum Report 1905*, HC 1906 [3164] xxxix, p. 138.
6. *Fifty Third Annual Asylum Report 1903*, HC 1905 [2262] xxxv, p. 129.
7. 'Hospital Building in Northern Ireland', in *The British Medical Journal* 1:5176 (Mar. 1960), p. 874; and *The Hospital*, 52:3, (Mar. 1956), pp 180–1, cited in https://historic-hospitals.com/northern-ireland/, accessed 22 Aug. 2020
8. John Hume, *The Open Door*. Londonderry Hospital Management Committee, c. 1965. Film. Available at https://digitalfilmarchive.net/media/the-open-door-1982, accessed 28 Oct. 2020.
9. Ironically, the comments were made by one of John Hume's political successors, SDLP Councillor Shaun Gallagher. Quoted in 'Gransha psychiatric hospital will soon be consigned to history', *Belfast Telegraph*, 8 Dec. 2011. www.belfasttelegraph.co.uk/news/northern-ireland/gransha-psychiatric-hospital-will-soon-be-consigned-to-history-28689708.html, accessed on 22 Aug. 2020.
10. If anything, their desire for healthy estuarial breezes may have been overdone, as implied by a later shelterbelt, which reduced its exposure at the expense of blocking the view.
11. Hume, *The Open Door*. Londonderry Hospital Management Committee, ca. 1965. Film. Available at https://digitalfilmarchive.net/media/the-open-door-1982, accessed 28 Oct. 2020.

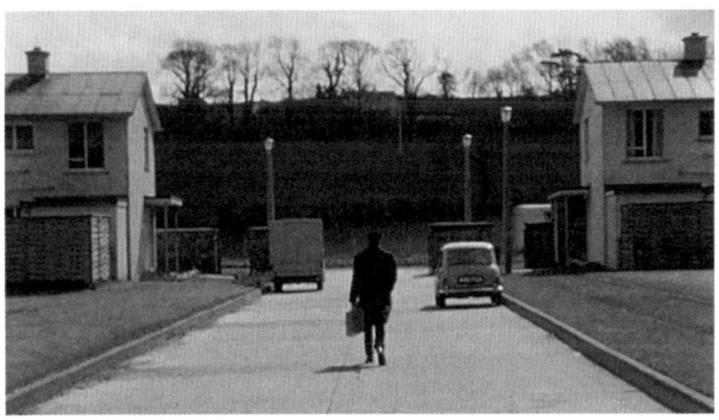

The closing sequence of the hospital's promotional film shows the recovered patient striding confidently back to society. *Image copyright of Terence McDonald Collection, reproduced by kind permission of the McDonald family and the IFI*

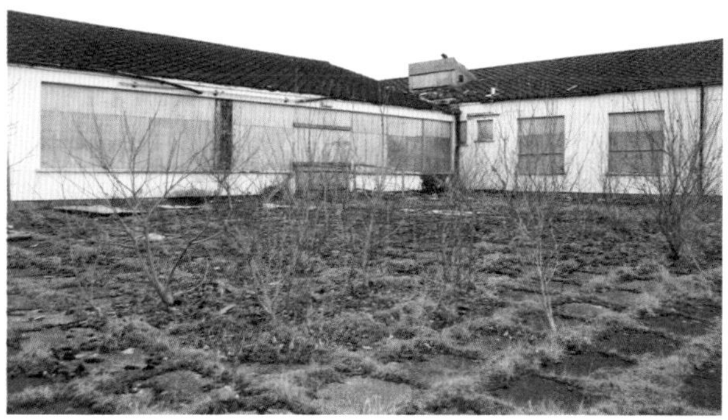

No such happy ending awaits Gransha's collection of redundant buildings, many built and abondoned in the decades since the film was made. *Photograph by the author, 2020.*

Bibliography

PRIMARY SOURCES

I. DRAWINGS, PHOTOGRAPHS, MANUSCRIPTS

Irish Architectural Archive, Ashlin & Coleman Collection, IAA: 76/1.

Irish Architectural Archive, TJ Cullen Collection, IAA: 85/74.

Irish Architectural Archive, Workhouse Drawings Collection, IAA: 85/138.

Irish Architectural Archive, Sligo Lunatic Asylum Collection, IAA: 89/11.

Irish Architectural Archive, Murray Collection, IAA: 92/46.

Irish Architectural Archive, WH Byrne Collection, IAA: 2006/142.

Irish Architectural Archive, Photographic Collections.

National Archives of Ireland, Chief Secretary's Office, NAI: CSO/RP.

National Archives of Ireland, Office of Public Works Collection, NAI: OPW/5HC/4.

National Library of Ireland, Eason Photographic Collection, NLI: Eas.

National Library of Ireland, Lawrence Photographic Collection, NLI: L_CAB_, L_ROY.

National Library of Ireland, Morgan Aerial Photographic Collection, NLI: MOR.

National Library of Ireland, Poole Photographic Collection, NLI: POOLEWP.

II. MAPS

Cork City Libraries: A Plan of the City & Suburbs of Cork according to the latest improvements by William Beauford, 1801, and Plan of the City and Suburbs of Cork, Surveyed and Drawn by Thomas Holt, 1832, www.corkpastandpresent.ie/mapsimages/corkcityinoldmaps/ accessed 30 Nov. 2020.

University of Dublin, Trinity Map Library: Historic Paper Maps for Island of Ireland, 1830s – 1960s.

Ordnance Survey of Ireland: Historic Map Viewer: Historic Maps for Republic of Ireland, 1840s – 1940s. www.map.geohive.ie, accessed 20 Jan 2021.

Public Records Office of Northern Ireland: Historic Map Viewer: Historic Maps for Northern Ireland, 1840s – 1960s. https://apps.spatialni.gov.uk/PRONIApplication/, accessed 20 Jan 2021.

University College Dublin Digital Library: Historic Town Plan Maps: large scale urban maps for Irish towns, 1830s – 1910s. https://digital.ucd.ie/view/ucdlib:40377, accessed 20 Jan 2021

III. CONTEMPORARY PRINTED BOOKS

Bentham, Jeremy, *Panopticon, or the Inspection-House* (Dublin, 1791).

Browne, William, *What Asylums Were, Are and Ought to Be* (Edinburgh: A&C Black, 1837).

Burdett, Henry C., *Hospitals and Asylums of the World: Volume 2: Asylum Construction, Plans and Bibliography* (London: J&A Churchill, 1891).

Burke, William, *A History of Clonmel* (Waterford: Harvey & Co, 1907).

Connolly, John, *The Construction and Government of Lunatic Asylums* (London: John Churchill, 1847).

De Barra, Eamon and John O'Sheehan, eds, *Oispideal na hÉireann: Ireland's Hospitals 1933–1950* (Dublin: Hospitals' Trust, 1956).

De Barra, Eamon, ed., *Irish Hospitals 1956–1971* (Dublin: Hospitals' Trust, 1971).

Kenny, Eyre E. C., *Short Hints and Observations on the Arrangement and Management of Lunatic Asylums* (Dublin: Hardy, 1848).

Hallaran, William Saunders, *An Inquiry into the Causes Producing the Extraordinary Addition to the Number of Insane* (Cork: Savage and Wallace, 1810)

__, *An Inquiry An Inquiry into the Causes and Cure of Insanity* (Cork: Edwards and Savage, 1818).

Stark, William, *Remarks on the Construction of Public Hospitals for the Cure of Mental Derangement: Read to a Committee of Inhabitants of the City of Glasgow* (Glasgow: Hedderwick & Son, 1810).

Swift, Jonathon, *Verses on the Death of Dr Swift* (Dublin: George Faulkner, 1739).

Tuke, Samuel, *Practical Hints on the Construction and Economy of Pauper Lunatic Asylums* (London: William Alexander, 1815).

IV. BILLS AND ACTS OF PARLIAMENT (selected)

Bill for establishing provincial asylums for lunatics in Ireland 1805, HC 1805 [61] i.

Act for the better Care and Maintenance of Lunatics, being Paupers or Criminals in England, 1808, 48 Geo. 3, c.96.

Richmond Lunatic Asylum (Ireland) Act 1815, 55 Geo. 3 c.107.

Lunatic Asylums (Ireland) Act 1817, 57 Geo. 3 c.106.

Dangerous Lunatics (Ireland) Act 1838, 1 & 2 Vic. c.27.

Central Criminal Lunatic Asylum (Ireland) Act 1845, 8 & 9 Vic. c.107.

County Asylums Act (England) 1845, 8 & 9 Vic. c.126.

Lunatic Asylums Repayment of Advances (Ireland) Act 1855, 18 & 19 Vic. c.109.

Lunacy (Ireland) Act 1867, 30 & 31 Vic. c.118.

Local Government (Ireland) Act 1898, 61 & 62 Vic. c.37.

Mental Treatment Act (NI) 1932, 22 & 23 Geo. 5 c.15.

Mental Treatment Act 1945, 1945 No. 19.

Health Act 1970, 1970 No. 1.

Mental Health Act 2001, 2001 No. 25.

V. PARLIAMENTARY AND DEPARTMENTAL REPORTS (selected)

Report from the Select Committee appointed to consider... making provision for the care of lunatics and idiots by Grand Jury presentments 1804, HC 1803-04 [109].

Report from the Committee on Madhouses in England, HC 1814–15 [296].

Report from the Select Committee on the Lunatic Poor in Ireland, HC 1817 [430] viii.

Report from the Select Committee of the House of Lords appointed to Consider the State of the Lunatic Poor in Ireland, HC 1843 [625] x.

Report of a Commission Inquiring into the Erection of District Lunatic Asylums in Ireland 1856, HC 1856 [9] liii.

Report of the Commissioners of Inquiry into the state of the Lunatic Asylums... in Ireland 1858, HC 1857–58 [2436-I].

Report of the Commission on the Relief of the Sick and Destitute Poor, Including the Insane Poor (Dublin: The Stationery Office, 1928).

Report of the Commission of Inquiry on Mental Handicap (Dublin: The Stationery Office, 1965).

Report of the Commission of Inquiry on Mental Illness (Dublin: The Stationery Office, 1966).

The Psychiatric Services – Planning for the Future: Report of a Study Group on the Development of Psychiatric Services (Dublin: The Stationery Office, 1984).

A Vision for Change: Report of the Expert Group on Mental Health Policy, (Dublin: the Stationery Office, 2006).

Final Report of the Commission to Inquire into Child Abuse (Dublin: Commission to Inquire into Child Abuse, 2009).

Report of the Inter-Departmental Committee to establish the facts of State involvement with the Magdalen Laundries (Dublin: Department of Justice, 2013).

Sharing the Vision: A Mental Health Policy for Everyone, (Dublin: Department of Health, 2018).

Final Report of the Commission of Investigation into Mother and Baby Homes (Dublin: Department of Children, 2021).

VI. ANNUAL REPORTS OF THE INSPECTORS OF PRISONS/LUNATIC ASYLUMS (selected)

Annual Report of the Inspectors-General of Prisons 1824, HC 1824 [294] xxii.

Fourth Report of the Inspectors-General of Prisons 1826, HC 1826 [173] xxiii.

Fifth Report of the Inspector of Prisons 1827, HC 1826–27 [471] xi.

Eighth Report of the Inspectors-General of Prisons 1830, HC 1830 [48] xxiv.

Fourteenth Report of the Inspectors-General of Prisons 1836, HC 1836 [118] xxxv.

Fifteenth Report of the Inspectors-General of Prisons 1837, HC 1837 [123] xxxi.

Sixteenth Report of the Inspectors-General of Prisons 1838, HC 1837–38 [186] xxix.

Twenty-first Report of the Inspectors-General of Prisons 1842, HC 1843 [462] xxvii.

Annual Asylum Report 1843, HC 1844 [567] xxx.

Annual Asylum Report 1844, HC 1845 [645] xxvi.

Annual Asylum Report 1845, HC 1846 [736] xxii.

Annual Asylum Report 1846, HC 1847 [820] xvii.

Annual Asylum Report 1848, HC 1849 [1054] xxiii.

Fifth Asylum Report 1851, HC 1851 [1387] xxiv.

Seventh Asylum Report 1855, HC 1854–55 [1981] xvi.

Eighth Asylum Report 1857, HC 1857 session 2 [2253] xvii.

Ninth Annual Asylum Report 1859, HC 1859 session 2 [2582] x.

Tenth Annual Asylum Report 1860, HC 1861 [2901] xxvii.

Eleventh Annual Asylum Report 1861, HC 1862 [2975] xxiii.

Fifteenth Annual Asylum Report 1866, HC 1866 [3721] xxxii.

Sixteenth Annual Asylum Report 1867, HC 1867 [3894] xviii.

Seventeenth Annual Asylum Report 1868, HC 1867–68 [4053] xxxi.

Eighteenth Annual Asylum Report 1869, HC 1868–69 [418] xxvii.

Nineteenth Annual Asylum Report 1870, HC 1870 [202] xxxiv.

Twentieth Annual Asylum Report 1871, HC 1871 [440] xxvi.

Twenty-First Annual Asylum Report 1872, HC 1872 [647] xxvii.

Twenty-Third Annual Asylum Report 1874, HC 1874 [1004] xxvii.

Twenty-Fourth Annual Asylum Report 1875, HC 1875 [1293] xxxiii.

Twenty-Eighth Annual Asylum Report 1879, HC 1878-79 [2346] xxxii.

Thirty-First Annual Asylum Report 1882, HC 1882 [3356] xxxii.

Thirty-Seventh Annual Asylum Report 1887, HC 1887 [5121] xxxix.

Forty-Third Annual Asylum Report 1893, HC 1894 [7466] xliii.

Forty-Fourth Annual Asylum Report 1894, HC 1895 [7804] liv.

Forty-Fifth Annual Asylum Report 1895, HC 1896 [8251] xxxix.

Forty-Sixth Annual Asylum Report 1896, HC 1897 [8639] xxxviii.

Forty-Seventh Annual Asylum Report 1897, HC 1898 [8969] xliii.

Forty-Eighth Annual Asylum Report 1898, HC 1899 [9479] xl.

Forty-Ninth Annual Asylum Report 1899, HC 1900 [312] xxxvii.

Fifty-First Annual Asylum Report 1901, HC 1902 [1265] xl.

Fifty-Second Annual Asylum Report 1902, HC 1903 [1762] xxvii.

Fifty-Third Annual Asylum Report 1903, HC 1905 [2262] xxxv.

Fifty-Fifth Annual Asylum Report 1905, HC 1906 [3164] xxxix.

Supplement to the Fifty-Fourth Report of the Inspector of Lunatics… being a special report on the alleged increase in insanity, HC 1906 [3126] xxxix.

Fifty-Seventh Annual Asylum Report 1907, HC 1908 [4302] xxxiii.

Fifty-Ninth Annual Asylum Report 1909, HC 1910 [5280] xli.

Sixty-Third Annual Asylum Report 1913, HC 1914 [7527] xl.

Sixty-Seventh Annual Asylum Report 1917, HC 1919 [32] xxv.

Sixty-Eighth Annual Asylum Report 1918, HC 1920 [579] xxi.

Sixty-Ninth Annual Asylum Report 1919, HC 1921 [1127] xv.

Report of the Inspector of Mental Hospitals, 1923.

Report of the Inspector of Mental Hospitals, 1929.

Report of the Inspector of Mental Hospitals, 1932.

Report of the Inspector of Mental Hospitals, 1942.

Report of the Inspector of Mental Hospitals, 1943.

Report of the Inspector of Mental Hospitals, 1946.

Report of the Inspector of Mental Hospitals, 1949.

Report of the Inspector of Mental Hospitals, 1950.

Report of the Inspector of Mental Hospitals, 1959.

Report of the Inspector of Mental Hospitals, 1977–1979.

Report of the Inspector of Mental Hospitals, 1988–1989.

Report of the Inspector of Mental Hospitals, 1990.

VII. OTHER PARLIAMENTARY PAPERS

Annual Reports of the Board of Public Works, Ireland, 1847–1900.

Annual Reports of the Local Government Board for Ireland, 1900–1920.

Copy of Treasury minute, dated 10 August 1855, appointing a commission for inquiring into the erection of district lunatic asylums in Ireland, HC 1856 (9) LIII.367.

Public Offices Site (Dublin) Act 1903, Account 1919–20, HC 1920 [3] xix.

Estimates for civil services for the year ending 31 March 1922, HC 1921 [41] xxii.

VIII. NEWSPAPERS/PERIODICALS

'The proposed new lunatic asylum for Monaghan', *The Dublin Builder*, 1 May 1863, p. 77.

'County of Donegal Lunatic Asylum', *The Dublin Builder*, 1 Mar. 1865, p. 62.

'Lunatic Asylum, Enniscorthy', *The Irish Builder*, 15 Jan. 1866, p. 20.

'Clare County Lunatic Asylum', *The Irish Builder*, 15 Mar. 1866, p. 71.

'Monaghan and Cavan new lunatic asylum', *The Irish Builder*, 1 June 1869, p. 135.

'The Portrane Asylum Competition', *The Irish Builder*, 15 Apr. 1895, p. 99.

'The latest development in asylum planning: The villa colony system', *The Irish Builder*, 10 Apr. 1901, pp 689–90.

'Mental Hospital at Monaghan: A worthy addition to Ireland's modern hospital buildings', *Irish Builder and Engineer,* 10 Apr. 1943, pp 141–2.

'Hospital building in Northern Ireland', *The British Medical Journal,* 19 Mar. 1960, p. 874.

'The scandal of the mental hospitals', *Magill*, 30 Oct. 1980.

'The Woods cover-up', *Magill*, 30 Dec. 1980.

IX. PARLIAMENTARY DEBATES

George Wyndham MP, House of Commons, 30 Jan. 1902, 4:101, cc. 1341.

Horace Plunkett MP, House of Commons, 16 May 1895, 4:33, cc. 1329.

Piaras Béalsaí TD, Dáil Éireann, 21 Jan. 1919, F:1.

Seán T. O'Ceallaigh TD, Dáil Éireann, 28 Apr. 1936, 61:12.

Seán Leamass TD, Dáil Éireann, 30 Jun. 1942, 87:17.

Seán McEntee TD, Dáil Éireann, 6 Nov. 1957, 164:4.

Barry Desmond TD, Dáil Éireann. 23 Oct. 1979, 316:3.

Charles Haughey TD, Dáil Éireann, 23 Oct. 1979, 316:3.

Barry Desmond TD, Dáil Éireann, 10 Apr. 1984, 349:9.

Michael Woods TD, Dáil Éireann, 12 Nov. 1980. 234:2.

Rory O'Hanlon TD, Dáil Éireann, 30 Jan. 1990, 394:8.

Mary O'Rourke TD, Dáil Éireann, 17 Apr. 1991, 407:1.

Enda Kenny TD, Dáil Éireann, 23 Apr. 2013, 799:4.

Helen McEntee TD, Dáil Éireann, 1 Feb. 2017, 937:1.

Mary Butler TD, Dáil Éireann, 15 Oct. 2020, 999:4.

X. SPEECHES / RECORDINGS / OTHER

Campbell, Aisling, Consultant psychiatrist, in panel discussion following *The Thomas Davis Lecture: Houses in Motion: Architecture and Patterns of Dwelling.* RTÉ Radio 1, first broadcast 16 Feb. 2020 (and conversation with author 12 May 2020).

Farrelly, John, Chief Executive Officer, Mental Health Commission, conversation with the author, 24 Jan. 2020.

Hume, John, *The Open Door*, Londonderry Hospital Management Committee, ca. 1965. Film. https://digitalfilmarchive.net/media/the-open-door-1982, accessed 28 Oct. 2020.

Kennedy, Harry, Executive Clinical Director, National Forensic Mental Health Service, conversation with the author, 17 Jun. 2019.

Powell, Enoch, MP, Address to the National Association of Mental Health Annual Conference, 9 Mar. 1961. https://navigator.health.org.uk/theme/enoch-powells-water-tower-speech, accessed 20 Jan 2021.

Reilly, Martin, Governor, Castlerea Prison, conversation with the author, 7 Jul. 2020.

St Brendan's Demolition, RTÉ Television, first broadcast 26 Nov. 1986, www.rte.ie/archives/collections/news/21232208-st-brendans-demolition, accessed on 28 Oct. 2020.

Sugrue, Una, Senior Architect, Grangegorman Development Agency, conversation with the author, 19 Aug. 2019.

SECONDARY SOURCES

I. PUBLISHED SOURCES

Allmond, Gillian, 'Light and darkness in an Edwardian institution for the insane poor – illuminating the material practices of the asylum age,' in *International Journal of Historical Archaeology*, 20:1, 2016, pp 1–22.

—, 'Liberty and the individual: The colony asylum in Scotland and England,' in *History of Psychiatry*; 28:1, Mar. 2017, pp 29-43.

—, '"Levelling Up the Lower Deeps": Rural and Suburban Spaces at an Edwardian Asylum,' in Georgina Laragy, Olwen Purdue and Jonathan Wright, eds, *Urban Spaces in Nineteenth-Century Ireland* (Liverpool: Liverpool University Press, 2018) pp 125–43.

Barry, Siobhan, Justin Brophy and Dermot Walsh, *The Lie of the Land: Psychiatric Service Land Disposal and Failures and Delays in Capital Development of Community Based Mental Health Services* (Blackrock: Irish Psychiatric Association, 2008).

Brennan, Damien, *Irish Insanity, 1800–2000* (Oxon: Routledge, 2014).

Brewer, John, Bill Lockhart and Paula Rodgers, 'Crime in Ireland since the Second World War,' in *Journal of the Statistical and Social Inquiry Society of Ireland*, 27:3, 1995–96, pp 135–75.

Butler, Richard J., *Building the Irish Courthouse and Prison: A Political History, 1750–1850* (Cork: Cork University Press, 2019).

Campbell, Jim, 'Mental health policy, care in the community and political conflict: The case of the integrated service in Northern Ireland', in Peter Bartlett and David Wright, eds, *Outside the Walls of the Asylum: The History of Care and Community 1750–2000* (London: Athlone Press, 1999) pp 227–43.

Casey, Christine and Alistair Rowan, *The Buildings of Ireland: North Leinster* (London: Penguin, 1993).

Casey, Christine, *The Buildings of Ireland: Dublin* (London: Yale University Press, 2005).

Cox, Catherine, *Negotiating Insanity in the Southeast of Ireland, 1820–1900* (Manchester: Manchester University Press, Palgrave, 2012).

Craig, Maurice, *The Architecture of Ireland from Earliest Times to 1880* (Dublin: Lambay Books, 1982).

Crooke, Emer, *White Elephants: The Country House and the State in Independent Ireland, 1922–1973* (Dublin: UCD Press, 2018).

Crossman, Virginia, *Politics, Pauperism and Power in Late Nineteenth-Century Ireland* (Manchester: Manchester University Press, 2006).

Dwyer, Dermot, ed., *St. Finan's Hospital Killarney: A Medical, Social & Sporting History 1852–2002* (Killarney: St Finan's Historical Society, 2002).

Edington, Barry, 'A space for moral management: The York Retreat's influence on asylum design', in Leslie Topp, James Moran and Jonathon Andrews, eds, *Madness, Architecture and the Built Environment* (New York & Oxon: Routledge, 2007) pp 85-104.

Evans, Robin, *The fabrication of Virtue: English Prison Architecture, 1750–1840* (Cambridge: Cambridge University Press, 1982).

Fennelly, Katherine, 'Out of sound, out of mind: Noise control in early nineteenth-century lunatic asylums in England and Ireland', in *World Archaeology*, 26:3, 2014, pp 416–30.

—, 'The Bedford Asylum: Building for the "industrious child" in early-nineteenth century Dublin', in Jane Eva Baxter and Meredith Ellis, eds, *Nineteenth Century Childhoods in Interdisciplinary and International Perspectives* (Barnsley: Oxbow Books, 2018).

Finnane, Mark, *Insanity and the Insane in Post-Famine Ireland* (London: Croom Helm, 1981).

Foucault, Michel, *Madness and Civilisation* (tr. Richard Howard; New York: Vintage, 1965).

Fuller, Louise, *Irish Catholicism since 1950: The Undoing of a Culture* (Dublin: Gill & McMillan, 2004).

Goffman, Erving, *Asylums: Essays on the Social Situation of Mental Patients and Other Inmates* (Chicago: Aldine Publishing Company, 1962).

Greally, Hanna, *Bird's Nest Soup* (Cork: Attic Press, 1987).

Grangegorman Development Agency, Grangegorman: *An Urban Quarter with an Open Future* (Dublin: GGDA, 2008).

Hamilton, Stephen and Hugh O'Donnell, *Purdysburn Hospital: The Legacy of a Villa Colony* (Belfast, 2013).

Hamilton, Stephen and David Martin, *The Burn, The Fever and Beyond* (Belfast, 2016).

Hickman, Clare, *Therapeutic Landscapes: A History of English Hospital Gardens since 1800* (Manchester: Manchester University Press, 2013).

Jones, Kathleen, *Asylums and After: A Revised History of the Mental Health Services from the Early 18th Century to the 1990s* (London: Athlone Press, 1999).

Kelly, Brendan, *Hearing Voices: The History of Psychiatry in Ireland* (Dublin: Irish Academic Press, 2014).

Kelly, Hugh, *St Senan's Hospital, Enniscorthy: The History 1860–2011* (Enniscorthy, 2011).

Kelly, Sean, *A Grand Old Lady, A History of the Downshire Hospital, 1869–2014* (Dundonald: South Eastern Health and Social Care Trust, 2012).

Loeber, Rolf, Hugh Campbell, Livia Hurley, John Montague and Ellen Rowley, eds, *Art and Architecture of Ireland, Volume IV* (Dublin: Royal Irish Academy, 2015).

Lonergan, Eamon, *St Luke's Hospital Clonmel 1834–1984* (Thurles: Tipperary Star, 1984).

–-, *The History of the South-Eastern Health Board, 1971–2004* (Kilkenny: South Eastern Health Board, 2004).

Malcolm, Elizabeth, *Swift's Hospital: A History of St Patrick's Hospital, Dublin, 1746–1989* (Dublin: Gill and Macmillan, 1989).

Markus, Thomas, 'The Sad, the Mad and the Bad', in Thomas Markus, ed., *Order in Space and Society: Architectural Form and its Context in the Scottish Enlightenment,* (Edinburgh: Mainstream Publishing, 1982) pp 25–114.

—, *Buildings and Power: Freedom and Control in the Origin of Modern Building Types* (Oxon; Routledge, 1993).

Mauger, Alice, '"Confinement of the Higher Orders": The social role of private lunatic asylums in Ireland, c. 1820–60', in *Journal of the History of Medicine and Allied Sciences,* 67:2, Apr. 2012, pp 281–317.

McCabe, Anton and Ciaran Mulholland, 'The red flag over the asylum: The Monaghan Asylum Soviet of 1919', in Pauline M. Prior, ed., *Asylums, Mental Health Care and the Irish 1800–2010* (Dublin: Irish Academic Press, 2012) pp 23-43.

McCullough, Niall, *Palimpsest: Change in the Irish Building Tradition* (Dublin: Anne Street Press, 1994).

McCullough, Niall and Valerie Mulvin, *A Lost Tradition: The Nature of Architecture in Ireland* (Kinsale: Gandon Editions, 1987).

McDermott, Joe, *St Mary's Hospital Castlebar: Serving Mayo Mental Health from 1866* (Castlebar: Western Health Board, 1999).

McLellan, Anne, Niamh Nic Ghabhann and Fiona Byrne, eds, *World Within Walls: From Asylum to Contemporary Mental Health Services* (Monaghan: Health Service Executive, 2015).

McClelland, Gillian, 'Speedwell Magazine: An insider view of Holywell Psychiatric Hospital, Antrim, 1959–1973', in Prior, *Asylums, Mental Health Care and the Irish*, pp 44-73.

McKinley, Robert, 'Tyrone and Fermanagh Hospital: A Chronological History' in Mitchell Haldane, ed., *Images of Omagh and District, Vol. 7* (Omagh: Rotary Club of Omagh, 1999), pp 64–83.

McParland, Edward, *Public Architecture in Ireland 1680–1760* (New Haven & London: Yale University Press, 2001).

Mental Health Commission, *Under the Clock Towers – An Overview of Remaining Nineteenth-Century Public Psychiatric Hospitals due for Closure* (Dublin: Mental Health Commission, 2011).

Millett, Kate, *The Loony-bin Trip* (New York: Simon and Schuster, 1990).

Moon, Graham, Robin Kearns, Alan Joseph, *The Afterlives of the Psychiatric Asylum: Recycling Concepts, Sites and Memories* (Farnham: Ashgate, 2015).

Mulholland, Marc, *To Comfort Always: 100 Years of Holywell Hospital, Antrim, 1898–1998* (Antrim: Homefirst Community Trust, 1999).

Mulligan, Kevin V., *The Buildings of Ireland: South Ulster* (London: Yale University Press, 2013).

Murphy, Donal, ed., *Tumbling Walls: The Evolution of a Community Institution, St Fintan's Hospital Portlaoise, 1833–1983* (Portlaoise: Midland Health Board, 1983).

North Western Health Board, *Reflecting on the North Western Health Board 1970–2004* (Manorhamilton: North Western Health Board, 2004).

O'Brien, Eoin, Lorna Browne and Kevin O'Malley, *The House of Industry Hospitals: The Richmond, Whitworth and Hardwicke (St Laurence's Hospital) – A closing memoir* (Dublin: Anniversary Press, 1988).

O'Dwyer, Frederick, *Irish hospital architecture: a pictorial history* (Dublin: Department of Health and Children, 1997).

—, *The Architecture of Deane and Woodward* (Cork: Cork University Press, 1997).

—, 'Hospital Architecture, 1922–2000' and 'Lunatic Asylums, 1800–1939', in Loeber, Campbell, Hurley, Montague and Rowley, *Art and Architecture of Ireland*, pp 209–214.

O'Hare, Aileen and Walsh, Dermot, *Irish Psychiatric Hospitals and Units 1981* (Dublin: Medico-Social Research Board, 1983).

Philo, Chris, *A Geographical History of Institutional Provision for the Insane from Medieval Times to the 1860's in England and Wales: This Space Reserved for Insanity* (Lewiston: Edwin Mellen Press, 2004).

Porter, Roy, *Mind-Forg'd Manacles: A history of madness in England from the Restoration to the Regency* (London: Athlone, 1987).

Power, Dermot, 'A History of the People's Park', in *The Waterford Archaeological and Historical Society Journal*, 52, 1996, pp 113-36.

Prior, Pauline M., *Mental Health and Politics in Northern Ireland: A History of Service Development* (Aldershot: Avebury Press, 1993).

—, 'Dangerous lunacy: The misuse of mental health law in nineteenth-century Ireland' in *The Journal of Forensic Psychiatry & Psychology*, 14:3, Dec. 2003, pp 525–53.

—, *Madness and Murder: Gender, Crime and Mental Disorder in Nineteenth Century Ireland* (Dublin: Irish Academic Press, 2008).

—, 'Overseeing the Irish asylums: The Inspectorate in Lunacy, 1845–1921', in Prior, *Asylums, Mental Health Care and the Irish*, pp 221–245.

—, 'Mental health law on the island of Ireland, 1800-2010', in Prior, ed, *Asylums, Mental Health Care and the Irish 1800 – 2010* (Dublin: Irish Academic Press, 2012), pp 316-334.

Prior, Pauline M. and David V. Griffiths, 'The "Chaplaincy Question" at Belfast District Asylum 1834–1870', in Prior, *Asylums, Mental Health Care and the Irish*, pp 167–184.

Reuber, Markus, *Staats- und Privatanstalten in Irland, Irre, Artze und Idioten 1600–1900* (Koln: Verlag Josef Eul, 1994).

—, 'The architecture of psychological management: The Irish asylums, 1801–1922', in *Psychological Medicine*, no. 26, 1996, pp 1179–89.

—, 'Moral management and the "Unseen Eye": Public lunatic asylums, 1800–1845', in Elizabeth Malcolm and Greta Jones, eds, *Medicine, Disease and the State in Ireland, 1650–1940*, (Cork: Cork University Press, 1999), pp 209–29.

Reynolds, Joseph, *Grangegorman: Psyschiatric Care in Dublin since 1815* (Dublin: Institute of Public Administration in association with Eastern Health Board, 1992).

Robins, Joseph, *Fools and Mad: A History of the Insane in Ireland* (Dublin: Institute of Public Administration, 1986).

Rowan, Alistair, *The Buildings of Ireland: North West Ulster* (London: Penguin, 1979).

Ryan, Annie, *Walls of Silence* (Callan: Red Lion Press, 1999).

Scull, Andrew, 'A convenient place to get rid of inconvenient people: the Victorian lunatic asylum', in Anthony D King, ed., *Buildings and Society: Essays on the Social Development of the Built Environment* (London: Routledge & Kegan Paul, 1980), pp 37–60.

Scull, Andrew, *The Most Solitary of Afflictions: Madness and Society in Britain, 1700–1900* (New Haven and London: Yale University Press, 1993).

—, *The Insanity of Place/The Place of Insanity: Essays on the History of Psychiatry* (Oxon: Routledge, 2006).

—, ed., *The Asylum as Utopia: W. A. F. Browne and the mid-nineteenth century consolidation of psychiatry* (Hove: Routledge, 2014).

Smith, C. J., Brendan Kelly and Harry Kennedy, 'A 25-year dynamic ecological analysis of psychiatric hospital admissions and prison committals: Penrose's Hypothesis updated', in *Irish Journal of Psychological Medicine*, pp 1–4. doi: 10.1017/ipm.2018.40.

Smith, James M, 'The politics of sexual knowledge: The origins of Ireland's containment culture and the Carrigan Report (1931)' in *Journal of the History of Sexuality*, 13:2, 200), pp 209–13.

Smith, Leonard, 'The architecture of confinement: Urban public asylums in England, 1750–1820', in Topp, Moran and Andrews, *Madness, Architecture and the Built Environment*, pp 41–62.

Southern Health Board, *Annual Report 1995* (Cork: Southern Health Board, 1995).

Stevenson, Christine, *Medicine and Magnificence: British Hospital and Asylum Architecture, 1660–1815* (New Haven: Yale University Press, 2000).

Sturdy, Harriet and William Parry-Jones, 'Boarding-out insane patients: The significance of the Scottish system 1857--1913', in Bartlett and Wright, *Outside the Walls of the Asylum*, pp 86–114.

Taylor, Jeremy, *Hospital and Asylum Architecture in England 1840–1914, Building for Health Care* (London: Mansell, 1991).

Thompson, John D. and Grace Goldin, *The Hospital: A Social and Architectural History* (New Haven & London: Yale University Press, 1975).

Topp, Leslie, *Freedom and the Cage: Modern Architecture and Psychiatry in Central Europe 1890–1914* (Pennsylvania: Pennsylvania State University Press, 2017).

Walsh, Dermot and Antoinette Daly, *Mental Illness in Ireland 1750–2002: Reflections on the Rise and Fall of Institutional Care* (Dublin: Health Research Board, 2004).

Walsh, Dermot, 'Mental health services in Ireland, 1959–2010', in Prior, *Asylums, Mental Health Care and the Irish*, pp 74–102.

Walsh, Oonagh, 'Lunatic and criminal alliances in nineteenth-century Ireland', in Peter Bartlett and Wright, *Outside the Walls of the Asylum*, pp 132–52.

—, '"Tales from the Big House": The Connacht District Lunatic Asylum in the Late Nineteenth Century', in *History Ireland*, 13:6, Nov-Dec. 2005, pp 21–5.

—, 'Landscape and the Irish asylum' in Úna Ní Bhroiméil and Glenn Hooper, eds, *Land and Landscape in Nineteenth Century Ireland* (Dublin: Four Courts Press, 2008), pp 156–72.

Williams, Jeremy, *A Companion Guide to Architecture in Ireland, 1837–1921* (Dublin: Irish Academic Press, 1994).

Williamson, Arthur P., 'Armagh District Lunatic Asylum: The First Phase', in *Seanchas Ardmhacha: Journal of the Armagh Diocesan Historical Society*, 8:1, 1975/1976, pp 111–20.

Yanni, Carla, *The Architecture of Madness: Insane Asylums in the United States* (Minneapolis: University of Minnesota Press: 2007).

II. UNPUBLISHED REPORTS AND THESES

Bolger, Teresa and James Hession, 'Grangegorman Dublin 7: Report on investigation and recording of structural remains at proposed site for Central Quad' (unpublished report, Rubicon Heritage, 2013).

Butterley, Lisa, 'Institutional reform in mental healthcare in Ireland: the establishment of the Ardee Mental Hospital, 1933, in its historical context' (unpublished PhD Thesis, NUI Maynooth, 2014).

Cogan, Denis, 'The Irish Workhouses: a study of their architectural legacy' (unpublished MUBC Thesis, University College Dublin, 1998).

Eastern Health Board, 'Draft proposal for the future of St Brendan's Hospital, Grangegorman' (Unpublished report, 1998).

Goslin, Bernadette, 'The Murray Collection of architectural drawings' (unpublished MA thesis, University of Dublin, 1990).

Grangegorman Development Agency Newsletter (Dec. 2019).

Gyves, Anthony, 'A History of St Otteran's Hospital' (unpublished MA thesis, University College Cork, 2010).

McKeith, Martin, 'The architectural development of the Irish diocesan major seminary – from 1782 to 1900' (unpublished MUBC Thesis, University College Dublin, 2012).

O'Dwyer, Frederick, 'Architectural heritage impact assessment report, St Senan's Hospital Enniscorthy' (unpublished report, 2019).

Quinlan, Patrick, 'Cure, Care and Containment: The architecture and landscape of Ireland's lunatic asylums, 1814–2014' (unpublished MUBC Thesis, University College Dublin, 2014).

Rutherford, Sarah, The landscapes of public lunatic asylums in England, 1808-1914' (unpublished PhD Thesis, DeMontford University, 2003).

III. WEBSITES AND ONLINE RESOURCES

Dictionary of Scottish Architects, 'Henry Thomas Wright', www.scottisharchitects.org.uk/architect_full.php?id=205393; accessed 27 Oct. 2019.

Daithi O'Corrain, 'Catholicism in Ireland, 1880–2016: Rise, Ascendancy and Retreat' (Unpublished draft paper, 2018), www.researchgate.net/publication/325486860_Catholicism_in_Ireland_1880-2015_Rise_Ascendancy_and_Retreat, accessed 2 Nov. 2020.

Dublin Institute of Technology, 'Speech by Minster of State for Mental Health, Kathleen Lynch TD, at the official opening of the Phoenix Care Centre at Grangegorman (28 Feb. 2013), www.dit.ie/newsandevents/news/archive2013/officialopeningofthephoenixcarecentreatgrangegorman/ Last accessed 11 May 2020.

Eurostat: Health Statistics, https://ec.europa.eu/eurostat/statistics-explained/index.php?title=File:Hospital_beds_%E2%80%94_psychiatric_care_beds,_2013_and_2018_(per_100_000_inhabitants)_Health20.png, accessed 29 Oct.2020.

Higher Education Authority, Higher Education Statistics, https://hea.ie/statistics-archive/, accessed 27 Dec. 2019.

Irish Architectural Archive, Dictionary of Irish Architects: individual entries for each institution, www.dia.ie, accessed 2 Jan. 2021.

Irish Examiner, 'Victorian building guiding just €6 a square foot at Enniscorthy,' 12 Jan. 2017, www.irishexaminer.com/property/victorian-building-guiding-just-euro6-a-square-foot-at-enniscorthy-438812.html, accessed 27 Dec. 2019.

Irish Penal Reform Trust, Irish Prison Statistics, 1970–2011, www.iprt.ie/prison-facts-2/, accessed 27 Dec. 2019.

Simon Communities of Ireland, 'Health Strategy 2001: Submission by the Simon Community of Ireland to the Department of Health on its review of the Health Service,' www.simon.ie/Portals/1/Docs/policies/submissions/archives/health_service_2001.pdf, accessed 10 Oct 2020.

Index

References to images are in italic

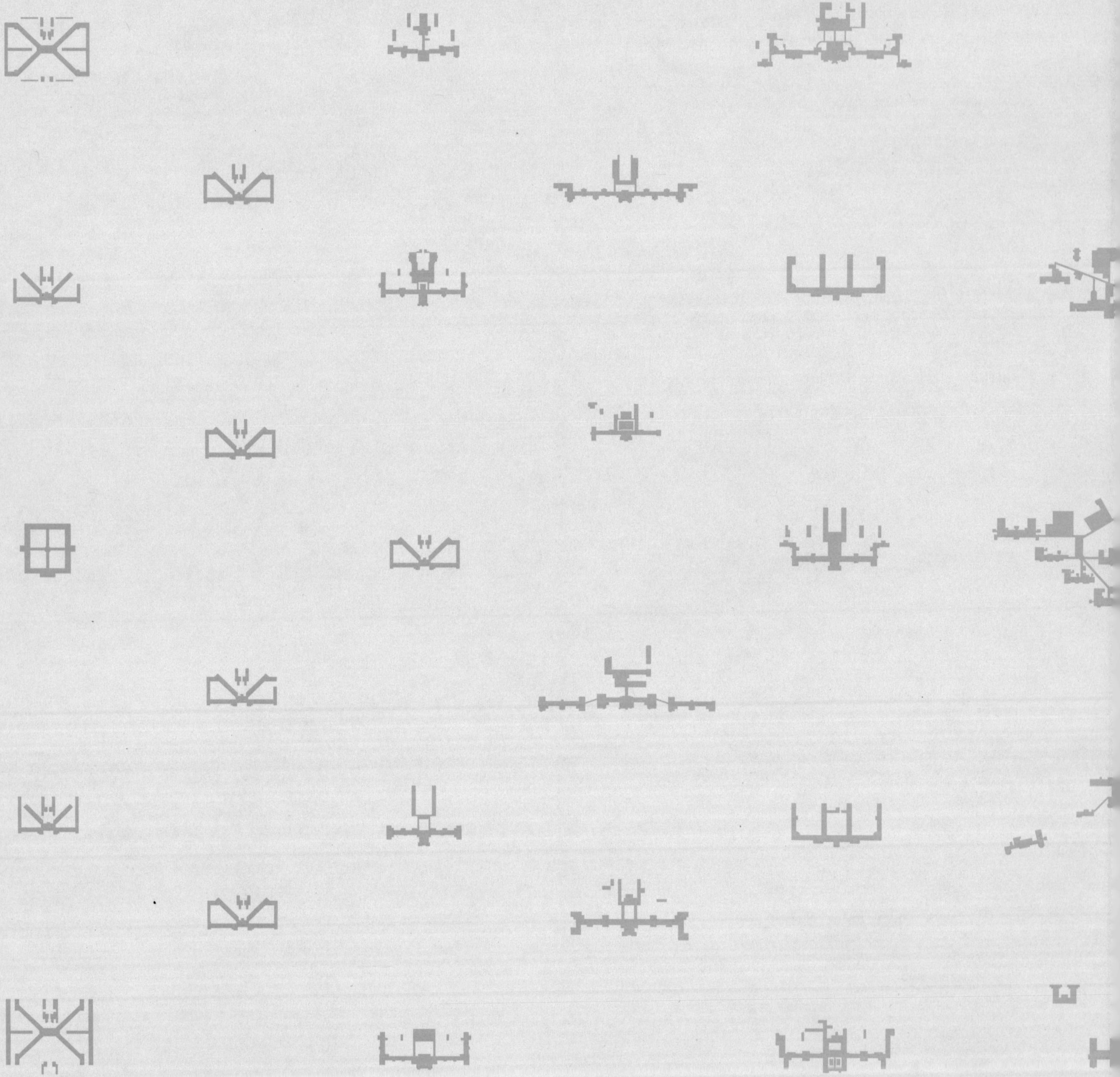